DIAGNOSTIC PROCEDURES FOR BACTERIAL INFECTIONS

Prepared under the auspices of the
Committee on Laboratory Standards and Practices
of the
American Public Health Association.

7th EDITION

Diagnostic Procedures For Bacterial Infections

Coordinating Editor

Berttina B. Wentworth, PhD

Editorial Board

Vickie S. Baselski, PhD - Gary V. Doern, PhD
Carole P. McArthur, PhD - J. Michael Miller, PhD
Cynthia A. Needham, PhD - David L. Sewell, PhD

APHA

American Public Health Association

Seventh Edition

AMERICAN PUBLIC HEALTH ASSOCIATION, INC.
1015 Fifteenth Street, NW
Washington, DC 20005

William H. McBeath, MD, MPH, Executive Director

Library of Congress Cataloging-in-Publication Data

Diagnostic procedures for bacterial infections.
Together with: Diagnostic procedures for mycotic and parasitic infections, constitutes a rev. ed. of: Diagnostic procedures for bacterial, mycotic, and parasitic infections. 6th ed. c1981.
Includes bibliographies and index.
1. Diagnostic bacteriology. I. Wentworth, Berttina B. II. Diagnostic procedures for bacterial, mycotic, and parasitic infections. III. title: Diagnostic procedures for mycotic and parasitic infections. [DNLM: 1. Bacterial Infections—diagnosis. WC 200 D536]
QR67.2.D53 1987 616.9′0475 87-19306
ISBN 0-87553-149-0

3M12/87

Printed and bound in the United States of America
Typography: Monotype Composition Company, Inc., Baltimore, Maryland
Set in: *Times Roman, Helvetica*
Text and Binding: Port City Press, Baltimore, Maryland
Cover Design: Donya Melanson Associates, Boston, Massachusetts

TABLE OF CONTENTS

SECTION 3 : ANTIMICROBIAL SUSCEPTIBILITY TESTING

SECTION 4 : DIRECT DETECTION METHODS

SECTION V : LABORATORY PRACTICE

PREFACE

So much new information about infectious diseases has accumulated since the publication of the 6th edition of *Diagnostic Procedures for Bacterial, Mycotic and Parasitic Infections* that the 7th edition has been divided into two volumes to accommodate this expansion in knowledge. The second volume, *Diagnostic Procedures for Mycotic and Parasitic Infections,* is in preparation.

This first volume on bacterial infections has new chapters on *Aeromonas* and *Plesiomonas, Branhamella,* plague and vaginosis, as well as expanded chapters on most other infections, such as miscellaneous gram-negative rod infections, enterobacterial infections and legionellosis. New areas in established chapters describe Lyme disease and cat scratch fever.

The section on antimicrobial susceptibility testing has been expanded to four chapters to include instrumented, automated, anaerobic and mycobacterial testing procedures. A new section on direct detection methods has been added with chapters on microscopy, microbial antigen detection, chromatography and nucleic acid probes.

Chapters offer not only the details of laboratory procedures, but also discussions of the clinical manifestations, therapy, epidemiology and public health significance of these infections.

As a service to readers, we have provided trade and proprietary names as sources of laboratory equipment and supplies, but such information does not constitute commercial endorsement by either the editors or the American Public Health Association. A list of the names and addresses of manufacturers cited appears on page 837.

The seven members of the Editorial Board have worked long and diligently to bring this volume to completion in a prompt and timely manner. While recognizing that no book can be completely up-to-date at the moment it appears, the Board hopes that this volume will contain the current information needed for its intended use: the laboratory diagnosis and further understanding of infectious diseases.

The Board wishes to thank all the authors for their prompt and excellent contributions to this book and the publications staff of APHA for their continuing support and encouragement.

We ask that readers who have questions regarding any material in this book please refer all inquiries to the Coordinating Editor, Berttina B. Wentworth, rather than to authors or other editors. Questions will then be referred to the appropriate person.

Berttina B. Wentworth

CONTRIBUTORS

Chapter 1: Cynthia A. Needham, Ph.D.
Section Head, Microbiology
Lahey Clinic Medical Center
Burlington, MA 01805

Chapter 2: Kenneth A. McPherson
Director, Market Analysis and Statistics
International Data Corporation
Framingham, MA 01701

Cynthia A. Needham, Ph.D.
Section Head, Microbiology
Lahey Clinic Medical Center
Burlington, MA 01805

Chapter 3: J. Michael Janda, Ph.D.
Research Microbiologist
Microbial Diseases Laboratory
California Department of Health Services
Berkeley, CA 94704

Chapter 4: Peter C. Appelbaum, M.D., Ph.D.
Director, Clinical Microbiology
Hershey Medical Center
Hershey, PA 17033

Chapter 5: Thomas A. Russo, M.D.
Fellow, Infectious Diseases
Department of Community Medicine
Tufts University School of Medicine
Boston, MA 02111

Sherwood L. Gorbach, M.D.
Professor, Community Health and Medicine
Tufts New England Medical Center
Boston, MA 02111

Chapter 6: Paul A. Granato, Ph.D.
Clinical Microbiologist
Department of Pathology
Crouse Irving Memorial Hospital
Syracuse, NY 13210-1699

Chapter 7: Ted L. Hadfield, Ph.D.
Chief, Microbiology Laboratory
Wilford Hall Medical Center
Lackland Air Force Base, TX 78236

Chapter 8: Charlotte D. Parker, Ph.D.
Associate Professor
Department of Microbiology
University of Missouri School of Medicine
Columbia, MO 65212

Beverley J. Payne, MPH
Microbiology Unit
Missouri Division of Health Laboratories
Jefferson City, MO 65101

Chapter 9: Karen Sue C. Kehl, Ph.D.
Director, Virology Section
International Clinical Laboratories, Inc.
Nashville, TN 37214

Chapter 10: Gary V. Doern, Ph.D.
Director, Department of Clinical Microbiology
University of Massachusetts Medical Center
Worcester, MA 01605

Chapter 11: Richard E. Winn, M.D.
Chief, Infectious Diseases
Wilford Hall Medical Center
Lackland Air Force Base, TX 78236

Chapter 12: Martin J. Blaser, M.D.
Chief, Infectious Disease Section
Veterans Administration Medical Center
Denver, CO 80220

Wen-lan L. Wang, Ph.D.
Chief, Microbiology Section
Veterans Administration Medical Center
Denver, CO 80220

Chapter 13: Jill E. Clarridge, Ph.D.
Chief, Microbiology Section
Laboratory Service
Veterans Administration Medical Center
Houston, TX 77211

Alice S. Weissfeld, Ph.D.
Director, Microbiology Specialists Incorporated
Houston, TX 77211

Chapter 14: J. J. Farmer, III, Ph.D.
Chief, Enteric Identification Laboratories
Enteric Bacteriology Section
Center for Infectious Diseases
Centers for Disease Control
Atlanta, GA 30333

Patricia M. Griffin, M.D.
Epidemiologic Intelligence Service Officer
Enteric Diseases Branch
Center for Infectious Diseases
Centers for Disease Control
Atlanta, GA 30333

I. Kaye Wachsmuth, Ph.D.
Chief, Enteric Bacteriology Section
Center for Infectious Diseases
Centers for Disease Control
Atlanta, GA 30333

Joy G. Wells, M.S.
Chief, Epidemiologic Investigations Laboratory
Enteric Bacteriology Section
Center for Infectious Diseases
Centers for Disease Control
Atlanta, GA 30333

Chapter 15: Judy A. Daly, Ph.D.
Assistant Professor
Department of Pathology
University of Utah
Salt Lake City, UT 84103

Chapter 16: Paul M. Mendelman, M.D.
Assistant Professor of Pediatrics
Division of Infectious Diseases
University of Washington
Seattle, WA 98105

Chapter 17: Washington C. Winn, Jr., M.D.
Professor, Department of Pathology
University of Vermont College of Medicine
Burlington, VT 05401

Chapter 18: Michael A. Saubolle, Ph.D.
Director, Microbiology Laboratories
Department of Pathology
Good Samaritan Medical Center
Phoenix, AZ 85062

Chapter 19: Mary J. R. Gilchrist, Ph.D.
Director, Clinical Microbiology
Children's Hospital Medical Center
Cincinnati, OH 48226

Chapter 20: James R. Greenwood, Ph.D.
Director, Public Health Laboratory
County of Orange
Santa Ana, CA 92702

Sydney M. Harvey, Ph.D.
Scientific Director
Nichols Institute Reference Laboratories
San Juan Capistrano, CA 92675

Chapter 21: Charles H. Zierdt, Ph.D.
Staff Microbiologist
Clinical Pathology Department
National Institutes of Health
Bethesda, MD 20892

Chapter 22: Wallace A. Clyde, Jr., M.D.
Professor of Pediatrics and Microbiology
Department of Pediatrics
University of North Carolina
Chapel Hill, NC 27514

Chapter 23: Stephen A. Morse, Ph.D.
Director
Sexually Transmitted Diseases Laboratory Program
Center for Infectious Diseases
Centers for Disease Control
Atlanta, GA 30333

Joan S. Knapp, Ph.D.
Chief, Bacteriology Research Branch
Center for Infectious Diseases
Centers for Disease Control
Atlanta, GA 30333

Chapter 24: Alfred E. Bacon, M.D.
Infectious Diseases Section
University Hospital
University of Michigan
Ann Arbor, MI 48109

Stephen C. Ross, M.D.
Infectious Diseases Section
University Hospital
University of Michigan
Ann Arbor, MI 48109

Chapter 25: Thomas J. Quan, Ph.D.
Research Microbiologist, Plague Branch
Division of Vector Borne Viral Diseases
Center for Infectious Diseases
Centers for Disease Control
Fort Collins, CO 80522-2087

Chapter 26: David L. Sewell, Ph.D.
Director, Microbiology Section
Clinical Pathology Service
Veterans Administration Medical Center
Portland, OR 97207

Chapter 27: James H Jorgensen, Ph.D.
Director, Clinical Microbiology Division
Department of Pathology
University of Texas Health Science Center
San Antonio, TX 78284

Wesley E. Kloos, Ph.D.
Department of Genetics
North Carolina State University
Raleigh, NC 27695

Chapter 28: Kathryn L. Ruoff, Ph.D.
Bacteriology Department
The Massachusetts General Hospital
Boston, MA 02114

Carol V. Garner, M.D.
Infectious Disease Unit
The Massachusetts General Hospital
Boston, MA 02114

Chapter 29: Sheila A. Lukehart, Ph.D.
Research Associate Professor
Division of Infectious Diseases
University of Washington
Seattle, WA 98195

Chapter 30: Cora E. Musial, Ph.D.
Postdoctoral Fellow
Department of Laboratory Medicine
Mayo Foundation
Rochester, MN 55901

Glenn D. Roberts, Ph.D.
Director
Clinical Mycology and Mycobacteriology Laboratories
Mayo Foundation
Rochester, MN 55901

Chapter 31: Michael Gelfand, M.D.
Director, Clinical Microbiology Laboratory
Methodist Hospitals
Memphis, TN 38104

Chapter 32: Carol A. Spiegel, Ph.D.
Director, Clinical Microbiology
University of Wisconsin Hospital and Clinics
Madison, WI 53791-9452

Chapter 33: David L. Tison, Ph.D.
Head, Clinical Microbiology Section
Multicare Medical Center
Tacoma, WA 98405

Chapter 34: Peter C. Fuchs, M.D., Ph.D.
Director of Microbiology
Department of Pathology
St. Vincent Hospital and Medical Center
Portland, OR 97225

Chapter 35: Steven D. Brown, Ph.D.
Director, Microbiology Laboratory
Department of Pathology
Good Samaritan Medical Center
Portland, Oregon 97210

Chapter 36: Ronald J. Zabransky, Ph.D.
Professor of Pathology & Laboratory Medicine
Mount Sinai Medical Center
Milwaukee, WI 53201

Chapter 37: Frederick S. Nolte, Ph.D.
Associate Director
Clinical Microbiology Laboratory
University of Rochester
Rochester, NY 14642

Chapter 38: Patrick R. Murray, Ph.D.
Co-Director, Clinical Microbiology Laboratory
Department of Microbiology
Barnes Hospital
St. Louis, MO 63110

Chapter 39: Richard C. Tilton, Ph.D.
Professor, Department of Laboratory Medicine
University of Connecticut School of Medicine
Farmington, CT 06032

Chapter 40: Robert Martin, Dr.P.H.
Chief, Division of Microbiology
Bureau of Laboratory and Epidemiological Services
Michigan Department of Public Health
Lansing, MI 48909

William A. Schneider, B.S.
Microbiologist, Diagnostic Microbiology Section
Bureau of Laboratory and Epidemiological Services
Michigan Department of Public Health
Lansing, MI 48909

Chapter 41: Stephen C. Edberg, Ph.D.
Associate Professor,
Department of Laboratory Medicne
Yale University School of Medicine
New Haven, CT 06510

Chapter 42: William M. Wagner, D.Sc.
Consulting Scientist
Training and Laboratory Program Office
Centers for Disease Control
Atlanta, GA 30333

Chapter 43: John H. Richardson, D.V.M.
Biosafety Officer
University Biosafety Office
Emory University School of Medicine
Atlanta, GA 30322

Chapter 44: Martin S. Favero, Ph.D.
Chief, Nosocomial Infections Laboratory Branch
Hospital Infections Program
Center for Infectious Diseases
Centers for Disease Control
Atlanta, GA 30333

Chapter 45: Richard H. Bell, Ph.D.
Director of Quality Engineering
Difco Laboratories Incorporated
Detroit, MI 48235

Section 1:
Specimen and Method Selection

CHAPTER 1

SPECIMEN COLLECTION

Cynthia A. Needham, Ph.D.

INTRODUCTION

The specimen is the beginning. All diagnostic information from the laboratory depends upon the knowledge by which specimens are chosen and the care with which they are collected and transported. Laboratorians are almost always removed from these events. Nonetheless, it remains their responsibility to insure that adequate instructions exist, that education is a continuing process and that mechanisms for quality assurance within the laboratory are defined and respected. Much has already been written on various aspects of this process. The goal of this chapter is to draw upon existing information and integrate it into a practical guide for specimen management.

SPECIMEN CHOICE AND COLLECTION

The site of the infection as well as the etiologic agent(s) suspected are two factors that determine which specimen(s) will have the highest diagnostic yield. A third consideration is the risk/benefit ratio of the collection procedure to the patient. In many situations, the optimum specimen is collected via an invasive procedure. It is imperative that the microbiologist be prepared to work with the clinician to provide guidance and alternatives when clinical circumstances do not justify the use of such procedures. Table 1:1 identifies specimen sources, details collection procedures for each and specifies appropriate containers for their transport to the laboratory.

Infections Involving Normally Sterile Body Fluids

It should be immediately apparent that infections which occur in normally sterile body sites present the least difficult decisions. If one wishes to

Table 1:1. Specimen Collection and Transport

Specimen	Type/Quantity	Collection	Transport Container
Catheter	Intravenous (arterial, cannula, central venous pressure, vascular, venous); 2-4 inch segment	Decontaminate skin surface; remove catheter, cut segment beneath skin surface	Sterile, screw-capped jar
	Urine (Foley)	Not appropriate for routine culture	
	Drainage Line (Penrose)	Same as above	
Ear	External	Cleanse external canal with mild detergent; collect surface scrapings or swab margin of inflammation	Scrapings in screw-capped tube; swab in aerobic transport container
	Internal	Cleanse external canal with mild antiseptic; collect drainage by tympanocentesis	Syringe; anerobic transport system
Eye	External		
	Conjunctiva	Cleanse skin around eye with mild antiseptic; do not use topical anesthetics; most specimens collected with a moistened swab; scrapings needed for diagnosis of viral or chlamydial infections	Sterile screwcapped tube for scrapings or swab in aerobic transport container; transport viral or chlamydial cultures in specific transport medium
	Corneal	Use topical anesthetics and collect scrapings with a platinum spatula	Inoculate specimens directly onto media and slide; use specific transport media for chlamydial and viral cultures
	Internal	Surgical procedure	Sterile, screw-capped tube
Fluids	Abdominal (Peritoneal, paracentesis, ascites); 1–5 mL per culture request	Decontaminate skin surface; aspirate with syringe	Syringe; sterile, screwcapped tube or jar; anaerobic transport system
	Amniotic; 1–2 mL per culture request	Aspirate with syringe avoiding vaginal contamination	Syringe; sterile screwcapped tube/jar or anaerobic transport system

Table 1:1. Specimen Collection and Transport (Continued)

Specimen	Type/Quantity	Collection	Transport Container
	Blood; 1–5 mL (child); 10–20 mL (adult); 3 samples per 24 hour period	Disinfect skin with 70% alcohol followed by 2% iodine	Vacuum tube with SPS or blood culture bottle
	Bone marrow; ≥ 1 mL	Disinfect skin as above and aspirate bone marrow	Same as above
	Cerebrospinal (CSF, ventricular); 1–2 mL per culture request	Disinfect skin as above and perform lumbar puncture or ventricular/suboccipital tap	Sterile, screw-capped tube, syringe, anaerobic transport system
	Chest (Empyema, thoracentesis, pleural); 1–5 mL per culture request	Decontaminate skin surface; aspirate with syringe	Same as above
	Cul de sac (Culdocentesis); 1–2 mL per culture request	Surgical procedure; aspiration through posterior vaginal vault	Same as above
	Ear (Tympanocentesis)	See ear, internal	
	Eye (Aqueous, Vitreous)	See eye, internal	
	Pericardial; 1–2 mL per culture request	Surgical procedure; sterile aspiration with syringe	Same as above
	Peritoneal dialysate; 100 mL	2 liter bag aseptically collected by patient on chronic ambulatory peritoneal dialysis (CAPD)	Same as above or dialysate collection bag
	Synovial (joint); 1–2 mL per culture request	Decontaminate skin surface; aspirate with syringe	Syringe; sterile, screwcapped tube; anaerobic transport system
Gastrointestinal	Bile, 1–2 mL per culture request	Aspirate with syringe during surgery or from drainage line (T-tube)	Same as above
	Gastric aspirate	Collect prior to ingestion of food	Sterile, screw-capped tube or jar, syringe

Table 1:1. Specimen Collection and Transport (Continued)

Specimen	Type/Quantity	Collection	Transport Container
	Rectal swab	Swab lesions of rectal wall during proctoscopy or sigmoidoscopy; not appropriate for stool culture; request voided specimen	Aerobic transport container; transport to lab immediately; if delayed more than 2–3 hours, use modified Cary-Blair or buffered-glycerol transport medium for bacteria/fungi and polyvinyl alcohol (PVA) fixative for parasites
	Stool, colostomy, ileostomy; minimum wt. 1 g; 3 consecutive specimens	Voided specimen	Same as above
Genital	Cervix	Use speculum and no lubricant; obtain exudate from endocervical glands by aspiration or swab under direct vision; culture specimens for *N. gonorrhoeae* at bedside; collect cervical scrapings for chlamydial or herpesvirus culture	*N. gonorrhoeae* culture medium (Jembec, transgrow, etc.); chlamydial or viral transport medium; anaerobic transport system for *Actinomyces* culture; swab container or syringe for other cultures
	Endometrium, uterus	Curetting or aspiration with syringe	Same as above
	Lymph node (inguinal)	Biopsy or needle aspiration	*Chlamydia* transport medium; aerobic transport container for *H. ducreyi*
	Products of conception (Lochia, placenta, membranes)	Tissue or aspirates	See cervix (above)
	Prostatic fluid	Digital massage through rectum	Sterile, screw-capped tube or jar
	Urethra	Swab urethral discharge; culture specimen for *N. gonorrhoeae* at bedside	*N. gonorrhoeae* culture medium (Jembec, transgrow, etc.); *Chlamydia* transport medium, swab container or screw-capped jar for other cultures

Table 1:1. Specimen Collection and Transport (Continued)

Specimen	Type/Quantity	Collection	Transport Container
	Vagina	Swab (calcium alginate or dacron swab) vaginal exudate; immediately examine microscopically for *Trichomonas* or fungal elements	Aerobic transport container
	Vulva	Examine serous exudate for *Treponema pallidum* by darkfield microscopy immediately after collection; collect sample at base of lesion for *H. ducreyi* or herpesvirus; collect lymph node aspirate for *Chlamydia*	Aerobic transport container; viral transport medium
Respiratory	Bronchial (brushing, washing, bronchial-alveolar lavage, biopsy)	Sample diseased part of lung with a telescoping, double-lumen, plugged bronchoscope; anesthetics toxic for bacteria and fungi	Sterile, screw-capped tube
	Epiglottis	Not recommended	
	Larynx	Swab inflamed area or posterior pharynx	Viral transport medium
	Lung aspirate or biopsy	Decontaminate skin; aspirate specimen through chest wall, transbronchoscopic needle biopsy; or thoracotomy	Sterile, screw-capped tube or jar
	Mouth	Rinse mouth; prep with dry sterile gauze; swab areas of exudation, or ulceration; avoid contact with tongue and saliva	Aerobic transport system
	Nasopharynx	Pass swab gently through nose into posterior nasopharynx and rotate	Aerobic transport container, syringe or sterile, screw-capped tube

Table 1:1. Specimen Collection and Transport (Continued)

Specimen	Type/Quantity	Collection	Transport Container
	Nose	Insert swab into nares and gently rotate against mucosal surface	Aerobic transport container
	Sinus aspirate	Aspirate specimen with syringe	Syringe or anaerobic transport container
	Sputum (expectorated)	Rinse mouth with water; collect lower respiratory tract secretions by deep cough; avoid salivary contamination	Sterile, screw-capped jar
	Tracheostomy site (endotracheal/tracheal aspirate)	Aspirate secretions using flexible tubing or catheter passed through tracheostomy	Same as above
	Throat (oropharynx)	Swab areas of exudation or inflammation; avoid contact with tongue, oral mucosa or saliva	Aerobic transport container
	Transtracheal aspirate	Aspirate exudate through small sterile catheter inserted into the trachea	Syringe or anaerobic transport system
Skin	Superficial (cellulitis, pyoderma)	Disinfect surface with 70% alcohol; aspirate of deepest portion of lesion preferable to swab; if vesicle is present, collect both fluid and cells from base of lesion	Syringe, sterile screwcapped tube or jar, swab in transport medium
	Extensive burns or decubiti (3–4 mm dermal punch)	Disinfect surface with 70% alcohol; collect by punch biopsy for quantitative culture	Sterile screwcapped jar
	Deep lesion (abscess, fistula, sinus tract, ulcer)	Disinfect surface with 70% alcohol; aspirate of deepest portion of lesion preferable to swab; avoid contamination by wound surface	Syringe, sterile screwcapped tube or jar, anaerobic transport system

Table 1:1. Specimen Collection and Transport (Continued)

Specimen	Type/Quantity	Collection	Transport Container
Tissue	Autopsy (5 cm^3 section)	Disinfect surface as above; homogenize tissue specimens before processing. Collect blood or other fluids by aspiration before the body cavity is opened	Sterile screwcapped tube or jar, blood culture bottle
	Surgical, biopsy	Surgical procedure, homogenize specimens before processing	Sterile screwcapped tube or jar, anaerobic transport system
Urine	Indwelling catheter, nephrostomy, ileal loop (1 mL for bacteria and fungi, 10–15 mL for mycobacteria	Disinfect tubing with 70% alcohol, aspirate urine with syringe; one specimen sufficient for diagnosis of bacterial or fungal infection. Three consecutive daily specimens needed for diagnosis of mycobacterial infection	Sterile screwcapped tube or jar
	Straight catheter (volumes as above)	Discard first 15–30 mL; one specimen is sufficient for diagnosis of bacterial or fungal infection; three consecutive daily specimens needed for diagnosis of mycobacterial infection	Same as above
	Clean voided midstream (volumes as above)	Same as above	Same as above
	Suprapubic aspirate (volumes as above)	Collected by needle aspiration; appropriate for anaerobic culture	Same as above

establish the etiologic agent of meningitis, spinal fluid is the only acceptable specimen. Although there is some risk associated with lumbar puncture, the consequences of inappropriate or inadequate antibiotic therapy far outweigh the risk of the collection process. Cerebrospinal fluid is sterile under normal circumstances and thus the only significant issue is contamination of the specimen with resident skin flora. Similar clinical settings include joint and intraocular infections, pericarditis, peritonitis and pleural space infection.

Where etiology is highly predictable, the risk of specimen collection becomes an increasingly important issue. For example, acute sinusitis can be treated empirically with a high success rate. Needle aspiration of the sinus cavity provides the only valid specimen for establishing a specific diagnosis, but the procedure is painful, risks introduction of other bacteria and will not usually alter therapy. Aspiration is necessary only if the disease progresses during therapy or an unusual pathogen is suspected. The same logic applies to otitis media. The infection can usually be treated empirically, but when a specific diagnosis must be reached, tympanocentesis must be performed. Attempts to use nasal or nasopharyngeal drainage to establish etiology for either of these infections should be strongly discouraged. Culture of these secretions does not accurately predict infectious etiology, although the specimen is easily obtained.[4,17]

The collection process is basically the same for all of these clinical settings and careful decontamination of the site of needle aspiration is the primary consideration. The skin must be meticulously disinfected to avoid contamination of the specimen as well as introduction of bacteria into a sterile site. The site of needle puncture should be cleaned first with 70% isopropyl or ethyl alcohol followed by disinfection with an iodine solution. Either a 1-2% solution of tincture of iodine or a 10% solution of povidone iodine (1% free iodine) is acceptable. The iodine should be allowed to dry for maximum effectiveness.

Intravascular Infections

Intravascular infections represent a slightly different situation in terms of specimen choice and collection. Specimen volume, the number of specimens collected and the temporal relationship of cultures will all influence the ultimate success of documenting a bacteremic event. Bacteremias can be divided into two groups. Those which have an intravascular focus, often referred to as primary bacteremia, generally result in the continual presence of bacteria in the bloodstream. The temporal relationship of specimen collection is far less important for infections of this type than for so-called secondary bacteremia where the focus of infection is extravascular. Bacteremic events are usually intermittent in the latter case and specimen collection should be timed to optimally coincide with a bacteremic event.

In practical terms, however, it is difficult to predict when a patient will become bacteremic. Consequently, blood should be collected at intervals no closer than 60 minutes and preferably at 3 to 4-hour intervals.

The optimal volume of blood for culture is 20 mL from adult patients. Most patients have small numbers of bacteria in their bloodstream. When quantitative studies have been performed, one-half or more of bacteremic patients have fewer than one bacterial cell per mL of blood.[8] In fact, evidence exists that increasing the volume of blood cultured from 10 mL to 20 mL increases the detection of clinically significant bacteremias by 38%.[9,20] Although children more frequently have higher numbers of bacteria than adults, a substantial percentage still have low-order bacteremias.[11] Total blood volume is reduced in pediatric-age patients, so a lower volume for culture is acceptable. Attempt collection of 1-2 mL from neonatal patients and 5-10 mL from older children.[20]

Three cultures should be performed over a 24-hour period if timing of collection and blood volume are appropriate. Even in patients who are intermittently bacteremic, approximately 80% of bacteremias can be documented with the first culture and 99% are detected when 3 cultures are performed.[23] Single blood cultures are not appropriate under any circumstances and the laboratorian should make every effort to insure that at least two cultures are performed on any patient. There are rare occasions when performing more than 3 cultures over a 24-hour period is appropriate, but they are limited primarily to patients who have a rapidly changing clinical status or who are receiving antimicrobial therapy. There are more effective alternatives available, however, even for the latter group (i.e., antimicrobial removal devices, resin containing bottles, etc.)

Although most blood culture systems in use today will allow recovery of the vast majority of organisms causing bacteremia, exceptions do exist. Examples include *Mycobacterium* spp., *Legionella* spp. and strains of pathogenic *Neisseria* which may be inhibited by the concentration of sodium polyanethol sulfonate present in blood culture media.[14] It is consequently important that the clinician be aware of the limitations of the system in routine use so that alternative methods can be employed when necessary.

The collection of blood for culture is similar to collection of all other sterile body fluids. Since contamination of the specimen with skin flora at the time of collection can create confusing results, meticulous disinfection of the venipuncture site is critical. Once a vein has been selected and the tourniquet put in place, the skin surface should be cleansed with 70% alcohol followed by an iodine-containing solution. If it is necessary to palpate the vein after disinfection, the phlebotomist should either decontaminate his or her fingers or wear sterile gloves. Increasing numbers of hospitalized patients have intravascular catheters which are used to monitor central venous pressure, deliver parenteral nutrition and chemotherapy, or simply to maintain venous access. The drawing of blood from these catheters should be discouraged, since they are usually in place long-term and are at greatly increased risk of infection. Blood specimens collected through such catheters yield results comparable to specimens collected by venipuncture, but their use for this purpose should be restricted to those patients in whom there is no alternative.[21]

Infections of the Urinary Tract

Urinary tract infections are among the most common infectious diseases seen in both outpatient and hospitalized patient populations. Urine is normally sterile. However, most specimen collection methods necessitate passage of urine over the colonized surfaces of the urogenital tract. Suprapubic aspiration eliminates any concern about contamination by avoiding contact with the colonized mucosal surfaces and represents the only acceptable specimen if anaerobic bacteriology is to be performed. However, a suprapubic tap is uncomfortable and unnecessary most of the time, thus is rarely performed.

Urine collected as a midstream, clean-voided specimen from a cooperative patient who has received adequate instruction will generally yield reliable results. In most institutions, clean-voided urine represents the majority of urine specimens submitted for culture. Urine obtained through catheterization avoids the problem of contamination, in part, but again is uncomfortable for the patient, risks introduction of bacteria into the bladder and can place the patient at risk for urosepsis resulting from manipulation of the urogenital structures. Consequently, catheterization should be performed only in specific circumstances. If the patient is to undergo catheterization for other reasons, then urine collected during the procedure may provide a better quality specimen for culture. Other situations in which a catheterized specimen may be justified include patients who are unable to cooperate (e.g., the extremely obese female patient) or the patient in whom a definitive diagnosis has not been reached using clean-voided specimens.

Patients who have long-term indwelling catheters are frequently colonized with microorganisms and there is limited value to the information gained by culturing their urine. If a specimen is to be collected for culture, the urine should be collected by needle puncture at the point of junction with the collecting tubing after the junction has been disinfected. Urine should never be sampled from the drainage bag nor should the catheter itself be submitted for culture.[7]

Diagnosis of an infection of the urinary tract relies upon a quantitative assessment of bacteria in the urine. Although a concensus does not exist as to the exact number necessary to establish infection, it is generally agreed that infection is characterized by large numbers of bacteria. There are several factors which can alter the number of organisms present in urine and these should be kept in mind when urine is being collected for culture.

Artificially low numbers of bacteria may occur if patients are urinating frequently, if they have consumed large volumes of fluid or if they have been hydrated intravenously. Collection of the first morning voided specimen will help to overcome these problems, since organisms tend to be concentrated in this specimen.

Artificially high numbers of bacteria may be present if the urine has not been collected carefully or if some problem has occurred in transport. While urine itself is usually sterile, the urethra and perineal regions are heavily colonized with bacteria. Therefore, careful instruction should be given to the patient prior to collection. Female patients should cleanse the urethral area by spreading the labia with one hand, using the other to wash themselves from front to back with soaped sponges. A separate sponge should be used for each stroke. The area should then be rinsed with clean wet sponges in the same manner. In male patients, the glans should be washed with soaped sponges and rinsed with clean wet sponges. Special care must be taken to retract the foreskin during the cleaning process if the patient is not circumcised. After cleansing, the patient should be instructed to void a little urine into the toilet and then to collect a portion of the midstream urine in a sterile cup.

Ordinary soap is recommended for cleaning the urethral area rather than disinfectants. The latter may be irritating and mechanical cleansing is the more important issue. In addition, if disinfectants are introduced into the urine during collection, they may be inhibitory to the growth of microorganisms.[15]

Catheterized specimens should be collected by cleansing the urethral area as described for a clean-voided specimen. After the catheter has been passed through the urethra and into the bladder, the first 15-30 mL of urine should be discarded and then a small amount collected into a sterile container for culture. Discarding the first urine helps to avoid contamination of the specimen with urethral flora.

Pediatric-age patients represent a special problem in terms of specimen collection. The collection of clean-voided specimens is complicated since it is difficult to give instructions which can be adequately followed. A taped on "pedi-bag" may serve as a useful alternative to more invasive procedures. The same precautions for cleaning the periurethral area should be carried out before the bag is taped in place. As soon as the child has voided, the bag should be removed and the specimen transported to the laboratory for processing.

A single clean-voided or catheterized specimen is usually sufficient to establish the etiologic agent of urinary tract infection. Exceptions include asymptomatic infection, infection characterized by low numbers of bacteria and diagnosis of disease caused by *Mycobacterium tuberculosis*, where two to three specimens may be necessary. The microbiologist should be familiar with some special procedures which result in nontraditional specimens. The four-cup method of Meares and Stamey[13] for diagnosing prostatitis, bladder washout for localizing the site of infection to upper versus lower[6] and use of the first voided urine specimen to diagnose gonococcal urethritis[16] are examples of such procedures.

Infections of the Lower Respiratory Tract

Bacterial infection of the lower respiratory tract offers a slightly different problem in terms of specimen choice. The structures of the lower respiratory tract are sterile. Unless an invasive procedure is used, most specimens must pass through the heavily colonized mucosal structures of the upper respiratory tract where they are subject to contamination with the colonizing microflora. However, the risk associated with needle aspiration, open lung biopsy or similar procedures clearly outweighs the benefits derived from such invasive procedures for most patients and they are infrequently performed. As with urinary tract infections, the preferred specimen is the one which can be most easily obtained, and in most instances will be an expectorated sputum. The clarity of instructions for collection and the patient's ability to understand and cooperate with these instructions will have significant impact on the quality of the material produced.

Nasopharyngeal aspiration may be useful in the obtunded patient or in pediatric-age patients. Children swallow their secretions and it is consequently difficult to obtain an expectorated specimen. Unfortunately, a nasopharyngeal aspirate is still subject to contamination with nasopharyngeal flora which may contain a variety of other potential pathogens. Endotracheal or tracheostomy aspirates may be collected from patients with a tracheostomy in place. However, there is still ample opportunity for upper airway contamination with this approach. In addition, the tracheostomy site becomes rapidly colonized with gram-negative bacilli following tracheostomy. They are present in large numbers in the exudate which typically accompanies the placement of an endotracheal tube and the diagnostic value of the specimen is the same as expectorated sputum.

Specimens collected at bronchoscopy offer some advantage over those already mentioned, although bronchoscopy is usually not necessary for the diagnosis of bacterial pneumonia. There is still significant opportunity for contamination with upper airway microflora as the bronchoscope must pass through the oropharynx. In addition, saliva may be aspirated during the collection process. Efforts to minimize salivary and oropharyngeal contamination have included positioning the patient's head below the lungs and the use of a bronchoscope with a telescoping double catheter protected with a distal polyethylene glycol plug. The inner catheter can be advanced once inserted into the mainstream bronchus, specimens collected and the inner catheter removed, theoretically shielding the specimen from contamination. Samples collected by this method can be reliably cultured for anaerobes.[24]

One of the primary difficulties with bronchoscopy is that the anesthetics used during the procedure are toxic to certain bacteria, including *Mycobacterium* species. Unfortunately, the diagnosis of tuberculosis is one of the situations when this procedure may be most useful. Toxicity can be minimized by limiting the time of exposure to the anesthetic once the specimen has been collected and by using a less toxic anesthetic, such as Lidocaine, whenever possible.[1]

Finally, it is possible to avoid the majority of upper airway contamination by using transtracheal aspiration, since the point of entry, the cricothyroid membrane, is below the level of mucosal colonization. Transtracheal aspiration, along with needle aspiration, open lung biopsy and sheathed bronchoscopy, provide the only acceptable specimens for anaerobic bacteriology.

Infections of the Upper Respiratory Tract

Although the majority of cases of pharyngitis are caused by viruses, bacteria still account for a significant number of infections, particularly in children. The most common bacteriologic agent is the Group A streptococcus. Specimens for culture should be collected under direct visualization by swabbing the tonsilar areas and the posterior pharynx, particularly where there is inflammation, ulceration or exudation. Care should be taken not to contaminate the swab with saliva during the collection process. The normal oral flora can inhibit the growth of the Group A streptococcus in vitro, and potentially give rise to falsely negative culture results. The swab should be either dacron, calcium alginate or non-toxic cotton.

Other bacterial pathogens which are occasional causes of pharyngitis include *Corynebacterium diphtheriae, C. haemolyticum* and *Neisseria gonorrhoeae*. The former should be considered if the patient has an incomplete history or no history of immunization, and the latter when the patient is infected at other sites or has a positive history for exposure via the practice of fellatio. Specimen collection is analogous to collection for Group A streptococcal infection. However, the laboratory should be alerted to the possibility of *C. diphtheriae* or *C. haemolyticum* as special conditions are necessary for their isolation. If *N. gonorrhoeae* is suspected, the specimen should be inoculated directly onto an appropriate selective medium immediately upon collection whenever possible.

Epiglottitis may have a bacterial or viral etiology. *Haemophilus influenzae* is the primary bacterial pathogen.[3] Two factors are significant when considering a patient with epiglottitis. The most important is that swabbing the involved area can precipitate edema with subsequent obstruction of the airway. Secondly, *H. influenzae* is a common colonizer of the oro- and nasopharynx and the clinical significance of its isolation is not clear.

Consequently, specimen collection should be restricted to blood (which is frequently positive) and the diagnosis made on clinical grounds otherwise.

Bordetella pertussis, the agent of whooping cough, is an uncommon cause of respiratory infection in the United States, but should be considered in children under the age of 6 months and in patients whose immunization status is unknown. The specimen of choice for diagnosing whooping cough is nasopharyngeal mucous, which can be collected either by aspiration through a thin catheter or with a calcium alginate swab passed through the anterior nares into the nasopharynx. Cough plates (an older approach to specimen collection) should not be used, since they are insensitive and a potential hazard to the health care worker collecting the specimen. As with the gonococcus, special conditions are necessary to insure recovery of *B. pertussis*, and an appropriate isolation medium or transport medium should be inoculated immediately (see Chapter 8, "Bordetella Infections.")

Finally, it should be kept in mind that disseminated forms of the systemic fungal diseases and tuberculosis can present with mucosal lesions in the oropharynx. A swab does not provide adequate material for documenting these infectious processes. A biopsy must be performed to provide both cultural and histopathologic confirmation of disease.

Infections of the Genital Tract

Both the site of infection and the likely agent must be considered when selecting specimens for diagnosis of infections of the genital tract. In the male, infection is restricted primarily to the urethra and external genitalia. In the female, vulvar, vaginal, cervical and urethral structures, as well as the structures of the upper genital tract, may be involved.

N. gonorrhoeae and *Chlamydia trachomatis* are the two most common bacterial causes of urethritis in both males and females. The appropriate specimen for culturing *N. gonorrhoeae* is urethral exudate, which can usually be expressed and collected onto a swab. In the absence of exudate, a small swab can be passed into the first 2-3 cm of the urethral canal and rotated. In either case, it is imperative that the specimen be inoculated onto a selective medium immediately or placed in an appropriate transport medium, such as Amies or Stuart's. Three environmental conditions will seriously compromise the recovery of the gonococcus. They are drying, low temperatures and exposure to an atmosphere which does not contain an elevated level of CO^2. Each of these factors should be considered whenever an attempt is made to recover *N. gonorrhoeae* and appropriate measures taken to insure that viability is maintained until the specimen is received in the laboratory. Direct inoculation of the specimen eliminates many of the effects of these environmental factors.[5]

C. trachomatis is an obligate intracellular organism which grows in the columnar epithelial cells lining the urethral canal. Demonstration of the organism relies upon the collection of an adequate number of these cells via urethral scraping. After removing any exudate, the specimen can be collected as described above. Examination of exudate is an insensitive procedure at best. Like the gonococcus, *C. trachomatis* is highly susceptible to environmental conditions and swabs should be placed in an appropriate transport medium for culture.

Microorganisms which cause vulvar lesions include *Treponema pallidum, Haemophilus ducreyi* and certain serotypes of *C. trachomatis*. The diagnosis of syphilis can be made by darkfield examination of serous fluid from a primary chancre. Specimens for darkfield microscopy are obtained by abrading the margin of the chancre and removing frank blood until serous material can be collected. A drop of serous fluid should be placed on a slide and examined immediately.

H. ducreyi, the bacterium responsible for chancroid or soft chancre disease, can be recovered in culture. Specimens are most easily collected by swabbing the base of the ulcer after gently cleaning surface debris from the lesion. Lymphogranuloma venereum (LGV) is rarely diagnosed at onset, which is characterized by the formation of a small, painless ulcer. The disease usually progresses to regional lymphadenopathy and a diagnosis is reached when the organism is recovered from a biopsied lymph node.

Although there is general acceptance that bacterial vaginitis (or vaginosis) does exist, the cause(s) remains controversial. *Gardnerella vaginitis*, a member of the normal vaginal flora in 10-40% of women, has been implicated as the etiologic agent of this syndrome.[22] Current evidence suggests that the syndrome may be due to a synergistic effect between certain components of the normal anaerobic flora and *G. vaginalis*.[18] Regardless of etiology, there is an association between the presence of large numbers of *G. vaginalis* and vaginosis, and the bacterium can be recovered in the laboratory. Specimens for culture should be collected by vigorously swabbing the surface of the vaginal mucosa with a dacron or calcium alginate swab. These specimens should not be cultured anaerobically.

Cervicitis is a clinical entity distinct from vaginitis in both symptoms and causative organisms. *N. gonorrhoeae* is one of the two most common agents. Specimens which are to be cultured for *N. gonorrhoeae* should be collected so as to avoid contact with vaginal secretions and are best obtained under direct visualization using a speculum which has been moistened with warm water. Lubricants may be toxic to the gonococcus and should not be used. The external cervix should be cleansed with a cotton-tipped swab to remove any vaginal secretions and the blades of the speculum used to compress the endocervix. Cervical exudate can then be collected using a dacron, calcium alginate or non-toxic cotton-tipped swab. The factors previously identified as significant for recovery of the gonococcus are operative with endocervical specimens as well.

The other common cause of cervicitis is *C. trachomatis*. Similar to urethritis, *C. trachomatis* inhabits the columnar epithelial cells lining the endocervix. Specimens collected for demonstration of the agent must contain adequate numbers of these cells, which can be obtained by first cleansing any cervical mucous or exudate from the site. Otherwise, the patient should be prepared as described previously, and the specimen collected by inserting a dacron, calcium alginate or non-toxic cotton-tipped swab into the endocervical canal and rotating it. The swab should be placed into an appropriate transport medium immediately if being submitted for culture.

Actinomyces infections of the endocervical area as well as the upper genital tract have been associated with the use of intrauterine devices. Infections can be documented by culture. Specimen collection should avoid any contact with the vaginal mucosa and material for culture should be submitted in an anaerobic transporter.

Infections of the Gastrointestinal Tract

Gastroenteritis is a common clinical syndrome which may be caused by a variety of infectious agents including viruses, parasites, bacteria and their toxins. The specimen of choice for diagnostic purposes is a freshly passed stool ideally obtained while the patient is still symptomatic. Specimens should be collected in a dry, leak-proof container with a tightly fitting lid. Alternatively, the stool specimen can be passed into a clean, dry bedpan or onto paper towels and then transferred to a container. The specimen should not be contaminated with urine or toilet paper. The latter is frequently impregnated with bismuth sulfate, which is toxic to some enteric pathogens. Since excretion of enteric pathogens is intermittent in many patients, more than one specimen should be submitted. Three stools collected over 2-3 days are believed to give the highest diagnostic yield. However, the same situation does not seem to be true for toxins, at least in the case of *Clostridium difficile*, where one stool specimen should be adequate to establish a diagnosis.

The use of rectal swabs for diagnosis of enteric infection should be discouraged. They do not provide sufficient material for culture and are consequently unreliable. The only setting in which rectal swabs may prove useful is in screening large populations for carriage of enteric pathogens where collection of a stool specimen may not be practical. Proctitis is an unusual complication of gonococcal infection which can be diagnosed by performing a rectal culture. A dacron or calcium alginate swab should be passed through the anal sphincter and the first few centimeters of rectal mucosa rubbed vigorously. Every effort should be made to avoid contamination with fecal material, since the presence of large numbers of gram-negative bacilli complicate the recovery of *N. gonorrhoeae*. The swab should be handled like all other specimens collected for culture for the pathogenic *Neisseria*.

Infection of the gall bladder (cholecystitis) is typically caused by members of the normal intestinal flora and may require surgical intervention. Bile should be obtained at the time of surgery. If the fluid is to be processed for anaerobic bacteriology, it should be placed in an anaerobic transporter or aspirated into a syringe for delivery to the laboratory. The practice of culturing T-tube drainage once a cholecystectomy has been performed is questionable at best since bacterial colonization occurs rapidly, and such requests should be discouraged.

The laboratory should be familiar with some unusual procedures which involve specimens collected from the gastrointestinal tract. Although the processing of fecal material for anaerobic bacteriology is in general of no use, one exception (in addition to recovery of *C. difficile*) does exist. Obstruction of the bowel can cause overgrowth of the small intestine with colonic anaerobes such as *Bacteroides* spp. The small bowel is normally colonized with acid-tolerant bacteria such as streptococci and lactobacilli. Thus, a small bowel aspirate can be processed for anaerobic bacteriology to determine if overgrowth with colonic flora has occurred.

Campylobacter pyloris has been implicated as the causative agent of gastritis.[12] It can be demonstrated either microscopically or in culture of gastric biopsies, which currently represents the specimen of choice. Although gastric aspirates are not useful for the recovery of most bacteria, they can be useful in the diagnosis of pulmonary tuberculosis, particularly in small children. Mycobacteria which are coughed up may be swallowed and can be recovered in culture from this site. Gastric aspiration should be performed before the ingestion of food and the specimen dispatched to the laboratory for immediate processing.

Requests for mycobacterial cultures of stool specimens are not useful in most circumstances. However, in severely immunocompromised patients where disseminated mycobacteriosis with intestinal invasion is suspected, processing should be attempted. Specimen requirements are analagous to those previously described for other enteric pathogens.

There are a variety of bacterial pathogens which can cause intestinal disease. Although specimen requirements are the same in most cases, it is unreasonable for the laboratory to attempt isolation of all of these agents. Thus, it is important for clinicians to be aware of which pathogens are routinely sought in the laboratory and equally important that they communicate with the laboratory when unusual or uncommon pathogens are suspected.

Infections of the Skin and Contiguous Tissues

Infections of the skin range from innocuous and self-limited processes to rapidly spreading disease which can result in significant morbidity and mortality. Specimen choice depends primarily upon the extent and character of the infection rather than organisms suspected. A significant problem in collecting specimens and interpreting culture results arises from the ease with which most open lesions are colonized with microflora that can be pathogenic. Thus, attention should be given to removing as much superficial material as possible before specimen collection is attempted.

Specimens to diagnose superficial infections such as impetigo or otitis externa can usually be collected by swabbing the involved area. Several factors should be considered, however, before the material is collected. Little information is obtained from culturing a dry and/or encrusted lesion. If there is no exudate present, then bacterial culture should probably not be attempted. When exudative lesions are present, superficial material should be removed and discarded, and the specimen taken from the interior of the wound. This approach applies to a variety of situations, including surgical wound infections, ruptured abscesses, decubiti and draining fistulae and sinus tracts. In skin infections involving relatively large areas, specimens are best collected from the leading margin rather than the central area of the wound. If cellulitis is present, a small amount of sterile Ringer's solution can be injected through the skin surface at the leading margin and then withdrawn. Careful skin decontamination should precede this procedure as well.

Specimens collected from unruptured abscesses do not pose the same problem in terms of superficial colonization that open wounds do. The skin overlying the abscess should be decontaminated in a fashion similar to that used for venipuncture and then the abscess aspirated with a syringe. Once the abscess has been incised and drained, it may be useful to submit a portion of the wall for culture as well. This is particularly true if the abscess is in deeper tissue and the specimen is collected at surgery. Such infections are not infrequently polymicrobial, so swabs should never be used in this setting as they do not provide adequate material for processing.

Burn wounds represent a particularly perplexing problem in terms of bacteriologic studies. If devitalized tissue is present, it is rapidly colonized with a variety of potential pathogens, but their presence generally does not signal tissue invasion. Quantitative bacteriology may have some role in monitoring the burn patient. However, to be at all meaningful, biopsy specimens must be collected only after extensive debridement of necrotic tissue. The preferred approach is to aggressively debride the burned tissue and monitor the patient with blood cultures if infection is suspected.

Infections of the Eye

Eye infections can be divided into external (i.e., conjunctivitis, keratitis) and internal. The appropriate specimen for establishing the etiology of conjunctivitis depends upon the bacterial pathogen suspected. *C. trachomatis* causes inclusion conjunctivitis in both neonates and adults. The pathology of infection is analagous to that in the genital tract, and the same specimen requirements apply. If *C. trachomatis* is suspected, the purulent discharge should be removed and the conjunctivae swabbed vigorously in order to obtain sufficient numbers of epithelial cells. For other bacterial causes of conjunctivitis, the organism is recovered from the purulent discharge, which can be collected with a swab. If *N. gonorrhoeae* is suspected, the specimen should be inoculated directly onto an appropriate selective medium.

Corneal infections represent a slightly different problem in terms of specimen collection. Application of a topical anesthetic is necessary in order to obtain corneal scrapings. However, these agents are toxic to bacteria. Proparacaine hydrochloride is recommended over other anesthetics if culture is attempted because it is less toxic than alternatives.[10] Corneal scrapings should be inoculated directly onto appropriate media, using the curette to make C- or S-shaped cuts into the agar surface.

Intraocular infections have been addressed under sterile body fluids.

Infections Requiring Surgical Biopsy

When deep tissue infections occur, it may be necessary to collect specimens for culture via a surgical procedure. Superficial contamination of the specimen with colonizing microflora is obviously avoided. However, all too frequently the amount of tissue submitted to the laboratory is insufficient for the tests requested. As large a sample as practical should be collected at surgery. If multiple foci of infection are evident, tissue samples should be collected from representative sites. If only a very small sample can be obtained, it is imperative that the laboratory work with the physician to prioritize the test requests.

SPECIMEN TRANSPORT AND PRESERVATION

There are a myriad of systems and devices into which specimens can be placed for transport to the laboratory. It is far better to limit the number of containers to a minimum so that personnel involved in specimen collection can choose from a small number of alternatives. Two sterile, screwcapped containers, one for small volumes and one for larger volumes, a collection/transport device for swabs which contains a non-nutritive transport medium such as Stuart's or Amies and an anaerobic transport system which contains a pre-reduced, non-nutritive transport medium such as Cary and Blair with an Eh indicator, will suffice for the majority of specimens. There are a limited number of specimens where inoculation directly onto the appropriate isolation medium is desirable. Examples include blood, specimens for isolation of *N. gonorrhoeae* and corneal scrapings.

Table 1:2. Storage and Preservation of Clinical Specimens if Processing is Delayed

Specimen	Preservative	Storage Temp 4°C	Storage Temp 25°C
Catheter, intravenous		X	
Ear			
External	Stuart's or Amies	X	
Internal	Nutritive transport medium		X
Eye			
Conjunctiva	Stuart's or Amies		X
Corneal Scraping	Direct plating		X
Internal (aqueous, vitreous humor	Direct plating		X
Fluids			
Abdominal	Anaerobic transport medium		X
Amniotic	Anaerobic transport medium		X
Blood	Direct inoculation of culture		X
Bone marrow	Direct inoculation of culture		X
Cerebrospinal			X
Chest			X
Cul-de-sac	Anareobic transport medium		X
Pericardial		X	
Synovial			X
Gastrointestinal			
Bile	Anaerobic transport medium		X
Gastric aspirate	Alkaline buffering system	X	
Stool, rectal swab			
Salmonella,	Buffered glycerol-saline		X
Shigella, Yersinia	Modified Cary-Blair	X	
Campylobacter	Modified Cary-Blair	X	
Vibrio	Modified Cary-Blair	X	
Genital			
Cervix			
Neisseria	Direct plating (eg., Jembec), Stuart's or Amies		X
Chlamydia	*Chlamydia* transport medium	X	
Actinomyces	Anaerobic transport medium		X
Endometrium	Same as cervix		
Prostatic fluid	Same as cervix		
Urethra	Same as cervix		
Vagina	Stuart's or Amies		X
Vulva	Stuart's or Amies		X
Respiratory			
Bronchial wash		X	
Lung aspirate	Anaerobic transport medium		X
Lung biopsy		X	
Mouth	Stuart's or Amies		X
Nasopharynx			
Group A streptococci	Stuart's or Amies (>24 hr, silica gel)		X
Corynebacterium	Loeffler or Pai slant (>24 hr, silica gel)		X
Neisseria	Direct plating (eg., Jembec), Stuart's or Amies		X
Bordetella	RL transport medium		X
Nose	Stuart's or Amies		X

Table 1:2. Storage and Preservation of Clinical Specimens if Processing is Delayed (Continued)

Specimen	Preservative	Storage Temp 4°C	Storage Temp 25°C
Sinus aspirate	Anaerobic transport medium		X
Sputum, tracheostomy		X	
Transtracheal	Anaerobic transport medium		X
Skin			
Superficial	Stuart's or Amies		X
Burn wound biopsy	Stuart's or Amies	X	
Deep lesion	Anaerobic transport medium		X
Tissue			
Autopsy		X	
Surgical biopsy	Anaerobic transport medium		X
Urine			
Clean-voided,		X	
Catheter, cystoscopic, etc.		X	
Suprapubic aspirate	Anaerobic transport medium		X

The time between specimen collection and laboratory processing should be kept to a minimum. It is generally accepted that specimens suffer significant deterioration within 1-2 hours after they have been collected, although there are surprisingly few studies which document this belief. If it is anticipated that transit time will be extended or if transport is unreliable, mechanisms for preservation must be defined and the appropriate materials made available. Table 1:2 lists recommendations for storage and preservation of specimens which cannot be processed within an acceptable time frame.

The temperature at which certain specimens should be stored until processed remains problematic. For example, expectorated sputum frequently contains small numbers of potential pathogens such as enteric gram-negative bacilli which are contaminants from the upper airway. If stored at room temperature for an extended period of time, the specimen may be overgrown with these bacteria. On the other hand, some of the common respiratory tract pathogens such as *H. influenzae* do not tolerate refrigerated temperatures well and their numbers will decline with time. Since there is no real alternative to storage at 4°C, every effort should be made to process such specimens as soon as technical staff becomes available. Guidelines should be provided to the laboratory personnel so that the most labile specimens are processed first, especially if they have been stored over an extended period.

Whenever possible, specimens which have been inoculated at the time of collection into a nutritive transport system (e.g., blood culture bottles, Jembec plates) should be placed at incubation temperatures as soon as they are delivered to the laboratory. The vast majority of bacterial pathogens grow optimally at 35-37°C, although viability can be adequately maintained at room temperature. Consequently, a positive culture will be recognized earlier if this growth requirement is met. Consideration may also be given to placing sterile body fluids at 35-37°C; since there is presumably no concern about overgrowth by contaminating bacteria, detection time may be decreased.

SPECIMEN QUALITY

Perhaps the most difficult issue for the laboratory is the assessment of specimen quality. Unfortunately, even highly sophisticated testing will not make up for an inappropriately collected, transported or preserved specimen. There are four facets to the laboratory's responsibility: (1) the provision of readily accessible and "user-friendly" guidelines for collection, transport and preservation of specimens for culture, (2) the establishment of and adherence to policies which define appropriate and inappropriate elements of specimen management, (3) constant education and reeducation of medical and support staff who are involved in specimen collection and (4) implementing screening procedures in the laboratory designed to detect specimens of poor quality.

Instructions for specimen management should be written in collaboration with representatives from the groups using them. The user's input is essential, since the format in which information is presented may determine whether the instructions are actively used. Issues such as bound manuals vs. rolodex card files, making the primary index based upon specimen source vs. test request, and the use of cross-indexing vs. information redundancy should all be presented and discussed so that a concensus can be reached. It cannot be overstressed that effective instructions are concise instructions. Although it may be intellectually satisfying to provide detailed information about WHY something is done, the essential information is HOW it is done.

The elements of specimen management have been the primary topic of this chapter and deserve no additional comment here. It should be remembered, however, that appropriate mechanisms must be put in place to identify specimens which have not been handled properly and that policies, once established, must be enforced.

Education of the medical staff and support personnel should be approached creatively and in an on-going program. Although formal presentations are the most common approach, they are probably the least effective. The use of audits to identify problem areas and focus educational efforts should be considered. Personal contact with specific individuals who have made inappropriate requests or violated good specimen collection procedures provides a continuum of information exchange. The laboratory report itself can provide a convenient vehicle for communication. Mistakes will always be made. It is the role of the laboratorian to keep the number to a minimum and view those that occur as opportunities for effective education.

The final facet, developing screening procedures in the laboratory to identify specimens of poor quality, remains a difficult and unresolved issue. Unfortunately, there is no easily recognizable sign that alerts the technical staff to potential problems. Microscopic examination of clinical material represents one approach which has been described and evaluated. This approach was first proposed for assessing expectorated sputum specimens.[2] It was based upon the assumption that inflammatory cells correlated with the presence of lower respiratory tract secretions and that squamous epithelial cells represented oropharyngeal contamination of the specimen. Several algorithms have since been developed using various combinations of these two cellular types to judge specimen quality. While no concensus exists as to which combination serves as the best predictor, it is generally agreed that some type of microscopic screen is valuable to eliminate sputum samples of questionable quality.

A similar assessment process has been proposed for a number of other specimen types. These include urine, superficial wounds and cervical specimens. Although such an approach is theoretically satisfying, there are no objective data to support the use of a microscopic screening procedure for specimen sources other than sputum. Even such factors as the relative survival rate of inflammatory and epithelial cells on swabs is uncharacterized. Neutrophil survival in fluids, at least, is known to be of limited duration.[19] Until such issues are evaluated, there are no alternatives. Thus, for the present, microscopic assessment of quality seems preferable to no assessment at all.

REFERENCES

1. Bartlett JG, Alexander J, Mayhew J, Sullivan-Sigler N, Gorbach SL. Should fiberoptic bronchoscopy aspirates be cultured? Am Rev Respir Dis 1976;114:73–8.
2. Bartlett RC. Medical microbiology: quality, cost and clinical relevance. New York: John Wiley, 1974.
3. Branefors-Helander P, Jeppsson P-H. Acute epiglottitis: a clinical, bacteriological and serological study. Scand J Infect Dis 1975;7:103–10.
4. Evans FO, Sydnor JB, Moore WEC, et al. Sinusitis of the maxillary antrum. N Engl J Med 1975;293:735–9.
5. Evans KD, Peterson EM, Curry JI, Greenwood JR, de la Maza LM. Effect of holding temperature on isolation of *Neisseria gonorrhoeae*. J Clin Microbiol 1986;24:1109–10.
6. Fairley KF, Bond AG, Brown RB, Habersberger P. Simple test to determine the site of urinary-tract infections. Lancet 1967;2:7513–14.
7. Gross PA, Harkavy LM, Barden GE, Kerstein M. Positive Foley catheter tip cultures - fact or fancy? JAMA 1974;228:72–3.

8. Henry NK, McLimans CA, Wright AJ, Washington JA II. Microbiological and clinical evaluation of the Isolator lysis-centrifugation blood culture tube. J Clin Microbiol 1983;17:864–9.
9. Ilstrup DM, Washington JA II. The importance of volume of blood cultured in the detection of bacteremia and fungemia. Diagn Microbiol Infect Dis 1983;1:107–10.
10. Jones DB, Leisegang TJ, Robinson NM. Cumitech 17. Laboratory diagnosis of ocular infections. Washington, DC: American Society for Microbiology, 1981.
11. LaScolea LJ, Dryja D, Sullivan TD, Mosovich L, Ellerstein N, Neter E. Diagnosis of bacteremia in children by quantitative direct plating and a radiometric procedure. J Clin Microbiol 1981;13:178–82.
12. Marshal BJ, Warren JR. Unidentified curved bacilli in the stomach of patients with gastritis and peptic ulceration. Lancet 1984:1068–9.
13. Meares EM, Stamey TA. Bacteriologic localization patterns in bacterial prostatitis and urethritis. Invest Urol 1968;5:492–518.
14. Rintala L, Pollock H. Effects of two blood culture anticoagulants on growth of *Neisseria meningitidis*. J Clin Microbiol 1978;7:332–6.
15. Roberts AP, Robinson RE, Beard RN. Some factors affecting bacterial counts in urinary infection. Br Med J 1967;1:400–3.
16. Schachter J. Urine as a specimen for diagnosis of STD. Am J Med 1983;28:93–7.
17. Schwartz R, Rodriguez WJ, Khan WN, et al. Acute purulent otitis media in children older than 5 years. Incidence of *Haemophilus* as a causative agent. JAMA 1977;238:1032–41.
18. Spiegel CA, Amsel R, Eschenbach D, et al. Anaerobic bacteria in non-specific vaginitis. N Engl J Med 1980;303:601–7.
18. Steele RW, Marmer DJ, O'Brien MD, Tyson ST, Steele CR. Leukocyte survival in cerebrospinal fluid. J Clin Microbiol 1986;23:965–6.
20. Tenney JH, Reller LB, Mirret S, Chang W-LL, Weinstein MP. Controlled evaluations of the volume of blood cultured in detection of bacteremia and fungemia. J Clin Microbiol 1982;15:558–61.
21. Tonnesen A, Peuler M, Lockwood WR. Cultures of blood drawn through catheters vs. venipuncture. JAMA 1976;235:1877-1926.
22. Vontuer LA, Eschenbach DA. The role of *Gardnerella vaginalis* in non-specific vaginitis. Clin Obstet Gynecol 1981;24:439–60.
23. Washington JA II. Blood cultures: principals and techniques. Mayo Clin Proc 1975;50:91–8.
24. Wimberly N, Faling LJ, Bartlett JG. A fiberoptic bronchoscopy technique to obtain uncontaminated lower airway secretions for bacterial culture. Am Rev Respir Dis 1979;119:337–43.

CHAPTER 2

METHOD EVALUATION AND TEST SELECTION

Kenneth A. McPherson, B.S. and Cynthia A. Needham, Ph.D.

INTRODUCTION

Test selection is the procedure which elevates laboratory analysis above the status of a costly way station between specimen collection and autoclaving. Test selection entered the laboratorian's realm most dramatically during the past ten years as the science of clinical microbiology migrated from an observational science to one which increasingly relies on inferences about probable disease states, given the existence of certain key test criteria. The laboratorian's objective in test selection is simply stated:

To identify the test procedure which best provides inferences about the disease state, given current technologies and laboratory facilities.

Defining "best" is the truly interesting element in appropriate test selection. Selecting appropriate tests involves weighing four key parameters:

1. How sensitive is the test in determining the true presence of a disease;
2. How selective is the test in excluding diseases which are truly absent;
3. What is the true prevalence of the disease among the population which the laboratorian will test; and
4. How significant are the benefits of a more efficient test relative to the increased cost of more efficient tests?

These four parameters interact in determining appropriate tests. The remainder of this chapter will examine these parameters and their interrelationships in four steps.

Step 1: to review and more explicitly define each of the parameters;

Step 2: to examine the overall relationship among the four parameters;

Step 3: to focus on isolating the effect of changes in each of the four parameters in turn while holding the remaining three parameters constant; and

Step 4: to identify specific techniques for evaluating tests and procedures in a clinical environment.

THE BASIC STATISTICS OF TEST SELECTION

The traditional departure point for detailed evaluation of test selection emphasizes quantitative definitions of key parameters. We will honor that sacred tradition by examining several key terms. As many predecessors have noted, a simple table diagram provides a clear basis for understanding the terms. Table 2:1 indicates the four possible combinations of disease states and test results.

Sensitivity: Measures the percent of trials in which the test indicates positive when the disease is present. In simple arithmetic:

Sensitivity = (A)/[(A) + (C)].

Specificity: Measures the percent of trials in which the test yields negative results when the disease is absent. In simple terms:

Specificity = (D)/[(B) + (D)].

Predictive value of a positive test result:[1] Predictive Value Positive (PVP) is the percentage of true test results which actually coincides with the presence of the disease, or:

PVP = (A)/[(A) + (B)].

Predictive value of a negative test result:[1] Predictive Value Negative (PVN)

Table 2:1. Disease States and Test Results

	Disease Present	Disease Absent
Test Positive	(A) True Positive	(B) False Positive
Test Negative	(C) False Negative	(D) True Negative

measures the percentage of negative test results which coincides with absence of the disease, or:

$$PVN = (D)/[(C) + (D)]$$

Efficiency:[1] An obvious measure is the number of times the test is correct, or:

$$\text{Efficiency} = [(A) + (D)]/[(A) + (B) + (C) + (D)].$$

Finally, test selection involves one measure which is essentially independent of specific tests. Prevalence is the proportion of population to be tested which actually has the disease. Test population prevalence may differ significantly from general population prevalence. The prevalence of sexually transmitted diseases at a venereal disease clinic typically greatly exceeds the prevalence of sexually transmitted diseases in the general population. Test selection at venereal disease clinics would reflect their higher prevalence.

Sensitivity and specificity are inherent properties of a given test. These two measures, once properly established, remain constant and are independent of the population tested. PVP, PVN and efficiency for any test depend upon both the inherent sensitivity and specificity of the test and upon the prevalence of the disease among the population being tested.

TEST UTILITY

Test utility is defined as the net benefit derived from a specific test. Test utility can be further defined as the sum of total expected net benefits for true positive and true negative reports less the total expected net costs of false negative and false positive reports. The test utility measure, therefore, incorporates the specificity and selectivity of the test, the prevalence of the disease within the test population and perceived benefits and costs for each of the possible outcomes.

We begin calculating test utility by determining the expected number of patients in each outcome cell, given the respective test population. The number of patients receiving true positive results (A) may be calculated as shown in Table 2:2. These four equations highlight the interactions among prevalence, sensitivity, specificity and expected test results.

Applying a given test in higher prevalence populations will increase the number of true positives, increasing the apparent value of the test. However, increased prevalence also increases the number of false negatives.

Applying a test in lower prevalence populations will increase the number

Table 2:2. Calculation of Test Utility

Number of Patients: True Positive = # People In Test Population × Prevalence of Disease in Test Population × Sensitivity

or,

$$(A) = [(A) + (B) + (C) + (D)] \times \frac{[(A) + (C)]}{[(A) + (B) + (C) + (D)]} \times \frac{(A)}{[(A) + (C)]}$$

Number of Patients: True Negative = # People In Test Population × 1 − Prevalence of Disease in Test Population × Specificity

or,

$$(D) = [(A) + (B) + (C) + (D)] \times \left[1 - \frac{[(A) + (C)]}{[(A) + (B) + (C) + (D)]}\right] \times \frac{(D)}{[(B) + (D)]}$$

Number of Patients: False Positive = # People In Test Population × 1 − Prevalence of Disease in Test Population × [1 − Specificity]

or,

$$(B) = [(A) + (B) + (C) + (D)] \times \left[1 - \frac{[(A) + (C)]}{[(A) + (B) + (C) + (D)]}\right] \times \left[1 - \frac{(D)}{[(B) + (D)]}\right]$$

Number of Patients: False Negative = # People In Test Population × Prevalence × 1 [− Sensitivity]

or,

$$(C) = [(A) + (B) + (C) + (D)] \times \left[\frac{[(A) + (C)]}{[(A) + (B) + (C) + (D)]}\right] \times \left[1 - \frac{(A)}{[(A) + (C)]}\right]$$

of true negatives, suggesting greater value to the test. However, lower prevalence yields more false positives.

These effects may be demonstrated using a simple example. Assume that a certain test has a sensitivity of 0.9 and a specificity of 0.8. Further, assume that two laboratories administer the test. The first laboratory has a test population with a 60% prevalence for the disease. The second laboratory has a test population with a 10% prevalence. The first laboratory should expect the results in Table 2:3 from 100 tests. For the second laboratory the expected results would be those shown in Table 2:4.

The first laboratory has generated 5 more false negatives from a total population of 100 than laboratory 2 generated using the same test. However, laboratory 2 generated 10 more false positives. In fact, laboratory 2 generated twice as many false positives as true positives (Table 2:5).

Now, assume that a second test becomes available with sensitivity 0.5 and a specificity of 0.8. The corresponding results would be those shown in Table 2:6. This comparison highlights several key points about these common measures.

1. Differing prevalence between the test populations had more impact on

Table 2:3. Expected Results For Laboratory 1 With 60% Prevalence

	Disease Present	Disease Absent	
Test Positive	54 True Positive	8 False Positive	62
Test Negative	6 False Negative	32 True Negative	38
	60	40	

Table 2:4. Expected Results For Laboratory 2 With 10% Prevalence

	Disease Present	Disease Absent	
Test Positive	9 True Positive	18 False Positive	27
Test Negative	1 False Negative	72 True Negative	73
	10	90	

Table 2:5. Comparison of Laboratory Results for Test 1.

	Lab 1	Lab 2		Lab 1	Lab 2
Prevalence	60%	10%	PVP	0.87	0.33
True Positive	54	9	PVN	0.84	0.99
True Negative	32	72	Efficacy	0.86	0.81
False Positive	8	18			
False Negative	6	1			

PVP and PVN than did differing sensitivities and specificities between the tests.

2. Positive test results provide less diagnostic value than negative test results in low prevalence populations. Test efficiency may be significantly influenced by disease prevalence as well as by the inherent characteristics of the test.
3. Low prevalence populations offer a significant challenge in developing test strategies. There are two approaches to test selection in low prevalence populations. The first strategy involves applying a screening test to initially enrich the population with respect to disease prevalence.

Table 2:6. Comparison of Tests With Differing Parameters in Different Populations

	Test One		Test Two	
Sensitivity	0.9		0.5	
Specificity	0.8		0.9	
	Lab 1	Lab 2	Lab 1	Lab 2
Prevalence	0.60	0.10	0.60	0.10
True Positive	54	9	30	5
True Negative	32	72	36	81
False Positive	8	18	4	9
False Negative	6	1	30	5
PVP	0.87	0.33	0.88	0.36
PVN	0.84	0.99	0.55	0.94
Efficiency	0.86	0.81	0.66	0.86

The reactive population can then be tested using a highly specific second test. The VDRL and FTA-ABS combination is an example of this test strategy. The alternative strategy is to employ a highly sensitive and specific initial test. Tests in this category tend to be relatively expensive. However, the additional cost may be fully justified for a low prevalence population.

The laboratorian must be careful to evaluate the predictive value of positive and negative test results within the context of a specific test population. Sensitivity and specificity in isolation are inadequate parameters for test evaluation.

TEST EVALUATION IN A CLINICAL ENVIRONMENT

The laboratorian should:

1. Review independent publications to obtain peer-reviewed measures of sensitivity and specificity for the test under evaluation and critically assess the validity of the studies establishing these values. Ransohoff and Feinstein[3] provide a clear discussion of potential bias in study design.
2. Determine test populations and establish realistic estimates of disease prevalence within the test population. Consider the possibility that introducing a new test may affect the nature of the test population.
3. Calculate predictive values and project estimates of true positives, true negatives, false positives and false negatives within the specified test population.
4. Develop estimates of the costs of false positives and false negatives, along with estimates of the benefits of true positives and true negatives. There is considerable debate in the literature about the feasibility of actually quantifying these costs and benefits. These estimates should

be viewed as guides to test selection rather than as deterministic absolutes which absolve the laboratorian of the need for judgment.[2]

This assessment should allow the laboratorian to determine if the test offers sufficient utility to be applied. Further, the assessment should provide guidance about whether the test should be used as a screen or as a definitive test.

REFERENCES

1. Galen RS, Gambino SR. Beyond normality: the predictive value and efficiency of medical diagnosis. New York: John Wiley, 1975.
2. Raiffa H. Decision analysis: Introductory lectures on choices under uncertainty. Reading, MA: Addison-Wesley, 1970.
3. Ransohoff DF, Feinstein AR. Problems of spectrum and bias in evaluating the efficacy of diagnostic tests. N Engl J Med 1978;299:926–30.

Section 2: Bacterial Diseases

CHAPTER 3

AEROMONAS AND *PLESIOMONAS* INFECTIONS

J. Michael Janda, Ph.D.

INTRODUCTION

Members of the genera *Aeromonas* and *Plesiomonas* are oxidase-positive, gram-negative, facultatively-anaerobic bacilli that sometimes infect both poikilothermic and homeothermic animals. Although these microorganisms are primarily commensals residing in fresh and saltwater environments, increased interest in them has recently occurred due to the heightened awareness that they are significant causes of disease in both normal and immunologically-compromised individuals. The original description of the genus *Aeromonas* is most commonly attributed to Sanarelli. In 1891, he isolated the gram-negative bacterium *Bacillus hydrophilus* from the blood of a frog suffering from "red leg" disease. In the intervening years this bacterium has been taxonomically-placed in a number of other genera including *Pseudomonas*; however, in 1936, Kluyver and van Neil proposed its inclusion in the genus *Aeromonas*, where it currently resides. The genus *Plesiomonas* was originally described by Ferguson and Henderson in 1947 (referred to as C27). These isolates were later included in the genus *Aeromonas*. Subsequent taxonomic and biochemical studies, however, indicate that these organisms are distinct from the aeromonads, and the plesiomonads have since been placed in their own genus.

Aeromonas

CAUSATIVE ORGANISMS

At present, four species are recognized within the genus: *A. salmonicida, A. hydrophila, A. sobria* and *A. caviae*. *A. salmonicida* is a nonmotile, indole-negative bacillus that fails to grow at 37°C, and is the causative agent of fish furunculosis. No human infection attributed to this bacterium has been reported. The latter three mesophilic aeromonads, all motile and indole-positive, are pathogens of man. Each of these species, however, contains more than one DNA hybridization group, which at present cannot be differentiated using simple biochemical tests.

CLINICAL MANIFESTATIONS

Aeromonas infections span the entire spectrum of diseases of man, being most commonly implicated in diarrhea, cellulitis and septicemia. *Aeromonas* gastroenteritis is usually a self-limiting illness of 1-7 days duration with symptoms appearing 24-48 hours after contact with the bacterium. The disease is found in both pediatric and adult patients, though generally more frequently in the former group. *Aeromonas* diarrhea may present in one of several ways, including an acute secretory gastroenteritis (most common), a dysenteric form resembling shigellosis, a chronic gastroenteritis of 10-14 days duration or longer, or as an infrequent cause of cholera-like illness or traveler's diarrhea.

Wound infections are the second most common disease produced by aeromonads.[1] These infections usually result from exposure of traumatized sites to contaminated water sources containing *Aeromonas* spp. The extent of this disease ranges from a mild cellulitis to a more fulminant myonecrosis.

Aeromonas bacteremia has, in the past, been principally a disease of patients with severe underlying illnesses such as hematologic malignancies, solid tumors or hepatobiliary disease as exemplified by Laennec's cirrhosis.[1] Recently, a number of reports have appeared documenting *Aeromonas* bacteremia in adults with no known underlying disease. Overall, a 28-59% mortality rate has been observed in septicemic patients, depending upon the population studied, severity of the underlying disease and method of treatment.

A final so-called "miscellaneous" category encompasses rare or unusual infections caused by *Aeromonas*,[1] such as meningitis, endocarditis, osteomyelitis, pneumonia, ocular and urinary tract infections.

THERAPY

Aeromonas spp. are usually susceptible to tetracycline, chloramphenicol, trimethoprim-sulfamethoxazole, the aminoglycosides and to third-generation cephalosporins.[9,10] Ineffective antimicrobial agents include penicillin and its semisynthetic derivates, ampicillin and first and second generation cephalosporins. Most *Aeromonas* gastroenteritis is self-limiting and does not require antimicrobial therapy. Therapy may be indicated for cases of severe dysentery, cholera-like disease or gastroenteritis of prolonged duration. The most commonly administered antibiotics in these instances have been tetracycline and trimethoprim-sulfamethoxazole. All other illnesses usually require treatment with broad spectrum agents or combinations of antibiotics.

EPIDEMIOLOGY

Aeromonas spp. are normal inhabitants of the aquatic biosphere and presumably can be recovered from soil also. Studies by Hazen and colleagues[3] suggest that most inland waters in the United States harbor these bacteria. Larger densities of these microorganisms, presumably due to the increase in water temperature, can be recovered during the summer months. This seasonal variation in aeromonad concentrations parallels the higher incidence of *Aeromonas* gastroenteritis observed over a similar time frame, suggesting that natural water sources (i.e., well water) are a potential source of infection.

PUBLIC HEALTH SIGNIFICANCE, PREVENTION AND CONTROL

Most *Aeromonas* infections occur sporadically and are community-acquired. At present there are no known reports of foodborne outbreaks of gastroenteritis, although until recently, many surveys failed to specifically look for this bacterium. With the increased recovery of *Aeromonas* spp. from a variety of food sources, the public health significance of such isolations and their relative concentrations in such products awaits further studies.

DIAGNOSTIC PROCEDURES

Primary Isolation and Culture

Aeromonas spp. produce luxuriant growth on most nonselective agars, and the isolation and identification of strains recovered from nonfecal sources is usually not a problem. Recovery of these bacteria from stool specimens can be difficult, since individual isolates have varying plating efficiencies on common enteric media,[2] and most fail to grow on agars designed for the isolation of *Vibrio* spp. It is therefore suggested that gastrointestinal specimens suspected of harboring *Aeromonas* should either be plated on several enteric media, inoculated onto a nonselective agar such as sheep blood, or streaked onto a selective medium designed specifically for the recovery of *Aeromonas* such as pril-xylose-ampicillin or xylose-sodium desoxycholate-citrate agars. For detection of *Aeromonas* in environmental samples or during transient colonization of man, alkaline peptone water (pH 8.5) has been found to be a satisfactory enrichment broth.[15]

The *Aeromonas*/*Plesiomonas* group can be presumptively identified by spot-testing colonies on nonselective media for indole and oxidase positivity. Strains positive for both characteristics can be tentatively identified as belonging to this group, while oxidase-positive colonies should be further evaluated using a larger battery of biochemical tests.[7] If nonselective media are not routinely used in the workup of fecal specimens, organisms that produce alkaline over acid slants on Kligler Iron Agar with or without gas may be screened for the oxidase reaction directly from this medium.[13]

Methods of Identification

The salient biochemical characteristics of the motile *Aeromonas* group are listed in Table 3:1. Isolates are usually easy to identify to the genus level, however, an occasional strain will generate a biochemical profile from conventional tests or from a miniaturized system consistent for either *Aeromonas* spp. or the phenotypically similar *Vibrio fluvialis*. This dilemma can be overcome by screening such isolates for lysine decarboxylase activity, salt tolerance, growth on thiosulfate-citrate-bile salts-sucrose (TCBS) agar and O/129 (2,4-diamino-6,7-diisopropylpteridine) sensitivity.[7] Besides identification to the genus level, larger laboratories and reference centers should probably determine the species status of each isolate since the biologic properties of each group differ significantly (Table 3:2).[6]

Markers of Epidemiology

Because of the variability in biochemical properties of mesophilic aeromonads, it is practical not only to determine the species of each strain, but

Table 3:1. Salient Features in the Identification of *Aeromonas* and *Plesiomonas*

Characteristic	*Aeromonas*	*Plesiomonas*
Metabolism	F*	F
Oxidase	+	+
Indole	+	+
Ornithine decarboxylase	−	+
Lysine decarboxylase	V†	+
Arginine dihydrolase	+	+
Acid from glucose	+	+
Acid from inositol	−	+
Gelatinase	+	−
Growth in nutrient agar with:		
0% NaCl	+	+
3% NaCl	+	+
6% NaCl	−	−
Sensitivity to O/129	−	+

* = fermentative
† = variable

Table 3:2. Biochemical Properties Useful in Determining the Species Status of *Aeromonas* Isolates

Characteristic	*A. hydrophila*	*A. sobria*	*A. caviae*
Esculin hydrolysis	+	−	+
Growth in KCN broth	+	−	+
Acid from salicin	+	−	+
Acid from arabinose	+	−	+
Lysine decarboxylase	+	+	−
Voges-Proskauer	+	+	−
Gas from glucose	+	+	−
H_2S (in GCF* medium)	+	+	−
Hemolysin (beta)	+	+	−
Gluconate oxidation	+	+	−

* Gelatin-Cysteine-Thiosulfate Medium.

to biotype the isolate in question, utilizing carbohydrate fermentation profiles and endproducts of metabolism. An alternative approach has been provided in a provisional serotyping scheme for motile *Aeromonas* spp. by Sakazaki and Shimada[11] based upon 44 distinct O somatic antigens.

Toxigenicity Tests

At present, the testing of individual *Aeromonas* spp. from clinical specimens for toxins should probably be attempted only by reference laboratories when conventional tests fail to demonstrate phenotypic markers suggestive of an enterotoxigenic isolate (lysine decarboxylase, Voges-Proskauer, beta-hemolysis), and the strain is suspected of causing diarrheal disease.

Evaluation of the Clinical Significance of Laboratory Tests

Besides determining the species designation of all *Aeromonas* recovered from infectious processes (Table 3:2), isolates from cases of gastrointestinal disease should be evaluated for biochemical markers associated with enterotoxigenicity or tested for cytotoxin or enterotoxin activity in appropriate models.[8]

Plesiomonas

CAUSATIVE ORGANISM

At present only one member of the genus is recognized (*P. shigelloides*). Hybridization studies indicate that this group is genetically homogeneous.

CLINICAL MANIFESTATIONS

The vast majority of infections reportedly due to *P. shigelloides* involve gastrointestinal disease. As with *Aeromonas*, the range of symptoms vary from an acute secretory form (most common) to a more severe colitis.[4] More recently, a number of extraintestinal infections caused by *P. shigelloides* have been documented, particularly in immunocompromised patients (neonates, sickle-cell disease). These latter infections include bacteremia, meningitis, cholecystitis, septic arthritis and ocular disease.

THERAPY

Recent studies by Reinhardt and George[10] indicate that most antimicrobial agents appropriate for use against enteric pathogens would be active against *P. shigelloides*. Drugs in this category include tetracycline, trimethoprim-sulfamethoxazole and the newer oxyquinolones. Other agents presumably active against a majority of *P. shigelloides* strains include chloramphenicol, the aminoglycosides and third-generation cephalosporins. Most isolates produce a beta-lactamase and are ampicillin-resistant.

EPIDEMIOLOGY

P. shigelloides is a common inhabitant of fresh and salt water environments and is commonly isolated from river and lake fish, sludge, and the feces of cats and dogs. In man, colonization rates appear to be extremely low (0.0087%) and most gastrointestinal isolates appear to be clinically significant. Three outbreaks of diarrhea reportedly due to *P. shigelloides* have been reported.[14] In two instances, potential sources for the outbreaks (tapwater, oysters) were identified. In extraintestinal disease where a potential source for *P. shigelloides* can be identified, it often involves consumption of seafood (i.e., crab).

PUBLIC HEALTH SIGNIFICANCE, PREVENTION AND CONTROL

Based on the data obtained from two outbreaks of *P. shigelloides*-associated gastroenteritis, the ingestion of large numbers of these micro-organisms was potentially related to undercooked or ''wet'' oysters and an inadequately-chlorinated water supply.[14] Since the exact incidence and concentration of *P. shigelloides* in foods (i.e., shellfish) and water supplies in the United States is unknown, recommendations regarding preventive measures and control of outbreaks will have to await further studies.

DIAGNOSTIC PROCEDURES

Primary Isolation and Culture

Plesiomonads can be isolated on most media commonly used for recovery of enteric pathogens. Since the incidence of *Plesiomonas*-associated diarrhea is apparently very low, the routine use of selective media designed specifically for the isolation of this organism is not warranted. In instances where an enteric pathogen is still being sought well after the acute phase of the illness, or for studies involving the carrier rate of *Plesiomonas* in defined populations, a selective medium may be required. Most studies suggest that inositol-brilliant green-bile salts agar is best suited for these purposes.[15]

Methods of Identification

P. shigelloides produces a characteristic biochemical profile typified by its lysine- and ornithine-decarboxylase activities, arginine-dihydrolase positivity, fermentation of inositol and failure to elaborate protease, gelatinase, lipase, hemolysin or deoxyribonuclease (Table 3:1). Because of this unusual phenotypic pattern, isolates are seldom misidentified if a preliminary oxidase test is performed.

Markers of Epidemiology

Since *P. shigelloides* is a phenotypically "tight" species and is susceptible to most antimicrobial agents, the use of biotypes or antibiograms as markers for tracing strains of epidemiologic significance is unproductive. Strains may, however, be separated by their serologic properties and at least 107 serovars (50 O groups, 17 H antigens) of *Plesiomonas* currently exist.[12]

Toxigenicity Tests

As yet most conventional assays designed to detect toxins potentially related to the pathogenesis of *P. shigelloides* have been negative. Some strains freshly isolated from stool specimens are invasive in HeLa cell assays, while others have been found to produce heat-labile and heat-stable toxins as detected in rabbit illeal loop and suckling mouse models.[5]

Serologic Tests

Many isolates react with antisera directed against *Shigella sonnei* (phase 1). Agglutinating antibodies against a strain of *P. shigelloides* have been demonstrated in the convalescent sera of a patient suffering from cholecystitis.

Evaluation of the Clinical Significance of Laboratory Tests

At present, studies aimed at determining the virulence-associated factors of *P. shigelloides* are inconclusive. Strains recovered from fecal specimens should be quantitated relative to the number of normal enteric flora present.

REFERENCES

1. Davis WA II, Kane JG, Garagusi VF. Human *Aeromonas* infections: a review of the literature and a case report of endocarditis. Medicine 1978;57:267-77.
2. Desmond E, Janda JM. Growth of *Aeromonas* species on enteric agars. J Clin Microbiol 1986;23:1065-7.
3. Hazen TC, Fliermans CB, Hirsch RP, Esch GW. Prevalance and distribution of *Aeromonas hydrophila* in the United States. Appl Environ Microbiol 1978;36:731-8.
4. Holmberg SD, Farmer JJ III. *Aeromonas hydrophila* and *Plesiomonas shigelloides* as causes of intestinal infections. Rev Infect Dis 1984;6:633-9.
5. Huq MI, Islam MR. Microbiological and clinical studies in diarrhoea due to *Plesiomonas shigelloides*. Indian J Med Res 1983;77:793-7.
6. Janda JM, Reitano M, Bottone EJ. Biotyping of *Aeromonas* isolates as a correlate to delineating a species-associated disease spectrum. J Clin Microbiol 1984;19:44-7.
7. Janda JM. Biochemical and exoenzymatic properties of *Aeromonas* species. Diagn Microbiol Infect Dis 1985;3:223-32.
8. Ljungh A, Wadstrom T. *Aeromonas* and *Plesiomonas* as possible causes of diarrhoea. Infection 1985;4:169-73.
9. Motyl MR, McKinley G, Janda JM. In vitro susceptibilities of *Aeromonas hydrophila, Aeromonas sobria* and *Aeromonas caviae* to 22 antimicrobial agents. Antimicrob Agents Chemother 1985;28:151-3.
10. Reinhardt JF, George WL. Comparative in vitro activities of selected antimicrobial agents against *Aeromonas* species and *Plesiomonas shigelloides*. Antimicrob Agents Chemother 1985;27:643-5.
11. Sakazaki R, Shimada T. O-serogrouping scheme for mesophilic *Aeromonas* strains. Japan J Med Sci Biol 1984;37:247-55.
12. Shimada T, Sakazaki R. New O and H antigens and additional serovars of *Plesiomonas shigelloides*. Japan J Med Sci Biol 1985;38:73-6.
13. Skillern JK, Overman TL. Oxidase testing from Kligler's iron agar and triple sugar iron agar slants. Curr Microbiol 1983;8:269-71.
14. Tsukamoto T, Kinoshita Y, Shimada T, Sakazaki R. Two epidemics of diarrhoeal disease possibly caused by *Plesiomonas shigelloides*. J Hyg Camb 1978;80:275-80.
15. Von Graevenitz A, Bucher C. Evaluation of differential and selective media for isolation of *Aeromonas* and *Plesiomonas* spp. from human feces. J Clin Microbiol 1983;17:16-21.

CHAPTER 4

ANAEROBIC INFECTIONS: NONSPOREFORMERS

Peter C. Appelbaum, M.D., Ph.D.

INTRODUCTION

During the last decade of the 19th century, Veillon and coworkers at the Faculty of Medicine in Paris initiated a series of important investigations on the role of nonsporeforming anaerobes in the pathogenesis of various human infections.[36] However, a hiatus of several decades passed during which nonclostridial anaerobic bacteriology lapsed into limbo. The pioneering work of Finegold and coworkers[36,111] and Holdeman, Moore and colleagues[55] led to a renaissance of interest in anaerobic bacteriology in the late 1960s and beyond: specimen transport and culture techniques were standardized, identification methods described and taxonomy, which until then had been confused and imprecise, was placed on a firm scientific base. Today, the role of anaerobic bacteria in the pathogenesis of human infections is clearly delineated[36,46] and clinical anaerobic bacteriology forms an integral part of a routine microbiology laboratory.

DEFINITION OF ANAEROBES AND MECHANISM OF OXYGEN-SENSITIVITY

It is surprisingly difficult to define an anaerobe and to explain why these organisms are killed by atmospheric oxygen. The relationship of anaerobic bacteria to oxygen is complex and toxicity may well be exerted in an indirect manner.[4]

Most clinically significant nonsporeforming anaerobic bacteria are obligate anaerobes, i.e., organisms which do not use, and whose growth is inhibited by, molecular oxygen. No growth occurs aerobically or microaerophilically on nutritionally complete media. According to Loesche,[72] obligate anaerobic bacteria may be divided into two groups: a) moderate obligate anaerobes–

organisms capable of growth at O_2 levels between 2-8%, representing most nonsporeforming anaerobes pathogenic for humans; b) strict obligate anaerobes that do not form colonies on agar after exposure to as little as 0.5% O_2, comprising many members of the normal indigenous flora of healthy humans but rarely isolated from ill patients.

According to Finegold,[36] a working definition of an anaerobe is a bacterium which requires reduced oxygen tension for growth and does not yield colonies on the surface of agar media in 10% CO_2 in air (18% oxygen). A few nonsporeforming anaerobes (mainly the gram-positive rods and cocci) may be microaerophilic, aerotolerant or even facultatively anaerobic.[4]

Exactly why anaerobes are inhibited or killed by oxygen is unclear. Multiple factors seem to be operational. It was originally hypothesized that anaerobes are killed by H_2O_2 and organic peroxides which accumulated because organisms could not produce catalases or peroxidases. However, several nonsporeforming anaerobes (including *Bacteroides fragilis* and *Propionibacterium acnes*) can produce catalase. Another theory suggested that anaerobes may be killed by accumulation of toxic superoxide anions, due to lack of superoxide dismutase, an enzyme which converts superoxide to less toxic O_2 and H_2O_2. However, it has been shown recently that several anaerobes, including some *Bacteroides* species, do produce varying amounts of superoxide dismutase. What other factors may mediate the harmful effects of oxygen on anaerobes are currently unknown.[4]

CLASSIFICATION, HABITATS AND ROLE AS NORMAL FLORA

Based on Gram stain morphology and other physicochemical characteristics, the nonsporeforming anaerobic bacteria may be broadly classified as listed in Table 4:1. Not all groups are significant human pathogens.

Nonsporeforming anaerobes occur throughout the body as normal indigenous flora. *Actinomyces* are mainly present in the mouth and upper respiratory tract, whereas bifidobacteria and lactobacilli colonize the mouth, intestine and vagina. Eubacteria may be encountered in the mouth and intestine, while propionibacteria occur on the skin, in the upper respiratory tract and in the vagina. *Bacteroides* and fusobacteria are found as normal flora in the upper respiratory tract, mouth, intestine, urethra, vagina and external genitalia. Gram-positive anaerobic cocci occur in all of these sites, while gram-negative anaerobic cocci occur in all sites except skin and external genitalia.[36]

HUMAN INFECTIONS DUE TO NONSPOREFORMING ANAEROBES

Because of improved techniques in anaerobic methodology and the increased use of immunosuppressive drugs and other forms of therapy that

Table 4:1. Classification of the Genera of Nonsporeforming Anaerobic Bacteria*

Gram-positive rods	Gram-negative rods
Actinomyces	*Anaerovibrio*
Arachnia	*Bacteroides*
Bifidobacterium	*Borrelia*
Eubacterium	*Butyrivibrio*
Lachnospira	*Desulfomonas*
Lactobacillus	*Fusobacterium*
Propionibacterium	*Leptotrichia*
Gram-positive cocci	*Selenomonas*
Coprococcus	*Succinimonas*
Gemmiger	*Succinivibrio*
Peptococcus	*Treponema*
Peptostreptococcus	*Wolinella*
Ruminococcus	Gram-negative cocci
Sarcina	*Acidaminococcus*
Staphylococcus	*Megasphaera*
Streptococcus	*Veillonella*

* Modified from Holdeman *et al*[55] and Koneman *et al.*[68]

compromise host resistance, there has been a rise in frequency of diagnosed nonsporeforming anaerobic infections during the past several years.[36,68] Most of these infections are endogenous; that is, the organisms are a part of the patient's own commensal flora. Exceptions are crepitant cellulitis, some benign superficial infections and infections following animal and human bites. Table 4:2 lists the most commonly encountered endogenous infections due to nonsporeforming anaerobes and Table 4:3 lists the relative incidence of anaerobic bacteria in various infections.

Infections, especially deep-seated abscesses and necrotizing lesions, are often polymicrobial and may contain sporeforming anaerobes, obligate aerobes, microaerophiles or facultative anaerobes. Predisposing factors for anaerobic infections include surgical and other trauma (e.g., automobile accidents, war, stab and gunshot wounds), decreased blood supply (e.g., trauma, arteriosclerosis), malignancy, tissue necrosis, immunosuppression, debilitating diseases and the concomitant presence of aerobes or facultative anaerobes in the tissues. All of the latter may lower the redox potential and/or oxygen tension, thus creating a favorable milieu for anaerobic growth. Additionally, anaerobes may produce endo- and exotoxins, enzymes, capsules and other virulence factors which may aid in their pathogenic potential.[4,36,68] Table 4:4 lists the nonsporeforming anaerobes most commonly encountered in human infections. Table 4:5 lists infections with which gram-positive and gram-negative nonsporeforming anaerobes have been causally associated. More information on these infections may be obtained by consulting the References.

Table 4:2. Endogenously Acquired Infections Due to Nonsporeforming Anaerobes*

Abscesses in any organ (brain, lung, hepatic, subhepatic, subphrenic)
Actinomycosis
Aspiration pneumonia
Complications of intra-abdominal infections (appendicitis; cholecystitis; post-trauma or post-surgical; following ruptured viscus; malignancy)
Cellulitis and other soft tissue infections
Dental and periodontal infection
Endocarditis, bacteremia, septicemia
Female genital tract infections (endometritis, tubo-ovarian abscess, post-abortal and postpartum infections)
Infected leg ulcers (decreased blood supply)
Meningitis
Necrotizing pneumonitis
Osteomyelitis (usually chronic)
Otitis media
Perineal infections
Peritonitis (generalized and pelvic)
Septic arthritis
Sinusitis (chronic)
Subdural empyema
Thoracic empyema

* Modified from Koneman *et al.*[68]

COLLECTION AND TRANSPORTATION OF SPECIMENS

Because collection of specimens for anaerobic culture involves techniques different from those commonly used for aerobes, clinical clues suggestive of anaerobic infection are of help in selecting the correct technique. These are presented in Table 4:6. It is important to realize, however, that these clues may not be present; if there is any suspicion of anaerobic infection, specimens should be selected and collected by methods that will optimize yields of both aerobic and anaerobic bacteria.[4,36]

Collection and Transport of Specimens for Anaerobic Culture

In general, all material from body areas not likely to be contaminated with normal flora should be cultured for both aerobic and anaerobic bacteria. Close collaboration between the clinical microbiology laboratory and the clinician is essential for the proper selection, collection and transport of specimens. The clinician should be notified in a spirit of cooperation that specimens contaminated with normal flora will not be routinely cultured for anaerobic bacteria.[4]

SPECIMEN PROCESSING

Once received in the laboratory, properly collected specimens should be processed and plated as soon as possible. Anaerobes are relatively fastidious

Table 4:3. Relative Incidence of Sporeforming and Nonsporeforming Anaerobic Bacteria in Various Infections*

Type of Infection	Incidence (%)
Bacteremia	10–20
Central nervous system	
Brain abscess	89
Subdural empyema	~50
Meningitis	Low†
Head and neck	
Chronic sinusitis	50
Chronic otitis media	†
Periodontal abscess	100
Other oral infections	†
Pleuropulmonary	
Aspiration pneumonia	85–90
Lung abscess	93
Necrotizing pneumonia	85
Empyema	76
Chronic bronchitis, bronchiectasis	†
Intraabdominal	
Peritonitis and abscess	90–95
Liver abscess	>50
Female genital tract	
Salpingitis, pelvic peritonitis	≥56
Tuboovarian abscess	92
Vulvovaginal abscess	74
Septic abortion and endometritis	73
Soft tissue	
Gas gangrene (myonecrosis)	100
Crepitant cellulitis	High†
Necrotizing fasciitis	High†
Urinary tract	
Cystitis	1
Urethritis	<1

* Adapted from Allen *et al.*[4]
† Percentage data not available.

and are at their most oxygen-labile during the period of transport, plating and initial growth on artificial media. In the laboratory, specimens which cannot be cultured immediately should be held at room temperature and not refrigerated. A lag period of a few hours will not significantly decrease the anaerobe yield from specimens submitted in anaerobic containers, but culture as soon as possible after receipt should be the rule. Specimens received aerobically should be plated within 30 min of receipt.

MEDIA FOR PRIMARY ANAEROBE ISOLATION

Primary isolation of anaerobes from clinical specimens requires the combined use of nonselective, selective and enrichment media.

Table 4:4. Major Nonsporeforming Anaerobes Encountered Clinically*

Gram-negative rods
Bacteroides fragilis
B.thetaiotaomicron
B.vulgatus
B.distasonis
B.melaninogenicus/asaccharolyticus/intermedius group
B.oralis group *(B.oralis, B.buccalis, B.veroralis)*
B.bivius/disiens
B.oris/buccae
B.ureolyticus
Fusobacterium nucleatum
F.necrophorum
F.mortiferum
F.varium
Gram-positive cocci
Peptostreptococcus magnus
Ps.asaccharolyticus
Ps.prevotii
Ps.anaerobius
Staphylococcus saccharolyticus†
Streptococcus intermedius‡
Gram-positive rods
Actinomyces spp. *(A.israelii; A.naeslundii; A.odontolyticus; A.viscosus)*
Arachnia propionica
Bifidobacterium spp.
Propionibacterium acnes
Eubacterium spp. *(E.lentum, E.limosum, E.alactolyticum)*

* Modified from Finegold[36] and Allen *et al.*[4]
† Varies in aerotolerance: some strains are obligate anaerobes, others are aerotolerant anaerobes.
‡ Not an obligate anaerobe.

Nonselective Media

Use of a nutritionally complete medium supplemented with vitamin K and hemin is of paramount importance. A good quality blood agar base, such as trypticase soy, brain heart infusion, Columbia, Brucella or Schaedler's agar base, is essential. The Centers for Disease Control (CDC) currently recommend a trypticase soy agar anaerobic blood plate supplemented with yeast extract, hemin, vitamin K_1, L-cystine and 5% sheep or rabbit blood. This medium supports better growth of *B. melaninogenicus, Fusobacterium necrophorum*, certain strains of *B. thetaiotaomicron, Actinomyces israelii* and some nutritionally dependent streptococci than does the previously recommended rabbit-blood trypticase soy agar medium.[4] Routine 5% sheep blood agar is unsatisfactory for anaerobic culture. Nonselective anaerobic blood plates are available commercially from a number of sources (BBL Microbiology Systems; Difco Laboratories; Scott Laboratories; Carr-Scarborough Laboratories; Regional Medical Laboratories; Gibco Laboratories) but plates prepared in-house offer improved yield and better growth than their commercial counterparts. After preparing plates, wrap them in cellophane bags and store them in the refrigerator at 2-4°C.[4] Plates in sealed bags may be stored for up to 6 weeks but growth is more luxuriant on plates stored for less than 4 weeks.[82] Before use, remove plates from refrigerator and dry the agar surfaces by warming the plates with lids ajar for 5 min at 35°C. Prereduce plates in an anaerobic jar or glove box for 6-24 h (optimally >24 h) before inoculation.[4,111]

Selective Media

Because anaerobic infections are often mixed, species present in small numbers, especially those of fastidious and slow-growing organisms, may be missed. Use of appropriate selective media is therefore necessary. Table 4:7 lists selective media for the isolation of specific groups. Most of the media are commercially available. Kanamycin, gentamicin or paramomycin may be used in selective anaerobic blood plates in combination with vancomycin. Some facultatively anaerobic gram-negative rods are occasionally resistant to kanamycin but susceptible to either gentamicin or paramomycin.[4] The selective media chosen depends on the individual needs of a specific laboratory, but most clinical laboratories will select kanamycin-vancomycin agar (with laked blood, for detection of black-pigmented *Bacteroides*) and phenylethyl alcohol agar as the media of choice.

Liquid Media

A liquid medium should always be used as a backup to solid media for primary isolation. Enriched thioglycolate medium without indicator, or chopped meat glucose medium, are both suitable for this purpose. Enriched thioglycolate broth is especially suitable for slow-growing organisms such as *A. israelii*, which may take several days to develop visible colonies on agar. Incubate tubes in an anaerobic system with caps slightly loosened to facilitate isolation of small numbers of organisms which may not grow if the medium is incubated in air. If a glove box is used for inoculation of tubes, tighten caps after gassing and place tubes in a regular incubator. Chopped meat is an excellent fluid medium which supports growth of most anaerobes. It is also a suitable medium for shipping cultures. Both thioglycolate and chopped meat media should be enriched with vitamin K and hemin. If liquid media are not gassed in an anaerobic environment during preparation, they should either be held overnight in an anaerobic atmosphere or heated 10 min in a boiling water bath to drive off oxygen and cooled before inoculation. Both types of liquid media are available commercially.[4,111]

If sulfur granules suggestive of actinomycosis are found on direct examination, wash them immediately with thioglycolate broth, grind with a small

Table 4:5. Infections Caused by Nonsporeforming Anaerobes

Site of Infection	Reference
HEAD AND NECK:	
Mouth and teeth: Dentoalveolar abscess, fistula formation with bacteremia, chronic periapical infection, pyogenic granuloma, dental cysts, post-extraction syndrome, dental actinomycosis, spread to lung and brain.	36
Infections of maxilla and mandible, including actinomycosis	36
Eye infections: Conjunctivitis, corneal ulcer, endophthalmitis, panophthalmitis, orbital cellulitis, lid infections, infections of lacrymal apparatus.	36
Infections of middle ear and mastoid: Chronic and rarely acute otitis media and mastoiditis, sinusitis (acute and chronic), with or without periorbital cellulitis, subperiosteal abscess, orbital cellulitis and abscess, cavernous sinus thrombosis, brain abscess.	36,110
Throat infections: Tonsillitis, peritonsillar abscess with or without pneumonitis, empyema, thrombophlebitis, bacteremia, pharyngitis, actinomycosis.	36
Diverse: Vincent's angina, stomatitis, cancrum oris, cheek infections, Ludwig's angina, salivary gland and thyroid infections, retropharyngeal abscess, parapharyngeal phlegmon, cellulitis of neck, mediastinitis.	10,36
CENTRAL NERVOUS SYSTEM	
Brain abscess, meningitis, sub- and extradural empyema, cerebritis, spinal epidural abscess, intramedullary abscess of spinal cord, osteomyelitis of the skull, ependymitis, septic venous thrombophlebitis, actinomycosis.	36,40,42
BACTEREMIA AND ENDOCARDITIS	
May be associated with jaundice, thrombophlebitis, septic shock, hematologic abnormalities. Pericarditis, myocarditis, infected vascular grafts.	36
RESPIRATORY TRACT INFECTIONS	
Pulmonary abscess with or without empyema or abscess	1,36
Necrotizing pneumonitis with or without empyema or abscess	17,36
Pneumonitis with or without empyema or abscess	36
Infected bronchogenic carcinoma cavity	36
Empyema in absence of parenchymal infection	1,36
Aspiration pneumonitis	36
Diverse: May play a role in bronchiectasis, septic pulmonary emboli secondary to septic thrombophlebitis, interstitial pneumonitis, acute bronchitis and tracheobronchial lymphadenitis, mediastinitis. Pulmonary actinomycosis.	36
ABDOMINAL AND PERINEAL INFECTIONS	
General abdominal: Post-operative and other wound infections, especially after large bowel surgery. Infections of abdominal wall, intra-abdominal abscess, especially in subphrenic and appendiceal areas, retroperitoneal abscesses, peritonitis, appendicitis and its complications, appendiceal actinomycosis, diverticulitis with or without bacteremia, infections of spleen and pancreas.	16,36,122
Liver and biliary tract: Liver abscess, chronic bacterial hepatitis, pylephlebitis, biliary tract infection with bactibilia.	13,36,37, 79,126
Perineum: Perineal sepsis with or without fistula formation and perirectal abscess, perianal and perineal hydradenitis suppurativa, actinomycosis.	14,36,131

Table 4:5. Infections Caused by Nonsporeforming Anaerobes (*Continued*)

Site of Infection	Reference
URINARY AND MALE GENITAL TRACTS	
Urinary tract: Urethritis, cystitis, ureteritis, pyelitis, pyelonephritis, renal abscess, metastatic renal infection with abscess formation, pyonephrosis, perinephric abscess, retroperitoneal renal abscess, post-operative wound infections, septic renal vein thrombophlebitis, perineal abscess, gas gangrene, actinomycosis.	36,94
Male genital tract: Acute or chronic prostatitis, prostatic abscess, periprostatic phlegmon, post-prostate biopsy sepsis, testicular abscess, balanoposthitis, scrotal sepsis.	9,27,36,52, 132
FEMALE GENITAL TRACT INFECTIONS	
Endometritis, pyometra	36,88,108, 117
Myometritis	
Parametritis	
Pelvic cellulitis, abscess	
Pelvic thrombophlebitis	
Peritonitis, intraabdominal abscess	
Bacteremia, with or without shock or intravascular hemolysis	
Metastatic infection, particularly of lung, liver, brain, heart valves, kidneys	
Wound infection or abscess	
Vulvar abscess	
Bartholinitis, Bartholin abscess	
Skenitis, Skene's abscess	
Paraclitoroidal abscess	
Non-specific vaginitis, abscess of vaginal wall, paravaginal abscess	
Salpingitis, tubal abscess	
Ovarian or tubo-ovarian abscess	
Abscesses of adjacent parts, groin, perirectal or ischiorectal areas, paraurethral, leg, abdominal wall	
SKIN, SOFT TISSUE, MUSCLE INFECTIONS	
Subcutaneous abscesses, perioral dermatitis, axillary abscess with or without hydradenitis suppurativa, periareolar breast abscess, paronychia, infected sebaceous, inclusion or pilonidal cysts, infected foot ulcers (diabetics, decreased blood supply), infected decubitus ulcers, tropical ulcer, anaerobic cellulitis, synergistic bacterial gangrene of the skin, chronic undermining ulcer ("Meleney's ulcer"), necrotizing fasciitis, Fournier's gangrene of the scrotum, myositis, myonecrosis, synergistic nonclostridial anaerobic myonecrosis, pyomyositis, infected vascular gangrene, human and animal bites, infected hematomas, burns, soft tissue infections in drug addicts, frostbite.	14,36,41,64, 70,71,80, 130
BONE AND JOINT INFECTIONS	
Osteomyelitis: Bones of skull and face, long bones, foot bones, especially in diabetics and patients with decreased blood supply, pelvic bones and sacrum, hand bones after bites, spinal bones, actinomycosis.	36,92
Arthritis	36
INTRAUTERINE/PEDIATRIC INFECTIONS	
Intrauterine: Chorioamnionitis with or without fetal bacteremia.	36,86
Neonate: Pneumonitis, bacteremia.	36
Older children: Same infections as adults.	36

Table 4:6. Clinical Suggestions of Possible Infection with Nonsporeforming and Other Anaerobes*

Foul-smelling discharge
Location of infection in proximity to a mucosal surface
Tissue necrosis or impaired blood supply
Abscesses
Penetrating wounds to the abdomen or pelvis
Aspiration
Gangrene, pseudomembrane formation
Gas in tissues or discharges
Endocarditis with negative routine blood cultures, with or without jaundice and thrombophlebitis
Infection associated with malignancy or other process resulting in tissue destruction
Infection related to the use of aminoglycosides (oral, parenteral or topical)
Septic thrombophlebitis
Infection following human or other bites
Black discoloration of blood-containing exudates; these exudates may fluoresce red under ultraviolet light (infections with black-pigmented *Bacteroides*)
Presence of sulfur granules in discharges (actinomycosis)
Clinical setting suggestive of anaerobic infection (e.g., septic abortion, infection following gastrointestinal surgery)
Classical clinical picture (actinomycosis, myonecrosis)

* Modified from Finegold[36] and Allen *et al.*[4]

volume of thioglycolate and plate, preferably on both anaerobic blood agar and on phenylethyl alcohol plates. Isolation of actinomycetes from heavily contaminated specimens is difficult to achieve, even when sulfur granules have been seen microscopically.[4] Traynor and colleagues[118] have described a procedure whereby the specimen is diluted in thioglycolate broth and aliquots plated on two horse blood agar plates, one nonselective, the other containing metronidazole to inhibit most other anaerobes. Plates are incubated anaerobically and examined after 4, 10 and 14 days.[118] Selective media have also been developed for isolation of *Actinomyces* species from dental sources.[4]

Selection of appropriate combinations of liquid and solid primary isolation media depends on the specimen collected and the needs of the individual laboratory, and should be clearly outlined in the laboratory's procedure manual. A guide for primary media selection is given in Table 4:8.

SPECIMEN INOCULATION[4,111]

Fluid Specimens

Inoculate tubes of liquid media near the bottom with 1-2 drops of material, then place 1-2 drops on each solid medium and streak for single colonies. Prepare a smear for Gram staining.

Table 4:7. Use of Selective Media in Isolation and Identification of Nonsporeforming Anaerobes*

Medium	Purpose and organisms isolated
Kanamycin/gentamicin/paramomycin-vancomycin blood agar	Selective for anaerobic Gram-negative rods and *Veillonella*
Laked kanamycin/gentamicin/paramomycin-vancomycin blood agar	Black-pigmented *Bacteroides* and other Gram-negative rods
Bacteroides bile esculin agar	*B.fragilis* group (grow on bile and hydrolyse esculin)
FRAG agar	Presumptive identification of *B.fragilis* group (D-glucuronic acid as fermentable C-source)
Fusobacterium egg yolk agar	*Fusobacterium; F.necrophorum* (lipase positive)
Rifampin blood agar	*F.mortiferum, F.varium;* certain *Eubacterium* spp.
Cadmium sulfate agar	*Actinomyces* spp.
Bifidobacterium agar	*Bifidobacterium* spp.
Lactobacillus agar	*Lactobacillus* spp.
Veillonella agar	*Veillonella* spp.
B.gingivalis agar	*B.gingivalis*
Phenylethyl alcohol blood agar	Gram-negative and -positive nonsporeforming and other anaerobes
Stiff blood agar (4–6% instead of usual 1.5-2% agar)	Prevention of swarming of clostridia

* Modified from Finegold;[38] Lyznicki *et al;*[76] Allen *et al;*[4] Hunt *et al;*[60] Sutter *et al.*[111]

Solid Specimens

Solid specimens may be first quickly dipped in boiling water to eliminate external flora. Mince tissue or other solid specimens with sterile scissors, adding one part enriched thioglycolate or buffered gelatin diluent to one part solid tissue, then grind the mixture with a sterile tissue grinder. Plates are then inoculated and Gram stains prepared as for fluid specimens.

Swabs

If 2 swabs are received as one specimen, use the first swab to inoculate 1/4 of each plate of agar medium and then to inoculate the liquid medium. Prepare a Gram stain with the second swab. If only one swab is received, prepare a suspension by scrubbing the material from the swab into approximately 0.5 mL thioglycolate and then proceed as described for liquid specimens (including preparation of a Gram stain).

ANAEROBIC INCUBATION PROCEDURES

Anaerobes vary in their oxygen tolerance. Therefore, care must be taken to avoid prolonged exposure to oxygen, especially on primary isolation. In

Table 4:8. Selection of Primary Isolation Media for Culture of Nonsporeforming Anaerobes in Clinical Specimens from Various Anatomic Sites

Specimen source	Primary isolation medium*
Central nervous system	AnBAP; THIO
Eye, ear, oropharynx	AnBAP; PEA; THIO
Pulmonary area	AnBAP; PEA (PV/GV/KV); THIO
Intraabdominal area	AnBAP; PEA; PV/GV/KV; THIO
Genitourinary area	AnBAP; PEA; PV/GV/KV; THIO
Muscle and other soft tissue	AnBAP; PEA; CMG
Bone marrow	AnBAP; THIO
Body fluids (other than blood and urine)	AnBAP; THIO

* Modified from Allen et al.[4]
AnBAP = non-selective anaerobic blood agar; THIO = enriched thioglycolate broth; PEA = phenylethyl alcohol blood agar; PV/GV/KV = paramomycin/vancomycin, gentamicin/vancomycin or kanamycin/vancomycin. Media in parentheses are optional.

a busy clinical laboratory, it is not always possible to incubate anaerobe plates immediately after plating. An alternative is the holding jar procedure which allows primary plating, inspection and subculture of colonies without undue exposure to oxygen. Three holding jars may be used: one for reduced uninoculated media, a second for freshly streaked plates awaiting incubation and a third for plates with colonies to be subcultured.[4] Rectangular boxes may be substituted for jars. A description of a convenient and inexpensive modification of the original holding jar method[4] as described by Martin[78] is illustrated in Fig.4:1.

(1) Hold uninoculated plates in an anaerobic glove box or jar for 6-24 h before inoculation. Commence the flow of gas with an initial 20-30 s flush with the regulator set at approximately 4 lb/in^2, followed by a decrease in flow rate to 1-2 bubbles/s. A gang valve with 3 outlets is convenient for regulating the gas flow to each jar. If CO_2 is used, the gas should be passed through a heated copper catalyst (Sargeant furnace) before use.[4]
(2) Place the reduced plating media in the first holding jar and flush continuously with inexpensive, commercial grade N_2 or CO_2.
(3) Inoculate the surface of each plate. Immediately after streaking, place the plate in the second jar and flush with gas as in (2).
(4) Use a third holding jar for any plates removed from a jar or glove box after incubation for subculture.
(5) After the holding jar is filled with freshly inoculated plates, remove the holding jar lid and incubate plates anaerobically.

Three common methods for anaerobic incubation are the anaerobe jar, anaerobic glove box and the roll streak system.

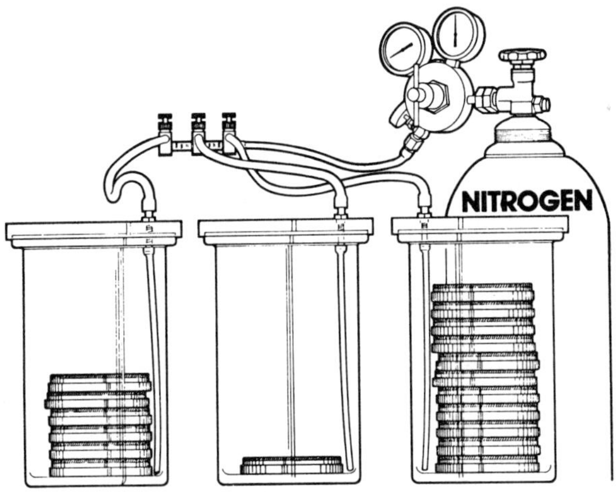

FIGURE 4:1. Schematic representation of a holding jar system with three jars which are continuously flushed with a gentle stream of nitrogen to minimize exposure of anaerobes to air during and after inspection and subculture of plates.

Anaerobe Jars

The anaerobe jar is a cylindrical container made of glass, metal or plastic. Metal or plastic lids are clamped to a flange at the top of the jar to create an airtight seal. Anaerobe jars utilize a cold catalyst consisting of palladium-coated aluminum pellets active at room temperature. Anaerobiosis may be achieved by evacuation and replacement (ER) with an anaerobic gas mixture or utilization of a disposable envelope which generates H_2 and CO_2. Although both methods are simple and effective, the ER method is more economical and establishes anaerobic conditions more rapidly than does the H_2-CO_2 generator. After sealing the jar, the H_2 that is generated combines with residual O_2 in the presence of the palladium catalyst attached to the lid to form water. Catalyst pellets, when used once, must be replaced or "rejuvenated" by heating in a dry-heat oven at 160-170°C for at least 2 h before reuse. Pellets should be stored at room temperature in a clean, dry container or dessicator.[4,111] Anaerobe jars are available from several manufacturers (Baltimore Biological Laboratories; Scott Laboratories; Oxoid USA).

ER Technique:

A suitable gas mixture (85% N_2, 10% H_2, 5% CO_2) is available commercially. Vacuum facilities are sufficient with or without a vacuum pump if evacuation to 51-61 cm Hg is achieved. Place fresh/rejuvenated catalyst in the lid of a jar holding materials to be incubated. Loosen the screwcaps of tubes to permit adequate gas exchange and place a methylene blue indicator in the jar. Fasten the lid and connect the vent to an ER device. Evacuate the jar to 51-61 cm Hg and refill with commercial grade N_2. Repeat this cycle twice. After evacuating the jar for the third time, fill it with the anaerobic gas mixture. Clamp off the rubber tubing attached to the jar, disconnect the jar from the vacuum and gas lines and incubate it.[4,111]

Envelope Generator Procedure:

The disposable envelope consists of a sealed foil envelope containing two pellets: one of citric acid and $NaHCO_3$, the other of sodium borohydride. On introduction of water into the envelope, the first pellet releases CO_2 the second H_2. To use the envelope, replace the catalyst, place materials in the jar and include the methylene blue indicator as for the ER procedure. Cut the corner of the envelope and add 10 mL of distilled water. Place the generator in an upright position in the jar, clamp the lid and incubate. If the jar is performing adequately, the lid with the catalyst on its undersurface should be warm to the touch and water of condensation should appear on the inside of the jar within 15-30 min after activation of the generator; otherwise, terminate the reaction by opening the jar and discarding the generator. The three most common causes of jar failure are failure to use an active catalyst, a faulty or defective gas generator and a poorly sealing gasket in the lid which allows escape of gas and influx of ambient air.[4,111] Redox indicators should always be included in the jar. Methylene blue indicators may be purchased in strip form or prepared in liquid form. The indicator is light blue when oxidized but colorless when reduced (after approximately 5 h of anaerobic incubation).[4]

Anaerobic Glove Box

An anaerobic glove box permits inspection and subculture of colonies without exposure to oxygen. The glove box is a gas-tight chamber with glove portals and an entry lock for transport of materials into and out of the chamber. An H_2-containing atmosphere is recirculated through a palladium catalyst to remove oxygen. Several types and sizes of chambers are commercially available,[4,111] such as that originally designed by Freter and associates[7] (Coy Laboratories). An unheated chamber in which a regular 37°C incubator is placed is probably superior to a heated chamber. The relative humidity within the chamber should be maintained at 70-85% by use of a silica gel dessicant. Anaerobic chambers should be regularly inspected for leaks, which usually occur in the glove ports.

The Roll Streak System

Moore and associates at the Anaerobe Laboratory of the Virginia Polytechnic Institute (VPI) and State University modified the roll-tube technique originally developed by Hungate and colleagues. The roll-streak system uses prereduced anaerobically sterilized (PRAS) media in tubes with butyl-rubber stoppers. After constituents of the medium are combined, boiled to remove air, tubed and autoclaved, they are stored in tubes under O_2-free CO_2. After autoclaving, tubes are cooled and allowed to solidify on a rolling machine such that the inner surfaces of the tubes are coated with a thin layer of the solidified medium. Both roll-streak agar and PRAS liquid medium require the addition of a reducing agent such as L-cysteine hydrochloride before sterilization. Both types of media are inoculated and subcultured in a stream of O_2-free CO_2 with the aid of a VPI gassing apparatus. Three types of CO_2 may be used: anaerobe-grade CO_2, commercial grade CO_2 rendered O_2-free by passing through a heated copper catalyst (Sargeant furnace), or a mixture of 97% CO_2 + 3% H_2 passed through a Deoxo H_2-purifier to remove traces of O_2 prior to use. The roll-streak system, like the glove box, allows manipulation of colonies without exposure to oxygen.[55]

In practical terms, the anaerobe jar and anaerobic glove box are the most commonly used methods. The jar technique is suitable for laboratories with limited space and relatively small numbers of cultures, while the glove box may be used by larger laboratories with heavier work loads.

Other Anaerobic Systems

The BioBag-A (Marion Scientific) consists of a gas-impermeable, transparent plastic bag containing catalyst and two ampules. When the ampules are crushed, one generates H_2, the other resazurin. The principle of O_2-binding is the same as that for the anaerobic jar and glove box. The method can be used as a transport device or for convenient inspection of colonies any time during incubation. Anagel (Baltimore Biological Laboratories) is a dehydrated agar-containing powder which, when hydrated and placed within the lid of a Petri dish, reduces the concentration of O_2, generates CO_2 and produces an atmosphere suitable for reduction of culture medium and growth of anaerobes.[4,111]

Incubation

Culture media should be incubated at 35°C. Ordinarily, inoculated media should be incubated in an anaerobe jar for at least 48 h before opening the jar.[4] However, studies by Rosenblatt[96] indicate that total recovery of anaerobes after incubation for 48 h in GasPak jars is not diminished by interruption of incubation after the first 24 h and exposure of cultures to room air or CO_2 for as long as 40 min. Plates incubated in a BioBag-A or in a glove box, or as roll-tubes, can be inspected daily for growth without exposing developing colonies to air. Primary isolation plates should be reincubated for 5-7 days. Liquid media should be held for a minimum of one week. Broth cultures from suspected actinomycosis, endocarditis, osteomyelitis or other serious infections should be held for at least 2, and preferably 4, weeks before being discarded as negative.[4,111]

Colonial morphology should be observed with a dissecting microscope, since distinctive colony characteristics are most helpful in differentiating many of these organisms. Plate reading with the unaided eye will miss important subtleties of distinctive colonial morphology. Laboratories should routinely observe and record a variety of characteristics that will aid in the identification of nonsporeforming anaerobes.

Fluid backup media should be subcultured (1) in all cases when growth is observed in liquid media but not on plate cultures, and (2) when Gram staining of fluid media reveals morphologic forms which do not grow on plates.

GRAM-NEGATIVE ANAEROBIC RODS

Table 4:9 lists the genera of gram-negative anaerobic rods that may be encountered in clinical specimens. *Bacteroides* and *Fusobacterium* are the most important of these. The other genera are relatively rare pathogens and infrequently encountered in clinical material.

General Characteristics

Gram-negative anaerobic rods are the most commonly encountered anaerobes in human clinical infections. The taxonomy of these organisms, especially of the genus *Bacteroides*, is still developing and has undergone several changes and additions in recent years (Table 4:10).[39] *B. fragilis* and *B. thetaiotaomicron* are the most prevalent species and of the greatest clinical significance. They are recovered from many intra-abdominal infections and from other sites. The *B. fragilis* group comprise the major part of the colonic flora, but are also found in smaller numbers in the female genital tract, but not usually in the mouth or upper respiratory tract.

The pigmented *Bacteroides* currently include 10 species, 8 of which may be found with varying degrees of frequency in human clinical material. *B. macacae* has thus far only been isolated from primates, and the exact taxonomic status of human isolates phenotypically similar to *B. levii* is unclear at present.[58] *B. denticola, B. gingivalis* and *B. loescheii* are part of the normal mouth flora and are important pathogens in oral and dental infections, sometimes producing infections of the head, neck and lower

Table 4:9. Differentiation of the Genera of Gram-negative Anaerobic Bacilli*

Characteristic	Genus
I. Nonmotile or peritrichous flagella	
A. Produce butyric acid (without isobutyric and isovaleric acids)	*Fusobacterium*
B. Produce major lactic acid	*Leptotrichia*
C. Produce acetic acid and hydrogen sulfide; reduce sulfate	*Desulfomonas*
D. Not as above (A, B, or C)	*Bacteroides*
II. Polar flagella	
A. Fermentative	
1. Produce butyric acid	*Butyrivibrio*
2. Produce succinic acid	
a. Spiral-shaped cells	*Succinivibrio*
b. Ovoid cells	*Succinimonas*
3. Produce propionic and acetic acids	*Anaerovibrio*
B. Nonfermentative; produce succinic acid from fumarate	*Wolinella*
III. Tufts of flagella on concave side of curved cells	
A. Fermentative	*Selenomonas*
B. Nonfermentative	*Mobiluncus*
IV. Bipolar tufts of flagella	*Anaerobiospirillum*

* Modified from Finegold and Edelstein.[39]

respiratory tract.[39] *B. endodontalis* is a newly recognized species which has been isolated from infected root canals.[119,120] The remaining pathogenic pigmented *Bacteroides* are common in the mouth, urogenital and gastrointestinal tracts, and are important in head, neck, mouth, dental, bite and pleuropulmonary infections.

The bile-sensitive saccharolytic *Bacteroides* group are found in the same settings as the pigmented group. *B. bivius* and *B. disiens* are mainly encountered in the female genital tract and oral infections. *B. oris* and *B. buccae*, formerly classified as *B. ruminicola*, are found in a variety of infections. *B. ureolyticus* has been isolated from many infections of head and neck, pulmonary, intra-abdominal, bone, soft tissue and urogenital sites.[39] *B. gracilis* is mainly found in periodontal infection but may be isolated from other sources.[62] *F. nucleatum* is commonly encountered in clinical infections similar to those associated with the pigmented *Bacteroides* group. *F. necrophorum* is a virulent organism which may cause disseminated infection commonly originating in a focus of membranous tonsillitis. Other gram-negative anaerobic rods may be encountered clinically but human infection is relatively rare and often in the form of opportunistic bacteremia in the immunocompromised host.[39] *Mobiluncus* species have been implicated in the pathogenesis of nonspecific vaginitis.[117]

Table 4:10. Recent Taxonomic Changes*

New nomenclature	Previous nomenclature
Bacteroides asaccharolyticus	*B.melaninogenicus* subsp. *asaccharolyticus*
B.gingivalis	*B.melaninogenicus* subsp. *asaccharolyticus*
B.intermedius	*B.melaninogenicus* subsp. *intermedius* (in part)
B.corporis	*B.melaninogenicus* subsp. *intermedius* (in part)
B.levii	*B.melaninogenicus* subsp. *levii*
B.macacae	New species
B.melaninogenicus	*B.melaninogenicus* subsp. *melaninogenicus*
B.loescheii	New species
B.denticola	New species
B.oris	*B.ruminicola,* human strains (in part)
B.buccae	*B.ruminicola,* human strains (in part)
B.veroralis	*B.oralis* (in part)
B.buccalis	*B.oralis* (in part)
B.zoogleoformans	Reinstated
B.endodontalis	New species
B.gracilis	New species
Fusobacterium periodonticum	New species
F.alocis	New species
F.sulci	New species
Wolinella succinogenes	New species (basonym, *Vibrio succinogenes*)
W.recta	New species
Clostridium symbiosum	*F.symbiosum*
Clostridium bullosum	*F.bullosum*
Eubacterium plautii	*F.plauti*

* Modified from Finegold;[38] Lyznicki *et al;*[76] Allen *et al;*[4] Hunt *et al;*[60] Sutter *et al.*[111]

Species Identification

Presumptive Identification:

Most clinically significant gram-negative rods may be placed in broad categories with the aid of a few tests (Table 4:11). Special-potency antibiotic disks can be used to differentiate between *Bacteroides* and *Fusobacterium* and to differentiate between some species in the same group.[39,111] An organism that pits agar, requires formate and fumarate for growth and is urease-positive, asaccharolytic and nitrate- or nitrite-positive may be presumptively identified as *B. ureolyticus*. Not all *B. ureolyticus* strains pit agar and smooth, spreading and pitting colonies may coexist in the same culture. Organisms that fluoresce brick-red or produce black pigment may be placed in the pigmenting *Bacteroides* group. An indole- and lipase-positive fluorescing or black-pigmented gram-negative coccobacillus may be identified as *B. intermedius*; lipase-negative strains require additional testing. A lipase-positive, indole-negative pigmenting *Bacteroides* is probably *B. loescheii*. The *B. fragilis* group may be presumptively identified by their special-potency disk susceptibility pattern (Table 4:11) and growth in bile-containing medium or on a bile esculin plate.[39,111] Differentiation between the major species may be conveniently achieved by catalase, indole, mannitol, rhamnose and trehalose reactions.[68] A thin indole-positive gram-negative rod with tapering ends that produces speckled, breadcrumb or smooth colonies is probably *F. nucleatum*. *F. necrophorum* is usually lipase-positive; pleomorphic gram-negative rods with rounded ends and occasional bizarre forms may be seen on Gram stain, and colonies are umbonate. Lipase-negative strains require additional testing. A bile-resistant *Fusobacterium* may be presumptively identified as *F. varium/F. mortiferum*, but other fusobacteria (e.g., *F. necrophorum*) may also grow in 20% bile.[39,111] Organisms not fitting into the *B. fragilis* group, pigmented *Bacteroides*, *B. ureolyticus* group or into *Fusobacterium* species may be termed *Bacteroides* species. The reader is referred elsewhere for details on identification of *Leptotrichia, Desulfomonas, Butyrivibrio, Succinivibrio, Succinimonas, Anaerovibrio, Wolinella, Selenomonas* and *Anaerobiospirillum*.[58]

Definitive Identification:

Definitive identification of most species requires additional biochemical testing and gas-liquid chromatographic (GLC) analysis of metabolic end-products (Table 4:12).[19,26,39,55,56,58,59,105,119,120,123]

Organisms of the *B. fragilis* group all grow on enriched blood agar as smooth, convex, gray-white colonies. All strains require hemin for growth. Cells may be pleomorphic or uniform, and some contain vacuoles. All strains grow well on or are stimulated by 20% bile (2% oxgall). However, *B. uniformis* does not grow as well in bile as do other members of the group. Three non-*B. fragilis* organisms are bile-resistant: *B. splanchnicus, B. eggerthii* and *B. multiacidus*. *B. multiacidus* is nitrate-positive: *B. splanchnicus* and *B. eggerthii* are sucrose-negative.[39,58] All three are uncommon clinical isolates. Colonies of the *B. fragilis* group grow on bile esculin agar and most produce blackening due to esculin hydrolysis; however, *B. vulgatus* may be esculin-negative. *B. fragilis* and *B. thetaiotaomicron* are catalase-positive, while *B. vulgatus, B. ovatus* and *B. uniformis* are usually catalase-negative.[39] *B. thetaiotaomicron* and *B. ovatus* may be difficult to separate: *B. ovatus* produces acid from xylan and is usually also salicin-positive, while *B. thetaiotaomicron* is negative for xylan and usually negative for salicin. Differentiation by means of a specific bacteriophage and by DNA homology is also possible. Additionally, *B. ovatus* is more ovoid on Gram stain than is *B. thetaiotaomicron*.[24,25,39] A hitherto unnamed *B. fragilis*, DNA homology group 3452A, closely resembles *B. distasonis* but is arabinose-positive and catalase- negative, whereas *B. distasonis* is arabinose-negative and usually catalase-positive.[39] Bile-resistant organisms which do not fit into any of the named species may be reported as *B. fragilis* group.

Bile-sensitive nonpigmenting *Bacteroides* comprise 3 groups: (1) Sac-

Table 4:11. Grouping Anaerobic Gram-Negative Rods*

Group and species	Kanamycin (1,000 μg)	Vancomycin (5μg)	Colistin (10 μg)	Growth in 20% bile	Catalase	Indole	Lipase	Slender cells with pointed ends	Growth stimulated by formate-fumarate	Nitrate reduction	Urease	Motility	Pitting of agar	Pigment	Brick-red fluorescence
B.fragilis group	R	R	R	$+^{-}$	V	V	−								−
Other *Bacteroides* spp.	R	R	V	−	−	V	−			$-^{+}$					
Pigmenting *Bacteroides* spp.	R	V	V	−	$-^{+}$	V	V							+	$+^{-}$
B.intermedius	R	R	S	−	−	+	$+^{-}$								
B.loescheii	R	R	V	−	−	−	V								
B.ureolyticus-like group	S	R	S	−	−	−	−		+	+	V	V	V		
B.ureolyticus	S	R	S	−	−	−			+	+	+	−	V		
B.gracilis	S	R	S	−	−	−			+	+	−	−	V		
Wolinella spp.	S	R	S	−	−	−			+	+	−	+	V		
Fusobacterium spp.	S	R	S	V	−	V	V	V							−
F.nucleatum	S	R	S	−		+	−	+							
F.necrophorum	S	R	S	$-^{+}$		+	$+^{-}$	−							
F.varium-mortiferum	S	R	S	+		V	−	−							

* After Finegold and Edelstein.[39]
R = resistant; S = susceptible; V = variable; + = positive reaction for majority of strains; − = negative reaction; $+^{-}$ = most strains positive; $-^{+}$ = most strains negative, some strains positive.
Compare the growth of the organism in an unsupplemented thioglycolate broth with growth in a broth supplemented with formate and fumarate.
Use the spot nitrate disk test.
Make a heavy suspension of the organism in 0.5 mL of sterile urea broth (Difco Laboratories). Incubate the suspension aerobically for up to 24 h. A bright pink or red is positive; this color usually appears within 15–30 min. If the indicator becomes reduced, add Nessler reagent to determine ammonia production (ammonia indicates a positive reaction).
Use the hanging-drop method with colonies from the isolation blood agar plate. If negative, check motility with a young broth culture supplemented with formate and fumarate.
Formate and fumarate should be added to test media for the *B.ureolyticus*-like group.

charolytic, (2) Saccharolytic and proteolytic and (3) Weakly or asaccharolytic. The saccharolytic organisms are divided into 2 groups by pentose fermentation reactions (arabinose and xylose are usually tested).[39,58] *B. oris* and *B. buccae* are pentose fermenters and may be differentiated by β-glucosidase testing or by polyacrylamide gel electrophoresis of cellular proteins. *B. oris* is usually more resistant to penicillin G (2 units) than is *B. buccae*.[39] *B. zoogleoformans*, another pentose-positive organism, is an oral strain rarely encountered clinically. It produces a viscous, tenacious (zoogleal) mass in broth.[19,39,58] Salicin and xylan fermentation may be used to differentiate between *B. oralis, B. veroralis* and *B. buccalis*, the three clinically encountered saccharolytic pentose nonfermenters.[39,58,105,123] *B. oralis* is salicin-positive and *B. veroralis* and *B. buccalis* salicin-negative; *B. buccalis* may be differentiated from *B. veroralis* by xylan fermentation (*B. veroralis* is positive, *B. buccalis* is negative).[39,105,123] Some strains of the *B. melaninogenicus* group may form pigment only after 21 days and some, especially *B. loescheii*, may resemble the *B. oralis* group. Salicin, xylan and gelatin will help differentiate these strains.[39]

B. bivius and *B. disiens* are both saccharolytic and strongly proteolytic. Gelatin and milk are usually digested within 2-3 days, but milk may take longer. *B. bivius* may be differentiated from *B. disiens* by lactose fermentation (*B. bivius* positive).[39,58] Under longwave ultraviolet (UV) light, colonies of both species may fluoresce light-orange to coral-pink. This should not be confused with the brick-red fluorescence of the pigmented *Bacteroides* group. Weakly saccharolytic or asaccharolytic, nonpigmented, bile-sensitive *Bacteroides* species are being increasingly isolated from clinical specimens: differentiation between these organisms is provided in Table 4:12.[39,58]

It should be noted that agar-pitting, formate/fumarate- requiring, anaerobic gram-negative rods have been reclassified into 4 groups: *B. ureolyticus, B. gracilis, Campylobacter concisus* and *Wolinella* spp. All 4 groups are sensitive to colistin (10 μg) and kanamycin (1000 μg) but resistant to a vancomycin 5 μg disk, catalase-negative, indole-negative, nitrate-positive, unable to grow in unsupplemented broth and stimulated by addition of formate/fumarate. Only *B. ureolyticus* is urease-positive, whereas only *C. concisus* and *Wolinella* spp. are motile.[62]

The degree and rapidity of pigment production by pigmented *Bacteroides* species depend mainly on the type of blood in growth plates. Laked rabbit blood agar is the best medium for this purpose. Two to 21 days may be required to detect pigment, which may vary from buff-tan to black. Some strains may not pigment before 21 days and may be confused with other *Bacteroides* species, as well as initially with strains of *A. odontolyticus*, which produce a red pigment. Pigmented *Bacteroides* may fluoresce pink, orange, chartreuse or brick-red. Brick-red is the only reliable color for presumptive identification since some nonpigmented *Bacteroides* may fluoresce coral-pink. Once pigment production occurs, fluorescence is masked.[39]

Table 4:12. Biochemical Reactions of *Bacteroides* Species Isolated from Human Sources*

	B.fragilis group						Bile-resistant non-*B.fragilis*		
	B.fragilis	*B.vulgatus*	*B.distasonis*	*B.ovatus*	*B.thetaiotaomicron*	*B.uniformis*	*B.multiacidus*	*B.splanchnicus*	*B.eggerthii*
Products from PYG	SAppa (ibivl)	SAp (ibivl)	SAppa (ibivl)	SAppa (ibiv1)	SAppa (ibivl)	Sapl (ibiv)	LSA (f)	SAP bibiv(l)	SAp (ibivl)
Hydrogen produced	2,3	1,3	–	2,1	1,3	±2	–±	4	–
Growth in 20% bile	4S	4S	4S	4S	4	2,4	4	2S	4
Esculin hydrolyzed	+	+–	+	+	+	+	+	+	+
Indole produced	–	–	–	+	+	+	–	+	+
Nitrate reduced	–	–	–	–	–	–	+	–	–
Gelatin digested	–w	+	–w	d	–w	–	–	+–	–
Milk reaction	c	c	c	c	c	c	c	c	c
Meat digested	–	–	–	–	–	–	–	–	–
Acid produced from									
Amygdalin	–+	–	+w	+–	+w	+	+–	–	–
Arabinose	–	+	–	+	+	+w	+	+	+
Cellobiose	–w	–	+	+	+	+w	+	–	–w
Dextrin	+	+	+	+	+	+	+	–	+
Esculin	+w	–	w+	w+	w+	+–	+–	–	–w
Fructose	+	+	+	+	+	+	+	d	–w
Glucose	+	+	+	+	+	+	+	+	+
Glycogen	+	+	–	+–	+	+–	–	–	+
Inositol	–	–	–	–	–	–	+	–	–
Inulin	d	+–	+	d	d	+w	–	–	–
Lactose	+	+	+	+	+	+	+	+	+
Maltose	+	+	+	+	+	+w	+	–	+
Mannitol	–	–	–	–+	–	–	+–	–	–
Mannose	+	+	+	+	+	+w	+	+	+
Melezitose	–	–	+	+–	d	–	w–	–	–
Melibiose	+w	+w	+	+	+	+w	+	–+	–
Raffinose	+	+	+	+	+	+	+	–	–
Rhamnose	–	+	+–	+w	+	–+	–+	–	w–
Ribose	–	–+	+–	+	+w	–+	+–	–	–

Salicin	–	–	+	+	– +	+ –	+	–	–
Starch	+	+	+	+	+	+	+	–	+ w
Sucrose	+	+	+	+	+	+ w	+	–	–
Trehalose	–	–	+	+	+	–	+ –	–	–
Xylose	+	+	+	+	+	+	+	–	+
Gas (PYG agar)	d	1,3	± –	1,2	1,2	1,2	1 –	1,4	– 2
Lipase	–	–	–	–	–	–	–	–	–
Catalase	+	– +	+ –	– +	+	– +	–	–	–

	Saccharolytic *Bacteroides*							
	Pentose fermenters			Pentose non-fermenters			Saccharolytic and proteolytic	
Characteristics	*B.oris*	*B.buccae*	*B.zoogleo-formans*	*B.oralis*	*B.veroralis*	*B.buccalis*	*B.bivius*	*B.disiens*
Products from PYG	SA (pibiv)	SA (fpivlfuibb)	SAP (ibiv)	SAf (l)	aS	AivS (l)	SAiV (ibf)	SA(ib ivfp)
Hydrogen produced	–	–	–	–	–	–	–	–
Growth in 20% bile	–	–	–	–	–	–	– 1	–
Esculin hydrolyzed	+	+	+	+	+	+	–	–
Indole produced	–	–	+ –	–	–	–	–	–
Nitrate reduced	–	–	–	–	–	–	–	–
Gelatin digested	+ –	+ w	d	+	–	+	+	+
Milk reaction	c	c	c	c	ac	c	p	p
Meat digested	–	–	–	–	–	–	+	+
Acid produced from								
Amygdalin	+ –	+ –	– w	+	–	w	–	–
Arabinose	+ –	+	d	–	–	–	–	–
Cellobiose	+ w	+	+ w	+	+	+	–	–
Dextrin	+	+	+	nt	nt	+	+	+
Esculin	+ –	d	–	+	w	–	–	–
Fructose	+	+	+ w	+	+	+	w	– w
Glucose	+	+	+ w	+	+	+	+	+
Glycogen	+	+	+ w	+	+	+	+	+
Inositol	–	–	–	–	–	–	–	–
Inulin	+	+ –	+	nt	+	+	–	–
Lactose	+	+	+ w	+	+	+	+	–

Table 4:12. Biochemical Reactions of *Bacteroides* Species Isolated from Human Sources* (*Continued*)

	Saccharolytic *Bacteroides*							
	Pentose fermenters			Pentose non-fermenters			Saccharolytic and proteolytic	
Characteristics	*B.oris*	*B.buccae*	*B.zoogleo-formans*	*B.oralis*	*B.veroralis*	*B.buccalis*	*B.bivius*	*B.disiens*
Products from PYG	SA (pibiv)	SA (fpivlfuibb)	SAP (ibiv)	SAf (l)	aS	AivS (l)	SAiV (ibf)	SA(ib ivfp)
Maltose	+	+	+w	+	+	+	+	+
Mannitol	–	–	–	–	–	–	–	–
Mannose	+	+	+w	+	+	+	+	–
Melezitose	–	–	–	–	–	–	–	–
Melibiose	d	+	d	+	w	+	–	–
Raffinose	+	+	+	+	+	+	–	–
Rhamnose	d	+ –	–	d	–	–	–	–
Ribose	d	d	–	–w	–	–	–	–
Salicin	+	+	d	+	–	–	–	–
Starch	+	+	+w	+	+	+	+	+
Sucrose	+	+	+	+	+	+	–	–
Trehalose	–	–	–	–	–	–w	–	–
Xylose	+	+	d	–	–	–	–	–
Gas (PYG agar)	–	–2	–1	– ±	– ±	–	–1	–1
Lipase	–	–	–	–	nt	–	–	–
Catalase	–	–	–	–	–	–	–	–

	Pigmented *Bacteroides* spp. Saccharolytic						Asaccharolytic		
Characteristics	*B.loescheii*	*B.denticola*	*B.mela-nino-genicus*	*B.corporis*	*B.inter-medius*	*B.levii*	*B.gingi-valis*	*B.asac-charo-lyticus*	*B.endo-dontalis*
Products from PYG	Sa (flpy)	SA (lfibiv)	SA (fibiv1)	SAibiv (b)	SAiv (ibpf)	ABp ibivs	BiV apibspa	AB iVSpib	AB pibivls
Hydrogen produced	–	–	–	–	–	1,3	–	d	–
Growth in 20% bile	–	–	–	–1	–	–	–	–	–

Esculin hydrolyzed	+	+	− +	−	−	−	−	−	−
Indole produced	−	−	−	−	+	−	+	+	+
Nitrate reduced	−	−	−	−	−	−	−	−	−
Gelatin digested	+	+	+	+	+	+	+	+	+
Milk reaction	c	c	c	pc	p	p	p	p	p
Meat digested	−	−	−	− +	+ −	+	+	+	+
Acid produced from									
Amygdalin	−	−	−	−	−	−	−	−	−
Arabinose	−	−	−	−	−	−	−	−	−
Cellobiose	+	−	−	−	−	−	−	−	−
Dextrin	+ −	+	+	+	+	−	−	−	−
Esculin	− +	+ w	−	−	−	−	−	−	−
Fructose	d	+	+	d	+ −	−	−	−	−
Glucose	+	+	+	+	+	+ w	−	−	−
Glycogen	+	+	+	+	+ −	−	−	−	−
Inositol	−	−	−	−	−	−	−	−	
Inulin	− +	+	+	−	+ −	−	−	−	−
Lactose	+	+	+	−	−	+ w	−	−	−
Maltose	+	+	+	+	+	−	−	−	−
Mannitol	−	−	−	−	−	−	−	−	−
Mannose	+ w	+	+	+ w	d	+ w	−	−	−
Melezitose	−	−	−	−	−	−	−	−	−
Melibiose	d	−	− +	−	−	−	−	−	−
Raffinose	+	+	+	−	d	−	−	−	−
Rhamnose	−	−	−	−	−	−	−	−	−
Ribose	−	d	−	−	−	−	−	−	−
Salicin	−	−	−	−	−	−	−	−	−
Starch	+ −	+	+	+	+ w	−	−	−	−
Sucrose	+	+	+	−	+	−	−	−	−
Trehalose	−	−	−	−	−	−	−	−	−
Xylose	−	−	−	−	−	−	−	−	−
Gas (PYG agar)	−	−	−1	−1	− ±	d	−	−	−
Lipase	+ −	−	−	−	+ −	−	−	−	−
Catalase	−	−	−	−	−	−	−	−	−

Table 4:12. Biochemical Reactions of *Bacteroides* Species Isolated from Human Sources* (*Continued*)

	Miscellaneous *Bacteroides* spp. Weakly saccharolytic/asaccharolytic								Saccharolytic		
									B.ruminicola		
Characteristics	*B.capillosus*	*B.furcosus*	*B.ureolyticus*	*B.praeacutus*	*B.gracilis*	*B.pneumosintes*	*B.putredinis*	*B.coagulans*	*ss ruminicola*	*ss brevis*	*B.hypermegas*
Products from PYG	sa (lfp)	La (fs)	SA (lf)	ABiV pibs(lf)	aS	a (sl)	SiV Paibb(l)	a (fpls)	SAF (pibiv)	SAfp (ibivbl)	PAl s(py)
Hydrogen produced	–	nt	1,2	–	1	–	2,4	–	–	–	–
Growth in 20% bile	–1	–2	–	d	–	–	–3	d	–	–	1,4
Esculin hydrolyzed	+	+–	–	–	–	–	–	–	+	+	+
Indole produced	–	–	–	–	–	–	+	+	–	–	–
Nitrate reduced	–	–	+	+–	+	–	–	–	–	–	–
Gelatin digested	–w	–w	+–	+w	–	–	+	+	+	+	–
Milk reaction	c	–	p–	–	–	–	p	cp	c	c	c
Meat digested	–	–	–+	–	–	–	d	–	–	–	–
Acid produced from											
Amygdalin	–	–	–	–	–	–	–	–	+	w	w–
Arabinose	–	–	–	–	–	–	–	–	+	+w	+
Cellobiose	–	–	–	–	–	–	–	–	+	+w	+–
Dextrin	–	–	–	–	–	–	–	–	r	+w	w–
Esculin	–	–	–	–	–	–	–	–	r	r	–
Fructose	–	w–	–	–	–	–	–	–	+w	+	+
Glucose	w–	w+	–	–	–	–	–	–	+	+	+
Glycogen	–	–	–	–	–	–	–	–	d	w+	–
Inositol	–	–	–	–	–	–	–	–	–	–	+–
Inulin	–	–	–	–	–	–	–	–	+	+w	+–
Lactose	–	–	–	–	–	–	–	–	+	+w	+

Maltose	−	−	−	−	−	−	−	−	+	+	+
Mannitol	−	−	−	−	−	−	−	−	−	−	+
Mannose	−	−	−	−	−	−	−	−	+	+	+
Melezitose	−	−	−	−	−	−	−	−	−	−w	−w
Melibiose	−	−	−	−	−	−	−	−	+	+	+
Raffinose	−	−	−	−	−	−	−	−	+	+w	+
Rhamnose	−	−	−	−	−	−	−	−	−	−	−+
Ribose	−	−	−	−	−	−	−	−	−	−	+w
Salicin	−	−w	−	−	−	−	−	−	+	r	d
Starch	−	−	−	−	−	−	−	−	+	d	−
Sucrose	−	−+	−	−	−	−	−	−	+	+	+
Trehalose	−	−	−	−	−	−	−	−	−	−	+
Xylose	−	−	−	−	−	−	−	−	+	−	+
Gas (PYG agar)	−3	−2	−1	−2	−	−	d	−2	−	−	2
Lipase	−	−	−	−	nt	−	−	−	−	−	−
Catalase	−	−	−w	−	−	−	+−	−	−	−	−

* Modified from References 19, 26, 39, 55, 56, 58, 59, 105, 119, 123; Cato, Van Winkelhoff (personal communications).
Products from 1% peptone-1% yeast extract-1% glucose (PYG) broth cultures: Capital letters indicate an average (from multiple cultures) of >1 meq of acid/100 mL broth; small letter = <1 meq/100 mL; A = acetic; B = butyric; F = formic; Fu = fumaric; iB = isobutyric; iV = isovaleric; L = lactic; P = propionic; Pa = phenylacetic; Py = pyruvic; S = succinic; products in parentheses ( ) may or may not be detected.
Hydrogen production (approximate concentration in headspace gas): ± = trace; 1 = 0.5%; 2 = 1%; 3 = 2%; 4 = 3% or more.
Growth in 20% bile: 1 = poor; 2 = moderate; 4 = excellent; S = stimulated (more growth than in the PYG control tube).
Milk: a = acid; c = curd; p = proteolyzed.
Sugars: + = pH below 5.5; − = pH 5.7 or above; w = weak reactions or pH 5.5 to 5.7.
Gas (PYG agar deeps): − = no gas detected; 2 = splits across agar; 3 = agar displaced; 4 = agar displaced to top of tube.
r = reported results vary between laboratories; nt = not tested.
Where two reactions given, the first is the more common.

Table 4:13. Characteristics of Species of the Genus *Fusobacterium* Isolated from Human Sources*

Characteristics	*F. nucleatum*	*F. gonidiaformans*	*F. varium*	*F. necrophorum*	*F. perfoetens*	*F. naviforme*	*F. russii*	*F. mortiferum*	*F. necrogenes*	*F. prausnitzii*	*F. periodonticum*	*F. alocis*	*F. sulci*
Products from PYG	Bap (FLs)	BAp (lfs)	BLap (s)	Bpa (ls)	Bap (L)	BLa (fps)	BLa (f)	Bap (sflv)	Bap (fsl)	BLF (s)	ABpls	ab	B a(s)
Propionate from:													
threonine	+	+	+	+	+	−	−	+	+	−	+	−	−
lactate	−	−	−	+	−	−	−	−	−	−	−	−	−
Hydrogen produced	−	4	4	4	4	−	−	4	4	−	−	4	1
Esculin hydrolyzed	−	−	−	−	−	−	−	+	+	+	−	−	−
Indole produced	+	+	d	+	−	+	−	−	−	−	+	−	−
Growth in 20% bile	±	−1	4,1	−4	−	−1	−1	4S	4,1	1−	−	−	−
Gelatin digested	−	−w	−	+−	−	−	−w	−	−	−	−	−	−
Milk reaction	−	−	−	cp−	−	−	−	−c	−	−a	a	−	−
Meat digestion	−	−	−	+−	−	−	−	−	−	−	−	−	−
Acid from:													
amygdalin	−	−	−	−	−	−	−	−w	−	−	−	−	−
cellobiose	−	−	−	−	−	−	−	w−	−w	−w	−	−	−
esculin	−	−	−	−	−	−	−	−	−	−w	−	−	−
fructose	−w	−	w+	−w	w	−	−	+w	w+	w−	+	−	−
glucose	−w	−	w+	−w	w	w−	−	+w	w+	w−	+	−	−

lactose	–	–	–	–	–	–	–	+w	–	w–	–	–	–
maltose	–	–	–	–	–	–	–	w–	–	w–	–	–	–
mannose	–	–	w+	–	–	–	–	+w	w+	–w	–	–	–
melibiose	–	–	–	–	–	–	–	w–	–w	–	–	–	–
raffinose	–	–	–	–	–	–	–	+w	–w	–	–	–	–
salicin	–	–	–	–	–	–	–	–w	–w	–w	–	–	–
starch	–	–	–	–	–	–	–	–w	–	–w	–	–	–
sucrose	–	–	–	–	w	–	–	+w	–w	–w	–	–	–
trehalose	–	–	–	–	–	–	–	–+	w–	–w	–	–	–
xylose	–	–	–	–	–	–	–	–w	–	–	–	–	–
Gas (PYG agar)	–2	4,2	4	4,2	3	–3	2–	4	4	–2	–	–	–
Lipase	–	–	–	+–	–	–	–	–	–	–	–	–	–

* Modified from Holdeman *et al*;[58] Cato *et al*;[20] Slots *et al*.[106]

Acid products from 1% peptone-1% yeast extract-1% glucose (PYG) broth cultures: Capital letters indicate an average (from multiple cultures) of >1 meq of acid/100 mL broth; small letters = <1 meq/100 mL. A = acetic; B = butyric; F = formic; P = propionic; S = succinic; V = valeric; products in parentheses ( ) may or may not be detected.

Hydrogen production (approximate concentrations in headspace gas): – = none detected; 4 = 3% or more.

Growth in 20% bile: – = no growth; ± = very poor; 1 = poor; 2 = moderate; 4 = excellent; S = stimulated (more growth than in the PYG control tube).

Milk reaction: a = acid; c = curd; p = proteolyzed.

Acid from sugars: + = pH below 5.5; – = pH 5.7 or above; w = weak reaction or pH 5.5 to 5.7.

Gas (PYG agar deeps): – = no gas detected; 2 = splits across the agar; 3 = agar displaced; 4 = agar displaced to the top of the tube.

Where two reactions are given, the first is the more common.

B. asaccharolyticus, B. gingivalis and *B. endodontalis* are phenotypically very similar; *B. gingivalis* produces phenylacetic acid and grows on *B. gingivalis* selective agar, while *B. endodontalis* may be differentiated by serology, absence of α-fucosidase, trypsin and *N*-acetyl-β-glucosamidase, inability to grow in an atmosphere of 95% N_2-5% H_2, a growth requirement for menadione and protein electrophoresis.[60,119,120] Other differentiating features of the pigmented *Bacteroides* group are referred to under Presumptive Identification and listed in Table 4:12.[39,58,119,120]

Organisms that do not fit into the described species are rarely encountered in clinical specimens and may be termed *Bacteroides* species (Table 4:12). It should be noted that most human isolates previously classified as *B. ruminicola* subspecies are in reality strains of *B. oris* and *B. buccae*.[58]

Fusobacteria, apart from their specific special-potency antibiotic susceptibility pattern (Table 4:13), produce major amounts of butyric acid without isobutyric or isovaleric acids. Most strains are weakly saccharolytic or asaccharolytic and nonproteolytic. Colonial morphology, as observed with the dissecting microscope, varies greatly from a speckled appearance for *F. nucleatum* to a fried-egg appearance for *F. mortiferum*. The most common clinical isolates, *F. nucleatum* followed in frequency by *F. necrophorum*, are both indole-positive; lipase production (*F. necrophorum* usually lipase-positive) and pattern of conversion of threonine and lactate to propionate are important in differentiation of these species. *F. mortiferum* produces bizarre pleomorphic rods and very large coccoid forms (round bodies).[39] *F. periodonticum, F. alocis* and *F. sulci* are 3 newly described oral isolates.[20,106] *F. periodonticum* may be differentiated from *F. nucleatum* by the former's ability to ferment galactose.[106] *F. alocis* and *F. sulci* are best differentiated from each other and from other nonreactive fusobacteria such as *F. russii* by polyacrylamide gel electrophoresis of soluble cellular proteins.[20] Properties and differentiation of the fusobacteria are listed in Table 4:13.[20,58,106]

ANAEROBIC COCCI

General Characteristics

The taxonomy of the anaerobic gram-positive cocci has recently undergone revision. All former species of *Peptococcus*, with the exception of *Peptococcus niger*, have been transferred to the genus *Peptostreptococcus*, which now includes *P. anaerobius, P. asaccharolyticus, P. indolicus, P. magnus, P. micros, P. prevotii* and *P. productus*. Additionally, a new species, *P. tetradius*, has been suggested to include organisms previously designated as "*Gaffkya anaerobia*."[34,98] Findings suggested that *P. niger* and *Peptostreptococcus parvulus* had similar guanine:cytosine ratios which were distinct from those of other gram-positive anaerobic cocci.[34] However, it has also been proposed that *P. parvulus* be transferred to the genus

Streptococcus.[18] Anaerobic gram-positive cocci have been reclassified into the genus *Streptococcus* if they produce major amounts of lactic acid from carbohydrate fermentation. This genus includes 3 other organisms which were formerly classified as peptococci or peptostreptococci: *Streptococcus intermedius, S. constellatus* and *S. morbillorum*. Many strains of these species are capnophiles which grow optimally, either initially or after one or more subcultures, in air + 5-10% CO_2; however, some are obligate anaerobes. Many strains may not grow in CO_2 or exhibit aerotolerance until several subcultures have been performed.[98] Some of these organisms are included in the British classification of *S. milleri*. The reader is referred to publications on the genus *Streptococcus* for further physicochemical descriptions of these organisms.[35]

The organism formerly known as *Peptococcus saccharolyticus* has been transferred to the genus *Staphylococcus*.[67,98] Most strains appear as obligate anaerobes in aerotolerance tests after 48 h incubation, but most will grow aerobically within 4-7 days. Other genera of anaerobic gram-positive cocci are *Ruminococcus, Gemmiger, Coprococcus* and *Sarcina*. These are infrequently encountered in clinical infections.[55,98]

The anaerobic gram-negative cocci comprise *Veillonella parvula* (synonymous with *V. alcalescens*), *V. atypica, V. dispar, Acidaminococcus fermentans* and *Megasphaera elsdenii*. These organisms are rarely implicated in human infections and account for a small minority of anaerobic cocci isolated from human sources. *V. parvula* is the only species isolated with any degree of frequency.[98]

Anaerobic gram-positive cocci are important human pathogens. The most common isolate is *P. magnus*, followed by *P. asaccharolyticus, P. anaerobius, P. micros* and *P. prevotii*. Infections in which anaerobic cocci have been implicated include abscesses of the breast (peri-areolar) and other soft tissues; infections involving the neck, dentoalveolar tissues, respiratory and female genital tracts; and infected surgical wounds. *P. magnus* is isolated from a variety of sites, most often as part of a mixed flora, but approximately 15% of the time in pure culture. These sites include bone and joint, intra-abdominal sepsis, soft tissue, blood, foot ulcers, pleural fluid, female genital tract, lung, sinuses and brain abscesses. *P. magnus* is particularly associated with bone and joint infections in the presence of foreign bodies. *P. indolicus* was recently isolated for the first time from a human infection (finger of a shepherd).[98] Lactate-producing streptococci are important human pathogens and are commonly isolated in mixed culture from intra-abdominal and biliary tract sepsis as well as from infections of the respiratory and female genital tracts.[35,98]

Identification

The anaerobic cocci may be divided microscopically into gram-positive and gram-negative groups. No unique characteristics are available to suggest

Table 4:14. Biochemical Reactions of Anaerobic Cocci*

	P. niger	*S.saccharolyticus*	*Ps.anaerobius*	*Ps.magnus*	*Ps.micros*	*Ps.indolicus*
Metabolic products from PYG	BC*iva*	A	ICA*ivib*	A (1s)	As1	BAp (1s)
Indole	–	–	–	–	–	+
Coagulase	–	–	–	–	–	+
Nitrate reduction	–	+	–	–	–	+
Propionate from lactate	–	–	–	–	–	+
Gas from PYG	w	+	+	–	–	+
Gelatin liquefaction	–	–	–	v	–	–
Catalase	–	+	–	+(–)	–	–
Urease	–	+	–	–	–	–
Starch hydrolysis	–	–	–	–	–	–
Esculin hydrolysis	–	–	–	–	–	–
Ammonia from glutamate	–	–	–	–	–	+
Ammonia from glycine	–	–	–	+	w	–
Carbohydrate fermentation						
Fructose	–	+	–	v	–	–
Maltose	–	–	w(–)	–	–	–
Mannose	–	+	–(w)	–	–	–
Sucrose	–	–	–(w)	–	–	–
Glucose	–	+	w(–)	–(w)	–	–
Cellobiose	–	–	–	–	–	–
Lactose	–	–	–	–	–	–
Xylose	–	–	–(w)	–	–	–

	P.asaccharolyticus homology group I	homology group II	homology group III (A-1)	*Ps.prevotii*	*Ps.tetradius*	*Ps.productus*	*S.parvulus*	*V.parvula*	*A.fermentans*	*M.elsdenii*
Metabolic products from PYG	Ba (p1)	BA (p1*ibiv*)	BLa(p)	Ba (p1s)	BLa (p)	As (1)	La	Ap (1s)	Ab(slp)	CB*ibvivas*(Fp)
Indole	+	+	+	−	−	−	−	−	−	−
Coagulase	−	−	−	−	−	−	−	−	−	−
Nitrate reduction	−	−	−	−	−	−	−	+	−	−
Propionate from lactate	−	−	−	−	−	−	−	+	−	+
Gas from PYG	+	+	+	+	+	+	−	+	+(−)	+
Gelatin liquefaction	−	−	−	−	−	−	−	−	−	−(w)
Catalase	v	v	v	+(−)	v	−	−	v	−	−
Urease	−	−	−	−(+)	+	d	−	−	−	−
Starch hydrolysis	−	−	−	−	−	−	−	−	−	−
Esculin hydrolysis	−	−	−	−(w)	−(w)	+	+	−	−(+)	−
Ammonia from glutamate	+	+	−	−	−	−	−	nt	nt	nt
Ammonia from glycine	−	−	−	−	−	−	−	nt	nt	nt
Carbohydrate fermentation										
Fructose	−	−	−	−(w)	+	+	+	−	−	+(−)
Maltose	−	−	−	w(−)	+	+	+	−	−	+(−)
Mannose	−	−	−	v	+	+	+	−	−	−(w)
Sucrose	−	−	−	−(w)	+	+	−	−	−	−(+)
Glucose	−	−(+)	+	w	+	+	+	−	−	+
Cellobiose	−	−	−	−	−	+	+	−	−	−
Lactose	−	−	−	−	−	+	+	−	−	−
Xylose	−	−	−	−	−	+	−(w)	−	−	−(w)

* Modified from Holdeman *et al*,[55] Ezaki *et al*,[34] Holdeman *et al.*[57]

Acid products form PYG: Capital letters indicate major products, and lower case letters indicate minor products; products in parentheses ( ) are occasional products; A/a = acetic; B/b = butyric; C/c = caproic; F/f = formic; IB/ib = isobutyric; IC/ic = isocaproic; IV/iv = isovaleric; L/l = lactic; P/p = propionic; S/s = succinic.

+ = positive; − = negative; w = weakly positive; v = variable; d = delayed; reaction in parentheses ( ) = occasional products.

that organisms are anaerobes rather than aerobes. Cells of *P. anaerobius* and *P. productus* are often elongated and in chains or pairs. Generally, peptococci occur singly or in small groups and are larger than peptostreptococci, which often appear in chains. However, these properties are not sufficiently specific to allow them to be used for taxonomic purposes.[98] *P. magnus* and *P. micros* can be differentiated by polyacrylamide gel electrophoresis[98] and microscopically by the larger cells of the former. Unusually large cocci, especially in groups or "packets," may suggest the presence of *Megasphaera, P. tetradius* or *Sarcina* spp.[98] Should the Gram stain yield equivocal results, gram-negative anaerobes may be separated from gram-positive ones by the KOH reaction[50] (see Table 4:21) and by the susceptibility of gram-negative anaerobes to colistin and resistance to vancomycin, when tested with special-potency susceptibility disks.[98,111]

Properties of the anaerobic cocci commonly encountered in clinical specimens are listed in Table 4:14.[34,55,57,98]anaerobic cocci on plates and in broth is relatively slow. Small colonies are not usually apparent on blood agar plates until after 48 h incubation. Colonies are usually small, convex and entire.[98] *V. parvula* fluoresces red under longwave UV light[22] and *P. niger* produces black colonies on blood agar plates.[98] Supplementation with Tween 80 and yeast extract may improve growth in fluid and semisolid media.[55,98,111] The non and weakly fermentative gram-positive cocci may be differentiated by Gram stain, gas-liquid chromatography (GLC), gelatin and indole production and nitrate reduction.[34,55,57,98,111] *P. anaerobius* may be identified by its unique susceptibility to sodium polyanethol sulfonate[134] (see Table 4:21), production of isocaproic acid[55,57,98] and production of *p*-hydroxyhydrocinnamic acid from tyrosine.[8] *P. indolicus* is unique in that it produces indole and coagulase and reduces nitrate.[34,98] *P. asaccharolyticus* is indole-positive and has been divided into 3 homology groups by DNA hybridization.[34] *P. productus* is more biochemically active than other anaerobic cocci, and *P. tetradius* is the only clinically encountered anaerobic coccus which is regularly urease-positive.[34,98] *V. parvula*, the only anaerobic gram-negative coccus of clinical importance, is inactive biochemically except for nitrate reduction and produces major amounts of acetic and propionic acids on GLC.[55,98]

GRAM-POSITIVE NONSPOREFORMING RODS

General Characteristics

The genera included here are *Actinomyces, Arachnia, Bifidobacterium, Eubacterium, Lachnospira, Lactobacillus* and *Propionibacterium*.[2,55,111] All organisms in this group are gram-positive to gram-variable rod-shaped cells. Morphology is highly variable. Most are obligate anaerobes but some are microaerophiles or facultative anaerobes. Most strains require 2-3 days of anaerobic incubation for visible growth on blood agar. *A. israelii* may require 2 or more weeks of incubation for primary isolation. Members of each genus are part of the normal flora of humans[36] and animals, and all potential pathogens also occur as normal flora.[2]

The morphology of gram-positive nonsporeforming anaerobic rods is influenced by the culture medium, length of incubation and other growth conditions, and may mimic aerobic/facultatively anaerobic groups such as *Clostridium, Bacillus, Corynebacterium, Erysipelothrix, Listeria, Nocardia* and *Streptococcus*. The pleomorphic cellular morphology and gram-variable nature of these organisms may lead to confusion in identification. Cells may be arranged in various patterns. Lactobacilli usually form chains of uniform rods but may be predominantly diphtheroidal. Some streptococci may form rod-shaped cells and some gram-positive anaerobic rods may form short coccoid forms. Oxygen-tolerance testing helps in separating aerobic/facultatively anaerobic genera from anaerobes with similar morphology.[2] Bifidobacteria usually form rods with bifurcated ends,[2,55,100] but this property is shared by other genera.[2] In addition, branching non-acidfast filaments of actinomycetes[2] may be confused with other genera. Certain clostridia, notably *Clostridium ramosum*, do not produce spores on the usual laboratory media and resemble the nonsporeformers morphologically.[2] Growth on egg yolk agar and other biochemical tests will help differentiate these groups (see Chapter 5, "Anaerobic Infections: Sporeformers").

Taxonomy and Differentiation

Genus differentiation of the gram-positive nonsporeforming rods is mainly on the basis of GLC and microscopic morphology.[2] *Actinomyces* species produce major or moderate peaks of acetic, plus either major succinic and lactic acids or major succinic acid only,[55,102,111] while propionibacteria and *Arachnia propionica* both produce major acetic and propionic acids[2,28,55,101] bifidobacteria produce major acetic and lactic peaks.[2,55,100] Lactobacilli produce major lactic acid peaks only,[2,55,65] while eubacteria yield chromatographic patterns which differ for individual species.[2,55,81] Only *Actinomyces* of clinical significance will be discussed here. Although 24 *Bifidobacterium* species were cited in the latest approved list,[100] their clinical significance in most cases is uncertain. Tests such as polyacrylamide gel electrophoresis of cellular proteins and DNA homology (which may be necessary for definitive identification and taxonomy) are not practical for clinical laboratories.[100] The latest approved list recognizes 34 *Eubacterium* species.[81] Only those isolated from human sites will be discussed. *Lachnospira multiparus*, a motile, weakly gram-positive, curved rod,[58] has been isolated from human intestinal material but not from human clinical specimens.[2]

Clinical Significance

The few members of this group that are of major clinical significance are the *Actinomyces* spp., *P. acnes* and occasionally *Eubacterium, Bifidobacterium* and *Lactobacillus*.[2] Propionibacteria, almost always *P. acnes*, are by far the most common clinical isolates.[2] Although most *P. acnes* isolates are contaminants,[2] clinical infections such as cerebrospinal fluid shunt infections, meningitis, endocarditis, hematogenous infections of joint prostheses and immune complex glomerulonephritis have been reported.[2,11,49,103,137]

Most *Eubacterium* species are isolated from polymicrobial infections and it is difficult to assess their significance.[2] Eubacteria, especially *Eubacterium lentum*, may be isolated from deep abscesses, wounds, blood, pulmonary and dental infections, and are rare causes of endocarditis. *E. brachy, E. timidum* and *E. nodatum* occur mostly in dental infections but may be implicated in infections at other sites.[2,54,81] Lactobacilli rarely cause disease, but endocarditis, endometritis, peritonitis, chorioamnionitis, dental abscess, septic arthritis and pneumonia have been attributed to these organisms.[75]

Bifidobacteria are also rare causes of disease. *Bifididobacterium dentium* (formerly known as *B. eriksonii* and *A. eriksonii*) is a normal inhabitant of the mouth and intestines and has been found in mixed infections of the lower respiratory tract, abscesses and human dental plaque.[100]

Human actinomycosis is most commonly caused by *A. israelii*, but also by *A. propionica, A. naeslundii, A. viscosus, A. odontolyticus, A. meyeri* and *B. dentium*.[2] Actinomycetes have also been implicated in the pathogenesis of periodontal disease and root caries.[2]

Direct Microscopic Examination

When actinomycosis is suspected, examine the tissue, body fluid, exudate, contraceptive device or gauze from draining wounds for sulfur granules. Granules are white/yellowish, irregularly shaped, hard, grain-like bodies $\leq$ 0.1-5 mm in diameter. They consist of masses of filamentous bacteria sometimes surrounded by hyaline clubs. Place granules on a slide in a drop of water, crush with another two slides and examine microscopically. The finding of thin ($\leq 1\ \mu m$) branched/unbranched filaments with peripheral clubs within a granule is excellent presumptive identification of one of the actinomycetes. Differentiation from aerobic filamentous branching rods may be done by a modified acid-alcohol-fast stain. Fluorescent antibody techniques have been developed for some actinomycetes, but these are not available commercially at this time.

Identification

Key characteristics for presumptive identification of the gram-positive anaerobic nonsporeforming rods are listed in Table 4:15[2] and specific characteristics in Tables 4:16-19.[21,23,28,81,100-102] Because these organisms are infrequently encountered in clinical specimens, laboratories with limited facilities may legitimately limit identification to the presumptive level indicated in Table 4:15 and send potentially significant organisms to a reference laboratory for definitive identification.[2]

Propionibacterium:

Most gram-positive, anaerobic, nonsporeforming rods isolated from human clinical material are *P. acnes*. This organism is part of the normal flora of hair follicles and sebaceous glands, and is also found in the mouth, nasopharynx, intestines and urogenital tract (including the male urethra). It is a common contaminant of body fluids such as blood and cerebrospinal fluid and must be differentiated from *Listeria monocytogenes* and other pathogens of like morphology. When sets of blood or other cultures are positive for *P. acnes*, thought must be given to its possible pathogenic potential. *P. acnes* strains are pleomorphic, exhibiting a diphtheroidal appearance with occasional branching and may be confused with actinomycetes. Most fresh strains grow as obligate anaerobes, but some may be facultatively anaerobic. *P. acnes* strains may be presumptively identified by their production of indole and catalase. Indole-negative strains may be confused with *A. viscosus* and catalase-negative strains with certain indole-positive eubacteria. In either case, additional testing is necessary for definitive identification.[2] Other propionibacteria are rare human pathogens. The biochemical characterization of the propionibacteria isolated from humans is given in Table 4:16.[28]

Eubacteria:

The second most commonly isolated nonsporeforming anaerobic rod is *E. lentum*. On Gram stain, this organism appears as a short gram-positive rod in pairs or short chains. It is inactive in most biochemical tests.[2] Characterization of *E. lentum* and other eubacteria from human sources is given in Table 4:17a,b.[81]

Actinomycetes:

Actinomyces israelii is rarely isolated from clinical material but is the most commonly isolated member of the *Actinomyces* and *Arachnia* group. On Gram stain, the organism may appear in the form of short diphtheroidal rods or as long, thin beaded filaments. Colonies may be smooth or rough. Rough colonies consist of thin, radiating filaments and develop a classic molar tooth appearance.[2] Biochemical differentiation of the actinomycetes is presented in Table 4:18.[101,102] *A. viscosus* is catalase-positive and can grow aerobically. *A. odontolyticus* may produce red colonies on anaerobic

Table 4:15. Some Key Differential Tests for Presumptive Identification of Gram-positive, Nonsporeforming Anaerobic Bacilli*

Species	Relationship to oxygen	Colonies on blood agar	Red pigment on blood agar	Appearance in enriched thioglycolate broth	Cellular morphology in enriched thioglycolate broth	Production of: Catalase	Production of: Indole	Glucose fermentation	Metabolic products in PYG† broth
Actinomyces israelii	M or OA	Rough	–	Granular or diffuse	Branching filaments or diphtheroidal	–	–	+	A,L,S
A.naeslundii	F	Smooth	–	Diffuse	Diphtheroidal, branching	–	–	+	A,L,S
A.odontolyticus	M or OA	Smooth	+	Diffuse	Diphtheroidal, branching	–	–	+	A,L,S
A.viscosus	F	Smooth	–	Diffuse	Diphtheroidal, branching	–	–	+	A,L,S
A.pyogenes	F	Smooth	–	Diffuse	Diphtheroidal, coccoidal	–	–	+	A,L,S
A.meyeri	OA,F	Smooth	–	Diffuse	Diphtheroidal, branching	–	–	+	A,L,S
Arachnia propionica	M or OA	Rough	–	Granular or diffuse	Branching filaments or diphtheroidal	–	–	+	A,P,(L),(S)
Bifidobacterium dentium	OA	Smooth	–	Diffuse	Thin rods, bifid ends, bulbous ends	–	–	+	A,L

Eubacterium alactolyticum	OA	Smooth	–	Diffuse	Thin rods, V-forms, cross-stick arrangements	–	–	+	A,B,C
E.lentum	OA	Smooth	–	Diffuse	Short coccoidal rods, diphtheroidal	–	–	–	(A)
E.limosum	OA	Smooth	–	Diffuse	Plump rods, bulbous and bifid forms	–	–	+	A,B
Lactobacillus catenaforme	OA	Smooth	–	Diffuse (granular)	Short rods in chains or singly	–	–	+	A,L
Propionibacterium avidum	F	Smooth	–	Diffuse	Diphtheroidal	+	–	+	A,P,(L),S
P.acnes	OA^F	Smooth	–	Diffuse (granular)	Diphtheroidal	$+^-$	$+^-$	+	A,P,L,S
P.granulosum	F	Smooth	–	Diffuse	Diphtheroidal	+	–	+	A,P,(L),S

* Modified from Allen.[2]

+ = Positive reaction for 90–100% of strains tested; – = negative reaction for 90–100% of strains tested; superscript = reaction shown with 11–25% of strains tested; F = facultatively anaerobic; M = microaerophilic; OA = obligately anaerobic.

Metabolic product analysis determined on peptone-yeast extract-glucose (PYG) broth cultures: A = acetic acid; B = butyric acid; C = caproic acid; L = lactic acid; P = propionic acid; S = succinic acid; parentheses ( ) = variable or, if produced, usually present only in trace amounts.

Table 4:16. Fermentations and Other Metabolic Reactions of Species of the Genus *Propionibacterium* Isolated from Humans*

Reaction	*P.jensenii*	*P.acnes*	*P.avidum*	*P.granulosum*	*P.lymphophilum*
Acid produced from:					
Adonitol	d+	d+	d+	−	+
Amygdalin	d+	−	−	d−	−
Arabinose	−	−	d+	−	−
Cellobiose	d−	−	−	−	−
Dulcitol	−	−	−	−	−
Erythritol	+	d+	+	−	+
Esculin	−	−	−	−	−
Fructose	+	d+	+	+	+
Galactose	+	d+	+	d−	−
Glucose	+	d+	+	+	+
Glycerol	+	d+	+	+	−
Glycogen	−	−	−	−	−
Inositol	d+	d−	d+	−	d+
Inulin	−	−	−	−	−
Lactose	d+	−	d+	−	−
Maltose	d+	−	+	d+	+
Mannitol	+	d−	d−	d+	−
Mannose	+	d+	+	+	−
Melezitose	d+	−	d+	d−	−
Melibiose	+	−	d+	d−	−
Raffinose	+	−	d+	d+	−
Rhamnose	−	−	−	−	−
Ribose	+	d+	d+	d−	+
Salicin	+	−	d+	−	−
Sorbitol	−	d+	−	−	−
Sorbose	−	−	−	−	−
Starch	−	−	−	−	d+
Sucrose	+	−	+	+	d−
Trehalose	+	−	+	d+	−
Xylose	d+	−	d−	−	−
Esculin hydrolysis	+	−	+	−	−
Starch hydrolysis	−	−	−	−	d−
Gelatin	−	+	+	d−	d+
Milk:					
Curd	d−	d+	+	+	−
Digestion	d−	d+	+	−	−
Indole produced	−	d+	−	−	−
Nitrate reduced	−	d+	−	−	d−
Catalase	d+	d+	+	+	d+
Gas	−,1	−,2	−,1	−,1	−,1
Acetoin	−	−	−	−	−
Growth in 20% bile	d+	2,1	d+	−,1	−,1

* Modified from Cummins and Johnson:[28] reactions determined by procedures given in Holdeman *et al.*[55]

\+ = positive reaction in 90–100% of strains or pH below 5.7 in 90–100% of strains; − = negative reaction in 90–100% of strains or pH 5.7 or above in 90–100% of strains; d− = reaction positive in 10–40% of strains; d+ = reaction positive in 40–90% of strains. Numbers refer to amount of gas produced (gas) or amount of growth (bile) on a 1–4 scale.

blood agar after plates have been held at room temperature for several days or after prolonged anaerobic incubation.[2]

Bifidobacteria and Lactobacilli:

B. dentium, the only *Bifidobacterium* species known to have pathogenic potential for humans, ferments a variety of sugars. Differentiation between it and other bifidobacteria isolated from human sources is given in Table 4:19.[100]

Good presumptive clues for recognizing lactobacilli include the appearance of slender gram-positive rods in chains which grow on *Lactobacillus* selective agar containing tomato juice and with a low pH. *L. catenaforme* is isolated most often from clinical specimens; it is indole-negative, hydrolyses esculin and starch and ferments several carbohydrates.[2] Detailed information on the differentiation of lactobacilli may be found in other publications.[55,65]

GENERAL LABORATORY IDENTIFICATION OF NONSPOREFORMING ANAEROBES

Direct Microscopic Identification

Direct specimen examination has been discussed in Chapter 38,"Microscopy." Other procedures include acridine orange staining, dark-field microscopy, fluorescent antibody testing, radioimmunoassay, coagglutination and countercurrent or crossed immunoelectrophoresis.[38,68,111]

Preliminary Identification

Not all anaerobes require extended biochemical testing for identification, and in most clinical laboratories it is not practical nor feasible to use the large number of tests required by standard manuals. Fortunately, certain characteristics (Table 4:20)[68] are useful in preliminary identification of many anaerobic isolates. Several "shortcuts" (Table 4:21) are available to facilitate preliminary identification of many groups. Over and above the preliminary tests, Dowell, Lombard and coworkers at the CDC have devised a modified conventional plate system (Presumpto method) for anaerobe identification. This commercially available method consists of a 3-plate system; each plate is divided into quadrants containing different components in Lombard-Dowell agar base. This method should be used together with a blood agar plate and a thioglycolate broth (Table 4:22). Identification tables for use with this system are available.[4,68,74] This method may be used also as a backup to other commercial methods.

Table 4:17a. Biochemical Reactions of Saccharoclastic Species in the Genus *Eubacterium* Isolated from Humans*

Characteristics	*E.aerofaciens*	*E.alactolyticum*	*E.biforme*	*E.budayi*	*E.contortum*	*E.cylindroides*	*E.eligens*	*E.formicigenerans*	*E.hadrum*	*E.hallii*	*E.limosum*	*E.moniliforme*	*E.multiforme*	*E.nitrotogenes*	*E.ramulus*	*E.rectale*	*E.saburreum*	*E.siraeum*	*E.tenue*	*E.tortuosum*	*E.ventriosum*
Cells motile	–	–	–	–	–	–	+	–	–	–	–	+	+–	–	–	d	–	–	d	–	–
Acid produced from:																					
Amygdalin	–	–	–	–	–w	–	–	–	–	–	–	–	–	–	–	A–	–	–	–	–	–A
Arabinose	–	–	–	–	Aw	–	–	d	–A	–	–A	–	–	–	–w	Aw	–	–	–	–	–
Cellobiose	A	–	–A	wA	A–	–w	A	–s	–w	–	–	–	w–	wA	A	Aw	–	wA	–	–w	–
Esculin	–A	–w	–w	–	–A	–	–	–	–	–	–	–	–	–	–	–	–	–	–	–	–A
Fructose	A	A	A	A	Aw	A	Aw	A	Aw	Aw	A	Aw	Aw	Aw	A	A	d	–w	–w	–A	A
Glucose	A	A	A	A	A	A	A–	A	Aw	Aw	A	A	Aw	A	A	A	Aw	–	w–	Aw	Aw
Glycogen	–	–	–	w–	–	–	–	–	–	–	–	–	–	–	–	a	–	–	–	–	–
Lactose	A–	–	d	A–	A–	–	A–	A–	A–	Aw	–	–	Aw	–w	A	A–	d	w–	–	–A	–A
Maltose	Aw	–	–	w	A	–	–s	A	–A	As	–w	–A	–	Aw	A–	A	d	w–	w–	–A	A
Mannitol	–	–A	d	–	–	–	–	–	–A	A–	A–	–	–	–	–A	–A	–	–	–	–	–
Mannose	A	–	A	A	d	A	–w	–s	Aw	Aw	–w	A	Aw	A	–w	–A	–A	w–	–	–	A
Melezitose	–	–	–	–	–	–	–	–	–	–	–	–	–	–	–	Aw	d	–	–	–	–
Melibiose	–	–	–	–	A–	–	–	–	–	–	–	–	–	–	Aw	Aw	–A	–	–	w–	–
Raffinose	–	–	–	–	Aw	–w	–	–	–	–	–	–	–	–	Aw	A	d	–	–	w–	–
Rhamnose	–	–	–	–	A–	–	–	–	–	–	–	–	–	–	–	–	–	–	–	–	–
Ribose	–	–	–	–	Aw	–	–	–A	–	–	Aw	–	–	–A	–	–	–	–	–	–	–A
Salicin	Aw	–	–A	–w	A	A–	–A	–	–A	–	–	–	–	d	d	Aw	–	–	–	w–	–
Sorbitol	–	–A	–	–	–	–	–	–	–A	As	–	–	–	–	w–	Aw	–	–	–	–	–
Starch	–	–	–	–w	–w	–w	w–	–s	–	–	–	–w	–	–w	–	Aw	–w	–w	–	–	d
Sucrose	A	–	–A	–	A	A–	–	–	Aw	–A	–	–	–	d	–w	A	A	–w	–	Aw	d
Trehalose	–A	–	d	–	–w	–	–	–	–	–	–	–	–	–A	–	d	d	–	–	–	–
Xylose	–	–	–	–	A–	–	A–	–A	Aw	–	d	–	–	–	–	Aw	d	–A	–	–	–
Esculin hydrolyzed	+–	–	d	+	+	+	–+	–	+–	–	+	–	+	+	+	+	+	+–	–	+	+
Starch hydrolyzed	–	–	–	–+	–	–+	–	–	–	–	–+	–	–	–	–	+	–	+–	–	–	–

Gelatin digested	–	–	–	–	–	–	–w	–	–	–	d	–w	–+	–w	–	–	–	–	+	–	–
Milk reaction	–c	–	–c	–	–c	–	c–	–c	–c	c–	–	–	c–	–c	c–	–c	c–	–c	dc	–c	c–
Meat digested	–	–	–	–	–	–	–	–	–	–	–	–	–w	–	–	–	–	–	+–	–	–
Indole produced	–	–	–	–	–	–	–	–	–	–	–	–	–	–	–	–	+	–	+	–	–
Nitrate reduced	–	–	–	+	–	–	–	–	–	–	–	v	+	+	–	–	–	–	–	d	–
H_2 produced	4	4	4,2	4	4	–,1	–	2,3	4	4	4	4	4	4	4	4	4	4	4	2,4	–
Butyrate produced	–	+	+	+	–	+	–	–	+	+	+	+	+	+	+	+	+	–	–	+	+
Other (see footnote)				†							‡	§		§					†		

* Modified from Moore and Holdeman.[81]

+ = positive reaction for 90–100% of strains; – = negative reaction for 90–100% of strains; ± = pH 6.0–7.0; A = acid (pH below 5.5); w = weak reaction (pH 5.5–5.9, sugars); d = 40–60% of strains positive; c = curd (milk); s = growth stimulated but pH usually not lowered; numbers (hydrogen) represent abundant to negative on a – to 4+ scale. When two reactions are given, the most common is listed first: A = 60–90% give pH below 5.5; Aw = 60–90% give weak acid; –A = 10–30% give pH below 5.5; and wA = 10–30% give weak acid.

Unless otherwise noted (in the footnotes), erythritol and inositol are not fermented and lecithinase is not produced.

† Lecithinase produced.

‡ Erythritol fermented.

§ Lecithinase may be produced.

Table 4:17b. Characteristics of Nonsaccharoclastic Species of *Eubacterium* Isolated from Humans*†

Characteristics	*E.brachy*	*E.combesii*	*E.dolichum*	*E.lentum*	*E.nodatum*	*E.timidum*
Carbohydrates fermented	–	–	–‡	–	–	–
Nitrate reduced	–	–	–	+	–	–
Gelatin hydrolyzed	–	+	–w	–	–	–
Esculin hydrolyzed	–	d	–	–	–	–
Hydrogen produced	2,4	4	–	–	–	–
Products§ (PYG cultures)	ic,iv,ib,(f,p,b,l,v)	A,B,iv,l,ib(p,f)	b(1,a)	(a,1,s)	b,a,(1,s)	(a,s)

* Modified from Moore and Holdeman.[81]

+ = positive reaction; – = negative reaction; w = weak reaction; d = variable; numbers (hydrogen) represent abundant to negative on a – to 4+ scale. When two reactions are given, the most common reaction is listed first. No acid produced from amygdalin, arabinose, cellobiose, erythritol, esculin, fructose, glucose, glycogen, inositol, lactose, maltose, mannitol, mannose, melezitose, melibiose, raffinose, rhamnose, ribose, salicin, sorbitol, starch, sucrose, trehalose, or xylose. Indole and lecithinase are not produced.

Growth may be stimulated in media containing certain carbohydrates.[81]

Capital letters represent an amount of product ≥1 meq/100 mL of culture; small letters represent an amount of product <1 meq/100 mL of culture; products in parentheses are not produced uniformly. a = acetate; b = butyrate; f = formate; ib = isobutyrate; ic = isocaproate; iv = isovalerate; l = lactate; p = propionate; s = succinate; v = valerate.

Table 4:18. Differentiation of actinomycetes and *Arachnia**

	A.israelii	*A.meyeri*	*A.naeslundii*	*A.viscosus*	*A.odontolyticus*	*A.pyogenes*	*Arachnia proponica*
Esculin hydrolysis	+	–	+	d	d	–	–
Gelatin hydrolysis	–	–	–	–	–	+	d
Starch hydrolysis	d	–	d	d	d	d	d
Nitrate reduction	d	–	+	d	+	–	+
Indole production	–	–	–	–	–	–	–
Milk reaction (curd)	d	d	d	d	d	+	d
Urease	–	–	+	d	–	–	–
Catalase	–	–	–	+	–	–	–
Fermentation of							
Glucose	+	+	+	+	+	+	+
Mannitol	d	–	–	–	–	–	+
Lactose	+	d	d	d	d	+	d
Sucrose	+	+	+	+	d	–	+
Maltose	+	+	+	+	d	d	+
Salicin	+	–	d	d	d	–	d
Glycerol	–	d	d	d	d	–	d
Xylose	+	+	d	–	d	d	–
Arabinose	d	d	–	–	d	d	–†
Galactose	+	d	+	d	d	+	d
Fructose	+	+	+	+	+	+	+
Raffinose	+	–	+	+	–	–	+
Ribose	+	+	d	d	d	+	d

* Modified from Schaal[101,102]; Cato *et al.*[21]; Collins and Jones.[23] Symbols as in Table 4:17.
† Strains of serovar 1 may produce acid.[101]

Table 4:19. Fermentative Characteristics Distinguishing the Species of the Genus *Bifidobacterium* Isolated from Humans*

	D-Ribose	L-Arabinose	Lactose	Cellobiose	Melezitose	Raffinose	Sorbitol	Starch	Gluconate	Xylose
B.bifidum	–	–	+	–	–	–	–	–	–	–
B.longum	+	+	+	–	+	+	–	–	–	d
B.infantis	+	–	+	–	–	+	–	–	–	d
B.breve	+	–	+	d	d	+	d	–	–	–
B.adolescentis	+	+	+	+	+	+	d	+	+	+
B.angulatum	+	+	+	–	–	+	d	+	d	+
B.catenulatum	+	+	+	+	–	+	+	–	d	+
B.pseudocatenulatum	+	+	+	d	–	+	d	+	d	+
B.dentium	+	+	+	+	+	+	–	+	+	+
B.globosum	+	d	+	–	–	+	–	+	–	d

* Modified from Scardovi.[100] Symbols: see Table 4:17.

	Mannose	Fructose	Galactose	Sucrose	Maltose	Trehalose	Melibiose	Mannitol	Inulin	Salicin
B.bifidum	–	+	+	d	–	–	d	–	–	–
B.longum	d	+	+	+	+	–	+	–	–	–
B.infantis	d	+	+	+	+	–	+	–	d	–
B.breve	+	+	+	+	+	d	+	d	d	+
B.adolescentis	d	+	+	+	+	d	+	d	d	+
B.angulatum	–	+	+	+	+	–	+	–	+	+
B.catenulatum	–	+	+	+	+	d	+	d	d	+
B.pseudocatenulatum	+	+	+	+	+	d	+	–	–	+
B.dentium	+	+	+	+	+	+	+	+	–	+
B.globosum	–	+	+	+	+	–	+	–	–	–

Table 4:20. Some Cardinal Identification Criteria of Nonsporeforming Anaerobes*

Relation to O_2
Colonial characteristics
Pigment
Hemolysis
Pitting of medium
Gram-stain reaction
Morphology
Motility
Flagella
Miscellaneous:
Growth in thioglycolate broth, catalase, reactions on milk medium; production of indole; hydrolysis of starch, esculin, and gelatin; reduction of nitrate; fermentation of key carbohydrates (e.g., glucose, mannitol, lactose, rhamnose); growth in presence of bile, penicillin, rifampin, and kanamycin; inhibition by sodium polyanetholsulfonate; metabolic products.

* Modified after Koneman *et al.*[68]

Definitive Identification

The "gold standard" for laboratory identification of nonsporeforming and other anaerobes includes reactions in a series of conventional sugars in combination with GLC.[55] Three anaerobic procedure manuals are available published by: Virginia Polytechnic Institute (VPI),[55] Centers for Disease Control (CDC)[31] and Wadsworth Anaerobic Laboratory.[111] The VPI manual utilizes PRAS media which may be prepared in-house or purchased commercially (Carr-Scarborough; Scott Laboratories). Originally, PRAS media were marketed in widemouthed tubes with butyl-rubber stoppers that had to be inoculated with a special gassing apparatus or in an anaerobic glove box.[55] Scott Laboratories has developed the PRAS II system in which tubes are shorter and narrower, and may be inoculated with a needle and syringe through a rubber stopper. In comparison with conventional and commercial systems, PRAS II has been found to correctly identify ≥93% of strains to genus or species levels.[15,66,99] Biochemical data can be interpreted with the aid of a computerized database. The CDC and Wadsworth Anaerobic Laboratory systems do not use PRAS sugars. It is very important, when using any one of these three manuals, to use the sugar bases recommended for the specific system. Failure to do so may invalidate results.[4]

Commercial Systems

The following methods are currently available.

a) API 20A (Analytab Products):

This system consists of a plastic strip with microtubules containing dehydrated substrates. Strips are inoculated with turbid suspensions of fresh growth and reactions read after 24 h anaerobic incubation. Sugar reactions are read after addition of a bromcresol purple indicator and are sometimes equivocal and difficult to read. Additionally, the system requires supplemental tests, including GLC, for correct identification of nonsaccharolytic/weakly saccharolytic organisms such as fusobacteria and anaerobic cocci. Results of published evaluations of API 20A are presented in Table 4:23.[6,66,83]

b) Minitek (BBL):

The Minitek anaerobe differentiation system utilizes paper disks impregnated with various biochemical substrates. Disks are dispensed into wells of specialized plastic plates. Dense inocula are prepared from fresh growth on agar plates. Reactions are read after 48 h anaerobic incubation. Color reactions of carbohydrate fermentation tests are sometimes difficult to read, but interpretation may be facilitated by addition of one extra drop of phenol red indicator to wells exhibiting equivocal reactions. As with API 20A, supplemental tests, including chromatography, are required for less reactive organisms. Published results for the Minitek system are given in Table 4:23.[6,12]

c) Microscan (American Microscan, Inc.):

This multiwell microtiter method has been adapted for anaerobe identification. Frozen trays with 24 wells containing different substrates are inoculated with a dense suspension of growth from plates and incubated anaerobically for 48 h. Results of one published study evaluating this system are presented in Table 4:23.[99] Microscan has recently replaced this 48 h system with a 4 h method.

d) Multiple-well microtube plate system:

Allen and coworkers[3,4] have recently developed a microtube plate system which permits the use of up to 50 differential tests for expanded biochemical characterization of anaerobes. A computerized database has been developed. Biochemical tests show a high degree of correlation with conventional procedures and the method may be combined with microdilution antimicrobial susceptibility tests. This system is suitable for laboratories with resources to prepare and store their own plates.[3,4]

e) Rapid Enzyme Systems:

An innovative new approach to clinical anaerobic bacteriology is the development of commercially available packaged microsystems for detection of preformed enzymes a few hours after inoculation.[97] API ZYM (Analytab) has been available for several years as a research tool. Recent studies have shown that enzyme profiles of clinically isolated and reference anaerobe

Table 4:21. "Short-cuts" for Preliminary Identification of Nonsporeforming Anaerobes

Method	Purpose	Reference
Special-potency antimicrobial susceptibility disks (kanamycin 1 mg; vancomycin 5 μg; colistin 10 μg; rifampin 15 μg; penicillin 2 Unit)	Preliminary differentiation between gram-positive and -negative non-sporeforming rods; differentiation between some *Bacteroides* and fusobacteria	111,112
Red fluorescence under long-wave (366 nm) ultraviolet light	Preliminary identification of *Veillonella*	22
Fermentation of glucose-1-phosphate	Screening for fermentative *Bacteroides* species	135
Susceptibility to phosphomycin (200–500 μg/ml)	Differentiation between *Bacteroides* (sensitive) and fusobacteria (resistant)	95
Polyanetholsulfonate disk test	Preliminary identification of *Pr.anaerobius* (resistant)	134
Bile and kanamycin disks	Preliminary identification of *B.fragilis* group	121
Disk test for nitrate reduction	Useful for all groups	133
Slide catalase with 15% H_2O_2 and added Tween 80	More sensitive for detection of catalase-positive organisms	51
Addition of 3% KOH to culture	Differentiation between gram-positive (no stringing) and gram-negative (stringing) organisms in cases when Gram stain yields equivocal results	50
Spot esculin test	Useful for all groups	91
Fluorescence with long-wave ultraviolet light	Preliminary differentiation between pigmented *Bacteroides*: *B.intermedius:* brilliant red; *B.melaninogenicus:* red-orange; *B.asaccharolyticus:* yellow or red; *B.gingivalis:* negative	107
Spot indole test with *p*-dimethylaminocinnamaldehyde (DMCA)	Useful for all groups	73
Rapid glutamic acid decarboxylase test	Preliminary identification of *B.fragilis, B.thetaiotaomicron, B.uniformis* (all positive), *B.distasonis, B.vulgatus* (some positive)	61
Lack of constitutive β-glucosidase (esculinase)	Typical of fusobacteria. *Bacteroides* possess the enzyme.	32
DNA probes	Identification of *Bacteroides* and fusobacteria	69

Table 4:22. Media and Characteristics of Cultures That Can be Determined Using the Differential Agar Media (Presumpto) System for Identifying Anaerobes*

Media	Characteristics
Blood agar	Relation to O_2,‡ colonial characteristics, hemolysis, pigment, fluorescence with ultraviolet light (Wood's lamp), pitting of agar, cellular morphology, Gram stain reaction, spores, motility (wet mount); inhibition by penicillin, rifampin, or kanamycin.
Enriched thioglycolate medium	Growth, rapidity of growth, gas production, odor, cellular morphology
Presumpto 1 plate	
LD† agar	Indole, growth on LD medium, catalase§
LD esculin agar	Esculin hydrolysis, H_2S, catalase
LD egg yolk agar	Lipase, lecithinase, proteolysis
LD bile agar	Growth in presence of 20% bile (2% oxgall), insoluble precipitate under and immediately surrounding growth
Presumpto 2 plate	
LD glucose agar	Glucose fermentation; stimulation of growth by fermentable carbohydrate
LD starch agar	Starch hydrolysis
LD milk agar	Casein hydrolysis
Ld DNA agar	Detection of deoxyribonuclease activity
Presumpto 3 plate	
LD mannitol agar	Mannitol fermentation
LD lactose agar	Lactose fermentation
LD rhamnose agar	Rhamnose fermentation
LD gelatin	Gelatin hydrolysis

* Modified from Koneman *et al.*[68]
† Lombard-Dowell agar.
‡ By comparing growth on anaerobe plate with blood agar (or chocolate agar) incubated in a 5% to 10% CO_2 incubator (or candle jar) or in room air.
§ The catalase test can be performed by adding 3% hydrogen peroxide to the growth on LD agar, but reactions after addition of H_2O_2 to catalase-positive cultures are more vigorous on LD esculin agar.

Table 4:23. Identification of Anaerobes with Commercial Methods*

Commercial method	Identification			
	Correct to species without extra tests	Correct to species with extra tests	Incorrect/no identification	
API 20A	57–71†	81–95	5–19	6,66,83
Minitek	70‡	86–90	6–10	6,12
Microscan	78	89	11	99
AnIdent	74–78	88–93	7–12	15,83,97
RapID ANA	76–86	92–95	3–8	5,15,83

* Data include clostridia.
† Range of published results, in percentage.
‡ When one percentage is given, only one published study was available for data analysis.

strains are well circumscribed and distinctive, but the method lacks a computerized database and is as yet not commercially available.[77] The An-Ident (Analytab)[15,83,97] and RapID ANA (Innovative Diagnostic Systems, Inc.)[5,15,83] systems are both commercially available 4-hour systems. Kits are inoculated with heavy suspensions of fresh growth from plates and incubated aerobically for 4 h. Both systems provide accurate identification of clinically encountered anaerobes, including weakly/nonsaccharolytic strains, without GLC. Additional tests required in some cases for accurate identification are simple and within the scope of the smaller microbiology laboratory. Both systems have a more taxonomically complete database than other commonly used commercial methods. Color reactions in both systems are sometimes difficult to interpret. This may account for the variance in results of some published studies.[5,15,83,97] With this proviso, however, both systems provide accurate anaerobe identification and both are suitable for routine use.

EXTENT OF ANAEROBE IDENTIFICATION IN THE CLINICAL LABORATORY

Wounds or abscesses often contain multiple species of aerobic and anaerobic bacteria. There are no clearcut rules as to how many isolates to identify in such cases. The relative proportion of epithelial cells to polymorphonuclear leukocytes and the relative number of different morphotypes in the Gram-stained smear help to determine specimen quality. When numerous morphological forms are seen but no pus cells are present, the physician should be contacted to discuss the clinical situation in an attempt to determine the specimen quality. In such cases, it is probably acceptable to limit the extent of workup and preliminary identification based on Gram stain and colonial morphology. When the direct smear suggests that the specimen is of poor quality, no useful information may be gained from extensive identification. In certain clinical situations, however (bacteremia; endocarditis; meningitis; liver, brain, tubo-ovarian and lung abscesses; serious skin, soft tissue, bone and joint infections; infections which do not respond to antimicrobial therapy), all anaerobes should be identified as fully as possible. Cultures reported preliminarily to group level should be held anaerobically for several days to allow for more complete identification should the need arise.[4]

GAS-LIQUID CHROMATOGRAPHY

GLC analysis for volatile and nonvolatile acids of broth cultures in peptone yeast glucose (PYG) or chopped meat carbohydrate (CMC) forms an integral part of the species identification of nonsporeforming and other anaerobes. The reader is referred to standard manuals for descriptions of the method.[55,111]

Recently, Thomann and Hill have suggested a safer solvent, methyl-*tert*-butyl-ether, for acid extractions.[116] Pankuch and Appelbaum have devised a method for direct extraction of volatile and nonvolatile acids. A block of agar with pure growth is removed, dissolved with acid and extracted by standard procedures with modified amounts of reagent. In 84% of cases, patterns of volatile and nonvolatile acids from agar corresponded with those in PYG and CMC. The majority of discrepancies were seen with organisms producing major lactate peaks (*Actinomyces, S. intermedius*), which produced trace or minor amounts on agar but major peaks in broth. With this caveat, direct GLC in conjunction with additional simple tests, such as Gram stain, colonial morphology, spot indole and catalase testing, may result in rapid preliminary genus and possibly species identification of most anaerobes.[85]

Direct extraction of acids from clinical specimens is feasible also and has been shown to be accurate in the rapid preliminary identification of organism groups. This procedure may be applied to purulent/serous specimens,[47,84,87,109,115,124,125,136] blood,[33] vaginal[108] and amniotic fluids.[48] The method has also been successfully applied to swabs.[93] Although the presence of volatile fatty acids in specimens is a reliable indicator of the presence of anaerobes, there is incomplete agreement concerning the presence of specific acids and their correlation with specific anaerobes.[47,84,87,109,115,124,125,136] Recently, Spiegel et al demonstrated chromatographic changes in vaginal fluid from patients with nonspecific vaginitis (NSV). Fluids from patients with NSV demonstrated higher succinate: lactate ratios ($\geq$0.4) than fluids from normal patients.[108] Gravett and coworkers have also used direct GLC of amniotic fluid as a method for rapid diagnosis of chorioamnionitis.[48]

IN VITRO ANTIMICROBIAL SUSCEPTIBILITY OF NONSPOREFORMING ANAEROBES

The antimicrobial susceptibility spectrum of nonsporeforming anaerobes has undergone changes in recent years. Several groups other than the *B. fragilis* group have developed resistance to penicillin. Resistance to clindamycin has gradually appeared, and it can no longer be assumed that anaerobes have a constant susceptibility pattern, as suggested a decade ago. The situation is further complicated by the recent proliferation of new broad-spectrum antimicrobial agents, many of which possess differing degrees of anti-anaerobic activity. Table 4:24 summarizes recent published information on the in vitro susceptibility of nonsporeforming anaerobes to a range of antimicrobial agents.[29,30,43-45,53,63,89,90,104,113,114,127-129] The choice of a specific anti-anaerobic agent will depend on the specific needs of the patient and the hospital setting.

Table 4:24. Antimicrobial Resistance Pattern of Non-sporeforming Anaerobes*

	B.fragilis group		*B.fragilis*		*B.thetaiotaomicron*		*B.ovatus*	
	MIC_{50}	MIC_{90}	MIC_{50}	MIC_{90}	MIC_{50}	MIC_{90}	MIC_{50}	MIC_{90}
Penicillin			32	32	32	64	8	32
Ampicillin	64	>256						
Amoxycillin	32	64–256	16	16–128				
Cefotetan			8	32				
Cefmetazole			16	64				
Cefoxitin	8–32	32–64	8–16	16–64	16–64	32–128	2–32	32–64
Moxalactam	2–16	32–128	0.5–8	4–32	32	≥64	1–32	128
Cefotaxime	8–16	128	8–32	16–256	16–32	32–>64	8	64
Cefoperazone	16–32	64–128	16–64	32–256	64	64	8	64
Ceftizoxime			32	128				
Cefmenoxime			32	64				
Ceftazidime			16	>128	>128	>128		
Ceftriaxone			64	512				
Cefpiramide	64	>256	64	>256	64	>256	32	128
Cefpirome			16	>128	64	>128		
Cefbuperazone	8–64	128–>256	4–16	8–32	64–128	>256	64–256	>256
Sch 34343	0.125	0.5	0.06	0.125				
Ticarcillin			32	512				
Piperacillin	8–32	64–128	4–16	32–128	16–256	32–>256	16	32
Mezlocillin	16	>128						
Azlocillin								
Apalcillin	64	>256	32	>256	64	>256	32	64
Amoxycillin-clavulanate	1	4	0.5	2				
Ampicillin-sulbactam	2	8						
Tetracycline	16	32						
Clindamycin	0.25–2	4–>256	0.5–1	2–4	2–4	4	0.5–1	2
Chloramphenicol	4–8	8–16	4	4	8	8	4	8
Metronidazole	0.5–2	1–4	0.5	1	0.5	1	0.5	1
Imipenem	≤0.06–0.5	0.25–1	≤0.062–0.5	0.125–1	0.25	0.5	0.125	0.5
Cinoxacin	512	>512	512	512				
Enoxacin	32	64	16	32				
Norfloxacin	128	256	16	32				
Ciprofloxacin	8	32	2–4	4–8				

Table 4:24. Antimicrobial Resistance Pattern of Non-sporeforming Anaerobes* (*Continued*)

	B.thetaiotaomicron/ B.ovatus		*B.vulgatus*		*B.distasonis*		*B.bivius*	
	MIC_{50}	MIC_{90}	MIC_{50}	MIC_{90}	MIC_{50}	MIC_{90}	MIC_{50}	MIC_{90}
Penicillin							16	64
Ampicillin								
Amoxycillin								
Cefotetan								
Cefmetazole								
Cefoxitin	16	32	4–16	16–32	8–32	32–64	2–4	4–8
Moxalactam	8	128	1–4	4–128	32–64	128–256	4–8	16–32
Cefotaxime	32	128	2–4	32–64	2–16	64–128	1–4	8–16
Cefoperazone	32	64	16	64	16	128	4	8
Ceftizoxime								
Cefmenoxime								
Ceftazidime			32	>128	32	>128		
Ceftriaxone								
Cefpiramide			32	256	128	>256		
Cefpirome			16	>128	32	128		
Cefbuperazone	32	256	4–32	16–128	128–>256	2–>256	8	16
Sch 34343								
Ticarcillin								
Piperacillin	8	64	4–16	128–256	8–16	32–>256	4–8	16–32
Mezlocillin								
Azlocillin								
Apalcillin			16	>256	64	>256		
Amoxycillin-clavulanate								
Ampicillin-sulbactam								
Tetracycline								
Clindamycin			1	>256	4	8	≤0.015–0.06	≤0.06
Chloramphenicol							2	2
Metronidazole							1	2
Imipenem							≤0.015	0.062
Cinoxacin								
Enoxacin								
Norfloxacin								
Ciprofloxacin								

	Black-pigmented Bacteroides		*B.melaninogenicus*		*B.intermedius*		*B.asaccharolyticus*	
	MIC_{50}	MIC_{90}	MIC_{50}	MIC_{90}	MIC_{50}	MIC_{90}	MIC_{50}	MIC_{90}
Penicillin			4	32			0.25	8
Ampicillin	0.25–0.5	16						
Amoxycillin	0.5	16						
Cefotetan								
Cefmetazole								
Cefoxitin	0.5	4–8	0.5–8	4–16	2	8	0.125	0.25
Moxalactam	0.25–4	8–16	0.25–16	8–32			≤0.062	1
Cefotaxime	0.25	2	0.25	8	0.5	4	≤0.062	0.5
Cefoperazone	2	8	2	4			≤0.062	0.5
Ceftizoxime								
Cefmenoxime								
Ceftazidime					2	16		
Ceftriaxone								
Cefpiramide								
Cefpirome					4	32		
Cefbuperazone	0.5	8	8	16				
Sch 34343								
Tircarcillin								
Piperacillin	0.25–1	8–16	16	32	≤2.0	16		
Mezlocillin								
Azlocillin								
Apalcillin								
Amoxycillin-clavulanate	0.25	0.5						
Ampicillin-sulbactam	0.25	1						
Tetracycline								
Clindamycin	≤0.06–0.062	<0.06–0.125	<0.015	0.031			≤0.015	≤0.015
Chloramphenicol	4	8	4	4			1	4
Metronidazole	1	2	2	4			0.125	1
Imipenem	≤0.06	≤0.06	0.031	0.062			≤0.015	≤0.015
Cinoxacin								
Enoxacin								
Norfloxacin								
Ciprofloxacin								

Table 4:24. Antimicrobial Resistance Pattern of Non-sporeforming Anaerobes* (*Continued*)

	Bacteroides spp. (non-pigmented, non-*B.fragilis* group)		Fusobacteria		*F.nucleatum*		Anaerobic cocci	
	MIC_{50}	MIC_{90}	MIC_{50}	MIC_{90}	MIC_{50}	MIC_{90}	MIC_{50}	MIC_{90}
Penicillin			0.125	1				
Ampicillin			2	16			0.25	0.5
Amoxycillin	4	32	0.12–0.5	1–16			0.12–0.25	0.25–1
Cefotetan								
Cefmetazole								
Cefoxitin	2–4	16	0.05–8	2–64	≤0.12	≤0.12	0.25–1	1–4
Moxalactam	0.25–2	8–32	0.25–8	4–64			0.25–2	4–16
Cefotaxime	≤0.5	64	≤0.12–8	0.25–16	0.12	0.5		
Cefoperazone	4	64	0.25–8	4–32				
Ceftizoxime			32	64				
Cefmenoxime			4	16				
Ceftazidime			≤0.12	2	1	2	0.5	4
Ceftriaxone								
Cefpiramide			2	8				
Cefpirome			≤0.12	2	≤0.12	0.5	0.25	2
Cefbuperazone	2–4	8–16	1–16	16–128			1–2	8–32
Sch 34343			0.125	1				
Ticarcillin								
Piperacillin	2–4	16	≤0.06–2	0.5–64	≤2.0	≤2.0	≤0.06–2	0.25–16
Mezlocillin			≤0.125	32			≤0.125	1
Azlocillin								
Apalcillin			.062	8				
Amoxycillin-clavulanate	0.5	1	0.12	4			0.12	0.25
Ampicillin-sulbactam			2	8			0.25	1
Tetracycline								
Clindamycin	≤0.06	4	≤0.06–0.5	0.25–16			<0.06–.25	0.5–2
Chloramphenicol			1–2	1–4			2	8
Metronidazole			0.06–0.5	0.25–1			0.5–1	1–>256
Imipenem	≤0.06	0.25	<0.06–0.125	0.25–1			<0.06	0.25
Cinoxacin			256	>512			128	512
Enoxacin			32	32			8	16
Norfloxacin			8	32			4	8
Ciprofloxacin			2	8–16			0.25–1	2–8

	Ps.anaerobius		*Ps.asaccharolyticus*		*Ps.tetradius*		*Ps.prevotti*		Gram-neg. cocci	
	MIC_{50}	MIC_{90}	MIC_{50}	MIC_{90}	MIC_{50}	MIC_{90}	MIC_{50}	MIC_{90}	MIC_{50}	MIC_{90}
Penicillin	0.125	8	≤0.015	0.25	≤0.015	0.5				
Ampicillin										
Amoxycillin										
Cefotetan										
Cefmetazole										
Cefoxitin	0.25	8	≤0.062–0.12	≤0.12–0.25	0.125	0.5	≤0.12	.25	1	4
Moxalactam	2	64	0.125	0.25	1	4			1	16
Cefotaxime	0.125	4	≤0.125	0.25	0.25	1	0.25	4	1	16
Cefoperazone	1	8	0.125	0.25	≤0.062	2			8	32
Ceftizoxime									8	16
Cefmenoxime									2	16
Ceftazidime			≤0.12	0.5			0.5	4		
Ceftriaxone										
Cefpiramide									4	8
Cefpirome			≤0.12	0.5			0.25	2.0		
Cefbuperazone									4–8	16–32
Sch 34343									0.125	0.5
Ticarcillin										
Piperacillin			≤2.0	≤2.0			≤2	≤2		
Mezlocillin										
Azlocillin										
Apalcillin									32	32
Amoxycillin-clavulanate										
Ampicillin-sulbactam										
Tetracycline										
Clindamycin	0.031	0.25	0.125	0.5	0.25	1			0.25	8
Chloramphenicol	1	1	1	2	2	4				
Metronidazole	0.125	0.25	0.5	1	0.5	1				
Imipenem	0.031	0.5	≤0.015	≤0.015	≤0.015	0.062			0.25	0.5
Cinoxacin										
Enoxacin										
Norfloxacin										
Ciprofloxacin									4	16

Table 4:24. Antimicrobial Resistance Pattern of Non-sporeforming Anaerobes* (*Continued*)

	Lactobacilli		Eubacteria		*Actinomyces*		Miscellaneous Non-sporeforming Gram-positive rods	
	MIC_{50}	MIC_{90}	MIC_{50}	MIC_{90}	MIC_{50}	MIC_{90}	MIC_{50}	MIC_{90}
Penicillin								
Ampicillin							0.5	2
Amoxycillin							0.12	0.5
Cefotetan								
Cefmetazole								
Cefoxitin	2–128	128–>256	4–32	8–64	4	8	0.25–4	2–16
Moxalactam	16	256	32	128–256			0.25–4	1–256
Cefotaxime	0.5		4–32	8–128			≤0.12	
Cefoperazone			16	128				
Ceftizoxime			32	128				
Cefmenoxime			16	128				
Ceftazidime	2		32	128			2	
Ceftriaxone								
Cefpiramide			128	128			0.5	0.5
Cefpirome	0.5		2	4			0.25	
Cefbuperazone	64–128	128–>256	4–32	64–128			1–4	2–64
Sch 34343	4	8	0.125	1			0.06	0.06
Ticarcillin								
Piperacillin	1–2	2	1–2	4–16			0.5–2	2–32
Mezlocillin							0.5	16
Azlocillin								
Apalcillin			16	32			1	2
Amoxycillin-clavulanate							≤0.06	0.25
Ampicillin-sulbactam							0.25	2
Tetracycline								
Clindamycin	1	4	1	8	0.25	1	≤0.06–0.25	0.25–128
Chloramphenicol							4	8
Metronidazole							4	≥128
Imipenem	4	4	0.125	1			0.06	0.125
Cinoxacin							256	>512
Enoxacin							16	32
Norfloxacin							4	64
Ciprofloxacin			8	16	2	8	1–2	8–16

* Compiled from references 29, 30, 43–45, 53, 63, 89, 90, 104, 113, 114, 127–129. Only work published between 1984 and 1986 is cited. Where ranges are given, data from >1 study are presented together.

REFERENCES

1. Alexander JC, Wolfe WG. Lung abscess and empyema of the thorax. Surg Clin N Am 1980;60:835-49.
2. Allen SD. Gram-positive, nonsporeforming anaerobic bacilli. In: Lennette EH, Balows A, Hausler WJ Jr, Shadomy HJ, eds. Manual of clinical microbiology. 4th ed. Washington, DC: American Society for Microbiology, 1985:461-72.
3. Allen SD, Siders JA, Johnson KS, Gerlach EH. Simultaneous biochemical characterization and antimicrobial susceptibility testing of anaerobic bacteria in microdilution trays. In: Tilton RC, ed. Proceedings of the third international symposium on rapid methods and automation in microbiology. Washington, DC: American Society for Microbiology, 1982:266-70.
4. Allen SD, Siders JA, Marler LM. Isolation and examination of anaerobic bacteria. In: Lennette EH, Balows A, Hausler WJ Jr, Shadomy HJ, eds. Manual of clinical microbiology. 4th ed. Washington, DC: American Society for Microbiology, 1985:413-33.
5. Appelbaum PC, Kaufmann CS, Depenbusch JW. Accuracy and reproducibility of a four-hour method for anaerobe identification. J Clin Microbiol 1985;21:894-8.
6. Appelbaum PC, Kaufmann CS, Keifer JC, Venbrux HJ. Comparison of three methods for anaerobe identification. J Clin Microbiol 1983;18:614-21.
7. Aranki A, Syed SA, Kenney EB, Freter R. Isolation of anaerobic bacteria from human gingiva and mouse cecum by means of a simplified glove box procedure. Appl Microbiol 1969;17:568-76.
8. Babcock JB. Tyrosine degradation in presumptive identification of *Peptostreptococcus anaerobius*. J Clin Microbiol 1979;9:358-61.
9. Bartlett JG, Gorbach SL. Anaerobic bacteria in suppurative infections of the male genitourinary tract. J Urol 1981;125:376-8.
10. Beck HJ, Salassa JR, McCaffrey TV, Hermans PE. Life- threatening soft-tissue infections of the neck. Laryngoscope 1984;94:354-61.
11. Beeler BA, Crowder JG, Smith JW, White A. *Propionibacterium acnes*: pathogen in central nervous system shunt infection. Report of three cases including immune complex glomerulonephritis. Am J Med 1976;61:935-8.
12. Bergan T, Vangdal M, Salveson A. Evaluation of Minitec and API as rapid diagnostic methods for anaerobic bacteria. Scand J Gastroenterol 1984;19(Suppl):103-11.
13. Bourgault A-M, England DM, Rosenblatt JE, Forgacs P, Bieger RC. Clinical characteristics of anaerobic bactibilia. Arch Intern Med 1979;139:1346-9.
14. Brenner DE, Lookingbill DP. Anaerobic microorganisms in chronic suppurative hidradenitis. Lancet 1980;2:921-2.
15. Burlage RS, Ellner PD. Comparison of the PRAS II, AN-Ident, and RapID-ANA systems for identification of anaerobic bacteria. J Clin Microbiol 1985;22:32-5.
16. Burney RE, Gudjonsson B, Cahow E, Spiro HM. Late appearance of intra-abdominal abscesses after total colectomy for inflammatory bowel disease. Arch Surg 1979;114:195–7.
17. Cameron EWJ, Appelbaum PC, Pudifin D, Hutton WS, Chatterton SA, Duursma J. Characteristics and management of chronic destructive pneumonia. Thorax 1980;35:340–6.
18. Cato EP. Transfer of *Peptostreptococcus parvulus* (Weinberg, Nativelle, and Prévot 1937) Smith 1957 to the genus *Streptococcus: Streptococcus parvulus* (Weinberg, Nativelle and Prévot 1937) comb. nov., nom. rev., emend. Int J Syst Bacteriol 1983;33:82-4.
19. Cato EP, Kelley RW, Moore WEC, Holdeman LV. *Bacteroides zoogleoformans* (Weinberg, Nativelle and Prévot 1937) corrig., comb. nov.: Emended description. Int J Syst Bacteriol 1982;32:271-4.
20. Cato EP, Moore LVH, Moore WEC. *Fusobacterium alocis* sp. nov. and *Fusobacterium sulci* sp. nov. from the human gingival sulcus. Int J Syst Bacteriol 1985;35:475-7.
21. Cato EP, Moore WEC, Nygaard G, Holdeman LV. *Actinomyces meyeri* sp. nov., specific epithet rev. Int J Syst Bacteriol 1984;34:487-9.

22. Chow AW, Patten V, Guze LB. Rapid screening of *Veillonella* by ultraviolet fluorescence. J Clin Microbiol 1975;2:546-8.
23. Collins MD, Jones D. Reclassification of *Corynebacterium pyogenes* (Glage) in the genus *Actinomyces*, as *Actinomyces pyogenes* comb. nov. J Gen Microbiol 1982;128:901-3.
24. Cooper SW, Pfeiffer DG, Tally FP. Evaluation of xylan fermentation for the identification of *Bacteroides ovatus* and *Bacteroides thetaiotaomicron*. J Clin Microbiol 1985;22:125-6.
25. Cooper SW, Szymczak EG, Jacobus NV, Tally FP. Differentiation of *Bacteroides ovatus* and *Bacteroides thetaiotaomicron* by means of bacteriophage. J Clin Microbiol 1984;20:1122–5.
26. Coykendall AL, Kaczmarek FS, Slots J. Genetic heterogeneity in *Bacteroides asaccharolyticus* (Holdeman and Moore 1970) Finegold and Barnes 1977 (approved lists, 1980) and proposal of *Bacteroides gingivalis* sp. nov. and *Bacteroides macacae* (Slots and Genco) comb. nov. Int J Syst Bacteriol 1980;30:559-64.
27. Cree GE, Willis AT, Phillips KD, Brazier JS. Anaerobic balanoposthitis. Br Med J 1982;284:859-60.
28. Cummins CS, Johnson JL. Genus I. *Propionibacterium* Orla-Jensen 1909, 337[AL]. In: Sneath PHA, Holt JG, eds. Bergey's manual of systematic bacteriology; vol 2. Baltimore: Williams and Wilkins, 1986:1346-53.
29. Del Bene VE, Carek PJ, Twitty JA, Burkey LJ. In vitro activity of cefbuperazone compared with that of other new β-lactam agents against anaerobic gram-negative bacilli and contribution of β-lactamase to resistance. Antimicrob Agents Chemother 1985;27:817–20.
30. Dias MBS, Jacobus NV, Gorbach SL, Tally FP. In vitro activity of cefbuperazone against *Bacteroides* spp. Antimicrob Agents Chemother 1985;27:968-70.
31. Dowell VR Jr, Hawkins TM. Laboratory methods in anaerobic bacteriology. CDC laboratory manual. Atlanta: Centers for Disease Control, 1977; Department of Health, Education and Welfare publication no. (CDC) 78-8272.
32. Edberg SC, Bell SR. Lack of constitutive β-glucosidase (esculinase) in the genus *Fusobacterium*. J Clin Microbiol 1985;22:435-7.
33. Edson RS, Rosenblatt JE, Washington JA II, Stewart JB. Gas-liquid chromatography of positive blood cultures for rapid presumptive diagnosis of anaerobic bacteremia. J Clin Microbiol 1982;15:1059-61.
34. Ezaki T, Yamamoto N, Ninomiya K, Suzuki S, Yabuuchi E. Transfer of *Peptococcus indolicus, Peptococcus asaccharolyticus, Peptococcus prevotii* and *Peptococcus magnus* to the genus *Peptostreptococcus* and proposal of *Peptostreptococcus tetradius* sp. nov. Int J Syst Bacteriol 1983;33:683-98.
35. Facklam RR, Carey RB. Streptococci and aerococci. In: Lennette EH, Balows A, Hausler WJ Jr, Shadomy HJ, eds. Manual of clinical microbiology. 4th ed. Washington, DC: American Society for Microbiology, 1985:154-75.
36. Finegold SM. Anaerobic bacteria in human disease. New York: Academic Press, 1977.
37. Finegold SM. Anaerobes in biliary tract infection. Arch Intern Med 1979;139:1338.
38. Finegold SM. Use of direct examination and selective media for rapid identification of clinically important anaerobes. In: Tilton RC, ed. Proceedings of the third international symposium on rapid methods and automation in microbiology. Washington, DC: American Society for Microbiology, 1982:254-7.
39. Finegold SM, Edelstein MAC. Gram-negative, nonsporeforming anaerobic bacilli. In: Lennette EH, Balows A, Hausler WJ Jr, Shadomy HJ, eds. Manual of clinical microbiology. 4th ed. Washington, DC: American Society for Microbiology, 1985:450-60.
40. Fischer EG, McLennan JE, Suzuki Y. Cerebral abscess in children. Am J Dis Child 1981;135:746-9.
41. Flanigan RC, Kursh ED, McDougal WS, Persky L. Synergistic gangrene of the scrotum and penis secondary to colorectal disease. J Urol 1978;119:369-71.
42. Garvey G. Current concepts of bacterial infections of the central nervous system. Bacterial meningitis and bacterial brain abscess. J Neurosurg 1983;59:735-44.

43. Goldstein EJC, Citron DM. Comparative in vitro activity of cefbuperazone against anaerobic bacteria isolated from community hospitals. Antimicrob Agents Chemother 1985;27:162-6.
44. Goldstein EJC, Citron DM. Comparative activity of the quinolones against anaerobic bacteria isolated at community hospitals. Antimicrob Agents Chemother 1985;27:657-9.
45. Goldstein EJC, Citron DM. Comparative in vitro activities of amoxycillin-clavulanic acid and imipenem against anaerobic bacteria isolated from community hospitals. Antimicrob Agents Chemother 1986;29:158-60.
46. Gorbach SL, Bartlett JG. Anaerobic infections. N Engl J Med 1974;290:1177-84;1237-45;1289-94.
47. Gorbach SL, Mayhew JW, Bartlett JG, Thadepalli H, Onderdonk AB. Rapid diagnosis of anaerobic infections by direct gas-liquid chromatography of clinical specimens. J Clin Invest 1976;57:478-84.
48. Gravett MG, Eschenbach DA, Speigel-Brown CA, Holmes KK. Rapid diagnosis of amniotic-fluid infection by gas-liquid chromatography. N Engl J Med 1982;306:725-8.
49. Groeneveld ABJ, Nommensen FE, Mullink H, Ooms ECM, Bode WA. Shunt nephritis associated with *Propionibacterium acnes* with demonstration of the antigen in the glomeruli. Nephron 1982;32:365-9.
50. Halebian S, Harris B, Finegold SM, Rolfe RD. Rapid method that aids in distinguishing gram-positive from gram-negative anaerobic bacteria. J Clin Microbiol 1981;13:444-8.
51. Hansen SL, Stewart BJ. Slide catalase. A reliable test for differentiation amd presumptive identification of certain clinically significant anaerobes. Am J Clin Pathol 1978;69:36-40.
52. Harris LF, Jackson RT, Breslin JA Jr, Alford RH. Anaerobic septicemia after transrectal prostatic biopsy. Arch Intern Med 1978;138:393-5.
53. Hill GB, Ayers OM. Antimicrobial susceptibilities of anaerobic bacteria isolated from female genital tract infections. Antimicrob Agents Chemother 1985;27:324-31.
54. Holdeman LV, Cato EP, Burmeister JA, Moore WEC. Descriptions of *Eubacterium timidum* sp. nov., *Eubacterium brachy* sp. nov., and *Eubacterium nodatum* sp. nov. isolated from human periodontitis. Int J Syst Bacteriol 1980;30:163-9.
55. Holdeman LV, Cato EP, Moore WEC, eds. Anaerobic laboratory manual. 4th ed. Blacksburg, VA: Virginia Polytechnic Institute and State University Anaerobe Laboratory, 1977.
56. Holdeman LV, Johnson JL. Description of *Bacteroides loescheii* sp. nov. and emendation of the descriptions of *Bacteroides melaninogenicus* (Oliver and Wherry) Roy and Kelly 1939 and *Bacteroides denticola* Shah and Collins 1982. Int J Syst Bacteriol 1982;32:399-409.
57. Holdeman Moore LV, Johnson JL, Moore WEC. Genus *Peptostreptococcus* Kluyver and van Niel 1936, 401[AL]. In: Sneath PHA, Holt JG, eds. Bergey's manual of systematic bacteriology; vol 2. Baltimore: Williams and Wilkins, 1986:1083-92.
58. Holdeman LV, Kelley RW, Moore WEC. Anaerobic Gram-negative straight, curved and helical rods. Family I. *Bacteroidaceae* Pribram 1933, 10[AL]. In: Krieg NR, Holt JG, eds. Bergey's manual of systematic bacteriology; vol 1. Baltimore: Williams and Wilkins, 1984:602-62.
59. Holdeman LV, Moore WEC, Churn PJ, Johnson JL. *Bacteroides oris* and *Bacteroides buccae*, new species from human periodontitis and other human infections. Int J Syst Bacteriol 1982;32:125-31.
60. Hunt DE, Jones JV, Dowell VR Jr. Selective medium for the isolation of *Bacteriodes gingivalis*. J Clin Microbiol 1986;23:441-5.
61. Jilly BJ, Schreckenberger PC, LeBeau LJ. Rapid glutamic acid decarboxylase test for identification of *Bacteroides* and *Clostridium* spp. J Clin Microbiol 1984;19:592-3.
62. Johnson CC, Reinhardt JF, Edelstein MAC, Mulligan ME, George WL, Finegold SM. *Bacteroides gracilis*, an important anaerobic bacterial pathogen. J Clin Microbiol 1985;22:799-802.

63. Jones RN, Gerlach EH. Antimicrobial activity of HR 810 against 419 strict anaerobic bacteria. Antimicrob Agents Chemother 1985;27:413-15.
64. Jones RB, Hirschmann JV, Brown GS, Tremann JA. Fournier's syndrome: necrotizing subcutaneous infection of the male genitalia. J Urol 1979;122:279-82.
65. Kandler O, Weiss N. Genus *Lactobacillus* Beijerinck 1901, 212[AL]. In: Sneath PHA, Holt JG, eds. Bergey's manual of systematic bacteriology; vol 2. Baltimore: Williams and Wilkins, 1986:1209-34.
66. Karachewski NO, Busch EL, Wells CL. Comparison of PRAS II, RapID ANA, and API 20A systems for identification of anaerobic bacteria. J Clin Microbiol 1985;21:122-6.
67. Kilpper-Bälz R, Schleifer KH. Transfer of *Peptococcus saccharolyticus* Foubert and Douglas to the genus *Staphylococcus: Staphylococcus saccharolyticus* (Foubert and Douglas) comb. nov. Zentral Bakteriol Mikrobiol Hyg I Abt Orig C 1981;2:324-31.
68. Koneman EW, Allen SD, Dowell VR Jr, Sommers HM. Color atlas and textbook of diagnostic microbiology. 2nd ed. Philadelphia: J.B. Lippincott, 1983:347-423.
69. Kuritza AP, Getty CE, Shaughnessy P, Hesse R, Salyers AA. DNA probes for identification of clinically important *Bacteroides* species. J Clin Microbiol 1986;23:343-9.
70. Leach RD, Eykyn SJ, Phillips I, Corrin B. Anaerobic subareolar breast abscess. Lancet 1979;1:35-7.
71. Leach RD, Eykyn SJ, Phillips I, Corrin B, Taylor EA. Anaerobic axilllary abscess. Br Med J 1979;2:5-7.
72. Loesche WJ. Oxygen sensitivity of various anaerobic bacteria. Appl Microbiol 1969;18: 723-7.
73. Lombard GL, Dowell VR Jr. Comparison of three reagents for detecting indole production by anaerobic bacteria in microtest systems. J Clin Microbiol 1983;18:609-13.
74. Lombard GL, Whaley DN, Dowell VR Jr. Comparison of media in the Anaerobe-Tek and Presumpto plate systems and evaluation of the Anaerobe-Tek system for identification of commonly encountered anaerobes. J Clin Microbiol 1982;16:1066-72.
75. Lorenz RP, Appelbaum PC, Ward RM, Botti JJ. Chorioamnionitis and possible neonatal infection associated with *Lactobacillus* species. J Clin Microbiol 1982;16:558-61.
76. Lyznicki JM, Busch EL, Blazevic DL. Medium for selective isolation and presumptive identification of the *Bacteroides fragilis* group. J Clin Microbiol 1982;15:123-9.
77. Marler L, Allen S, Siders J. Rapid enzymatic characterization of clinically encountered anaerobic bacteria with the API ZYM system. Eur J Clin Microbiol 1984;3:294-300.
78. Martin WJ. Practical method for isolation of anaerobic bacteria in the clinical laboratory. Appl Microbiol 1971;22:1168-71.
79. McDonald MI, Corey GR, Gallis HA, Durack DT. Single and multiple pyogenic liver abscesses. Natural history, diagnosis and treatment, with emphasis on percutaneous drainage. Medicine 1984;63:291-302.
80. Meislin HW, Lerner SA, Graves MH, et al. Cutaneous abscesses. Anaerobic and aerobic bacteriology and outpatient management. Ann Intern Med 1977;87:145-9.
81. Moore WEC, Holdeman Moore LV. Genus *Eubacterium* Prévot 1938, 294[AL]. In: Sneath PHA, Holt JG, eds. Bergey's manual of systematic bacteriology; vol. 2. Baltimore: Williams and Wilkins, 1986:1353-73.
82. Murray PR. Growth of clinical isolates of anaerobic bacteria on agar media: effects of media composition, storage conditions and reduction under anaerobic conditions. J Clin Microbiol 1978;8:708-14.
83. Murray PR, Weber CJ, Niles AC. Comparative evaluation of three identification systems for anaerobes. J Clin Microbiol 1985;22:52-5.
84. Nord C-E. Diagnosis of anaerobic infections by gas-liquid chromatography. Acta Pathol Microbiol Scand B 1977;259(Suppl):55-9.
85. Pankuch GA, Appelbaum PC. Agar medium for gas-liquid chromatography of anaerobes. Am J Clin Pathol 1986;85:82-6.

86. Pankuch GA, Appelbaum PC, Lorenz RP, Botti JJ, Schachter J, Naeye RL. Placental microbiology and histology and the pathogenesis of chorioamnionitis. Obstet Gynecol 1984;64:802-6.
87. Phillips KD, Tearle PV, Willis AT. Rapid diagnosis of anaerobic infections by gas-liquid chromatography of clinical material. J Clin Pathol 1976;29:428-32.
88. Platt LD, Yonekura ML, Ledger WJ. The role of anaerobic bacteria in postpartum endomyometritis. Am J Obstet Gynecol 1979;135:814-7.
89. Prabhala RH, Rao B, Marshall R, Bansal MB, Thadepalli H. In vitro susceptibility of anaerobic bacteria to ciprofloxacin (Bay o 9867). Antimicrob Agents Chemother 1984;26:785–6.
90. Prabhala RH, Thadepalli H, Rao B, Bansal MB, Marshall R. In vitro activity of cefbuperazone, a new cephamycin, against anaerobic bacteria. Antimicrob Agents Chemother 1985;27:640-2.
91. Qadri SMH, Johnson S, Smith JC, Zubairi S, Gillum RL. Comparison of spot esculin hydrolysis with the PathoTec strip test for rapid differentiation of anaerobic bacteria. J Clin Microbiol 1981;13:459-62.
92. Raff MJ, Melo JC. Anaerobic osteomyelitis. Medicine 1978;57:83-103.
93. Reed PJ, Sanderson PJ. Detection of anaerobic wound infection by analysis of pus swabs for volatile fatty acids by gas-liquid chromatography. J Clin Pathol 1979;32:1203-5.
94. Ribot S, Gal K, Goldblat MV, Eslami HH. The role of anaerobic bacteria in the pathogenesis of urinary tract infections. J Urol 1981;126:852-3.
95. Rodriguez JAG, Prieto JP, Sanchez JEG, Gonzalez MCS, Luengo FM. Susceptibility to phosphomycin as a differential character for gram negative anaerobic bacilli. J Appl Bacteriol 1976;41:251-4.
96. Rosenblatt JE. Reevaulation of current methods for incubation of anaerobes. In: Tilton RC, ed. Proceedings of the third international symposium on rapid methods and automation in microbiology. Washington, DC: American Society for Microbiology, 1982:271-4.
97. Rosenblatt JE. Anaerobic identification systems. Clin Lab Med 1985;5:59-65.
98. Rosenblatt JE. Anaerobic cocci. In: Lennette EH, Balows A, Hausler WJ Jr, Shadomy HJ, eds. Manual of clinical microbiology. 4th ed. Washington, DC: American Society for Microbiology, 1985:445-9.
99. Savuto PS, Ellner PD. Evaluation of a microtiter system for identification of anaerobic bacteria. J Clin Microbiol 1984;20:81-3.
100. Scardovi V. Genus *Bifidobacterium* Orla-Jensen 1924, 472^{AL}. In: Sneath PHA, Holt JG, eds. Bergey's manual of systematic bacteriology; vol. 2. Baltimore: Williams and Wilkins, 1986:1418-34.
101. Schaal KP. Genus *Arachnia* Pine and Georg 1969, 269^{AL}. In: Sneath PHA, Holt JG, eds. Bergey's manual of systematic bacteriology; vol. 2. Baltimore: Williams and Wilkins, 1986:1332-42.
102. Schaal KP. Genus *Actinomyces* Harz 1877, 133^{AL}. In: Sneath PHA, Holt JG, eds. Bergey's manual of systematic bacteriology; vol. 2. Baltimore; Williams and Wilkins, 1986:1383-1418.
103. Schlesinger JJ, Ross AL. *Propionibacterium acnes* meningitis in a previously normal adult. Arch Intern Med 1977;137:921-3.
104. Shafran SD, Wong J, Chow AW. In vitro activity of Sch 34343 and cefbuperazone against anaerobic bacteria. Antimicrob Agents Chemother 1985;27:749-52.
105. Shah HN, Collins MD. *Bacteroides buccalis*, sp. nov., *Bacteroides denticola*, sp. nov., and *Bacteroides pentosaceus*, sp. nov., new species of the genus *Bacteroides* from the oral cavity. Zentral Bakteriol Mikrobiol Hyg I Abt Orig C 1981;2:235-41.
106. Slots J, Potts TV, Mashimo PA. *Fusobacterium periodonticum*, A new species from the human oral cavity. J Dent Res 1983;62:960-3.
107. Slots J, Reynolds HS. Long-wave UV light fluorescence for identification of black-pigmented *Bacteroides* spp. J Clin Microbiol 1982;16:1148-51.

108. Spiegel CA, Amsel R, Eschenbach D, Schoenknecht F, Holmes KK. Anaerobic bacteria in nonspecific vaginitis. N Engl J Med 1980;303:601-7.
109. Spiegel CA, Malangoni MA, Condon RE. Gas-liquid chromatography for rapid diagnosis of intra-abdominal infection. Arch Surg 1984;119:28-32.
110. Sugita R, Kawamura S, Ichikawa G, Goto S, Fujimaka Y. Studies on anaerobic bacteria in chronic otitis media. Laryngoscope 1981;91:816-21.
111. Sutter VL, Citron DM, Edelstein MAC, Finegold SM. Wadsworth anaerobic bacteriology manual. 4th ed. Belmont, CA: Star Publishing, 1985.
112. Sutter VL, Finegold SM. Antibiotic disk susceptibility tests for rapid presumptive identification of gram-negative anaerobic bacilli. Appl Microbiol 1971;21:13-20.
113. Sutter VL, Kwok Y-Y, Bulkacz J. Comparative activity of ciprofloxacin against anaerobic bacteria. Antimicrob Agents Chemother 1985;27:427-8.
114. Tally FP, Cuchural GJ Jr, Jacobus NV, et al. Nationwide study of the susceptibility of the *Bacteroides fragilis* group in the United States. Antimicrob Agents Chemother 1985;28:675-7.
115. Thadepalli H, Gangopadhyay PK. Rapid diagnosis of anaerobic empyema by direct gas-liquid chromatography of pleural fluid. Chest 1980;77:507-13.
116. Thomann WR, Hill GB. Modified extraction procedure for gas-liquid chromatography applied to the identification of anaerobic bacteria. J Clin Microbiol 1986;23:392-4.
117. Thomason JL, Schreckenberger PC, Spellacy WN, Riff LJ, LeBeau LJ. Clinical and microbiological characterization of patients with nonspecific vaginosis associated with motile, curved anaerobic rods. J Infect Dis 1984;149:801-9.
118. Traynor RM, Parratt D, Duguid HLD, Duncan ID. Isolation of actinomycetes from cervical specimens. J Clin Pathol 1981;34:914-6.
119. Van Steenbergen TJM, van Winkelhoff AJ, Mayrand D, Grenier D, De Graaff J. *Bacteroides endodontalis* sp. nov., an asaccharolytic black-pigmented *Bacteroides* species from infected dental root canals. Int J Syst Bacteriol 1984;34:118-20.
120. Van Winkelhoff AJ, Van Steenbergen TJM, Kippuw N, De Graaff J. Further characterization of *Bacteroides endodontalis*, an asaccharolytic black-pigmented *Bacteroides* species from the oral S cavity. J Clin Microbiol 1985;22:75-9.
121. Vargo VL, Korzeniowski M, Spaulding EH. Tryptic soy bile-kanamycin test for the identification of *Bacteroides fragilis*. Appl Microbiol 1974;27:480-3.
122. Wang SMS, Wilson SE. Subphrenic abscess. The new epidemiology. Arch Surg 1977;112:934-6.
123. Watabe J, Benno Y, Mitsuoka T. Taxonomic study of *Bacteroides oralis* and related organisms and proposal of *Bacteroides veroralis* sp. nov. Int J Syst Bacteriol 1983;33:57-64.
124. Watt B, Geddes PA, Greenan OA, Napier SK, Mitchell A. Can direct gas-liquid chromatography of clinical samples detect specific organisms? J Clin Pathol 1982;35:706-8.
125. Watt B, Geddes PA, Greenan OA, Napier SK, Mitchell A. Gas-liquid chromatography in the diagnosis of anaerobic infections: a three year experience. J Clin Pathol 1982;35:709-14.
126. Weinstein L. Bacterial hepatitis: a case report on an unrecognized cause of fever of unknown origin. N Engl J Med 1978;299:1052-4.
127. Wexler H, Carter WT, Harris B, Finegold SM. Comparative in vitro activities of cefpiramide and apalcillin against anaerobic bacteria. Antimicrob Agents Chemother 1984;25:162-4.
128. Wexler H, Carter WT, Harris BH, Finegold SM. In vitro activity of cefbuperazone against anaerobic bacteria. Antimicrob Agents Chemother 1985;27:674-6.
129. Wexler HM, Harris B, Carter WT, Finegold SM. In vitro efficacy of sulbactam combined with ampicillin against anaerobic bacteria. Antimicrob Agents Chemother 1985;27:876-8.

130. Whitehead SM, Eykyn SJ, Phillips I. Anaerobic paronychia. Br J Surg 1981;68:420-2.
131. Whitehead SM, Leach RD, Eykyn SJ, Phillips I. The aetiology of perirectal sepsis. Br J Surg 1982;69:166-8.
132. Whitehead SM, Leach RD, Eykyn SJ, Phillips I. The aetiology of scrotal sepsis. Br J Surg 1982;69:729-30.
133. Wideman PA, Citronbaum DM, Sutter VL. Simple disk test for detection of nitrate reduction by anaerobic bacteria. J Clin Microbiol 1977;5:315-9.
134. Wideman PA, Vargo VL, Citronbaum D, Finegold SM. Evaluation of the sodium polyanethol sulfonate disk test for the identification of *Peptostreptococcus anaerobius*. J Clin Microbiol 1976;4:330-3.
135. Wilkins TD, Walker CB. Fermentation of glucose-1-phosphate: a screening test for fermentative *Bacteroides* species. Appl Environ Microbiol 1976;31:320-1.
136. Wüst J. Schnelldiagnose anaerober Infektionen mit der direkten gaschromatographischen Untersuchung von klinischem Material. Schweiz Med Wschr 1980;110:362-9.
137. Yocum RC, McArthur J, Petty BG, Diehl AM, Moench TR. Septic arthritis caused by *Propionibacterium acnes*. J Am Med Assoc 1982;248:1740-1.

CHAPTER 5

ANAEROBIC INFECTIONS: SPOREFORMERS

Thomas A. Russo, M.D. and Sherwood L. Gorbach, M.D.

INTRODUCTION

The genus *Clostridium* comprises the sporeforming anaerobic rods of clinical significance. To date, over 80 species have been defined biochemically and metabolically, while numerous others await future characterization. Clostridia are ubiquitously distributed throughout nature and are residents of body flora of numerous animals, including man. In humans, these organisms normally inhabit the gastrointestinal and female genital tracts and occasionally the skin and oropharynx.

Though these organisms usually reside in peaceful coexistence with their host, when given the proper circumstances their pathogenic potential can be realized. Various clostridia are capable of endogenous and exogenous infection, as well as toxin-related disease. Bacteriologic isolation represents a spectrum from asymptomatic colonization to overwhelming sepsis and, rarely, death.

Clostridium perfringens has the greatest propensity for virulence and is a frequent isolate from clinical specimens, although other clostridia have been associated with the full range of clinical disease as well. The process of bacteriologic culture and identification of nonperfringens clostridial species, like that of many anaerobes, is a time-consuming and expensive task. Since the presence of clostridia may represent only normal flora, it is essential to correlate clinical data with the culture result. Such cooperation between microbiologist and clinician will allow for optimal patient management as well as avoidance of unnecessary work and expense on the part of the clinical laboratory.

HUMAN INFECTIONS

Clostridium perfringens and the Histotoxic Clostridia

The histotoxic clostridia are widely distributed in nature and are present in the gastrointestinal tract of humans and many animals. Their clinical manifestations are diverse. Bacteriologic isolation is not necessarily synonymous with illness, but requires clinical correlation to assess its true significance. Clinical manifestations are listed in Table 5:1.

C. perfringens can produce 11 different toxins. On the basis of major toxins (alpha, beta, epsilon and iota)[23] the various strains have been classified into 5 toxin types; A, B, C, D and E (Table 5:2). Type A and occasionally type C strains are primarily responsible for human disease. Toxin typing is accomplished by injecting culture supernates, with and without specific antitoxin, intraperitoneally into mice and observing them overnight for death.

Table 5:3 lists the clostridial species that have been isolated from human soft tissue infections and Table 5:4 summarizes the antimicrobic susceptibility data for commonly isolated clostridia.

Toxin-producing Clostridia

An outline of the clinical syndromes produced by *C. botulinum, C. tetani* and *C. difficile* is summarized in Table 5:1.

DIAGNOSTIC PROCEDURES

Collection and Transport

Appropriate collection and transport of clinical specimens containing clostridia is vital to maximize their isolation. Some virulent species are rather aerotolerant, whereas others are very sensitive to the lethal effects of oxygen, and improper handling will preclude their isolation. Details relevant to individual clostridial species are discussed below.

Microscopic Examination

Gram stain examination is perhaps the most important step in the processing of a clinical specimen for clostridia. The isolation and identification of some clostridia can take up to 7 days. Microscopic examination of the specimen may be the only information available to the clinician during the initial 24-48 hours.

Clostridia stain gram-positive although some species have a tendency to be gram-variable or gram-negative. Spores are generally not seen in clinical specimens. *C. perfringens* appear as fat, "boxcar," gram-positive rods; other species display a full range of morphology, making distinction from each other and from other gram-positive rods difficult.

Nonetheless, the value of Gram stain examination cannot be understated. It can demonstrate organisms that may not be successfully cultured due to

Table 5:1. Clinical Manifestations of Clostridial Infections

Organism	Disease	Comment
C. perfringens	Food poisoning[6]	Enterotoxin produced after ingestion of inadequately cooked meat and meat products. Caused mostly by toxin type A Infectious dose 10^8.
	Enteritis necroticans[15]	Uncommon in U.S. Consumption of undercooked pork. Caused by type C High morality
Histotoxic clostridia[15,21]	Localized skin/soft tissue infection *C.perfringens* *C.ramosum* *C.septicum* *C.novyi*	Often polymicrobial and generally nonfulminant
	Suppurative visceral infection	
	Diffuse spreading cellulitis/ fasciitis	50% mortality. *C. perfringens, C. ramosum, C. septicum* usual pathogens
	Myonecrosis (gas gangrene)	Usually related to trauma/surgery Fulminant disorder *C. perfringens* causes 80% Surgical debridement lifesaving
	Nontraumatic myonecrosis	Variant of gas gangrene without apparent source Strong association with silent colon cancer *C. perfringens* and occasionally *C. septicum* responsible
	Bacteremia	Clinical sepsis not necessarily present; Clinical correlation required *C. septicum* asociated with malignancy[18]
C. botulinum[7,10,12]	Botulism Food-borne	Now a rare disease in U.S. Ingestion of food containing preformed paralytic neurotoxin Caused by type A, B, E, and rarely F
	Wound	Rare Toxin absorbed from local production Mostly caused by type A and B
	Infant	Most common form in U.S. Intestinal colonization results in in vivo toxin production(?) Caused by type A and B
C. tetani[7,32]	Tetanus Local Generalized Neonatal	Now rare in U.S. but common in developing countries. Disease due to protein toxin called tetanospasmin.
C. difficile	Pseudomembraneous colitis[2,3,25] Antimicrobic-associated diarrhea	Toxin must be demonstrated. Toxin A (enterotoxin) and Toxin B (cytotoxin)

Table 5:2. Toxins of Clostridium Perfringens

	A	B	C	D	E
Toxins:	alpha	alpha beta epsilon	alpha beta	alpha epsilon	alpha iota

Table 5:3. Species of *Clostridium* Isolated from Soft Tissue Infections in Humans*

Species	Number of Isolates
Clostridium perfringens	20
Clostridium ramosum	15
Clostridium bifermentans	5
Clostridium sphenoides	4
Clostridium sporogenes	3
Clostridium innocuum	3
Clostridium difficile	3
Clostridium butyricum	3
Clostridium sordellii	3
Clostridium limosum	2
Clostridium subterminale	2
Clostridium septicum	2
Clostridium novyi	2
Clostridium tertium	1
Clostridium baratii	1
Clostridium cadaveris	1
Clostridium beijerinckii	1
Clostridium fallax	1
Clostridium carnis	1
Clostridium pseudotetanicum	1
Clostridium ghonii	1
Unclassified	12
Total	87

* From Gorbach and Thadepalli.[16]

the presence of antibiotics. Observation of organisms suspicious for clostridia should lead to culture of the specimen on Nagler Egg Yolk Agar for a presumptive diagnosis of *C. perfringens* overnight. In the setting of gas gangrene or rapidly progressive cellulitis and fasciitis, a smear demonstrating the presence of gram-positive rods in the absence of inflammatory cells is highly suggestive of clostridial infection and appropriate management can be initiated immediately.

Isolation

The primary isolation of clostridia from clinical specimens is accomplished with the use of fresh, appropriately supplemented media. A variety of blood

Table 5:4. Compiled Susceptibility of Clostridial Species to Antimicrobial Agents*

	C. perfringens	*C. difficle*	*C. septicum*	*C. botulinum*	*C. ramosum*	*C. bifermentans*
Penicillin (1 μg/ml)	93%† (134)‡	92% (84)	100% (33)	95% (224)	49% (49)	100% (4)
Metronidazole (4 μg/ml)	73% (33)	99% (84)	100% (33)	100% (224)	50% (48)	—
Clindamycin (4 μg/ml)	99% (134)	77% (84)	100% (33)	94% (224)	30% (49)	100% (4)
Cephalothin (16 μg/ml)	100% (58)	49% (84)	100% (33)	98% (224)	—	—
Cefoxitin (16 μg/ml)	100% (65)	15% (84)	100% (23)	99% (224)	—	—
Cefotaxime (16 μg/ml)	—	—	100% (33)	—	—	—
Imipenem (4 μg/ml)	100%§ (11)	0%§ (17)	—	—	—	—
Vancomycin (4 μg/ml)	—	99% (84)	100% (23)	88% (224)	49% (49)	—
Chloramphenicol (16 μg/ml)	99% (134)	93% (89)	100% (23)	100% (224)	100% (49)	100% (4)

* Data from References, 1,4,13,14,26,29,30,31.
† = percent susceptible, ‡ = number of strains, § = personnel communication, N. Jacobus.

agar (BA) plates are effective, commonly supplemented with vitamin K, hemin and yeast extract. Phenylethyl alcohol (PEA) blood agar can be employed to facilitate isolation when swarming colonies overgrow; anaerobic blood plates with 4-6% agar can also be used in this setting.[11] If initial Gram stain or clinical circumstances indicate a possible clostridial infection, a Nagler Egg Yolk Agar plate should be plated initially to aid in more rapid laboratory detection of *C. perfringens*. Inoculation of thioglycolate broth should always be performed to serve as a backup.

Several selective methods can be employed to isolate only clostridia.[28] Treatment of freshly inoculated chopped meat broth for 10 min at 80°C prior to plating eliminates the majority of nonsporeforming organisms. Suspending culture material in 50% ethyl alcohol for 1 h at room temperature is another spore selection method. Media containing sulfite and iron, which blackens clostridial colonies,[24] or the addition of neomycin (100 μg/mL) to BA or Egg Yolk Agar (EYA) can be used as semi-selective plate media. Selection techniques also are available for the isolation of *C. botulinum* or *C. difficile* from stool specimens.

Identification

Clostridium perfringens and other Histotoxic Clostridia:

Rapidly growing *C. perfringens* may be apparent on culture plates after overnight incubation, but the majority of clostridial species appear on BA within 48 hours and an occasional strain may take longer. Establishing an organism's identity in the genus *Clostridium* requires that it be oxygen intolerant, be a gram-positive rod and have spores.

Aerotolerance testing excludes facultative anaerobes that can mimic clostridia; however, some clostridial species (e.g., *C. tertium*) are capable of microaerophilic growth. Potential confusion with *Bacillus* species can be resolved by catalase testing; *Bacillus* species are usually catalase-positive whereas clostridia rarely are.

Certain clostridial species may stain gram-negative (e.g., *C. clostridioforme*) which may create confusion as to their true genus. This can be clarified by testing for vancomycin (5 μg) and colistin (10 μg) susceptibility on a BA plate with taxo discs. A pattern of vancomycin susceptibility and colistin resistance is usually seen with clostridial species.

The presence of spores in a confirmed anaerobe identifies it as a clostridial species. If spores cannot be demonstrated initially, a plate held aerobically at room temperature may precipitate their formation. Ethanol or heat-spore tests can also be used.[28] Because it is often difficult to demonstrate sporulation with *C. perfringens, C. ramosum* and *C. clostridioforme*, spore demonstration is not usually considered mandatory for their identification in clinical laboratories.

C. perfringens can be recognized by its gray spreading colonies that often produce a characteristic double zone of hemolysis on blood agar, depending on the isolate and the culture media. Typical fat, "boxcar," gram-positive rods, a double zone of hemolysis, demonstration of lethicinase production and a positive Nagler test lend support to the identification. The Nagler reaction is demonstrated by smearing one-half of an egg yolk blood plate with type A antitoxin and streaking the clostridia in a straight line across the plate. Nagler test-positive species produce an opulescence only on the half not containing antitoxin. If an isolate produces only a single zone of β-hemolysis, it can be presumptively identified as *C. perfringens* using the above criteria; however, *C. baratii, C. sordellii* and *C. bifermentans* are also Nagler test-positive and can produce β-hemolysis and lethicinase. Further biochemical testing is needed (Table 5:5). Nonhemolytic, nonlethicinase-producing *C. perfringens* occur infrequently. These organisms require more extensive biochemical testing and gas liquid chromatography (GLC) evaluation for final identification.

Though a microbiologist experienced in anaerobic taxonomy can presumptively identify many nonperfringens species by colonial appearance, Gram stain morphology and limited biochemical testing, definitive speciation usually requires more extensive biochemical testing and GLC analysis of acid endproducts.

Several methods are available for biochemical testing. Carbohydrate fermentation media have been most extensively used in characterizing clostridial species (e.g., PRAS II). These tests are growth-dependent and require sufficient substrate metabolism for interpretation. This may take several days with fastidious organisms. Careful observation of individual manufacturer's instructions is necessary for optimal accuracy in evaluating results.

Several growth-dependent miniaturized systems also are available (e.g., API 20A, Minitek) for identification of clostridia. These systems require a heavy inoculum and test interpretation can be difficult with slower growing organisms.

Table 5:5. Characteristics of Nagler Positive-Clostridium Species

	β-Hemolysis				
	double zone	single zone	indole	gelatin	urease
C. perfringens	±*	±	−	+	−
C. barati	−	±	−	−	−
C. sordelli	−	±	+	+	−
C. bifermentans	−	±	+	+	±

* ± = variable reaction.

Recently, rapid micromethods that are nongrowth-dependent have been marketed. Conventional and chromogenic tests are employed to provide results after 4 h of aerobic incubation. Presently, further testing on the reliability of these systems is needed.

GLC is an analytical system which permits identification of volatile and nonvolatile acid endproducts of bacterial metabolism. Each species demonstrates a characteristic pattern of acid production, roughly equivalent to a fingerprint. GLC, used in combination with biochemical testing, is the "gold standard" for clostridial speciation, short of DNA analysis.

Many laboratories have neither the time, money nor equipment to perform this level of clostridial identification. Individual laboratories should examine their goals and decide what level of speciation is appropriate for their needs.

Clostridium perfringens, "Food Poisoning"

Confirmation of this diagnosis requires demonstration of 10^5 organisms per gram of suspected food and 10^6 *C. perfringens* spores per gram of feces obtained within 48 hours of the onset of symptoms. Food or fecal specimens forwarded to reference laboratories should be shipped at 4°C, not frozen. Since both heat-resistant and heat-sensitive strains can produce enterotoxin and cause disease, a heat-spore selection should not be used. An egg yolk-free tryptose-sulfite-cycloserine agar is recommended; clostridia appear as black colonies. Serotyping has been used as an epidemiologic tool in investigating outbreaks. However, only 40% of strains evaluated in the United States are typable, and this approach is presently not felt to be helpful. [27] While various enterotoxin assays have been developed, their accuracy in diagnosing disease and investigating outbreaks needs further evaluation.[22]

Clostridium botulinum

A diagnosis of botulism can be confirmed by demonstrating the presence of botulinum toxin in the serum or intestinal contents of the patient or in suspect food. *C. botulinum* is rarely present in the feces of normal individuals or in asymptomatic wounds; therefore, its isolation from these sites is strong presumptive evidence for disease. Identification of *C. botulinum* from suspect food samples is useful but toxin should be demonstrated to incriminate the food as the source of botulism.

Botulinum toxins are extremely potent, and minute quantities, absorbed percutaneously, by ingestion or inhalation, can result in death. All suspect material and clinical specimens must be handled with maximum precautions. Specimens for evaluation should include intestinal contents, serum and suspect food in foodborne disease; wound drainage, debrided tissue, serum and stool in wound botulism; and feces and serum in infant botulism.

Ideally, 10-15 mL of serum and 25-50 g of feces should be obtained. Suspect food should either be left in its original container or placed in a sterile, unbreakable container. Since most laboratories are not equipped to process such specimens, immediate assistance for processing is always available from state laboratories or the Centers for Disease Control (CDC). All specimens, except those from wounds, should be refrigerated and shipped as quickly as possible. Wound specimens should be placed in anaerobic transport devices.

Toxin demonstration is more rapid (48 hours) and specific than isolation and identification of *C. botulinum* itself. The mouse neutralization assay is the most sensitive and specific method available for toxin detection. Several more rapid in vitro assays have been developed but are less sensitive and specific and require further investigation.

Isolation and identification is best performed by spore selection techniques. Details of both toxin assay and bacteriologic isolation and identification are available in a CDC publication on this topic.[5]

Clostridium tetani

The diagnosis of tetanus is based primarily on the characteristic clinical picture. No laboratory tests are available to confirm the presence of disease. However, a positive serum toxin-neutralizing titer is usually sufficient evidence to rule out tetanus. *C. tetani* can be cultured from a wound by usual anaerobic isolation techniques. The presence of the organism does not necessarily prove the diagnosis since it has frequently been demonstrated in contaminated wounds in the absence of clinical symptoms. Furthermore, even in the setting of clinical tetanus, C. *tetani* can be recovered from only 1/3 of wounds.[8]

Clostridium difficile

Toxin assays are presently the most sensitive and specific means of diagnosing *C. difficile*-related intestinal disorders. The cytotoxicity assay remains the "gold standard" for detection of *C. difficile* toxins. Several cell culture lines undergo "actinomorphic" changes after exposure to either toxin A or B, although the latter is decidely more active. Changes can be seen as early as 3 hours; the test is read at 18 hours for typical cytotoxicity. These effects are commonly neutralized with *C. sordellii* antitoxin. This assay is 95% sensitive and 100% specific.[9]

When the cytotoxin assay is performed at a reference laboratory, at least 5 g of stool should be forwarded. If processing can occur in less than 4 hours, transport at room temperature will suffice; for a delay of 4 hours to 4 days the specimen should be shipped at 4°C; if a delay of greater than 4 days is anticipated, the specimens should be frozen. Although cytotoxicity assays have been performed generally by reference laboratories, commercial assay kits are now available, though their reliability has not been absolutely established.

A recently marketed rapid latex test appeared to work well in some investigations, although the mechanism of action is being studied. This latex reagent was shown in one study to react with an antigen, apparently distinct from toxin A or B, which is present in both toxigenic and nontoxigenic strains of *C. difficile*.[20] Counterimmunoelectrophoresis using the antiserum presently available has an unacceptably high rate of false-positive and false-negative reactions.[17] Enzyme immunoassays for detection of toxins A and B seem to be specific and sensitive. A recent report described an assay with a combined sensitivity of 95%.[19] This ELISA test may prove to be a suitable alternative to the cytotoxicity assay.

Culture detection of *C. difficile* can be achieved with either spore selection techniques or preferably with a selective medium (cycloserine-cefoxitin-egg yolk-fructose-agar). Because *C. difficile* is present in 1-3% of the general population, and in some asymptomatic individuals who have received antibiotics, and has been reported in up to 30% of hospitalized patients without a history of antibiotic usage or clinical manifestations, a positive fecal culture in the absence of toxin should be interpreted with caution. For practical purposes, a positive fecal toxin test in the appropriate clinical circumstances is sufficient for the diagnosis of antibiotic-associated diarrhea.

REFERENCES

1. Appelbaum PC, Chatterton SA. Susceptibility of anaerobic bacteria to ten antimicrobial agents. Antimicrob Agents Chemother 1978;14:371–6.
2. Bartlett JG, Chang TW, Gurwith M, Gorbach SL, Onderdonk AB. Antibiotic-associated pseudomenbranous colitis due to toxin-producing clostridia. N Engl J Med 1978;298:531–4.
3. Borriello SP, Larson HE, Welch AR, Barclay F, Stringer MF, Bartholomew BA. Enterotoxigenic *Clostridium perfringens*: a possible cause of antibiotic associated diarrhea. Lancet 1984;1:305–7.
4. Brown WJ, Waatti PE. Susceptibility testing of clinically isolated anaerobic bacteria by an Agar Dilution Technique. Antimicrob Agents Chemother 1980;17:629–35.
5. Centers for Disease Control. Botulism in the United States, 1899–1977. Handbook for epidemiologists, clinicians and laboratory workers, 1979.
6. Center for Disease Control. Foodborne Disease Outbreaks, Annual Summary, 1981. Atlanta: Centers for Disease Control, 1983.
7. Center for Disease Control. Annual Summary 1983: reported morbidity and mortality in the United States. Morbid Mortal Weekly Rep 1984;32:114.
8. Centers for Disease Control. Tetanus Surveillance U.S. Department Health, Education and Welfare. Report No. 4. Atlanta: Centers for Disease Control, 1984:11.
9. Chang TW, Lauermann M, Bartlett JG. Cytotoxicity assay in antibiotic-associated colitis. J Infect Dis 1979;140:765–70.
10. Chia JK, Clark JB, Ryan CA, Pollack M. Botulism in an adult associated with food-borne intestinal infection with *Clostridium botulinum*. New Engl J Med 1986;315:239–40.

11. Dowell VR Jr, Hawkins TM. Laboratory methods in anaerobic bacteriology, CDC laboratory manual. Atlanta: Centers for Disease Control; DHEW publication no. (CDC)78-8272.
12. Dowell VR Jr. Botulism and tetanus: selected epidemiologic and microbiologic aspects. Rev Infect Dis 1984;6(suppl 1):202–7.
13. Dzink J, Bartlett JG. *In Vitro* susceptibility of *Clostridium difficile* isolates from patients with antibiotic-associated diarrhea or colitis. Antimicrob Agents Chemother 1980;17:695–8.
14. Gabay EL, Rolfe RD, Finegold SM. Susceptibility of *Clostridium septicum* to 23 antimicrobial agents. Antimicrob Agents Chemother 1981;20:852–3.
15. Gorbach SL. Other *Clostridium* species including gas gangrene. In: Mandell GC, Douglas RG Jr, Bennett JE, eds. Principles and practice of infectious diseases. 2nd ed. New York: John Wiley, 1985:1362–8.
16. Gorbach SL, Thadepalli H. Isolation of *Clostridium* in human infections. J Infect Dis 1975;131(suppl):581–5.
17. Jarvis W, Nurez-Montiel O, Thompson F, Dowell V, Town M, et al. Comparison of bacterial isolation, cytotoxicity and counterimmunoelectrophoresis for the detection of *Clostridium difficile* and its toxin. J Infect Dis 1983;147:778.
18. Koransky JR, Stargel MD, Dowell VR. *Clostridium septicum* bacteremia. Its clinical significance. Am J Med 1979;66:63–6.
19. Langhou BE, Viscidi RP, Gdovin SL, Yolken RH, Bartlett SG. Enzyme immunoassays for detection of *Clostridium difficile* toxins A and B in fecal specimens. J Infect Dis 1984;149:781–8.
20. Lyerly DM, Wilkins TD. Commercial latex test for *Clostridium difficile* toxin A does not detect toxin A. J Clin Microbiol 1986;23:622–3.
21. MacLennan JD. The histotoxic clostridial infections of man. Bacterial Rev 1962;26:177–274.
22. McClane BA, Strouse RJ. Rapid detection of *Clostridium perfringens* type A enterotoxin by enzyme-linked immunosorbent assay. J Clin Microbiol 1984;19:112–15.
23. McDonel JL. *Clostridium perfringens* toxins (type A, B, C, D, E). Pharm Ther 1980;10:617–55.
24. Mossel DAA. Enumeration of sulfite reducing clostridia occurring in foods. J Sci Food Agr 1959;10:662–9.
25. Mulligan ME. Epidemiology of *Clostridium difficile* induced intestinal disease. Rev Infect Dis 1984;6:222–8.
26. Schwartzman JD, Reller LB, Wang WL. Susceptibility of *Clostridium perfringens* isolated from human infections to twenty antibiotics. Antimicrob Agents Chemother 1977;11:695–7.
27. Shandera WX, Tacket CO, Blake PA. Food poisoning due to *Clostridium perfringens* in the United States. J Infect Dis 1983;147:167–70.
28. Sutter VL, Citron DM, Edelstein MAC, Finegold SM. Wadsworth Anaerobic Bacteriology Manual. 4th ed. St. Louis: C.V. Mosby, 1985.
29. Sutter VL, Finegold SM. Susceptibility of anaerobic bacteria to 23 antimicrobial agents. Antimicrob Agents Chemother 1976;10:736–52.
30. Swenson JM, Thornsberry C, McCroskey LM, Hatheway CL, Dowell VR. Susceptibility of *Clostridium botulinum* to thirteen antimicrobial agents. Antimicrob Agents Chemother 1980;18:13–19.
31. Tally FP, Armfield AY, Dowell VR, Kwok Y, Sutter VL, Finegold SM. Susceptibility of *Clostridium ramosum* to antimicrobial agents. Antimicrob Agents Chemother 1974;5:589–93.
32. Weinstein L. Tetanus. New Engl J Med 1973;289:1293–6.

CHAPTER 6

ANTHRAX AND OTHER *Bacillus* INFECTIONS

Paul A. Granato, Ph.D.

INTRODUCTION

Bacillus anthracis, the etiologic agent of anthrax, is regarded as the major pathogen within the genus *Bacillus*, and has been responsible for pandemics of human and animal disease throughout recorded time.[11] Anthrax was introduced into the United States through the Mississippi Delta in the early 1700s, with the earliest reported cases occurring in animals. The first human case, reported in 1824, was a Kentucky cattle tender. Koch proved the etiology of anthrax in 1877 when "Koch's postulates" were demonstrated for the first time. Several years later, Pasteur produced an effective animal vaccine using an attenuated strain of the anthrax bacillus.[11]

Although *B. anthracis* is known as the primary pathogen within this genus, other members of this group have emerged as potential agents of human disease, usually as opportunistic pathogens. Nonanthrax *Bacillus* species have been implicated in serious infections associated with immunosuppression, traumatic wounds and burns, parenteral drug abuse and hemodialysis. *Bacillus cereus* is recognized as an important cause of food poisoning.

CAUSATIVE ORGANISMS

The genus *Bacillus* includes aerobic, gram-positive rods that produce spores and are catalase-positive.[7] The structure and location of the endospore within the vegetative cell are useful taxonomic characteristics (Table 6:1). Spores may be oval or spherical, and may be located centrally, subterminally or terminally. In some species, the presence of the spore causes the vegetative cell to swell. Capsules are present in some species, particularly *B. anthracis*.

Table 6:1. Characteristics of Members of the Genus *Bacillus**

	Morphology					Biochemical												
Species	Spore location†	Spore swells sporangium	Vacuoles	Motility	Rods 1 μm or wider	Catalase	Anaerobic growth	Glucose	Mannitol	Arabinose & xylose	Starch hydrolysis	V-P	$NO_3 \rightarrow NO_2$	Growth in 7% NaCl	Growth at 50°C	Lecithinase	Citrate	Gelatin liquefaction
B. anthracis	c	−	+	−	+	+	+	+	−	−	+	+	+	+	−	+	V	+
B. cereus	c	−	+	V	+	+	+	+	−	−	+	+	+	+	−	+	+	+
B. mycoides	c	−	+	−	+	+	+	+	−	−	+	+	+	+	−	+	+	+
B. thuringiensis	c	−	+	V	+	+	+	+	−	−	+	+	+	+	−	+	+	+
B. megaterium	c	−	−	V	+	+	−	+	V	V	+	−	V	+	−	−	+	+
B. subtilis	c	−	−	+	−	+	−	+	−	+	+	+	+	+	+	−	+	+
B. pumilus	c	−	−	+	−	+	−	+	+	+	−	+	−	+	+	−	+	+
B. licheniformis	c	−	−	+	−	+	+	+‡	+	+	+	+	+	+	+	−	+	+
B. firmus	c	−	−	V	−	+	−	+	+	V	+	−	+	+	−	−	−	+
B. circulans	cts	+	−	V	−	+	V	+	+	+	+	−	V	V	+	−	V	+
B. polymyxa	cts	+	−	+	−	+	+	+‡	+	+	+	+	+	−	−	−	−	+
B. laterosporus	c	+	−	+	−	+	+	+	+	−	−	−	+	−	+	+	−	+
B. brevis	cts	+	−	+	−	+	−	+	V	−	−	−	V	−	+	−	V	+
B. sphaericus	t	+	−	+	V	+	−	−	−	−	−	−	−	V	−	−	V	V
B. alvei	cts	+	−	+	V	+	+	+	−	−	+	+	−	−	−	−	−	+
B. stearothermophilus	cts	V	−	+	V	+	−	+	V	V	+	−	V	−	+	−	V	V
B. coagulans	cts	V	−	+	V	+	+	+	V	V	+	V	V	−	+	−	V	−
B. macerans	t	+	−	+	−	+	+	+‡	V	+	+	−	+	−	+	−	V	+

* Key: +, greater than 90% of isolates positive; −, less than 10% of isolates positive; V, variable reactions, 10 to 90% of isolates positive; V-P, Voges-Proskauer reaction.
† c represents central; t, terminal; and s, subterminal.
‡ gas is also produced.

Bacillus species are divided into two groups based upon the size of the vegetative cell (Table 6:1). In small-cell species, the bacterium has a width of 0.6 to 0.8 μm and a length of 1.5 to 3.0 μm; in large-cell species, the width is 1.0 to 1.5 μm and the length is 2.0 to 5.0 μm. Some species produce vacuoles in the vegetative cell. Although *Bacillus* species are gram-positive, some species show a variable Gram reaction when samples in the later stages of growth are stained.

The various *Bacillus* species have an enormous range of colonial morphologies that vary according to the composition of the medium. Isolated colonies may be quite rough and may spread over the surface of the medium, particularly when the agar surface is moist. Yellow, pink, red or even black pigmented colonies may be observed.

When grown in vitro, *B. anthracis* produces long chains that resemble bamboo rods. When seen in vivo, the chains are shorter and single bacilli or diplobacilli are commonly seen. When grown in culture, *B. anthracis* does not produce a capsule unless it is cultivated under increased carbon dioxide tension. Capsules around bacteria, however, are readily apparent when smears from infected material are examined.

CLINICAL MANIFESTATION

Anthrax

Human anthrax may present as a cutaneous, pulmonary or gastrointestinal disease, depending upon the portal of entry. Cutaneous anthrax is the most common form of the disease (95-98% of human cases) and results from the handling of infected animals or their byproducts.[21] Following an incubation period of 1 to 12 days, a small, painless papule appears that develops within a few more days into a vesicle filled with a dark, bluish-black fluid. The vesicle ruptures to produce a lesion, often called a "malignant pustule," that is characterized by a black eschar at the base surrounded by a prominent ring of inflammation. The "malignant pustule" usually occurs on the hand, forearm or head, and rarely is found on the trunk or lower extremities.

Pulmonary anthrax, also known as "woolsorters" disease, typically occurs in individuals who handle raw wool, hides or horse hair. These individuals acquire their disease by inhalation of spores. The patient's symptoms are typical of a respiratory infection with fever, malaise, myalgia and a nonproductive cough. Within several days, the infection becomes severe, with the development of marked respiratory distress, cyanosis and death within 24 hours.

Gastrointestinal anthrax occurs rarely, is rapidly fatal and results from the ingestion of contaminated meat. The anthrax bacillus invades the gastrointestinal mucosa producing ulcerations and symptoms of fever, generalized abdominal pain, nausea and vomiting, with blood loss through the stool or through hematemesis. Profound prostration results with the eventual development of shock and death.

Regardless of the portal of entry, untreated anthrax appears to follow a similar course after the initial stage. In the early systemic phase of the disease, the organism is transported by macrophages to the mediastinal lymph nodes and other tissues where spore germination, bacterial growth and toxin production occur. The late systemic phase is characterized by septicemia and widespread exotoxin production with resultant thrombosis, circulatory failure, cyanosis and death. The septicemic phase may also produce a usually fatal anthrax meningitis.

Therapy

Most strains of *B. anthracis* are exquisitely susceptible to penicillin (0.03 units/mL or less), the treatment of choice for anthrax.[8] In cutaneous anthrax, early diagnosis and treatment allow for a 100% cure rate. In mild, uncomplicated cases, oral penicillin (500 mg q 6 h) is quite effective, while in more serious disease, higher doses (4-6 million units/day) given intravenously or intramuscularly may be required. In the penicillin-allergic patient, erythromycin, tetracycline or chloramphenicol have been shown to be curative.

Pulmonary anthrax requires high-dose, intravenous penicillin therapy (18-24 million units/day) with the possible addition of streptomycin (1-2 g/day). Therapy early in the course of the disease is usually curative. High-dose penicillin therapy has also been suggested for the treatment of gastrointestinal anthrax although clinical experience is limited, due to the infrequency of the disease.

Food Poisoning

B. cereus food poisoning occurs as two separate and distinct clinical syndromes[23] caused by two different enterotoxins. The more common diarrheal syndrome has the longer incubation period (6 to 24 h) and produces lower gastrointestinal tract symptoms of diarrhea, abdominal cramps and nausea with little vomiting or fever, similar to *Clostridium perfringens* food poisoning. The emetic form of the disease is more severe, has a shorter incubation period (1 to 6 h) and is characterized by predominantly upper gastrointestinal tract symptoms similar to staphylococcal food poisoning. The illness is characterized by nausea, vomiting and abdominal cramps with little or no diarrhea or fever.

Laboratory diagnosis of *B. cereus* food poisoning is rarely attempted unless an outbreak occurs. Laboratory confirmation of an outbreak of *B.*

cereus requires isolating at least 10^5 organisms per gram from implicated food, from the stools of ill persons or from both. Because the symptoms of *B. cereus* food poisoning are usually mild, self-limited and mediated by enterotoxin, antibiotic therapy is not indicated.

Opportunistic Bacilli

Nonanthrax *Bacillus* species recovered from clinical specimens are usually regarded by many laboratorians as skin or air contaminants. However, with the increased use of immunosuppressant drugs and organ transplants, *Bacillus* species, previously considered harmless commensals, have emerged as potential human pathogens. Nonanthrax *Bacillus* species are generally associated with three types of infection: (a) local infections of a closed space such as the eye, with a history of preceding trauma or manipulation; (b) mixed infections with other organisms; and (c) disseminated infections including bacteremia, endocarditis and meningitis.[6,9,18,22,24,25] The *Bacillus* species most commonly associated with these infections include *B. cereus, B. circulans, B. macerans, B. coagulans, B. brevis, B. pumilis, B. sphaericus, B. thuringiensis* and *B. subtilis*.

Although there is no single criterion for assessing the clinical relevance of a *Bacillus* isolate, suspicion should be aroused by certain circumstances. These include: (a) colonies located only on the original streak lines; (b) an isolate recovered from a normally sterile body site such as blood or spinal fluid; (c) repeated recovery of the same organism from more than one specimen; (d) the presence of gram-positive rods on primary smears of clinical material; and (e) recovery of an organism from a compromised host or mainline drug addict.

EPIDEMIOLOGY

Anthrax

All *Bacillus* species, including *B. anthracis*, are ubiquitous in the environment, where they are found in decaying organic matter, dust, soil, vegetables and water. Some species are part of the normal flora of humans. *B. anthracis* is a saprophytic bacterium that can become a facultative parasite. The bacteria can survive indefinitely in soil where they continually undergo cycles of germination and sporulation, depending upon conditions of the microenvironment. Infected animals contaminate the soil with excrement and blood containing vegetative cells. These organisms will sporulate in an aerobic environment outside the body. Spores form when the weather becomes dry. If they are ingested inadvertently by grazing animals, an outbreak of anthrax can occur.

Anthrax primarily afflicts herbivorous animals and is a major livestock disease worldwide, involving thousands of cattle, goats, sheep and horses annually. Carnivorous animals can be infected secondarily if they feed on infected carcasses, but the disease is not spread from animal to animal. Europe accounts for about one-third of the cases of anthrax in animals, while the major portion of infections occur in Asia and Africa. In the United States, sporadic cases occur in the Gulf coast, midwestern states and California. Man is largely responsible for introducing anthrax into new areas by transporting hair, hides, bristles and bone (especially bone meal as fertilizer) from infected animals. Man is infected by contact with infected animals or animal products containing anthrax spores. About 7,000 cases per year are reported in the world, but estimates suggesting 20,000 - 100,000 cases per year are more reasonable, because many countries do not report the disease.[2] The incidence is highest in underdeveloped countries and only a few cases are reported in the United States each year.

Food Poisoning

The diarrheal type of gastroenteritis caused by *B. cereus* is associated with a wide range of foods, including meat products, soups, vegetables, puddings and sauces, whereas the emetic disease is associated with boiled and fried rice. Several serotypes of *B. cereus* are found in outbreaks of the diarrheal form, whereas emetic disease is most commonly caused by Serotype 1. Since the Serotype 1 spore is more resistant to heat than others, it may survive better in cooked rice. Outbreaks of *B. cereus* food poisoning have been reported throughout the world but the disease is uncommonly reported in the United States, where it may be underreported due to confusion with food poisoning caused by *C. perfringens* and staphylococci.

PREVENTION AND CONTROL

Control of anthrax requires eliminating or reducing contact with infected animals. Animals infected with anthrax should be treated; the exposed herd quarantined and vaccinated with the viable spore vaccine. Animals that die of anthrax should be cremated or buried deeply in the ground with lime to prevent contamination of pastures. Active immunization is the only known method of preventing anthrax in herbivors that graze in pastures contaminated with spores. In comparing the living vaccine with an alum-precipitated protective antigen vaccine, the living vaccine provided good protection but caused some local disease in animals.[10] The use of the protective antigen vaccine, however, produced only a short-term immunity in animals for several months. The use of both vaccines simultaneously provides a marked increase in the level of resistance and is the recommended procedure for animal immunization. The alum-precipitated, protective-antigen vaccine has been used in humans to protect workers in high risk environments, but antibody titers declined rapidly and booster doses of the vaccine are suggested at 6 to 12 month intervals to maintain immunity.

DIAGNOSTIC PROCEDURES

Safety Considerations

Extreme care and strict safety precautions must be adhered to in handling specimens and/or cultures suspected of containing *B. anthracis*. Perform specimen processing and cultural work in a biological safety cabinet; wear protective clothing, gloves and mask; and exercise extreme caution to prevent aerosolization or self-inoculation. Disinfect bench surfaces with 1% (wt/vol) sodium hypochlorite and autoclave or soak all discarded and contaminated items in hypochlorite disinfectant.

Clinical Specimens

The isolation of *B. anthracis* from human specimens depends upon the collection of the sample prior to the administration of antibiotics. Penicillin administered six hours before collection of a specimen, or a broad-spectrum antibiotic given several days earlier eliminates the organism from vesicular lesions.[8] Blood cultures are of limited diagnostic value in the early stages of disease because the organism does not appear in the blood until several hours before death.

Prepare several smears for microscopic examination from the clear vesicular fluid of the macular-papular lesions of man or animals and from noncoagulated blood from the carcasses of animal bodies. Transport the slides to the laboratory in an airtight container, such as a sealed Petri plate, to minimize environmental contamination. Saturate swab specimens for culture in vesicular or body fluid and place in sterile, screwcapped tubes for transit to the laboratory. Place blood samples collected in the terminal stages of disease or tissue samples of lymph node, spleen or peritoneal exudate obtained at biopsy or necropsy in sterile containers. Specimens that will be delayed in transport should be refrigerated or frozen. A variety of environmental samples including hides, hair, bone, fertilizer, soil, water, etc., may also be collected for laboratory analysis. Use aseptic technique in collecting these environmental samples and employ care in their transport to avoid infecting handlers or contaminating the environment.

Microscopic Examination of Smears

Fix smears for microscopic examination in 10% formalin for 10 min or in Zenker's fluid for 5 min to inactivate *B. anthracis* and its spores. Routine flame or heat fixation of smears will not inactivate anthrax spores.[3] Prepare at least 2 smears from each specimen and inactivate them. Gram stain one smear and stain the other smear using a fluorescent antibody procedure for detecting *B. anthracis* capsule, if available. Fluorescein conjugates of polyclonal sera and monoclonal antibody to capsule are available from the Centers for Disease Control (CDC). Otherwise, any capsular staining procedure, such as the modification of Leifson's method,[20] can be used. If the laboratory receives only one smear for examination, the capsular stain should be performed.

On microscopic examination of Gram stained smears, anthrax bacilli appear as large, gram-positive rods (3-10 μm by 1.3 μm) with flattened ends. Vegetative cells appear singly or in short chains but spores are rarely observed in fresh clinical material. When present, however, spores are oval, located centrally to subterminally and produce no observable cellular swelling. The presence of this cellular morphology along with the presence of encapsulated rods supports the tentative diagnosis of anthrax.

Cultural Examination of Clinical Specimens

Any routinely used noninhibitory medium, such as 5% sheep blood agar, is suitable for the recovery of *B. anthracis* from clinical specimens. Specimens that are heavily colonized with normal flora, such as feces and sputa, should also be inoculated onto Knisely's selective medium;[12] however, some strains of *B. anthracis* may be partially or totally inhibited by this medium.

The identification of *B. anthracis* poses a special problem, because, as shown in Table 6:1, the routinely performed morphologic and biochemical tests may not distinguish *B. anthracis* from the closely related species of *B. cereus, B. mycoides* and *B. thuringiensis*. Therefore, specialized confirmatory identification tests that are generally unavailable in most clinical laboratories must be performed. Several growth characteristics and screening tests, however, are useful in determining whether confirmatory identification testing is indicated.

Screening Tests

Colonial morphology, hemolytic activity, motility and penicillin susceptibility are useful screening tests for the presumptive identification of *B. anthracis*. However, closely related species may share these same characteristics. Although hemolytic activity is not a totally reliable indicator for identification, colonies that are strongly beta-hemolytic have never been reported to be *B. anthracis*. After 36 hours of incubation, colonies of *B.*

anthracis have a rough texture (ground glass appearance) with a serrated edge and occasionally form peripheral projections to produce the classical medusa-head morphology. However, *B. cereus, B. mycoides* and *B. thuringiensis* may also produce medusa-head colonies.[17]

A useful and reliable procedure for the preliminary screening of suspect *B. anthracis* is the motility test. All isolates of *B. anthracis* are nonmotile. To determine motility, inoculate the test organism into an enriched broth medium, such as Penassay broth, that is shaken aerobically at 35°C. Remove a sample of the broth during exponential growth to determine motility by the hanging-drop method. Examine motility determinations promptly after removal from culture because motility depends on an energized membrane. Any *Bacillus* isolate that is motile may be safely assumed to be a nonanthrax species.

B. anthracis is generally extremely susceptible to penicillin whereas *B. cereus, B. mycoides* and *B. thuringiensis* are resistant. *B. anthracis* will show a clearly defined zone of inhibition around a 10-unit penicillin disc when grown on Mueller-Hinton or 5% sheep blood agar. However, interpretive standards for zone diameters have not been established. Any *Bacillus* species that has a medusa-head colonial morphology, is nonhemolytic, nonmotile and is susceptible to penicillin may be *B. anthracis* and requires confirmatory identification.

Confirmatory Tests

An important characteristic for confirming the identity of *B. anthracis* is its ability to produce a capsule when grown on an enriched medium incubated in a carbon dioxide environment.[14] Subculture suspect colonies onto a nutrient or brain heart infusion agar containing 0.5% sodium bicarbonate and incubate at 35°C in a candle jar or in 5% CO_2. Virulent strains become encapsulated and produce a mucoid colony that is characteristic only of *B. anthracis* (no other *Bacillus* species does this). The presence of the capsule can be detected by using fluorescein-conjugated antibody or by the M'Fadyean capsular stain[15] in which the bacterial cell stains blue and the capsule pink.

Other tests used for confirming the identity of *B. anthracis* include: (a) detecting the presence of a plasmid-mediated tripartite toxin;[16] (b) detecting a quantitative increase in alpha-glycosidase activity;[19] (c) selective bacterial agglutination using various lectin assays;[4] and (d) susceptibility to gamma bacteriophage. In general, these specialized confirmatory identification tests for *B. anthracis* are performed only in reference laboratories and are described in greater detail elsewhere.[5]

Laboratory Diagnosis of *B. cereus* Food Poisoning

The laboratory diagnosis of *B. cereus* food poisoning is usually made by quantitatively determining the number of organisms present per gram of suspect food or fecal material. The recovery of low numbers of *B. cereus* from a fecal sample is not sufficient evidence to establish a diagnosis because the organism may be present as part of the normal flora. Generally, the recovery of at least 10^5 organisms per gram of clinical sample is required to establish the diagnosis of *B. cereus* food poisoning.

The following procedure is recommended for the isolation and presumptive identification of *B. cereus* from foodstuffs, vomitus, stool and environmental samples.

1. Macerate samples in sterile 0.5% (wt/vol) peptone broth. Prepare serial dilutions and plate 0.1 mL volumes onto a blood agar medium containing 25 U/mL polymyxin.[1]
2. After overnight incubation of this medium at 35°C, enumerate suspect colonies and inoculate a mannitol-egg yolk agar plate[13] by stabbing various sites to a depth of 4-6 mm. Incubate this plate overnight and examine it for halos around the sites of inoculation and for evidence of fermentation, i.e., a change in the violet background to yellow.
3. Any *Bacillus* isolate that is lecithinase-positive and mannitol fermentation-negative may be presumptively identified as *B. cereus*. Confirmatory tests for the identification of *B. cereus* (Table 6:1) may be performed, but most *Bacillus* isolates that grow on the blood agar base-polymyxin medium and give appropriate reactions on the mannitol-egg yolk agar are *B. cereus*.

Laboratory Diagnosis of Other *Bacillus* Infections

Nonanthrax *Bacillus* species are readily recovered on a variety of conventional media after 18-24 h incubation. The confirmatory identification of these isolates is achieved by observing microscopic morphologies and performing appropriate biochemical tests as shown in Table 6:1.

REFERENCES

1. Bouwer-Hertzberger SA, Mossil DAA. Quantitative isolation and identification of *Bacillus cereus*. In: Corry JEL, Roberts D, Skinner FA, eds. Isolation and identification methods for food poisoning organisms. London: Academic Press, 1982:255-9.
2. Brachman PS. Anthrax. In: Hobby G, ed. Antimicrobial agents and chemotherapy. Ann Arbor, MI: American Society for Microbiology, 1966:111-14.
3. Buravtseva NP. Effect of fixing smears over a flame on the viability of anthrax spores (Transl. from Russian). In: Osobo opasnye infektsii na Kavkaze Stayropol, 224, 1966. From: Biol Abstr 1968;49:Entry No. 57451.
4. Cole HB, Ezzell JW Jr, Keller KF, Doyle RJ. Differentiation of *Bacillus anthracis* and other *Bacillus* species by lectins. J Clin Microbiol 1984;19:48-53.
5. Doyle RJ, Keller KF, Ezzell JW. *Bacillus*. In: Lennette EH, Balows A, Hausler WJ Jr, Shadomy HJ, eds. Manual of clinical microbiology. 4th ed. Washington, DC: American Society for Microbiology, 1985:211-15.

6. Farrar W. Serious infections due to "non-pathogenic" organisms of the genus *Bacillus*. Am J Med 1963;34:134-41.
7. Gibson T, Gordon RE. Genus I. *Bacillus*. In: Buchanan RE, Gibbons NE, eds. Bergey's manual of determinative bacteriology. 8th ed. Baltimore: Williams and Wilkins, 1974:529-50.
8. Gold H. Treatment of anthrax. Fed Proc 1967;2:1563-8.
9. Ihde DC, Armstrong D. Clinical spectrum of infections due to *Bacillus* species. Am J Med 1973;55:839-45.
10. Klein F, DeArmon IA Jr, Lincoln RE, Mahlandt BG, Fernelius AL. Immunity against *Bacillus anthracis* from protective antigen live vaccine. J Immunol 1962;88:15-17.
11. Klemm DM, Klemm WR. A history of anthrax. J Am Vet Assoc 1959;135:458-62.
12. Knisely RF. Selective medium for *Bacillus anthracis*. J Bacteriol 1966;92:784-6.
13. Kramer JM, Turnbull PCB, Munshi G, Gilbert RJ. Identification and characterization of *Bacillus cereus* and other *Bacillus* species associated with food poisoning. In: Corry JEL, Roberts D, Skinner FA, eds. Isolation and identification methods for food poisoning organisms. London: Academic Press, 1982:261-86.
14. Meynell E, Meynell GG. The role of serum and carbon dioxide in capsule formation by *Bacillus anthracis*. J Gen Microbiol 1964;34:153-64.
15. M'Fadyean J. A peculiar staining reaction of the blood of animals dead of anthrax. J Comp Pathol 1903;16:35-41.
16. Mikesell P, Ivins E, Ristroph JD, Dreier TM. Evidence for plasmid-mediated toxin production in *Bacillus anthracis*. Infect Immun 1983;39:371-6.
17. Parry JA, Turnbull PCB, Gibson JR. A color atlas of *Bacillus* species. London: Wolfe Medical Publications, 1983.
18. Pearson HE. Human infections caused by organisms of the *Bacillus* species. Am J Clin Pathol 1970;53:506-15.
19. Sadler DF, Ezzell JW Jr, Keller KF, Doyle RJ. Glycosidase activities of *Bacillus anthracis*. J Clin Microbiol 1984;19:594-8.
20. Soltys MA. A new method of demonstrating capsulated *Bacillus anthracis*. J Clin Pathol 1960;13:526-7.
21. Taylor LT, Carslaw RW. Cutaneous anthrax. Lancet 1967;1:1214-15.
22. Tauzon CU, Murray HW, Levy C, Solny MN, Curtin JA, Sheagren JN. Serious infections from *Bacillus* sp. JAMA 1979;241:1137-40.
23. Terranova W, Blake PA. *Bacillus cereus* food poisoning. N Engl J Med 1978;298:143-4.
24. Turnbull PC, Jorgensen BD, Kramer JM, Gilbert RJ, Parry JM. Severe clinical conditions associated with *Bacillus cereus* and the apparent involvement of exotoxins. J Clin Pathol 1979;32:289-93.
25. Weinstein L, Colburn C. *Bacillus subtilis* meningitis and septicemia. Arch Intern Med 1950;86:585-6.

Chapter 7

BARTONELLOSIS, CAT SCRATCH DISEASE AND RAT-BITE FEVER

Ted L. Hadfield, Ph.D.

BARTONELLOSIS

INTRODUCTION

In 1870, an outbreak of fever occurred among laborers transported into Peru to build a railway from Lima to Oroya. Approximately 7000 deaths were attributed to fever and the malady became known as Oroya Fever.[19] In 1885, Daniel Carrion, a Peruvian medical student, injected himself with verrugamatous material and died of Oroya fever, establishing a link between the two clinically distinct diseases.[9,18,19] In 1909, Barton described organisms in blood of patients with Oroya fever.[13] In 1926, Noguchi[12] cultured *Bartonella bacilliformis* from patients and produced both Oroya fever and verruga peruana in animals. Reproduction of both diseases in rhesus monkeys firmly established *B. bacilliformis* as the etiologic agent of the two dramatically different clinical entities. Again, in 1938, an outbreak of fever occurred in Columbia with 4000 deaths.[18] Although not reported from this area previously, the disease was identical to Oroya fever. Small outbreaks have occurred as recently as 1959. Until 1966, bartonellosis was regarded as the only hemotropic bacterial infection in man. Since then, there have been reports of infections from Thailand,[20] Sudan,[19] Connecticut,[11] Illinois,[7] Niger[5] and Virginia.[1] None of the reports described *Bartonella* but the patients in Sudan had skin lesions resembling verruga peruana.[19] Although these reports all describe hemotropic organisms, the microbiologic, epidemiologic and pathologic data is sparse, leaving questions about validity in some instances.

CAUSATIVE ORGANISM

Bartonella bacilliformis is a small, pleomorphic rod or coccobacillus with unipolar flagella. The organism stains reddish-purple with Giemsa stain and is gram-negative, but retains counter stain poorly. It is seen in clusters of small bacillary forms, slightly curved, 0.25-0.5 μm in diameter by 1-3 μm long.[2,13] *Bartonella* grows best at 28-30°C in semisolid nutrient agar containing fresh rabbit serum and rabbit hemoglobin.[13] Cultures may be incubated at 37°C but organisms lose viability faster.[18]

CLINICAL MANIFESTATIONS

In the nonimmune person, acute bartonellosis may be insidious or abrupt in onset and usually results in the manifestations of Oroya fever. The incubation period is approximately 3 weeks,[17,18] but may be longer. When onset is insidious, patients experience intermittent fever, malaise, and headache for 2-7 days. When onset is abrupt, the patient experiences high fever with chills, severe nausea, myalgia, vomiting, diarrhea, lymphadenopathy, rapid respirations, vertigo and headache, followed by severe anemia.[16] The rapidly evolving anemia is hemolytic and macrocytic. Howell-Jolly bodies, basophilic granulations, nucleated erythrocytes (RBCs) and immature myeloid cells are present in the peripheral blood.[15,16] The erythrocyte count may fall from normal to less than 10^6 RBCs/mm^3 in 4-5 days.[18] The severity of the anemia is only exceeded by hemorrhage. The sudden drop in erythrocytes causes a peculiar color in the skin, due to slight jaundice combined with pallor. At this stage, muscle pain, joint pain and headache may be severe, and the patient may develope dyspnea, insomnia, delirium and in terminal cases, coma. Patients recovering from Oroya fever may have bone, joint and muscle pain and a markedly enhanced erythropoietic response as the infection subsides.

The rapid drop in the RBC count is due to the shortened life span of the RBCs because of bacterial attachment and subsequent invasion, hyperactivity of the spleen and a decreased erythropoietic response.[3,12,15] Bacteria are easily seen on peripheral blood films during the acute phase of the disease. Reticuloendothelial cells phagocytize and destroy infected RBCs and contain many bacteria.[16] Although organisms seem to penetrate erythrocytes in vivo, only adherence has been demonstrated in vitro.[10,20] The number of organisms in the blood is low or undetectable by microscopy when onset is insidious and during recovery.[14] The mortality rate of acute Oroya fever approaches 40% in untreated patients. However, patients with Oroya fever frequently have concomitant salmonellosis, amebiasis, malaria, tuberculosis or other enteric pathogen infections that may contribute to the high mortality rate. After a variable latent period, patients recovering from

Oroya fever develop a chronic benign cutaneous form of bartonellosis called verruga peruana.[16]

The cutaneous eruptive lesions of verruga peruana may follow Oroya fever or develop without prior symptoms. Nodules develop over 1-2 months and may persist for months to years. Verrugas are most notable on the exposed parts of the body. Serous membranes may become inflamed, with *Bartonella* present in leukocyte effusions. The verruga vary from red to purple in color and appear in crops; lesions in all stages of growth and regression may be seen in the same patient. The verrugas may be sessile, miliary nodular, pedunculated or confluent and may reach 1-2 cm in diameter.[2] Verrugas are not tender unless secondarily infected. Organisms may be cultured from cutaneous lesions and occasionally from the blood and bone marrow.

EPIDEMIOLOGY AND PUBLIC HEALTH SIGNIFICANCE

Bartonellosis is strictly limited to areas in or near the river valleys on the western slopes of the Andes mountains, between an elevation of 2,000 and 8,000 feet, in Peru, Ecuador and Columbia.[6] The disease is endemic in these regions. Five to ten percent of the population represent asymptomatic cases and long term carriers which serve as reservoirs of infection.[10] The geographic restriction of the infection is most likely due to the limited habitats of its sandfly vector, *Phlebotomus verrucarum*, a documented vector in Peru, where *P. pescei* is a suspected vector. The suspect species in Columbia is *P. colombianus*. Sandflies become infected after taking a blood meal from an infected human.[21]

PREVENTIVE MEASURES

Prevention of infection requires control of sandflies, generally done by spraying interiors and exteriors of dwellings with insecticides and by the use of insect repellents and netting. There is no effective immunization.

COLLECTION AND PROCESSING OF SPECIMENS

Oroya Fever

Blood for culture and thin films are optimally collected prior to antibiotic therapy. The organism grows quickly when erythrocyte infection is high and culture may be positive during recovery from the infection, when bacteria are not detectable in blood films. Blood cultures should be repeated over several days if initially negative. At autopsy, portions of the spleen, liver and enlarged lymph nodes should be collected aseptically for culture and microscopic examination.

Verruga Peruana

B. bacilliformis may be cultured from the cutaneous lesion, blood or bone marrow in this stage of the disease. Blood cultures may be positive throughout the eruptive phase before antibiotics are given. Although *Bartonella* can be cultured from verrugous lesions, cultures are often contaminated with skin flora and bacteria are not evident in older fibrotic lesions.[6]

DIAGNOSTIC PROCEDURES

Bartonellosis is a long-lasting infection. No item is more important for diagnosis than a history of travel to an endemic zone or a positive culture. Distinctive collections of bacilli on red blood cells and in vascular endothelial cells, especially in liver, lymph nodes and spleen, are pathognomonic of Oroya fever. Identification of *B. bacilliformis* from cultures is required for diagnosis when pathognomonic features are not observed.

Microscopic Examinations

Most RBCs carry 1-6 or more bacteria. Infections are less severe before and after the anemia peaks and after therapy. The presence of bacteria on and within the RBCs is a characteristic feature of bartonellosis, but some forms may not be recognizable and culture will be required.

Primary Culture Media

B. bacilliformis grows best in semisolid nutrient agar containing fresh rabbit serum and rabbit hemoglobin or in fresh leptospiral medium; it can also be grown on 5% sheep blood agar. Media are incubated at 25°C and colony development takes 2-4 weeks. In liquid media, bartonellae grow in rounded clumps about 5mm below the surface of the medium. They are not hemolytic on blood agar[10] when grown at a 25°C or 37°C. Giemsa stains of microcolonies show distinctly stained rods around a densely stained central mass. *B. bacilliformis* retains Gram stain poorly and no distinctive biochemical tests have been described for it. Colonies of *B. bacilliformis* may occur as two colonial types on solid media. One type appears small, dark and round, has an entire edge and is friable. The other type colonies are larger and lighter in color, have irregular edges and are not friable. Both colony types appear to have a bubble in the center of the colony.[20]

Identification Procedures

A Giemsa-stained blood film showing a majority of RBCs (up to 90%) infected with numerous bacteria suggests a presumptive diagnosis of bartonellosis (Oroya fever). The intracytoplasmic development of *Bartonella* in rounded masses detected at autopsy or in biopsy specimens has not been described in any other disease. Verruga are also distinctive in their histology but may be confused with a number of other clinical entities, including Kaposi's sarcoma.[4]

Serology

Commercial antisera are not available for rapid identification of *Bartonella*. However, Knoblock, Soland, Alvarez et al.[8] reported the use of enzyme-linked immunosorbent assay (ELISA), fluorescent antibody and hemagglutination techniques for detecting antibodies to *B. bacilliformis*. Serologic assays showed that 63.6% of the population in the endemic zone had antibody. ELISA was the most sensitive test. IgM specific antibody was detected by a fluorescent antibody technique.

Treatment of acute bartonellosis with chloramphenicol, penicillin, tetracycline or streptomycin produces a dramatic clinical response. The choice of antibiotic is often dictated by the presence of secondary infection. Cutaneous verrugal lesions show a variable response to antibiotic therapy; larger and secondarily infected nodules may require surgical excision.[13]

REFERENCES

1. Archer GL, Coleman PH, Cole RM, et al. Human infection from an unidentified erythrocyte associated bacterium. N Engl J Med 1979;301:897-900.
2. Dooley JR. Bartonellosis. In: Binford CH, Connor DH, eds. Pathology of the tropical and extraordinary diseases: An atlas; vol 1. Washington, DC: Armed Forces Institute of Pathology, 1976;190-3.
3. Dooley JR. Haemotropic bacteria in man. Lancet 1980;11:1237-9.
4. Garcia FU. Tissue reactions in Bartonellosis may suggest Kaposi's sarcoma. Arch Pathol Lab Med 1985;109:703-4.
5. Gretillat S, Konarcewski B. Presence d'un procaryote du genere Haemobartonella, Tyzzer et Weinmann 1939, dans le Sang des Nigeriens de la region de Niamey. Bull Soc Pathol Exot 1978;71:412-16.
6. Howe C. Carrion's disease: Immunologic studies. Arch Intern Med 1943;72:147-9.
7. Kallick CA, Levin S, Reddi KT, et al. Systemic lupus erythematosis associated with hemobartonella-like organisms Nature 1972;236:145-6.
8. Knobloch J, Soland L, Alvarez O, Delgado E. Antibodies to *Bartonella bacilliformis* as determined by fluorescence antibody test, indirect haemagglutination and ELISA. Trop Med Parasitol 1985;36:183-5.
9. Knoblock J. Hundreth anniversary of Carrion's death. Trop Med Parasitol 1985;36:183.
10. Kreier JP, Ristic M. The biology of hemotrophic bacteria. Ann Rev Microbiol 1981;35:325-38.

11. Metler NE. Isolation of a *microtatobiotye* from patients with hemolyticuremic syndrome and thrombocytopenic purpura and from mites in the United States. N Engl J Med 1969;281:851-64.
12. Noguchi H. The etiology of Oroya fever. J Exp Med 1926;43:851-64.
13. Norbert J, Roberts JR. *Bartonella bacilliformis* (Bartonellosis). In: Mandell GL, Douglas RG, Bennett JE, eds. Principles and practice of infectious diseases. 2nd ed. New York: John Wiley, 1985:1378.
14. Peters D, Wigand R. *Bartonellaceae*. Bacteriol Rev 1955;19:150-62.
15. Reynadarje C, Ramos J. The hemolytic anemia of human bartonellosis. Blood 1961;17:562-78.
16. Ricketts WE. Clinical manifestations of Carrion's disease. Arch Intern Med 1949;84:751-4.
17. Ricketts WE. Carrion's disease. A study of the incubation period in thirteen cases. Am J Trop Med Hyg 1947;27:657-62.
18. Schultz MG. A history of bartonellosis (Carrion's disease). Am J Trop Med Hyg 1968;17:503-15.
19. Strong RP, Tyzer EE, Sellards AW, Brues CT, Gastiaburu JC. Report of first expedition to South America. 1913. Cambridge, MA: Harvard Univ Press, 1915.
20. Walker TS, Winkler HH. *Bactonella bacilliformis*: Colonial types and erythrocyte adherence. Infect Immun 1981;31:480-4.
21. Weinman D. Bartonellosis and anemias associated with *Bartonella*-like structures. In: Balows A, Hausler WJ Jr, eds. Diagnostic procedures for bacterial, mycotic and parasitic infections. 6th ed. Washington, DC: American Public Health Association, 1981:235-48.

CAT-SCRATCH DISEASE

INTRODUCTION

Cat-scratch disease (CSD) was first recognized by Robert Debr'e at the University of Paris in the early 1930s.[3] He described a 10-year old boy with many scratchs on his arms and epitrochlear lymphadenitis. No cause could be established. A draining fistula closed and the swollen node resolved within a few weeks. Debr'e saw several additional cases over the years, and in his first published report in 1950 he coined the term cat-scratch disease.[7] Simultaneously, Molleret recognized the disease process at the Louis Pasteur Institute.[4] Other investigators, including Hanger and Foshay, described the disease and confirmed its association with cats.[4] Today, the illness is referred to as cat-scratch disease, cat-scratch fever, benign inoculation lymphoreticulosis or nonbacterial regional lymphadenitis.

Although the disease had been described, an association with cats firmly established, the histopathology reported and a skin test developed, the causative agent remained a mystery until 1983 when Wear, Margileth, Hadfield et al[35] described the presence of small gram-negative bacilli in lymph nodes of patients with CSD. This report was followed by a description of the bacteria in primary inoculation sites[23] and in conjunctival granulomas of children with the oculoglandular syndrome of Parinaud.[36] These reports convincingly established the etiology of CSD.

CAUSATIVE ORGANISM

The bacilli are small (0.15-0.25μm x 0.5-1.0μm), pleomorphic and gram-negative when stained with the Brown-Hopps tissue Gram stain. They are so small that their presence is easily overlooked in tissue Gram stains. When stained with a Wharthin-Starry silver impregnation stain, the bacilli appear much larger and are easily recognized. The organisms frequently appear in clumps around capillaries and lymphatic vessels, and may also be found free in lymphatic sinuses and necrotic debris in early lesions. Organisms are not acidfast; do not stain with Gomori-methenamine silver stain nor with periodic acid schiff stain.[34] (Fig. 7:1. See color plate.)

CLINICAL MANIFESTATION

The clinical manifestation of CSD begins 3-5 days after exposure as a primary inoculation lesion, usually on the extremities although occasionally on the neck, face or trunk. The primary inoculation lesion is located in a scratch, or rarely a bite site, and develops into a papule or pustule. The pustule may be present for a few days or persist for 8 weeks. The primary lesion may be healed by the time regional lymphadenopathy develops and the patient seeks medical attention. Surprisingly, lymphangitis is not a feature of CSD.[6,25] Regional lymphadenopathy usually develops within 2 weeks after the scratch, but may develop after 3-50 days.

Despite impressive lymphadenopathy, the patient is rarely acutely ill. Lymphadenopathy is seen in all patients with CSD and 50% of the patients have adenopathy as the only sign or symptom. Tender nodes are present in 80% of patients and are usually found in the head, neck, axilla or inguinal areas. Less frequently, epitrochlear, femoral or popliteal nodes are involved. Multiple site involvement occurs in approximately 40% of the cases. Lymph node enlargement ranges in size from 1-8 cm and suppuration occurs in 14% of patients. Lymphadenopathy persists for a few weeks to 4 months in most patients but may persist for up to 2 years in rare cases,[6,22,24,25] where CSD has been mistaken for more serious diseases such as lymphoma.[14,20] Additional signs and symptoms that may occur include splenomegaly (14%), rashes (4%), encephalopathy (2%), and rarely seizures, pleural effusions, hepatomegaly, hepatitis, atypical pneumonia and breast nodules.

Fever (38.3-42.1°C) is the second most common sign (33%) and may persist for up to 28 days. Fatigue and malaise (27%), anorexia (12%), headache (11%) and sore throat (11%) are seen less often. Ocular granuloma with conjunctivitis occurs in 5.7% of patients and is the hallmark of Perinaud's oculoglandular syndrome, the most prevalent unusual manifestation.[25] Other unusual manifestations include encephalitis,[32] skin rashes (maculopapular, petechial, erythema multiforme, or erythema nodosum),[22] osteolytic lesions,[5,15] cerebral arteritis,[2,8] thrombocytopenic purpura,[3] atypical pneumonia,[28] erythema nodosum,[22] radiculitis,[26] breast tumor,[5] anicteric hepatitis,[19] pleural effusion,[16,19] anemia, hepatosplenomegaly[10,27] and sepsis.[1,18]

Central nervous system (CNS) involvement presenting as encephalopathy, meningitis, radiculitis, polyneuritis or myelitis with paraplegia occurs in 1-2% of patients.[13,16] The onset of neurologic symptoms is sudden, usually accompanied by fever and occurs 1-6 weeks after the adenopathy. Neurologic examination may show focal or diffuse CNS dysfunction. Focal or generalized seizures are common. Cerebrospinal fluid analysis usually reveals minimal or no pleocytosis, slightly elevated protein and negative cultures. In most patients with neurologic systems, electroencephalograms are normal for one to several months. Severe manifestations last for 1-2 weeks with gradual recovery.[21]

THERAPY

At present, the best therapy for CSD is reassurance that the lymphadenopathy is benign and in most cases will subside spontaneously within 2-4 months. Successful management includes aspirin or acetaminophen for pain, node aspiration if the node becomes fluctuant and repeated examinations to ensure the adenopathy is decreasing in size.[24] Excisional biopsy is frequently done to rule out more serious diseases[8,11] and may be done in selected patients to relieve persistent pain. However, surgical removal of an involved node is not recommended unless a diagnosis cannot be made by other means,[3,17,22] even though removal quickly ends the disease.[22,30] Antimicrobial drugs are not recommended because patients with CSD characteristically do not respond to them. Because the disease is bacterial, not responsive to antibiotics and self-limited, the use of steroids is not recommended.

EPIDEMIOLOGY

Cat-scratch disease is transmitted only from animals, usually cats, to man. There are no documented cases of person-to-person transmission. CSD is a distinctly pediatric disease: 80% of cases occur in persons under 21 years of age.[6] More than 90% of all cases are transmitted by cat scratches, bites, or licks; and about 70% of cases are associated with newly acquired kittens rather than long-time household pets. Family clustering occurs in 5% of cases and suggests a common source of infection.[22] Other rare sources of CSD have been described, including scratches or punctures by rose thorns, porcupine quills, monkeys, rabbits and dogs. Although Warwick[33] reported small outbreaks of CSD, it is unlikely any epidemics have occurred. CSD occurs in every country, in all races, and predominately in males, who tend to be more aggressive with animals. It occurs year around but appears to be more frequent during the fall, winter and spring months in the northern climates[22,23] and in spring, summer and fall months in the southern climates. This corresponds with periods when household pets and humans are more likely to be indoors. Survey data[6] received from 211 hospitals around the country for a 10-year period showed about 1425 patient discharges with a diagnosis of CSD.

PUBLIC HEALTH SIGNIFICANCE, PREVENTION AND CONTROL

Prevention of CSD is difficult since there are approximately 50 million cats in the United States. Some cases of CSD even involved cats that were declawed. The organism may be a transient member of the normal feline oral or genital flora; the bacilli could easily be transmitted to the claws during grooming. If true, declawing should help reduce the overall incidence of CSD. In addition, avoiding bites and not allowing cats to lick open wounds would also reduce the risk of infection. Because the cat is invariably well at the time of transmission, one cannot determine which cat will transmit bacilli. Inability to culture the organism has prevented epidemiologic studies as well as development of rapid tests for diagnosis of CSD.

DIAGNOSTIC PROCEDURES

Many diseases have signs and symptoms similar to CSD; thus the diagnosis can be puzzling if the primary inoculation site has healed or is inapparent and a history of animal contact is not elicited. The differential diagnosis for chronic lymphadenitis includes a variety of infectious agents and noninfectious etiologies (Table 7:1). There is no single diagnostic test available for diagnosis of CSD. In many instances this may be a diagnosis by exclusion. However, in typical cases of CSD, four of the following five criteria will confirm the diagnosis. In an atypical presentation of CSD, all five criteria are necessary:

(1) a history of animal contact plus a scratch, primary inoculation site or eye lesion; (2) a positive CSD skin test; (3) negative laboratory studies for other causes of infectious lymphadenopathy; (4) characteristic histopathology of a biopsied lymph node; and (5) the presence of typical silver-staining bacteria in histopathologic sections of lymph nodes, primary inoculation site or eye lesions.

Table 7:1. Differential Diagnosis for Lymphadenopathy of Unknown Origin

Bacterial	Fungal-Parasitic	Viral	Noninfectious
Lymphogranuloma venereum	Coccidiomycosis	Kawasaki's syndrome	Hodgkin's disease
Cat scratch disease	Histoplasmosis	Infections due to:	Non-Hodgkins lymphoma
Brucellosis	Sporotrichosis	Epstein-Barr virus	Leukemia
Infections due to:	Toxoplasmosis	Cytomegalovirus	Histiocytosis
Staphylococcus aureus	Chaga's Disease	Adenovirus	Sarcoidosis
β-hemolytic streptococci		Enterovirus	
Mycobacteriun tuberculosis		Herpes simplex virus	
Mycobacteria other than *M. tuberculosis*		Rubella virus	
Treponema pallidum		Varicella-zoster virus	
Streptobacillus moniliformis			
Francisella tularensis			

Pathology

Although surgical excision of lymph nodes is not recommended for diagnosis or therapy of CSD, nodes may be removed to rule out lymphoma, leukemia, sarcoid or other causes of lymphadenopathy. For whatever reason, some lymph nodes from patients with CSD will be removed and examined histogically. The histopathology shows a wide range of features and was described first by Molleret[4] and again by Campbell.[2] Campbell[2] described three phases of changes in the lymph node. The early phase consists of lymphoid hyperplasia with thickening of the capsule, hypertrophy of germinal centers, swelling of lymphatic capillaries and formation of microabscesses. Early stage changes may be similar to changes associated with sarcoid or lymphoma. Phase 2 consists of necrosis with tangible histiocytes. The microabscesses expand and may coalesce with adjacent microabscesses. Granulomas begin to form with invasion of large lymphocytes and epithelial cells. Necrosis develops in the areas of the abscesses and early granulomas consist of necrotic cells with karyorrhectic nuclei, acidophilic debris and fibrin. Dilated capillaries may be thrombosed. Pericapsular inflammation with edema is present and Langhan's giant cells may be present. In the third stage, granulomas with palisading epitheloid cells and a stellate configuration are evident. This is the stage most frequently observed on histiologic examination. The center of the granuloma is infiltrated with neutrophils but may show a caseous necrosis similar to a *Mycobacterium tuberculosis* infection. Also, the changes seen in the third stage closely resemble those seen in tularemia, lymphogranuloma venereum and brucellosis.

Warthin-Starry stains are most likely to demonstrate organisms in the early or first stage. Organisms are seen in clumps around swollen vessels and in histiocytes. They are abundant in areas of microabscess formation before necrosis is evident. As the microabscess enlarges, necrosis becomes more prominent, granulomas begin to form and the bacilli are increasingly more difficult to find. They may be found in small clusters, singly in histiocytes or free in the necrotic debris. Bacilli rarely are seen in granulomas with suppurative centers and a mantle of palisading epitheloid cells. Aspiration biopsy also may be an acceptable way to make the diagnosis of CSD.[30]

Microscopy

CSD bacilli are small gram-negative rods seen most frequently in early lesions in lymph node, skin or ocular granulomas. They are best seen when stained with the Warthin-Starry silver impregnation stain (See color plate Figure 7:1). They are occasionally seen in stellate granulomas in lymph nodes. They have not been seen in aspirated suppurative material by routine Gram or acridine orange stains.

Primary Isolation And Culture

Many investigators have tried to culture the etiologic agent of CSD. The most consistent finding in CSD nodes has been the presence of small bacilli. They have been identified in lymph node tissue sections, ocular granulomas and primary skin lesions of patients who fulfilled all the criteria for CSD. Nodes, containing bacilli in histologic sections, have been inoculated on a variety of artificial media, into several tissue culture systems and into animals[13] without success to date.

Serologic Tests

There are no specific serologic tests for diagnosis of CSD. A skin test antigen is the most reliable noninvasive diagnostic test; however, CSD skin test antigen is not readily available. The skin test antigen is prepared by the method of Rose.[2] Pus from nodes of patients who fulfill the diagnostic criteria for CSD is diluted 1:4 with normal saline, heated to 60°C for 3 days and dispensed into sterile ampules. After having been tested for hepatitis B antigen, human immunodeficiency virus (HIV/HTLV-III/LAV) and sterility, the antigen is ready for use in skin testing. New preparations are compared with a standard skin test antigen for potency and specificity. Warwick[33] reported 5% false-positive and 5% false-negative reactions. It is possible that the false-positive reactions represent subclinical or undiagnosed infections.[4] False-negative reactions may occur early in the course of the disease. Often, patients skin tested a second time 60 days later are positive.

REFERENCES

1. Black JR, Herrington DA, Hadfield TL, Wear DJ, Margileth AM, Shigekawa B. Life-threatening cat-scratch disease in an immunocompromised host. Arch Intern Med 1986;146:394–6.
2. Campbell J. Cat-scratch disease. Pathology 1977;12:277–92.
3. Carithers HA, Carithers CM, Edwards RO Jr. Cat-scratch disease: Its natural history. JAMA 1969;207:312–16.
4. Carithers HA, Carithers CM, Edwards RO Jr. Cat-scratch disease: Notes on its history. Am J Dis Child 1970;119:200–3.
5. Carithers HA. Cat-scratch disease associated with an osteolytic lesion. Am J Dis Child 1983;137:968–70.
6. Carithers HA. An overview based upon a study of 1200 patients. Am J Dis Child 1985;139:1124–33.
7. Debr'e R, Lamy ML, Jammet L, et al. La maladie des griffes de chat. Bull Mem Soc Med Hop Paris 1950;66:76–80.
8. Emmons RW, Riggs JL, Scachter J. Continuing search for the etiology of cat-scratch disease. J Clin Microbiol 1976;4:112–14.
9. Gerber MA, Sedgwick AK, MacAlister TJ, et al. The aetiological agent of cat-scratch disease. Lancet 1985;1:1236–9.
10. Greenbaum B, Nelson P, Marchildon M, Donalson M. Hemolytic anemia and hepatosplenomegaly associated with cat-scratch fever. J Pediatr 1986;108:428–30.
11. Hadfield TL, Malaty RH, VanDellen A, Margileth AM. Electron microscopy of cat-scratch disease bacillus. J Infect Dis 1985;152:643–5.
12. Hadfield TL, Wear DJ, Margileth AM, English CK. Is *Rothia dentocariosa* the cause of cat-scratch disease. Lancet 1985;11:720.
13. Hadfield TL, Schlagel CJ, Margileth AM. Stalking the cause of cat-scratch disease. Diag Med 1985;8:1–5.
14. Hendricks WM, Rosenthal M. Infectious mononucleosis presenting as cat-scratch disease. N Carolina Med J 1983;44:433–44.
15. Johnson JF, Lehman RM, Shiels WE, Blaney SM. Osteolysis in cat-scratch fever. Radiology 1985;156:373–4.
16. Katner HP, Treen B, Pankey GA, Glasgow S, Cortez LM, Dalovisio J. Pleural effusion and anicteric hepatitis associated with cat-scratch disease. Chest 1986;89:302–3.
17. Knight PJ, Muline AF, Vassey LE. When is lymph-node biopsy indicated in children with enlarged peripheral nodes? Pediatrics 1982;69:391–6.
18. Korbitz B. Systemic cat-scratch disease with hepatosplenomegaly, multiple lymphadenopathy, and hepatic dysfunction. Rocky Mt Med J 1973;70:23–7.
19. Lambert H, Hausser E. Anicteric hepatitis. A new possible complication of cat-scratch disease. Rev. Med Suisse Romande 1965;85:689–93.
20. Luddy RE, Sutherland JC, Levy BE. Cat-scratch disease simulating malignant lymphoma. Cancer 1982;50:584–94.
21. Lyon LW. Neurologic manifestations of cat-scratch disease. Arch Neurol 1971;25:23–7.
22. Margileth, AM. Cat-scratch disease: nonbacterial regional lymphadenitis. The study of 145 patients and a review of the literature. Pediatrics 1968;42:803–18.
23. Margileth AM, Wear DJ, Hadfield TL. Cat-scratch disease: Bacteria in skin at the primary inoculation site. JAMA 1984;252:928–31.
24. Margileth AM. Cervical adenitis. Pediatr Rev 1985;7:13–24.
25. Margileth AM, Zawolsky PM. Chronic lymphodenopathy in children and adolescents. Am Fam Physician 1985;31:166–80.
26. Miller P, Bell WE. Cat-scratch disease with encephalopathy. Clin Pediatr 1980;19:233–5.
27. Rocco VK, Roman RJ, Eigenbrodt EH. Cat-scratch disease. Gastroenterology 1985;89:1400–6.
28. Selby G, Walker GL. Cerebral arteritis in cat-scratch disease. Neurology 1979;89:1413–18.

29. Sheldon GC, Smellie H. Cat-scratch disease with pneumonia. Br Med J 1957;2:446–7.
30. Silverman, JF. Fine needle aspiration cytology of cat-scratch disease. Acta Cytol 1985;29:542–7.
31. Small WT, Sniffen RC. Nonbacterial regional lymphadenitis (cat-scratch fever). Evaluation of surgical treatment. N Engl J Med 1956;255:1029.
32. Torres JR, Sanders CV, Strub RL. Cat-scratch disease causing reversible encephalopathy. JAMA 1978;240:1628–9.
33. Warwick WJ. The cat-scratch syndrome, many diseases or one disease? Prog Med Virol 1967;9:256–7.
34. Verhoff FH. Parinaud's conjunctivitis; a mycotic disease due to a hitherto undescribed filamentous organism. Arch Ophthalmol 1913;42:345–51.
35. Wear DJ, Margileth AM, Hadfield TL. Cat-scratch disease: A bacterial infection. Science 1983;221:1403–5.
36. Wear DJ, Malaty RH, Zimmerman LE, et al. Cat-scratch disease bacilli in the conjunctiva of patients with Parinaud's oculoglandular syndrome. Ophthalmology 1985;92:1282–7.

RAT-BITE FEVER

INTRODUCTION

Rat-bite fever is a systemic illness that occurs worldwide and is typically acquired by direct contact with infected rats or other small rodents. Rat-bite fever is caused by infection with either *Streptobacillus moniliformis* or *Spirillum minor*, both commonly found in the oropharyngeal flora of rodents.[13,15] Human infections with *S. moniliformis* resulting from ingestion of milk to which rats have had access have been reported as Haverhill fever or erythema arthriticum epidemicum. Rarely, the disease occurs after traumatic injury. Infection with *S. minor* is found worldwide but predominately in Asia, where it is known as Sodoku. There has been only one reported case of *S. minor* infection in the United States in the past 28 years.[7]

CAUSATIVE ORGANISMS

Streptobacillus moniliformis is a nonmotile, gram-negative aerobic bacillus. The organism is highly pleomorphic, is usually less that 1μm wide by 1-5μm long, with rounded or pointed ends, but may form curved or looped filaments as long as 150μm. In young cultures, the filaments appear to consist of single cells. As the culture ages, fine granules and alternate light and dark bands appear in the filaments. Fragmentation into irregular, coccobacillary elements occurs. Filaments may consist of a series of oval to elongated bulbous swellings, each 1-3μm in diameter, giving the appearance of a string of beads. True branching does not occur. Cell membrane-associated, extracellular oil-like droplets are very characteristic. Streptobacilli occur as bacterial-phase organisms or as cell wall deficient L-forms.[8]

Bacterial-phase organisms have been isolated and maintained on trypticase soy agar or in trypticase soy broth supplemented with 20% horse or rabbit serum and incubated in 8-10% CO_2. Brain-heart infusion cysteine broth supplemented with 2.5% papain digest of ox liver (Panmede, Payne and Byrne, Ltd., Greenford, England) or commercially available, fastidious anaerobe broth have been shown to be superior media for isolation of *S. moniliformis*.[24] In broth media, diagnostic "puff ball" colonies appear after 2-6 days. Under anaerobic conditions, the organism may resemble *Bacteroides* species or *Fusobacteria* species. *S. moniliformis* may spontaneously develop into L-forms in vivo and in vitro.[13]

CLINICAL MANIFESTATIONS

The onset of rat-bite fever caused by *S. moniliformis* is abrupt, usually within 10 days of rodent exposure or bite, and is ushered in by high fever and shaking chills. Headache, vomiting, myalgias and muscle tenderness accompany the fever. The white blood cell count may be normal but is often elevated to as high as 30,000/mm^3 with a left shift. Coagulopathy with thrombocytopenia may develop.[17] Two to four days after onset of symptoms, 90% of patients develop a rash similar to that of Rocky Mountain spotted fever[17] and 50% experience joint symptoms. Like CSD, the wound heals without suppuration or local lymphangitis. The rash is generalized and may consist of discrete erythematous macules with some petechial hemmorrhages or it may be morbiliform. The rash is most prominent on the palms and soles, and may become confluent. Other lesions, at various stages of development, include painful papules, vesicles, discharging pustules and scabs.[23] Arthralgias are common and may progress to full-blown mono-or polyarticular arthritis with effusions.[9] The knees, wrists and elbows are most often involved. Sore throat often follows the development of arthralgias. After 3-5 days of acute disease, fever spontaneously decreases and symptoms resolve within 2 weeks. In the absence of treatment, the disease may occasionally assume a relapsing course with episodes of fever occurring at irregular intervals for weeks or months. A predominant feature of *S. moniliformis* infection is development of chronic arthritis which persists for years. Complications include severe arthritis,[10] endocarditis, [12] pneumonia, periods of remission and exacerbation,[2] pericarditis,[3] septic infarcts and abscess formation including brain abscesses,[5,14] periarteritis nodosa[18] and amnionitis. [6]

DIAGNOSIS

In people with fever, rash and a history of rat-bite or close rodent contact, the differential diagnosis may be narrowed to leptospirosis, *S. moniliformis* or *S. minor* infection. Otherwise, the differential diagnosis will include Rocky Mountain spotted fever, meningococcal septicemia, erythema multiforme, Coxsackie virus and other viral infections. *S. minor* is suggested by suppuration at the bite site, a more lengthy incubation period and little or no joint symptoms. Precise diagnosis of rat-bite fever rests on identifying *S. moniliformis* by culture or *S. minor* by dark field examination or animal inoculation. Specific agglutinating antibody to *S. moniliformis* can develop in 10 days; titers of 1:80 are considered diagnostic. Agglutinin titers peak at 1-3 months and may persist for up to 2 years. Fluorescent antibody and complement fixation tests are available.[13] The marked pleomorphism of the organism may be observed directly in clinical specimens and can provide a clue to the diagnosis of *S. moniliformis* infection.[22]

THERAPY

Both etiologic agents of rat-bite fever are susceptible to penicillin, the drug of choice. Tetracycline, streptomycin, erythromycin, chloramphenicol and cephalothin have also been used with success. Tetracycline and streptomycin are active against L-forms of *S. moniliformis*.[5,6]

EPIDEMIOLOGY AND PATHOGENESIS

Up to 50% of healthy wild and laboratory rats harbor *S. moniliformis* in the oronasopharynx.[25] The organism has been isolated also from infected turkeys and guinea pigs, and found in consumable products such as raw milk (Haverhill fever). [7,14,17]

The incidence of rat-bite fever is highest in urban areas with poor sanitation and large rat populations. Children are more often infected than adults; those working in laboratories with rodents are also at risk.[1,19] Of the 13 cases reported between 1958 and 1983, 6 were associated with bites of laboratory rats. An outbreak among school children in Britain appears to be due to contaminated milk, but inability to isolate the organism from dairy products used at the school cast doubt on milk as the source.[16]

Infection is associated with the bite of a rat, mouse or other small rodent, with direct transmission of the organism through the break in the skin. Rat-bite fever has also been reported following close contact with cats, dogs, pigs, squirrels, and live or dead rats.[4,5] Other cases have no definite history of rodent or animal exposure and may represent examples of consuming food or liquids contaminated by rats, mice or other infected animals. Turkeys acquire the organisms after being exposed to or feeding on rats or mice and become potential foodborne sources of infection. Once having breached the skin, or the bowel in cases of ingestion-related infection, *S. moniliformis* replicates in situ, and, if not halted by local defense mechanisms, spreads hematogenously to virtually any distant site of the body.[13]

PUBLIC HEALTH SIGNIFICANCE, PREVENTION AND CONTROL

Rat-bite fever is an uncommon disease and, in the United States, generally occurs in laboratory personnel who handle rodents. Man is a dead-end host for the organism. Unpasteurized milk may be another source of *S. moniliformis*. In both major epidemics associated with *S. moniliformis* (Haverhill fever and the boarding school epidemic in Chelmsford, Essex, Britain), nonpasteurized milk likely contaminated with rat urine was consumed.[14] Preventive measures begin with rodent control programs, and consumption of raw milk should be avoided.

DIAGNOSTIC PROCEDURES

Selection and Processing of Specimens

Collect blood aseptically and mix with an equal volume of sterile 2.5% sodium citrate in a small sterile flask. Prepare blood films and stain with Gram, Wayson, Giemsa or acridine orange stain. Aseptically transfer the contents of the flask to sterile tubes and centrifuge for 30-45 min to pack the cells. Discard the supernatant. Use the sedimented cells to inoculate a freshly poured, solidified agar medium containing 15% rabbit serum. If ascitic fluid or serum enriched media are not available for primary isolation, use routine blood culture media and increase the volume of patient's blood to 20%.[11] However, blood culture media should not contain sodium polyanethol sulfonate. Put 0.1 mL of the sedimented cells in an equal volume of broth and transfer 0.1 mL of this cell suspension to the surface of the blood agar. Distribute the inoculum over the agar surface by tilting the plate. Inoculate two tubes of trypticase soy, tryptose phosphate or thioglycolate broth with the remaining cells. Incubate inoculated media in a candle jar or CO_2 incubator for 2-3 days at 35°C. If no growth is apparent, transfer 1 mL to fresh broth daily for 3 days. If growth is observed, remove a "puff ball" for subsequent transfer and microscopic examination.

Joint fluids should be citrated as for blood. Inoculate 2 tubes of broth with 1 mL or more of joint fluid per tube. Inoculate 0.1 mL of fluid onto fresh agar plates as for blood. Pus or exudate from a wound, cutaneous eruption or abscess should be examined microscopically and inoculated into broth and onto fresh agar plates as for joint fluids.

Microscopic Examination

Microscopic examination of clinical specimens with Brown-Hopp's tissue Gram stain, Giemsa, Gram or Wayson stains may demonstrate characteristic pleomorphism and provide a clue to the diagnosis of *S. moniliformis*. Examination of colonies from broth or agar plates may show short rods, long beaded filaments, chains of bacilli and coccobacillary forms.

Culture Procedures

In broth, growth appears as white granules referred to as "puff balls" or "bread crumbs." The growth is usually at the bottoms of the tube as discrete particles suspended in the broth or on the surface of sedimented red blood cells in blood cultures.[8] Daily subculture is required to maintain viability of the organisms. Young broth cultures or stock strains can be suspended in defibrinated blood, quick frozen and stored at -70°C.

Growth on solid media may take 1-2 weeks. High humidity in the incubation chamber is critical for survival of the organisms. Although subcultures may grow well aerobically and anaerobically, an increased concentration of CO_2 is generally required for primary isolation. Organisms remain viable for 3-7 days on solid media. Bacterial colonies may be seen on serum enriched media after 2-3 days of incubation. The bacterial colonies are 1-3 μm in diameter and tend to be round, smooth, white, glistening and butyrous in consistency. Surface colonies on sheep blood agar are similar in appearance and are nonhemolytic. L-phase colonies appear spontaneously several days after appearance of primary bacterial colonies and may be found within, adjacent to or beneath a primary colony. L-phase colonies are embedded in the agar and have a fried-egg configuration, with a dark center surrounded by a translucent zone containing swollen bodies and oil-like globules. L-phase colonies are indistinguishable from other L-phase, mycoplasmal or ureaplasmal colonies.

Growth And Biochemical Characteristics

S. moniliformis is aerobic and facultative. Blood, serum or ascitic fluid is required for growth. Growth does not occur and cannot be sustained in infusion, nutrient or other broths and agars unless they are supplemented with one of these body fluids. The optimal pH of media is 7.5. Growth does not occur at 23°C.

Biochemical tests for identification of streptobacillus require serum supplementation. The following reactions are positive: esculin may be hydrolyzed slightly; slight amounts of H_2S produced with lead acetate; alkaline phosphatase is produced; methylene blue is reduced anaerobically; and potassium tellurite and 2,3,5-triphenyltetrazolium chloride are reduced aerobically and anaerobically. Negative biochemical tests include gelatin liquification, casein or serum digestion, indole, acetylmethyl carbinol production, phenylalanine deamination, urea hydrolysis, nitrate reduction, oxidase, catalase, benzidine reactions and gluconate oxidation. Fermentation reactions are as follows: acid but no gas from glucose, maltose, dextran, glycogen and starch. Negative fermentation tests include: adonitol, cellobiose, dulcitol, glycerol, inositol, inulin, mannitol, melibiose, raffinose, rhamnose, sorbitol, sorbose and trehalose. [8,22]

Rowbotham[21] reported rapid identification of streptobacilli using fatty-acid profiles obtained by gas-liquid chromatography. The major peaks were palmitic (C16:0), linoleic (C18:2), oleic (C18:1) and stearic (C18:0).

SEROLOGY

Agglutinins may be detected in sera of patients with *S. moniliformis* infections. Acute and convalescent sera should be collected at least one week apart. Interpretation of agglutination tests may be difficult because of spontaneous clumping. Strain ATCC 14647 may be used for preparation of an agglutinogen or as antigen for preparation of rabbit antiserum. Consistent low titers of approximately 1:80 are not diagnostic of a recent infection because titers in this range may persist for at least two years.[2] L-phase varients share an antigen with the bacterial cell form but lack a second antigen present in the bacillary form.

Spirillum minor

Spirillum minor is also found in the blood, infected eye discharges and oropharynx of approximately 25% of rats. Cats, pigs and other animals that feed on rats may subsequently become infected and transmit the disease by bite or scratch. *S. minor* is a gram-negative, tightly coiled organism, 0.5 μm wide and 1.7 μm long, with 2-6 spirals and bipolar tufts of flagella. It is recognized by its morphology, characteristic darting motility on darkfield examination and pathogenicity for laboratory animals.[13,24]

CLINICAL MANIFESTATIONS

Clinical manifestations are similar to streptobacillary rat-bite fever. After an incubation period of 1-4 weeks, symptoms begin abruptly with fever and chills. Unlike streptobacillary rat-bite fever, myalgias are infrequent. The rodent bite heals by the time the patient is seen, but often regresses, becomes inflamed and proceeds to ulcerate. Both lymphangitis and local lymphadenopathy develop coincident with the onset of fever, headache, nausea, vomiting and myalgia. The rash associated with *S. minor*-induced rat-bite fever is usually generalized, with large reddish brown or blotchy purple macules and may appear as roseolar or urticarial lesions. The rash may spread from the area of the bite. Arthritis is rare. Fever subsides within hours but may return after a few days for short periods. Such episodes may continue for months or even years,[20] but in most patients, infection usually resolves spontaneously within 1-2 months, even after 6-8 of these brief relapses. In untreated cases, up to 6.5% of patients may die from this disease.[20]

Diagnosis

S. minor has not been isolated on artificial media but can be seen by darkfield microscopic examination of material from the local bite area, skin lesions, draining lymph nodes or blood. Animal inoculation is usually required for diagnosis. *S. minor* can be demonstrated in the blood or body fluids of mice, rats, guinea pigs or monkeys 1-3 weeks after intraperitoneal injection of clinical specimens from infected patients.[8] When organisms are scarce or not demonstrable in peritoneal fluid or blood, impression films of heart muscle stained with a spirochete silver impregnation stain may reveal numerous organisms. Specific serologic tests for diagnosis are not available.

S. minor is susceptible to penicillin; tetracycline may be used as an alternative drug for penicillin-sensitive individuals.[20]

REFERENCES

1. Anderson LC, Leary SL, Manning PJ. Rat-bite fever in animal research laboratory personnel. Lab Animal Sci 1983;33:292-4.
2. Brown TM, Nunemaker JC. Rat-bite fever. A review of the American cases with reevaluation of etiology; report of cases. Bull Johns Hopkin Hosp 1942;70:201-327.
3. Carbeck RB, Murphy TF, Britt EM. Streptobacillary rat-bite fever with massive pericardial effusion. JAMA 1967;201:703-4.
4. Cole JS, Stroll RW, Bulger RJ. Rite-bite fever. Ann Intern Med 1969;71:979-82.
5. Dijkmans BAC, Thomeer RTWM, Vielvoye GJ, Lampe AS, Mattie H. Brain abscess due to *Streptobaccillus moniliformis* and *Actinobacterium meyerii*. Infection 1984;12:262-4.
6. Faro S, Walker C, Pierson RL. Amnionitis with intact amniotic membranes involving *Streptobacillus moniliformis*. Obstet Gynecol 1980;55(Suppl):9-11.
7. Lambe DW, McPhedran AM, Mertz JA, et al. *Streptobacillus moniliformis* isolated from a case of Haverhill fever. Am J Clin Pathol 1973;60:854-60.
8. Rogesa M. *Streptobacillus moniliformis* and *Spirillum minor*. In: Lennette EH, Balows A, Hausler WJ Jr, Shadomy HJ, eds. Manual of clinical microbiology. 4th ed. Washington, DC: American Society for Microbiology, 1985:400-6.
9. Levaditi C, Selbie FR, Delorme M. Mode of transmission of infectious polyarticular rheumatism caused by *Streptobacillus moniliformis*. Crit Rev Soc Biol 1931;107:501-6.
10. Mandel DR. Streptobacillary fever, an unusual cause of infectious arthritis. Cleveland Clin 1985;51:203-5.

11. Martone WJ, Patton CM. Rat-bite fever. In: Balows A, Hausler WJ Jr, eds. Diagnostic procedures for bacterial, mycotic and parasitic infections. 6th ed. Washington, DC: American Public Health Association, 1981:581-6.
12. McCormack RC, Kaye D, Hook EW. Endocarditis due to *Streptobacillus moniliformis*. JAMA 1967;200:77-9.
13. Murray HW. *Streptobacillus moniliformis* (rat-bite fever). In: Mandell GL, Douglas RG, Bennett JE, eds. Principles and practice of infectious disease. 2nd ed. New York: John Wiley, 1985:1305-6,1349.
14. Oedig P, Alarson H. Streptothrix muris ratti (*Streptobacillus moniliformis*) isolated from a brain abscess. Arch Pathol Microbiol Scand 1950;27:436-9.
15. Parker F, Hudson NP. The etiology of Haverhill fever (erythema arthriticum epidemicum). Am J Pathol 1926;2:357-61.
16. Pilsworth R. Haverhill fever. Lancet 1983;2:336-7.
17. Portnoy BL, Satterwhite TK, Dyckman JK. Rat-bite fever misdiagnosed as Rocky Mountain spotted fever. South Med J 1979;72:607-9.
18. Prouty M, Schafer EL. Periarteritis nodosa associated with rat-bite fever due to *Streptobacillus moniliformis* (erythema arthriticum epidemicum). J Pediatr 1950;36:605-13.
19. Raffin BJ, Freemark M. Streptobacillary rat-bite fever: A pediatric problem. Pediatrics 1979;64:214-17.
20. Roughgarden JW. Antimicrobial therapy of rat-bite fever. Arch Intern Med 1965;116:39-54.
21. Rowbotham TJ. Rapid identification of *Streptobacillus moniliformis*. Lancet 1983;2:567-8.
22. Savage NL, Joiner GN, Florey DW. Clinical, microbiological and histological manifestations of *Streptobacillus moniliformis*-induced arthritis in mice. Infect Immun 1983;34:605-9.
23. Shanson DC, Gazzard BG, Midgley J, et al. *Streptobacillus moniliformis* isolated from blood in four cases of Haverhill fever. First outbreak in Britain. Lancet 1984;2:92-4.
24. Shanson DC, Pratt J, Greene P. Comparison of media with and without "Panmead" for the isolation of *Streptobacillus moniliformis* from blood cultures and observations on the inhibitory effect of sodium polyanethol sulphonate. J Med Microbiol 1985;19:181-6.
25. Strangeways WT. Rats as carriers of *Streptobacillus moniliformis*. J Pathol Bacteriol 1933;37:47-9.

CHAPTER 8

BORDETELLA INFECTIONS

Charlotte D. Parker, Ph.D. and Beverley J. Payne, M.P.H.

INTRODUCTION

Bordetella pertussis is a small, fastidious, gram-negative coccobacillus which parasitizes the human respiratory tract and causes whooping cough. This bacterium was first cultivated by Bordet and Gengou in 1906 on potato infusion agar containing blood and glycerol and Bordet-Gengou (BG) medium remains in wide use today. *B. pertussis* remains difficult to isolate and exacting in its cultural requirements. Whooping cough caused by *B. pertussis* may be a serious or sometimes fatal illness, especially in infants under one year of age. *B. parapertussis* may also cause whooping cough.

CAUSATIVE ORGANISMS

Genus *Bordetella* consists of three closely related species, *B. pertussis*, *B. parapertussis* and *B. bronchiseptica*,[23] and the less closely related *B. avium*.[17] These organisms are obligate aerobes characterized by an inability to attack sugars, a requirement for nicotinic acid or nicotinamide, and a 61-70 mol% guanine plus cytosine (G+C) ratio. Laboratory identification is based on morphology, growth properties, serologic properties and biochemical tests. *B. pertussis* and *B. parapertussis* are usually identified by direct fluorescent antibody (DFA) techniques, if growth characteristics, microscopic appearance and colonial morphology are typical. *B. bronchiseptica* and *B. avium* are nonfermentative bacilli, best identified by techniques standard for that group.

CLINICAL MANIFESTATIONS

The human respiratory tract is the only site from which *B. pertussis* and *B. parapertussis* have been isolated. By contrast, *B. bronchiseptica* is found most commonly in the respiratory tract of domestic and wild animals, although it may cause wound infections and may be transmitted to man.[23] *B. avium*, as proposed by Kersters et al[17] incorporates the *B. bronchiseptica*-like organisms. This species causes rhinotracheitis in turkeys, but has yet to be implicated in human infections.

Whooping cough is a localized infection of the upper respiratory tract, although pneumonia may occur. Following an incubation period of about one week, infected persons develop symptoms of a mild upper respiratory tract infection. This catarrhal stage persists about 1-2 weeks, with gradual development of more severe cough characteristic of the paroxysmal stage. Properly performed cultures are almost always positive at this time.[18] After 2-4 weeks the cough begins to subside, and a lengthy convalescent stage (weeks to several months) begins. Cultures are usually positive early in the paroxysmal stage, but become negative for 50-90% of persons by the end of this stage and are rarely positive during the convalescent stage. No evidence supports the existence of long term carriers, but inapparent infections in adults and in partially immune individuals may play a role in transmission.[13,14,20,21]

THERAPY

Antibiotics are useful in the treatment of whooping cough to reduce infectivity and thus break the transmission cycle, to possibly relieve symptoms and for prophylaxis in contacts. Antibiotics may shorten the course of disease if used early, but have little effect on symptoms if used late.[4,5] The most useful antimicrobials for treatment and prophylaxis are erythromycin and trimethoprim-sulfamethoxazole,[5,16] both because they can be given to infants and children and because of excellent activity against *B. pertussis*. Recent reports of failure of erythromycin to effect a bacteriological cure probably result from the use of forms of erythromycin other than the estolate ester or treatment for less than 14 days.[5] Several newer cephalosporins (cefoperazone and ceftriaxone) and imipenem may also be useful, according to in vitro studies.[3]

EPIDEMIOLOGY

The epidemiology of whooping cough has altered since near universal vaccination in infancy became standard practice.[21] Current vaccines are about 85% effective in preventing disease in children exposed in the home and ameliorate the severity of the illness in immunized children who become symptomatic. The recent experience of several European countries, however, suggests that when vaccine coverage of children declines, epidemics of whooping cough, including severe disease, follow.[13]

Reported cases of pertussis in the United States have averaged about 2000 per year,[7,10] but increased to nearly 4000 cases in 1985.[11] Whooping cough is almost entirely a childhood disease in unimmunized populations, but in the United States, significant numbers of cases occur in adults.[21] Infections are transmitted by the respiratory route and are limited to humans. Nearly all susceptible children exposed in an intimate setting, such as at home or in a nursery school class, will become infected and most will develop typical disease. Infection in adults may be typical, atypical or inapparent. In recent outbreaks, significant numbers of *B. parapertussis* have been recovered, often associated with *B. pertussis*.

PUBLIC HEALTH SIGNIFICANCE

Epidemic whooping cough is easily recognized because large numbers of typical cases occur in children. Laboratory confirmation, even of only a few cases, allows rapid intervention by health authorities. Vaccination campaigns, appropriate antibiotic therapy and prophylaxis, case finding, allocation of specific health resources and other standard public health approaches can then be applied. Large epidemics strain public health resources, however, and in the absence of adequate vaccination, control may not be possible.[13] Because deaths, serious sequelae and severe illnesses requiring hospital care occur during epidemics, prevention is a major public health consideration.

Endemic whooping cough presents a different set of problems for public health workers because diagnosis and laboratory confirmation can be difficult. Case finding and followup of sources of infection are slowed by the usual requirement of one week or more for confirmatory diagnosis by culture. Clinical diagnosis may be delayed by a low index of suspicion or by the nonspecific symptoms of mild and atypical whooping cough cases. The disease may be recognized only when children develop typical coughing paroxysms. The success of health authorities in detecting endemic whooping cough is strongly correlated with both the appropriateness of their techniques and their interest in the problem.

DIAGNOSTIC PROCEDURES

Selection and Processing of Specimens

Successful laboratory confirmation of a clinical diagnosis of pertussis is directly related to the suitability of the respiratory tract samples. The specimen of choice in most settings for both direct fluorescent antibody (DFA) tests and culture is duplicate pernasal nasopharyngeal swabs (Fig.

8:1). These specimens are obtained with tiny calcium alginate swabs on fine flexible wire (Ultrafine Calgiswab, Inolex Corp. or equivalent). Cotton-tipped swabs are known to be detrimental to pertussis organisms and should not be used.

The specimen is obtained by immobilizing the patient's head, gently inserting the swab into the nostril until it reaches the posterior nares and allowing it to remain there a few seconds. The tickling sensation of the

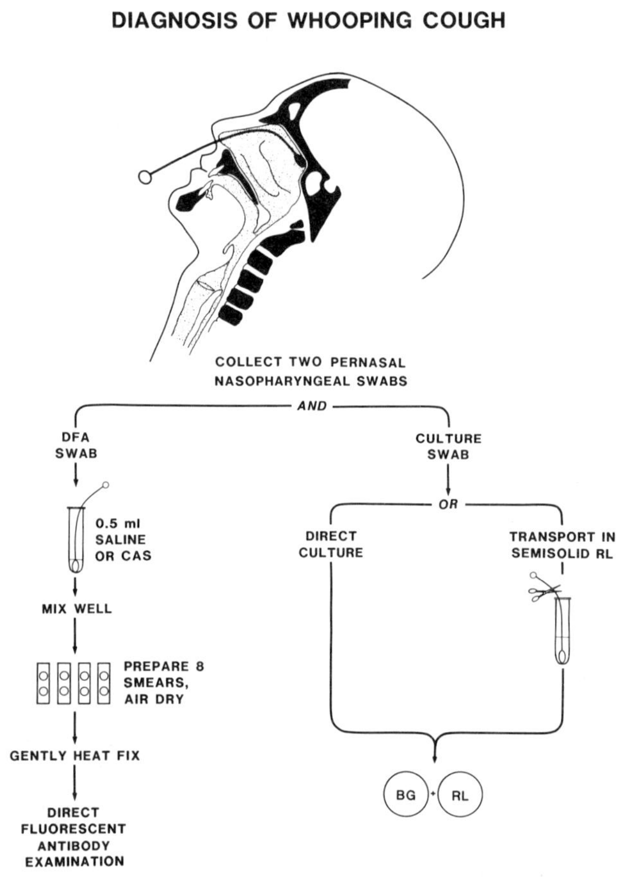

FIGURE 8:1. Recommended protocol for diagnosis of whooping cough. The proper placement of the swab for collection of a nasopharyngeal specimen is shown, although the size of the calcium alginate tip is exaggerated for clarity. Two swabs should be obtained, one for DFA examination and one for culture. BG = Bordet-Gengou medium; CAS = 1% casein hydrolysate; DFA = direct fluorescent antibody technique; RL = Regan-Lowe plating or transport medium. (Modified from reference 22, with permission.)

swab will usually induce a cough. If resistance is encountered during insertion of the swab, the other nostril should be tried. One of two swabs collected should be used for preparation of DFA slides and the other for culture.

Although the collection of throat swabs at the time nasopharyngeal swabs are taken has been shown to increase the number of positive cultures, throat swabs should not be used in place of nasopharyngeal swabs. Bronchial or nasopharyngeal secretions obtained by washings or aspiration, transtracheal aspirates, etc., may be superior specimens.[22] However, by far the more adaptable technique for specimen collection is pernasal nasopharyngeal swabs, and these should be substituted when "cough plates" are requested.

Time of Collection:

The earlier in the course of the disease specimens can be obtained the better the chances for laboratory confirmation by DFA, culture or both. Decreases in the percentage of positive laboratory results occur after the initial 3 weeks of illness or after antibiotics have been instituted.[8,14,18] In our experience, specimens transported in Regan-Lowe medium are rarely positive by culture if the patient has received prior antibiotic treatment.

Transport of Specimens for Culture:

If at all feasible, direct plating of specimens at bedside onto freshly made BG and Regan-Lowe (RL) plates is the most reliable culture technique. This is especially important for patients previously treated with antibiotics. However, if bedside culturing is not feasible, transporting the swab to the laboratory in RL transport medium has been very successful.[22,24]

The specimen swab is pushed into the soft agar and left submerged during transport to the laboratory.[24] Full strength RL in slant form has also been used successfully for transport.[25]

The relative success of holding inoculated transport media at various temperatures (35°C, room temperature, 4°C) is not known with certainty. However, room temperature appears to be the most detrimental to the survival of *B. pertussis*. Ideally, specimen transport for up to 48 h at 4°C will preserve viable *B. pertussis* and minimize overgrowth by other organisms.

Specimens for Microscopy:

Place a second nasopharyngeal swab in 0.25-0.5 mL of 1.0% casein hydrolysate to be used to prepare smears for microscopy.

Rapid Methodology

Direct fluorescent antibody (DFA) microscopy is the most rapid laboratory test available and has proven valuable for diagnosis in children with severe upper respiratory illness. However, because results (both positive and negative) are presumptive, DFA should be used in conjunction with culture. The use of DFA in parallel with cultural procedures will greatly enhance the chances of a positive result.[9,10,25] While the sensitivity of culturing is strongly dependent on sampling and transport conditions, the success of DFA is more directly related to the experience of the microscopist. Pertussis DFA stains are inherently difficult to interpret; therefore, laboratories not routinely performing this procedure should prepare smears and refer them to an experienced laboratory.[6,15]

The nasopharyngeal swab transported in casein hydrolysate should be agitated with a vortex mixer or shaken vigorously for 20 s before being used to prepare smears. Prepare 4-8 smears. Drops of fluid may be added repeatedly to the slide and dried down to increase the amount of material examined. The fluid should be applied so that the smear is visible but not opaque upon drying. Smears that are too thin may yield false negative results, but very thick smears are extremely difficult to read. After smears have air-dried and are heat-fixed, they are then ready for either staining or mailing to a reference laboratory. Smears may be stored desiccated in the cold for up to 6 months.

Some laboratories prefer to prepare smears directly from the nasopharyngeal swabs (personal communication, T. Kurzynski). This method has the advantage of placing mucus strands directly on the slide and often *B. pertussis* cells are attached to these strands. However, it also limits the numbers of smears that can be prepared and allows less control of the thickness of the smear.

For DFA staining, use both *B. pertussis* and *B. parapertussis* antisera. (Difco Laboratories' antisera is the only commercially available sera in the United States in March, 1987. Other commercial antisera may become available but should be thoroughly tested before being put into use.) Fluorescein isothiocyanate-conjugated negative control antiserum is unavailable, but because both fluoresceinated anti-*B. pertussis* (pertussis-conjugate) and fluoresceinated anti-*B. parapertussis* (parapertussis-conjugate) antisera show a high degree of specificity, routinely read the pertussis-conjugate stained smear against the parapertussis-conjugate stained smear as the control for nonspecific fluorescence. Each conjugate should be titered against thin smears of stock *B. pertussis* and *B. parapertussis* to obtain the correct working dilution, following directions in the package insert. The following techniques may need to be modified for use with other antisera. The protocol for performing DFA stains is as follows (adapted from reference 22, with permission):

1. Add a drop of the working dilution of the appropriate conjugate to each smear and spread the conjugate to cover. Stain two patient smears with pertussis-conjugate (to permit examination of adequate material) and one patient smear with parapertussis-conjugate).

2. Place slides in a moist chamber for 30 min.
3. Tap off excess conjugate, rinse gently with phosphate-buffered saline, and allow slides to stand for 10 min in individual containers of phosphate-buffered saline, pH 7.6. (Coplin jars work well to prevent cross-contamination.)
4. Remove slides, rinse both sides gently with distilled water, and allow to air-dry.
5. Add 1 drop of mounting fluid, pH 9.0, and a cover slip to each smear and examine under oil immersion.
6. Hold duplicate smears for possible Gram stain, repeat DFA, or both. Directions for preparing phosphate-buffered saline and mounting fluid are found in the Appendix, Chapter 45, "Media, Reagents and Stains."

Thin smears of quality control strains of *B. pertussis* and *B. parapertussis* should be included in each run as controls. *B. pertussis* smears are stained with pertussis-conjugate and parapertussis-conjugate, while *B. parapertussis* smears are stained with parapertussis-conjugate only. For a valid test, both *B. pertussis*/pertussis-conjugate and *B. parapertussis*/parapertussis-conjugate slides must be strongly positive and the *B. pertussis*/parapertussis conjugate slide must be negative.

Morphological characteristics most closely resembling those typically found in clinical material are observed when stock strains of *B. pertussis* and *B. parapertussis* are grown on antibiotic-free BG medium for 24 hours. (A number of control smears may be prepared at one time and stored desiccated in the cold. Preferred quality control strains of *B. pertussis* and *B. parapertussis* are recent clinical isolates, transferred only a few times, and maintained by lyophilization or freezing at −70°C in blood.)

Patient smears are methodically examined under oil immersion with a fluorescence microscope for brightly fluorescing, very small coccobacilli that may occur singly, in pairs or occasionally in small clusters. Both *B. pertussis* and *B. parapertussis* fluoresce a bright yellow-green with clean-cut periphery and dimly stained to unstained centers (ovoid doughnut appearance). DFA showing organisms with questionable morphology and/or fluorescence, or organisms that fluoresce with both conjugates are reported as "*B. pertussis* or *B. parapertussis* not found." Questionable morphology can, at times, be resolved with a Gram stain of one of the remaining smears. Nonspecific staining with gram-negative diplococci, gram-positive cocci, *Haemophilus*, and diphtheroids has been observed[22] (personal observations).

Primary Isolation and Culture

Because of its specialized growth requirements, we recommend two specific media for culture of *B. pertussis*. Bordet-Gengou (BG) has been the medium of choice for many years. However, in 1977, Regan and Lowe reported the use of selective charcoal media for the transport and isolation of *B. pertussis* and *B. parapertussis*.[24] Workers in the United States and Canada have had good results with the Regan-Lowe formulation, both for isolation and for transport.[15,24,25] (personal communications, E. Dodd; T. Kurzynski; M. Wallace)

The use of two media, BG without antibiotics and RL with antibiotics, provides the broadest capabilities for the isolation of *B. pertussis*. One study comparing isolation on RL to that with commercially prepared BG showed RL to be vastly superior to BG (25/25 positive with RL vs 4/25 positive with BG).[12] However, the experience of others with freshly prepared BG and RL has shown these media to be almost equivalent, although occasional isolates will grow on one medium and not the other[1] (personal communications, T. Kurzynski; M. Wallace). Some formulations of commercial BG base include peptones which inhibit growth of clinical isolates of *B. pertussis*, or these formulae lack sufficient potato extract to reproducibly support growth of clinical isolates. Additionally, use of Oxoid charcoal agar (CM119) is required for success with RL medium. (See recommended BG and RL formulations in Chapter 45, "Media, Regents and Stains.") BG should be freshly poured just before use to minimize drying. A practical suggestion might be to purchase or to prepare tubes of appropriate BG base medium which can be held refrigerated, then melted, cooled and supplemented with blood for preparation of plates as cultures are requested. This technique offers the advantage of long shelf life and acceptible isolation rates. *B. pertussis* and *B. parapertussis* colonies are more easily differentiated from other growth on BG because of their partial hemolysis.

RL plates have longer shelf life than BG; however, colonies of *B. pertussis* and *B. parapertussis* on RL are more difficult for the inexperienced bacteriologist to recognize. A transparent medium which lacks blood and charcoal but incorporates methylated beta-cyclodextrin has recently been reported by Japanese workers to be useful,[2] but has yet to be evaluated in the United States.

B. pertussis is very fastidious and its successful isolation from clinical material can be affected by a number of factors. Improper sampling, either by technique or timing, transport delay, drying and exposure to improper temperatures are among the most critical problems. If transport and processing of the sample is rapid (no more than one hour), the swabs can be immersed in 0.25-0.5 mL sterile casein hydrolysate and kept cold. When received in the laboratory, specimens are agitated and 0.1 to 0.2 mL of fluid is streaked onto BG and RL media. Plates are then incubated upright for 24 h to allow the fluid to be absorbed. When specimens will be in transport longer than an hour, the swab should be submerged in RL transport medium and maintained at 4°C. In the laboratory, the swab is removed from the soft agar, streaked onto BG and RL plates, then returned to the transport medium. The swab in transport medium is incubated for 48 h at 35°C for enrichment and then replated on BG and RL plates.

All plates should be incubated in an atmosphere of increased humidity at 35°C. Although elevated CO_2 has no effect on growth, candle jars provide the necessary humidity in a convenient manner. Because *B. pertussis* grows so slowly, plates should be examined for 7 days before being discarded. Isolation is more rapid on nonselective media such as BG, but selective media like RL are invaluable for situations where small numbers of organisms would be quickly overgrown. *B. parapertussis* will grow slowly on blood and nutrient agars, whereas clinical isolates of *B. pertussis* will not. *B. bronchiseptica* and *B. avium* are even less fastidious, growing more rapidly and being easily isolated on routine laboratory media.

No matter which approach a laboratory chooses, it is important to use two primary plates, one with and one without antibiotics. Selective plates used in conjunction with RL transport medium should contain the same antibiotic. Some laboratories have reported an 8-10% increase in positive cultures when RL transport medium is incubated for 48 h at 35°C and replated,[24] (personal communication, T. Kurzynski), but other laboratories have recovered few or no additional isolates from 48 hours of enrichment (personal communications, J. Barbaree; E. Dodd; M. Wallace). For maximum productivity, laboratories forced to economize on culture protocols should retain two primary plates (BG and RL) and discontinue the second plating.

Methods of Identification

Microscopic colonies of *B. pertussis* may appear as early as 48 h on nonselective media but rarely are clinical isolates visible to the naked eye before the 3rd day. To insure as rapid a report as possible, plates should be examined with a dissecting microscope under oblique illumination. Colonies characteristically appear 1-2 days later on media containing antibiotics than on nonselective media. Colonies of *B. pertussis* on BG are tiny and glistening, resembling a bisected pearl, and usually have a hazy zone of hemolysis. On RL plates, colonies are round, domed, shiny, compact and may exhibit a tendency to run together slightly.

B. parapertussis and *B. bronchiseptica* colonies resemble *B. pertussis* colonies on BG medium but appear earlier and develop more quickly. Once developed, *B. parapertussis* colonies are duller and have a more distinct beta hemolysis than *B. pertussis*, and may show a slight brownish color. On RL, *B. parapertussis* colonies are grayer and less domed. Colonies of *B. bronchiseptica* on BG develop macroscopically in 24 h. Colonies are well developed at 48 h, and exhibit a rough surface that is pitted like beaten metal. *B. bronchiseptica* grows rapidly on RL, exhibiting large colonies with a nonhomogeneous appearance and putrid odor.

Typical colonies on BG or RL media should be Gram stained. Bordetellae are gram-negative coccobacilli, 0.2-0.5 μm by 0.5-2.0 μm, that exhibit a slow uptake of safranin. It is recommended that the safranin counterstain be left on for 2 min to increase resolution of the cells.[23] Cells occur singly, in pairs or small clumps, and may appear more pleomorphic (with filaments or thick bacillary forms) from old cultures or media containing antibiotics. *B. pertussis* is small and usually more coccobacillary, while *B. parapertussis* is usually more rod-shaped and may exhibit palisading. On Gram stains, *B. bronchiseptica* and *B. avium* more closely resemble enteric rods. Because bordetellae are relatively inert biochemically, identification of *B. pertussis* and *B. parapertussis* is usually confirmed by serologic tests (such as fluorescent antibody staining) and growth characteristics. Table 8:1 summarizes the pertinent biochemical differences between the species.[17,22,23]

Serologic Tests

Serologic tests useful for clinical diagnosis are not available. Both agglutination tests and enzyme immunoassays using pure antigens for antibody detection may be performed,[19] but standardization and availability of reagents is poor and interpretation is difficult.

Table 8:1. Properties of *Bordetella* Species*

Characteristic	*B. pertussis*	*B. parapertussis*	*B. bronchiseptica*	*B. avium*
Involved in respiratory infections	+†	+	+	+
Recovered from wounds	−	−	+	NK
Visible growth on:‡				
BG	3–6 days	1–3 days	1–2 days	1–2 days
CA/BA/IA	−	1–3 days	1–2 days	1–2 days
MAC	−	−	+	+
Christensen urea	−	+ (24 h)§	+ (4 h)§	−
Triple sugar iron	No change	No change	No change	No change
Motility	−	−	+	+‖
Nitrate	−	−	+	−¶
Simmons citrate	−	+	+	+
Brown pigment on Heart Infusion-tyrosine agar**	−	+	−	−

* Key identifying features to differentiate *Bordetella* spp. are given.[17,22,23] Other tests negative for all species include anaerobic growth, carbohydrate fermentation, gelatin, esculin, indole production, phosphatase, and starch and casein hydrolysis. Catalase is variable for *B. pertussis*, but positive for the other species, while oxidase by the sensitive Kovac's method is negative only for *B. parapertussis*.

† + = positive; − = negative; NK = not known.

‡ BG = Bordet-Gengou agar; CA = chocolate agar with 5–7% CO_2; BA = blood agar; IA = infusion agar; MAC = MacConkey agar.

§ Indicates hours required for positive test using a heavy inoculum.

‖ Motility better at 25°C.

¶ Nitrate positive only if media supplemented with serum and/or NAD.

** Heart Infusion Tyrosine agar is commercial heart infusion agar supplemented with 1 g/liter L-tyrosine.

EVALUATION OF LABORATORY FINDINGS

Considerable judgment is involved in evaluating laboratory reports regarding diagnosis of pertussis. The only diagnostic absolute is culture positivity. For a variety of reasons (including adequacy of specimens, availability of suitable transport media, availability and freshness of plating media, time since symptoms appeared, previous antibiotic treatment, vaccination status), negative cultures do not rule out pertussis. Controversy exists as to whether children with typical symptoms and negative cultures have pertussis or viral infections. Direct evidence to resolve this issue may be hard to obtain, but culture of the parents and all contacts with symptomatic upper respiratory tract infections is recommended. One or more of these persons will have a positive culture if the illness is whooping cough. With the current availability of adequate transport medium, cultural diagnosis should become routine.

Serological diagnosis suffers from many of the same problems and drawbacks as cultural diagnosis. In antigen detection tests, such as DFA, both false-positive and false-negative tests may occur; but error is minimized by referring smears to experienced readers. Some sources of error are intrinsic in the method. Animal sera may react with normal flora organisms of the nasopharynx, either immunospecifically or through nonspecific binding of immunoglobulins, to give false positives. False-negative DFA tests approach 40%, and may result from small numbers of organisms in the specimens, previous antibiotic therapy or the general insensitivity of this method.

REFERENCES

1. Ahmad F, Calder MA. Isolation of *Bordetella pertussis*: benefits of using both Bordet-Gengou and charcoal agar media. J Clin Pathol 1984;37:1071-7.
2. Aoyama T, Murase Y, Iwata T, et al. Comparison of blood-free medium (cyclodextrin solid medium) with Bordet-Gengou medium for clinical isolation of *Bordetella pertussis*. J Clin Microbiol 1986;23:1046-8.
3. Bannatyne RM, Cheung R. Susceptibility of *Bordetella pertussis* to cephalosporin derivatives and imipenem. Antimicrobial Agents Chemother 1984;26:604-5.
4. Baraff LJ, Wilkins J, Wehrle PF. The role of antibiotics, immunization and adenoviruses in pertussis. Pediatrics 1978;61:224-30.
5. Bass JW. Pertussis: current status of prevention and treatment. Pediatr Infect Dis 1985;4:614-19.
6. Broome CV, Fraser DW, English WJ II. Pertussis-diagnostic methods and surveillance. In: Manclark CR, Hill JC, eds. International symposium on pertussis. Bethesda, MD: U.S. Department of Health, Education and Welfare 1979:19-22; publication no. (NIH)79-1830.
7. Centers for Disease Control. Pertussis surveillance, 1979-1981. Morbid Mortal Weekly Rep 1982;31:333-6.
8. Centers for Disease Control. Pertussis-Maryland, 1982. Morbid Mortal Weekly Rep 1983;32:297-300.

9. Centers for Disease Control. Pertussis outbreak-Oklahoma. Morbid Mortal Weekly Rep 1984;33:2-10.
10. Centers for Disease Control. Pertussis-United States, 1982 and 1983. Morbid Mortal Weekly Rep 1984;33:573-5.
11. Centers for Disease Control. Pertussis surveillance-United States, 1984 and 1985. Morbid Mortal Weekly Rep 1987;36:168-71.
12. Chan F, Rossier E, MacKenzie A, Camus A. Superiority of charcoal-cephalexin-blood agar for the isolation of *Bordetella pertussis* [Abstract]. Annual meeting of the American Society for Microbiology. Washington, DC: American Society for Microbiology, 1983:355.
13. Cherry JD. The epidemiology of pertussis and pertussis immunization in the United Kingdom and the United States: a comparative study. Curr Problems in Pediatr 1984;14:7-77.
14. Field LH, Parker CD. Pertussis outbreak in Austin and Travis County, Texas, 1975. J Clin Microbiol 1977;6:154-160.
15. Gilligan PH, Fisher MC. Importance of culture in laboratory diagnosis of *Bordetella pertussis* infections. J Clin Microbiol 1984;20:891-3.
16. Immunization Practices Advisory Committee (ACIP). Diphtheria, tetanus and pertussis: guidelines for vaccine prophylaxis and other preventive measures. Morbid Mortal Weekly Rep 1985;34:405-26.
17. Kersters K, Hinz K-H, Hertle A, et al. *Bordetella avium* sp. nov., isolated from the respiratory tracts of turkeys and other birds. Int J Syst Bacteriol 1984;34:56-70.
18. Linneman CC, Bass JW. *Bordetella* infections. In: Balows A, Hausler WJ Jr., eds. Diagnostic procedures for bacterial, mycotic and parasitic infections. 6th ed. Washington, DC: American Public Health Association, 1981:249-60.
19. Manclark CR, Meade BD, Burstyn DG. Serological response to *Bordetella pertussis*. In: Rose NR, Friedman H, Fahey JL, eds. Manual of clinical laboratory immunology. Washington, DC: American Society for Microbiology, 1986:388-94.
20. Mertsola J, Kuronen T, Turunen A., et al. Diagnosis of pertussis. J Infect 1984;8:149-56.
21. Nelson JD. The changing epidemiology of pertussis in young infants: The role of adults as reservoirs of infection. Am J Dis Child 1978;132:371-3.
22. Parker CD, Payne BJ. *Bordetella*. In: Lennette EH, Balows A, Hausler WJ Jr, Shadomy HJ, eds. Manual of clinical microbiology. 4th ed. Washington, DC: American Society for Microbiology, 1985:394-9.
23. Pittman M. Genus *Bordetella*. In: Krieg NR, Holt JG, eds. Bergey's manual of systematic bacteriology; vol 1. Baltimore: Williams and Wilkins, 1985:388-93.
24. Regan J, Lowe F. Enrichment medium for the isolation of *Bordetella*. J Clin Microbiol 1977;6:303-9.
25. Shayegani M, Brisebois PR, Schoonmaker DJ, Masley-Hannett ME. *Bordetella pertussis* in New York state, 1972-1982. New York State J Med 1986;86:129-32.

CHAPTER 9

BORRELIOSIS

Karen Sue C. Kehl, Ph.D.

CAUSATIVE ORGANISM

Borrelia spp. are members of the family *Spirochaetaceae*, order *Spirochaetales*.[17] *Borrelia recurrentis* is carried by the body and head lice, *Pediculus humanus corporis* and *P. humanus capitis*, and causes epidemic relapsing fever in man. Tickborne or endemic relapsing fever is caused by *Borrelia* carried by *Ornithodoros* (soft-shelled) ticks. Species identification of these *Borrelia* is difficult. Their ability to undergo antigenic variation precludes serologic diagnosis and the inability to culture the organism has until recently, prevented biochemical identification. Their morphologic characteristics are also similar, therefore species identification has been based upon the vector. Table 9:1 lists common *Borrelia* species, their vectors and geographic locations.[17] Relapsing fever is endemic in the western United States and is caused by *Borrelia hermsii, B. parkeri* and *B. turicatae* whose vectors are *Ornithodoros hermsi, O. parkeri* and *O. turicata*, respectively.[8] Recent determination of DNA base contents (guanine plus cytosine) and DNA homology for these three species of *Borrelia* suggest that they are actually a single species,[12] local variants of which have adapted to different hosts. At this time, however, *Borrelia* are still identified to species level according to their tick vector.

Borrelia burgdorferii is a newly described species of *Borrelia* which causes Lyme disease in man.[5,14,21] Analysis of DNA base contents and DNA homology studies have shown that this is indeed a new and distinct species.[12,18] It is also tick-borne, being carried by the *Ixodes* (hard-shelled) tick.

Nonvector-borne *Borrelia* have been isolated from the mucous membranes of man. *Borrelia vincentii* is believed to cause fusospirochaetal infections, one of which is Vincent's angina. *Borrelia buccalis* has also been isolated

Table 9:1. Relapsing Fever *Borrelia*

Borrelia	Vector	Geographic Location
B. recurrentis	*Pediculus humanus corporis* *P. humanus capitis*	Cosmopolitan
Crocidurae Group *B. crocidurae* *B. merionesi* *B. microti*	*Ornithodoros erraticus*	Central Africa Turkey Iran
B. duttonii	*O. moubata*	Africa
B. hermsii	*O. hermsii*	Western USA and Canada
B. hispanica	*O. erraticus erraticus*	Spain, Portugal, N. Africa
B. mazzottii	*O. talaje*	South America
B. parkeri	*O. parkeri*	Western USA
B. persica	*O. tholozani*	Central Asia
B. turicatae	*O. turicata*	Southwestern USA
B. venezuelensis	*O. rudis*	Central and South America

from the mucous membranes of the mouth and *Borrelia refringins* from the genitalia. These latter organisms are not believed to be pathogenic for man.[8]

Borrelia are 10-20 μm in length and 0.2-0.5 μm in width with sharply pointed ends (Figure 9:1). They have 5-10 coarse uneven, irregular spirals with a wavelength of 2-3 μm and an amplitude of 1 μm.[17] The cells are surrounded by two triple-layered membranes; a foamy elastic envelope consists of protein and lipids.[11] The specific antigen responsible for serotype specificity and capable of undergoing antigenic variation is located in the outer envelope.[1,15,24] The inner cytoplasmic membrane consists of glucosamine, galactosamine and muramic acid.[8]

Fifteen to 20 parallel fibrils (flagella) are inserted subterminally, coil around the body and intertwine in the middle causing a corkscrew-like motility. They are located between the cytoplasmic membrane and the outer envelope.[17] The flagellar structure is similar to that of other spirochetes and gram-positive bacteria.[13]

The cytoplasm contains ribosomes, mesosomes and a nuclear region. The organisms have no mitrochondria and no undulating membrane. Cell division occurs by transverse fission.[17]

Only recently has it been possible to cultivate a few of the species of *Borrelia*.[16] These organisms cannot synthesize long-chain fatty acids and

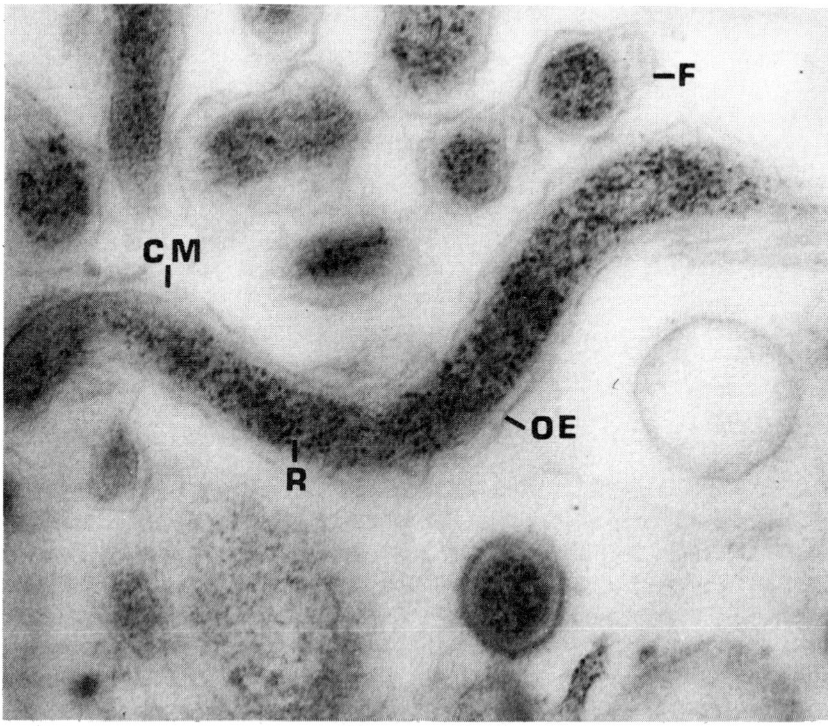

FIGURE 9:1. Electron micrograph of *Borrelia turicatae* (X37,200). CM = cell membrane, OE = outer envelope, F = flagella, R = ribosomes.

thus require them for growth. Energy metabolism occurs via glycolysis with lactic acid as the sole major product of glucose metabolism. Some species have been shown to ferment maltose, starch and trehalose in addition to glucose.[13] *Borrelia* are microaerophilic and grow optimally at 28-30°C in Kelly's medium or one of its numerous modifications. The most recent modification of BSK medium allows the growth of the North American borreliae as well as *B. burgdorferii*.[2,3,15]

CLINICAL MANIFESTATIONS AND EPIDEMIOLOGY

Relapsing Fever

Several species of *Borrelia* cause disease in man known as relapsing fever. The clinical course consists of an incubation period, the first attack phase and relapses. The incubation period is 2-15 days with an average of

5-9 days for both louseborne and tickborne disease. Disease is characterized by sudden onset of shaking chills, high fever, headache, aching muscles and joints and abdominal pain, the latter being associated with a rapidly enlarging liver and spleen. There is some dizziness, thirst, cough and difficult breathing.

Laboratory results at this time are indicative of liver damage. There is thrombocytopenia and anemia. The prothrombin and partial thromboplastin times are increased. Transient proteinuria, hematuria and red blood cell casts indicative of renal damage may be present.

The initial period of fever is terminated within 7 days by crisis, characterized by abrupt onset of chills, sweating and weakness. The temperature and blood pressure drop; hypotensive shock is not uncommon. *Borrelia* are found in the blood during the attack phase and disappear with the onset of crisis. This Jarisch-Herxheimer-like reaction is believed to be due to the release of endogenous pyrogens from leukocytes as they engulf spirochetes killed by either antibodies or antibiotics.

The temperature and blood pressure return to normal within 8 hours. After a 5-9 day period of normalcy, a relapse with return of fever and other clinical manifestations occurs. Relapses are of shorter duration and decreasing severity. They too terminate in crisis. Complications are common and include cardiac and hepatic failure, cerebral edema, shock and disseminated intravascular coagulation (DIC).[8,20]

Louseborne relapsing fever is characterized by febrile phases of longer duration and few, if any, relapses. The lice cannot transmit *B. recurrentis* to their progeny but they pass the organism from man to man.[8] This disease has been reported from all over the world except Antarctica, and is associated with crowding, lack of cleanliness, poor housing and undernourishment. These conditions are evident during wars and natural disasters, which explains the occurrence of epidemics at such times.[19]

Tickborne relapsing fever has febrile phases of short duration and as many as 4-5 relapses. Tickborne disease is more severe and prolonged than louseborne, lasting 3 weeks to 7 months.[8] Ticks conserve the *Borrelia*, passing them transoverially to their progeny. It is believed that tickborne *Borrelia* were originally parasites of small rodents and were transferred by ticks to man, thus man is an accidental host. The infection is restricted to visitors of tick-infested areas. In the United States, the disease is endemic in Arizona, Colorado, California, Oregon, Texas, and possibly Utah, Montana and Washington.[7]

Lyme Disease

Lyme disease is an immune-mediated, inflammatory disorder which occurs after the bite of the *Ixodes* (hard-shelled) tick. The incubation period ranges from 3 to 30 days. The disease begins with a characteristic skin lesion;

erythema chronicum migrans (ECM). In some patients, the disease remains localized to the skin lesion; however, in most patients it disseminates. Secondary lesions, meningeal irritation, migratory musculoskeletal pain, hepatitis and lymphadenopathy are seen. Regardless of treatment, these symptoms fade within 3-4 weeks. Weeks to months later, neurologic and cardiac abnormalities may occur. Meningitis, cranial neuropathy and peripheral radiculoneuropathy lasting several months are seen in about 15% of patients. About 8% of patients develop cardiac involvement, most commonly, some degree of heart block which lasts several weeks. Weeks to years later, 60% of patients develop arthritis. Early in the disease, it is manifest as migratory musculoskeletal pain. Months after the onset of illness, frank arthritis is seen. The clinical manifestations of Lyme disease vary from mild disease with skin lesions alone to severe disease involving skin, nerves, heart and joints simultaneously.[22]

European erythema migrans disease, lymphocytoma and acrodermatitis chronica are associated with the bite of *Ixodes ricinus* ticks and resemble Lyme disease. Patients may experience cardiac, nervous and joint abnormalities as well.[25] Many patients demonstrate high antibody titers to the *Ixodes dammini* spirochete, *B. burgdorferii*.[4]

Lyme disease transmitted by *I. ricinus* has been reported in the Scandinavian countries, England, Scotland and all of the countries of western Europe. In the United States, it is endemic in 16 states including Connecticut, New York, New Jersey, Maryland, Minnesota and Wisconsin, where it is transmitted by *I. dammini*. In California, Oregon and Utah, Lyme disease is transmitted by *I. pacificus*.[6]

TREATMENT AND PREVENTION

Relapsing Fever

Prompt defervescence and prevention of relapse can be accomplished through the use of a variety of antibiotics; tetracycline and chloramphenicol being the most effective. The usual recommended dosage is 0.5 g every 6 h for 5-10 days.[13,20]

A Jarisch-Herxheimer-like reaction with chills, fever and a drop in blood pressure usually occurs within 2 hours of treatment and corresponds to the clearing of spirochetes. This same reaction is seen during the crisis of untreated patients and after the treatment of primary and secondary syphilis.

Prevention of epidemic relapsing fever requires elimination of the vector. Good personal hygiene, avoidance of overcrowding and delousing procedures have worked in the past to eliminate the lice. Prevention of the spread of lice by enforcing sanitary measures is essential.

Prevention of endemic relapsing fever requires avoidance of the *Ornitho-*

dorous ticks. Their varied hosts and geographic location make eradication almost impossible. Avoidance of known tick infested areas and the use of insect repellant on persons and clothing may decrease the chance of exposure.

Lyme Disease

Tetracycline, 250 mg four times a day, is the drug of choice for adults with early Lyme disease. Phenoxymethyl penicillin, 500 mg 4 times a day and erythromycin, 250 mg 4 times a day are alternative choices. In each instance, the drug should be continued for 10 days or up to 20 days if symptoms persist. ECM resolves sooner and there are fewer relapses in tetracycline- or penicillin-treated patients than in those given erythromycin.[22] Major late complications (myocarditis, meningoencephalitis and recurrent arthritis) have not been seen in patients treated with tetracycline, whereas 8% of penicillin-treated patients and 14% of erythromycin-treated patients did develop major complications. Treatment of major late complications with high doses of intravenous penicillin has been effective. Minor late complications (headache or pain in joints, tendons or muscles) have been seen in nearly half of all patients regardless of treatment.[22]

Immature ticks (nymphs) feed primarily in May through June and transmit the spirochete at this time. The larvae feed in August and are infected with the spirochete during feeding. The nymphal stage of the tick is primarily responsible for disease transmission. The adult ticks prefer the white-tailed deer as a host. The increased frequency of Lyme disease has been linked to the increased abundance of deer.

In one study, removal of the preferred adult host, the deer, did not show a corresponding decrease in the number of larvae or infected nymphs the following spring.[27] Therefore, prevention of Lyme disease requires avoidance of the *Ixodes* tick. The use of insect repellant as well as prompt tick-removal before attachment may decrease the likelihood of disease transmission.

DIAGNOSTIC PROCEDURES

Specimen Collection

Specific diagnostic procedures are essential to confirm the diagnosis of relapsing fever and Lyme disease. Specimens must be collected before appropriate therapy has been initiated. *Borrelia* are present in the blood stream in large numbers during the initial attack of relapsing fever; relapses show a decreasing number of organisms. The organisms are not present during afebrile periods while bizarre forms are found during crisis. Therefore, blood should be collected during the initial attack phase and successive relapses. Blood (heparinized or citrated) should be collected for thick and thin smears and for culture of the organism. Serum, cerebrospinal fluid and joint fluid (if indicated) should also be collected. Tissue specimens, including spleen, lymph nodes, liver and central nervous system tissue, should be collected during relapses.[19,20]

Due to a lack of knowledge regarding the presence and location of *B. burgdorferii* during the course of Lyme disease, multiple samples from involved areas should be collected. Blood (heparinized or citrated) collected during the first few days of illness, cerebrospinal fluid and joint fluid are appropriate samples for laboratory analysis. Biopsy of ECM lesions is usually unrewarding.[23] In addition, serum should be collected for serologic study.

Microscopy

Citrated blood or body fluid may be examined directly by darkfield illumination for the presence of *Borrelia*. Movement of red cells disturbed by *Borrelia* aid in locating the organisms. The organisms are easily recognized by their morphology and by their twisting and rotating motion. Alternatively, blood can also be collected in heparinized microhematocrit tubes,[10] sealed and allowed to stand vertically until the red cells settle. The plasma is then examined for *Borrelia* using darkfield illumination. This serves to concentrate the organisms, remove interfering red blood cells and allow easier identification.

Thick and thin blood smears should be prepared and stained for *Borrelia*. Thick smears are prepared and dehemoglobinized with distilled water as is done for identification of malarial parasites. They are then washed with 0.01 M phosphate buffered saline, pH 6.8. The thin smears are fixed with acetone for 1 min or methanol for 3 min. *Borrelia* can be stained with aniline dyes and a variety of stains are acceptable; Wright, May-Grunwald and Giemsa stains are most commonly employed.

Direct fluorescent antibody techniques for the diagnosis of relapsing fever are not practical due to the ability of the organisms to undergo antigenic variation[24] and the absence of commercially available antiserum to *Borrelia*. Direct fluorescent antibody techniques for the diagnosis of Lyme disease are also not recommended, since *Borrelia* have not been found upon direct examination of blood or other body fluids. *Borrelia* may be visualized with a variety of silver stains; however, only rarely have relapsing fever *Borrelia* been demonstrated in the brain, spleen and lymph nodes of infected animals and man.[8] Similarly, *B. burgdorferii* has been demonstrated by silver stain in the edge of ECM lesions in only 12% of the patients examined.[23] Therefore, direct examination of tissue does not appear to be practical for the diagnosis of relapsing fever and Lyme disease.

Primary Isolation and Culture

One of the major advances in *Borrelia* research occurred in 1971 with the advent of Kelly's medium for the cultivation of pathogenic borreliae. This artificial culture medium required large numbers of organisms as an inoculum, was tedious to prepare and supported the growth of only a few strains of *Borrelia*. Modifications by Stoenner, Barbour and Steere have served to improve Kelly's original media. [2,3,21,23,24] The most recent modification, BSK II, requires only a small inoculum (1 or 2 organisms), and achieves spirochete densities of 1-4 x 10^8 per mL with a generation time of 11-12 hours.[3] This medium supports the growth of the N. American borreliae: *B. hermsii, B. parkeri* and *B. turicatae*, as well as *B. burgdorferii*.[2,3,15]

Blood culture for *Borrelia* can be performed in several ways. Citrated or heparinized whole blood, 0.5 mL, is used to inoculate tubes containing 10 mL BSK II medium. Plasma collected using the microhematocrit techniques described above or pellets prepared by centrifugation of the plasma (12,000 X g for 20 min) may also be used as an inoculum. Tissue for culture is ground in 1 mL of BSK II medium and 0.1 mL of the emulsion used as an inoculum. The broth is incubated at 33°C and examined for *Borrelia* weekly for one month by darkfield microscopy. Blind subculture of each tube (0.1 mL) to a second tube of BSK II medium may serve to increase the sensitivity of culture. Body fluids may be cultured by inoculating 0.5 mL of specimen into 10 mL of BSK II medium.

SEROLOGIC PROCEDURES

Relapsing Fever

Numerous serologic procedures detecting agglutinating, complement-fixing, borreliocidal and immobilizing antibodies have been employed to diagnose relapsing fever. Agglutination procedures[7] using a known *Borrelia* suspension and serum diluted with phosphate-buffered saline are often difficult to interpret due to autoagglutination. Complement-fixing antibodies have been detected using either saponin-treated antigens[8] or antigens from organisms grown in chick embryos.[28] However, this test is not practical because of the difficulty in preparing antigens. Immobilizing and borreliocidal tests have been most commonly employed. A suspension of live *Borrelia* is mixed with dilutions of serum and after incubation, lysis or death of *Borrelia* is ascertained by darkfield microscopy. Using this procedure, high antibody titers were detected in convalescent sera when the appropriate species of *Borrelia* was used as the target antigen.[20] The necessity of maintaining live *Borrelia* of the appropriate species, however, diminishes the practical utility of this procedure. An indirect immunoenzyme test[9] was developed to circumvent the need for live *Borrelia*. *Borrelia* fixed on a slide are allowed to react with the patient's serum. Anti-human immunoglobulin conjugated with horseradish-peroxidase is used to stain the borreliae. Results obtained with this procedure have been shown in one study to be comparable to those obtained with the immobilizing test.[9]

These serologic procedures are, however, of little value in making the diagnosis of infection during the acute stages of illness since detectable antibody is present only in convalescent sera. Also, due to the phase variation of the organism, antibody detection is difficult and false-negative reactions occur. Furthermore, the tests are difficult to perform and interpret, and cross reactions are seen with sera from patients with typhus, syphilis and leptospirosis.

Lyme Disease

Isolation of *B. burgdorferii* from patients with Lyme disease has proven difficult; therefore standardized serologic tests are employed for diagnosis. An indirect immunofluorescent assay (IFA) and an enzyme-linked immunosorbent assay (ELISA) have been used to demonstrate antibodies that bind to *B. burgdorferii*.[26] Peak IgM titers occur 3 to 6 weeks after the onset of ECM. Peak IgG titers occur months later in patients with arthritis.[26] Either test can be used with a high degree of sensitivity and specificity for complicated Lyme disease; however, crossreactions have been observed with sera from patients with treponemal diseases.

REFERENCES

1. Barbour AG, Tessier SL, Stoenner HG. Variable major proteins of *Borrelia hermsii*. J Exp Med 1982;156:1312-24.
2. Barbour AG, Burgdorfer W, Hayes SF, Peter O, Aeschliman A. Isolation of a cultivable spirochete from *Ixodes ricinus* ticks of Switzerland. Curr Microbiol 1983;8:123-6.
3. Barbour AG. Isolation and cultivation of Lyme disease spirochetes. Yale J Biol Med 1984;57:521-5.
4. Barbour AG. Immunochemical analysis of Lyme disease spirochetes. Yale J Biol Med 1984;57:581-6.
5. Burgdorfer W, Barbour AG, Hayes SF, Benach JL, Grunwaldt E, Davis JP. Lyme disease —a tick-borne spirochetosis? Science 1983;216:1317-19.
6. Burgdorfer W. Discovery of the Lyme disease spirochete and its relation to tick vectors. Yale J Biol Med 1984;57:515-20.
7. Felsenfeld O. Borreliae, human relapsing fever and parasite vector-host relationships. Bacteriol Rev 1965;29:46-74.
8. Felsenfeld O. *Borrelia* strains, vectors, human and animal borreliosis. St. Louis: Warren H. Green, 1971.
9. Felsenfeld O, Wolf RH. The indirect immunoenzyme test for the detection of antibodies against North American *Borrelia*. Am J Clin Pathol 1974;61:839-43.

10. Goldsmidt JM, Mahomed K. The use of the microhematocrit technic for the recovery of *Borrelia duttonii* from the blood. Am J Clin Pathol 1972;58:165-9.
11. Hougen KH. Electron microscopy of *Borrelia merionesi* and *Borrelia recurrentis*. Acta Pathol Microbiol Immunol Scand 1974;82:799-809.
12. Hyde FW, Johnson RC. Genetic relationship of Lyme disease spirochetes to *Borrelia, Treponema*, and *Leptospira* spp. J Clin Microbiol 1984;20:151-4.
13. Johnson RC. The biology of parasitic spirochetes. New York: Academic Press, 1976.
14. Johnson RC, Schmid GP, Hyde FW, Steigerwalt AG, Brenner DJ. *Borrelia burgdorferii* sp Nov.: Etiologic agent of Lyme disease. Int J Syst Bacteriol 1984;34:496-7.
15. Kehl, KSC. Analysis of the antigens of *Borrelia hermsii, B. parkeri* and *B. turicatae* and their relationship to the relapse phenomenon (Dissertation). Milwaukee: The College of Wisconsin, 1984.
16. Kelly R. Cultivation of *Borrelia hermsii*. Science 1971;173:443-4.
17. Krieg NR, Holt JG, eds. Bergey's manual of systematic bacteriology; vol 1. Baltimore: Williams and Wilkins, 1984:57-62.
18. Schmid GP, Steigerwalt AG, Johnson SE, et al. DNA characterization of the spirochete that causes Lyme disease. 1984;20:155-8.
19. Schuhardt VT, ed. Symposium on relapsing fever in the Americas. Am Assoc Adv Sci Monogr 1942;18:58-66.
20. Southern PM, Sanford JP. Relapsing fever, a clinical and microbiological review. Medicine 1969;48:129-49.
21. Steere AC, Godzicki RL, Kornblatt AN, et al. The spirochetal etiology of Lyme disease. N Engl J Med 1983;308:733-40.
22. Steere AC, Malawista SE, Bartenhagen NH, et al. The clinical spectrum and treatment of Lyme disease. Yale J Biol Med 1984;57:453-61.
23. Steere AC, Grodzicki RL, Craft JE, Shrestha M, Kornblatt A, Malawista SE. Recovery of Lyme disease spirochetes from patients. Yale J Biol Med 1984;57:557-60.
24. Stoenner HG, Dodd T, Larsen C. Antigenic variation of *Borrelia hermsii*. J Exp Med 1982;156:12971311.
25. Weber K, Schierz G, Wilski B, Preac-Mursic V. European erythema migrans disease and related disorders. Yale J Biol Med 1984;57:465-71.
26. Wilkinson HW. Immunodiagnostic tests for Lyme disease. Yale J Biol Med 1984;57:567-72.
27. Wilson ML, Levine JF, and Spielman A. Effect of deer reduction on abundance of the deer tick (*Isodes dammini*). Yale J Biol Med 1984;57:697-705.
28. Wolstenholme B, Gear JHS. A complement fixation test for the diagnosis of relapsing fever. Trans Roy Soc Trop Med Hyg 1948;41:513-17.

CHAPTER 10

BRANHAMELLA INFECTIONS

Gary V. Doern, Ph.D

INTRODUCTION

Prior to 1975, despite sporadic reports of *Branhamella catarrhalis* endocarditis, meningitis and bronchopulmonary infections, this organism was generally regarded as a harmless commensal of the upper respiratory tract of healthy humans. During the last decade, however, *B. catarrhalis* has been recognized with increasing frequency as a significant human pathogen. It is not clear whether this increased awareness of *B. catarrhalis* infections represents an actual change in disease incidence or whether *B. catarrhalis* infections are simply being recognized more often due to technologic advances in clinical and laboratory medicine. Irrespective of the answer to this question, *B. catarrhalis* must now be considered an important, if not common, cause of a wide variety of human infectious diseases.

CAUSATIVE ORGANISM

Previously referred to as *Micrococcus catarrhalis* and then as *Neisseria catarrhalis, Branhamella catarrhalis* received its current genus designation in 1970, when genetic, physiologic and antigenic characterizations determined that this organism was taxonomically distinct from *Neisseria* species.[5] Subsequent analysis of guanine plus cytosine content, DNA homology studies and characterization of cell envelope proteins and lipopolysaccharide support this separation.[10,12] At the present time, *B. catarrhalis* is the only species of the *Branhamella* genus that is of consequence to humans as a cause of disease.

Branhamella catarrhalis is an aerobic, oxidase-positive, gram-negative diplococcus, morphologically indistinguishable from *Neisseria* species.[7] The organism grows best at a temperature of 35-37°C in an atmosphere of 5-7%

CO_2; however it may also be propagated in ambient atmospheric air. On sheep blood agar, greyish flat entire colonies, 3-5 mm in diameter, are observed after 24 h incubation. On enriched chocolate agar, colonies are similar in size and shape, but a light tan appearance is usually seen. Growth on solid media selective for pathogenic *Neisseria*, e.g., Thayer-Martin medium, is variable. *Branhamella catarrhalis* fails to ferment glucose, maltose, sucrose or lactose, but reduces both nitrate and nitrite and produces an extracellular DNAse. *B. catarrhalis* does not produce gamma glutamylaminopeptidase nor prolylaminopeptidase, two enzymes often used for the rapid characterization of *N. meningitidis* and *N. gonorrhoeae*.

CLINICAL MANIFESTATIONS AND EPIDEMIOLOGY

Branhamella catarrhalis has been associated with a broad spectrum of human infectious diseases.[5] These include endocarditis, meningitis, septic arthritis, conjunctivitis, keratitis, acute urethritis and sepsis without a focus of infection in patients with underlying lymphoproliferative disorders. These diseases are, however, relatively uncommon. In contrast, *B. catarrhalis* is a frequent cause of acute otitis media, maxillary sinusitis and bronchopulmonary infections, particularly in patients with antecedent compromised lung function.

Although precise incidence figures do not exist, *B. catarrhalis* is probably the third most common bacterial cause of otitis media and maxillary sinusitis, exceeded only by *Haemophilus influenzae* and *Streptococcus pneumoniae*. Similarly, in individuals with underlying impaired lower respiratory tract function, *B. catarrhalis* is probably the third most common cause of bacterial bronchopulmonary infections, exceeded only by the same two organisms. Indeed, there exists a striking similarity between the disease spectrum of *B. catarrhalis* and that associated with nontypable strains of *H. influenzae*.

Branhamella bronchopulmonary infections represent a continuum of disease. At one extreme, *B. catarrhalis* is commonly associated with acute exacerbation of chronic bronchitis characterized principally by cough and purulent sputum production. Chest x-rays are usually unremarkable; constitutional manifestations are usually absent. At the other extreme, *B. catarrhalis* is an important cause of frank bacterial pneumonia. Typically, patients manifest fever, dyspnea, tachycardia, increased respirations and productive cough. Pleuritic chest pain is variable. Ausculation varies from diffuse wheezes and rhonchi to localized signs of consolidation. Chest x-rays may reveal bronchopulmonic infiltrates or, more commonly, alveolar consolidation. Pleural effusion with empyema and bacteremia are both uncommon but have been reported.

Nearly all patients with *B. catarrhalis* bronchopulmonary infections have some form of predisposing functional abnormality of the lower respiratory tract. The most common is chronic obstructive pulmonary disease. The vast majority of all infections arise following endobronchial seeding of the lungs. This reflects mucosal carriage of *B. catarrhalis* as part of the normal bacterial flora of the upper respiratory tract and oral cavity. Hematogenous seeding of the lungs probably does not occur. The same is true of direct human-to-human droplet transmission. A comprehensive review of *B. catarrhalis* infections was recently published.[6]

THERAPY

The majority of clinically significant isolates of *B. catarrhalis* produce a beta-lactamase and are thus resistant to penicillin and other penicillinase-susceptible beta-lactam antimicrobials such as ampicillin and amoxicillin.[8,14,17] The *B. catarrhalis* beta-lactamase is probably not plasmid-associated; it is produced constitutively and remains strongly cell-associated. Its activity is abrogated by beta-lactamase inhibiting compounds such as clavulanate and sulbactam. Analysis of isoelectric points indicates that the *B. catarrhalis* beta-lactamase probably exists in several forms. Irrespective of isoelectric points, however, all enzymes have higher substrate affinity for penicillin than for ampicillin or amoxicillin, thus explaining why ampicillin minimum inhibitory concentrations (MIC's) are usually 5- to 10-fold lower than pencillin MIC's for beta-lactamase-producing strains.[8] Despite their relatively low MIC's, beta-lactamase-positive strains should be considered resistant to ampicillin and amoxicillin since therapeutic failures have been noted when these antimicrobials have been used to treat *B. catarrhalis* infections caused by beta-lactamase-positive strains.[6] The *B. catarrhalis* beta-lactamase possesses diminished cephalosporinase activity. Not surprisingly, therefore, second and third generation cephalosporins are uniformly inhibitory at low concentrations.[2] Similarly, Augmentin (a combination of amoxicillin and clavulanic acid) is highly active due to inactivation of the *B. catarrhalis* beta-lactamase by clavulanic acid.

Other antimicrobials with extensive in vitro activity against *B. catarrhalis* include erythromycin, chloramphenicol, tetracycline, trimethoprim-sulfamethoxazole and the aminoglycosides.[6] Antimicrobials with little or no activity against *B. catarrhalis* include vancomycin, clindamycin and methicillin.[6] The drugs of choice for non-life-threatening *Branhamella* infections in which oral therapy is indicated are cefaclor, erythromycin, tetracycline, Augmentin and trimethoprim-sulfamethoxazole. Serious infections in which parenteral therapy is warranted may be treated with parenteral second and third generation cephalosporin antimicrobials.

DIAGNOSTIC PROCEDURES

Discussion of the role of the laboratory in the diagnosis of *Branhamella* infections will be restricted to otitis media, maxillary sinusitis and bronchopulmonary infections. The specimens of choice in otitis media are typanocentesis fluid or myringotomy aspirates; in maxillary sinusitis, sinus aspirates are the preferred specimens. In patients suspected of having *Branhamella* bronchopulmonary infections, expectorated sputum is usually satisfactory, since it has been shown that such specimens yield results equivalent to those obtained from transtracheal aspirates.[1]

Specimens should first be Gram stained. Gram-stained smears typically reveal numerous polymorphonuclear leukocytes (PNM's) and large numbers of gram-negative diplococci, both intracellular and extracellular (See color plate Figure 10:1). The importance of Gram-stained smears as a simple, rapid, inexpensive, sensitive and specific means for making the diagnosis of *Branhamella* infections cannot be overstated. Middle ear fluid from patients with *B. catarrhalis* otitis media, sinus aspirates from patients with *B. catarrhalis* maxillary sinusitis and expectorated sputa from patients with *B. catarrhalis* bronchopulmonary infections almost always yield typical Gram-stained smears. Furthermore, *Neisseria* species rarely cause these diseases. As a result, a Gram-stained smear similar to that depicted in Figure 10:1 is nearly pathognomonic for *Branhamella* infections.[6] Specimens should be inoculated onto media containing 5% defibrinated sheep blood and onto enriched chocolate agar. In addition, expectorated sputa should be inoculated onto a *Neisseria* selective medium since many if not the majority of strains of *B. catarrhalis* will grow on such media.[7] Use of *Neisseria* selective medium will serve to minimize over-growth of *Branhamella* by oral pharyngeal bacterial flora commonly found in even the highest quality expectorated sputa. Plates should be incubated at 35-37°C in 5-7% CO^2 for a total of 3 days and examined daily for the presence of colonies consistent with *B. catarrhalis*.

Gram-stained smears and an oxidase test should be performed on suspicious colonies. Colonies which yield oxidase-positive, gram-negative diplococci should be further characterized for fermentation of glucose, maltose, lactose and sucrose as well as the ability to reduce nitrate. Organisms which reduce nitrate but fail to ferment these four carbohydrates may be identified as *B. catarrhalis*. Tests for carbohydrate fermentation may be performed using any of the following basal media: cystine-trypticase agar,[3] NYC fermentation media,[9] cystine proteose peptone agar[16] or proteose peptone agar containing NaCl and K_2HPO_4.[13] Use of miniaturized kit systems for the identification of *B. catarrhalis* is problematic. One 4-hour chromogenic substrate micromethod (API NeIdent, Analytab Products) did not effectively identify *B. catarrhalis*.[11] A second 4-hour chromogenic substrate micromethod (Rapid NH System, Inovative Diagnostics System) correctly identified 23 of 24 strains of *B. catarrhalis*.[16]

Clinically significant isolates of *B. catarrhalis* should be examined for production of beta-lactamase. Either the iodometric[4] or chromogenic cephalosporin[15] method should be employed. Isolates found to produce beta-lactamase should be considered resistant to penicillin, ampicillin and amoxicillin. Given the uniform activity of a variety of other antimicrobials versus *B. catarrhalis*, there is little need to perform susceptibility tests other than a beta-lactamase assay. However, if such supplemental tests are determined to be warranted, a quantitative dilution method should be used. Disk diffusion susceptibility tests have not been standardized for *B. catarrhalis*.

At the current time, there exist no serologic procedures that are of practical value in making the diagnosis of *Branhamella* infections, nor are there any immunochemical methods to assist in the laboratory identification of this organism.

REFERENCES

1. Aitken JM, Thornley PE. Isolation of *Branhamella catarrhalis* from sputum and tracheal aspirates. J Clin Microbiol 1983;18:1262-6.
2. Alvarez S, Jones M, Holtsclaw-Berk S, Guarderas J, Berk SL. In vitro susceptibilities and beta-lactamase production of 53 clinical isolates of *Branhamella catarrhalis*. Antimicrob Agents Chemoth 1985;27:646-50.
3. Brown WJ. A comparison of fermentation methods for the confirmation of *Neisseria gonorrhoeae*. Health Lab Sci 1975;13:54-8.
4. Catlin BW. Iodometric detection of *Haemophilus influenzae* beta-lactamase: rapid presumptive test for ampicillin resistance. Antimicrob Agents Chemoth 1975;7:265-9.
5. Catlin BW. Transfer of the organism named *Neisseria catarrhalis* to *Branhamella* gen. Nov. Int J Syst Bacteriol 1970;20:155-9.
6. Doern GV. *Branhamella catarrhalis* - An emerging human pathogen. Diagn Microbiol Infect Dis 1986;4:191-201.
7. Doern GV, Morse SA. *Branhamella (Neisseria) catarrhalis*: criteria for laboratory identification. J Clin Microbiol 1980;11:193-5.
8. Doern GV, Siebers KG, Hallick LM, Morse SA. Antibiotic susceptibility of beta-lactamase-producing strains of *Branhamella (Neisseria) catarrhalis*. Antimicrob Agents Chemoth 1980;17:24-9.
9. Faur VC, Weisburd MH, Wilson ME, May PS. A new medium for the isolation of pathogenic *Neisseria* (NYC medium), I. Formulation and comparisons with standard media. Health Lab Sci 1973;10:44-9.
10. Henrikson SD. *Moraxella, Neisseria, Branhamella* and *Acinetobacter*. Ann Rev Microbiol 1976;30:63-83.
11. Janda WM, Morello JA, Bohnkoff M. Use of the API NeIdent system for identification of pathogenic *Neisseria* spp. and *Branhamella catarrhalis*. J Clin Microbiol 1984;3:338-41.
12. Johnson KG, McDonald JJ, Perry MA. Studies on the cellular and free lipopolysaccharides from *Branhamella catarrhalis*. Can J Microbiol 1976;22:460-7.
13. Knapp JS, Holmes KK. Modified oxidation-fermentation medium for detection of acid production from carbohydrates by *Neisseria* spp and *Branhamella catarrhalis*. J Clin Microbiol 1983;18:56-60.
14. McLeod DT, Power JT, Calder MA, Seaton A. Bronchopulmonary infection due to *Branhamella catarrhalis*. Br Med J 1983;287:1446-52.

15. O'Callaghan CH, Morris A, Kirby S, Shingler AH. Novel method for detection of beta-lactamase by using a chromogenic cephalosporin substrate. Antimicrob Agents Chemoth 1972;1:283-6.
16. Robinson MJ, Oberhofer TR. Identification of pathogenic *Neisseria* species with the Rapid NH System. J Clin Microbiol 1983;17:400-5.
17. Shurin PA, Marchant CD, Kim CH, Hare GF, Johnson CE, Tutikasi MA, Knapp LJ. Emergence of beta-lactamase-producing strains of *Branhamella catarrhalis* as important agents of acute otitis media. Pediatr Infect Dis 1983;2:34-9.

CHAPTER 11

BRUCELLOSIS

Richard E. Winn, M.D.

INTRODUCTION

In 1887, Bruce reported the first isolation of a bacterium later shown to be one of the causative agents of brucellosis, known then as undulant fever. In addition, he was able to transmit the disease to a primate. In 1885, Bang had isolated what proved to be the same organism from abortive material of cattle. In the early 1920s, the seminal work of Bruce was recognized with the designation of *Brucella* as the genus name for this group of bacteria.

Since that time brucellosis has been determined to be a worldwide disease producing enzootic infections in commercial livestock (cattle, sheep, goats and swine) and more recently in dogs. Infection in man occurs principally through occupational exposure (abattoir-workers, veterinarians, laboratory workers and livestock handlers). Acquisition may occur through direct contact with infected materials or indirectly through ingestion of animal products such as milk or cheese.

CAUSATIVE ORGANISMS

Brucella are small, pleomorphic, nonmotile, nonsporulating, coccal-to-coccobacillary gram-negative bacteria. They range in size from 0.5-0.7 μm by 0.5-1.5 μm and are arranged singly or in pairs and short chains. There are six recognized species, four of which have been shown to be pathogenic for man. *Brucella abortus* (cattle), *B. melitensis* (sheep and goats), *B. suis* (swine) and *B. canis* (dogs) are recognized human pathogens. *Brucella neotomae*, which is found in the desert wood rat and *B. ovis*, which causes ram epididymitis in Australia and New Zealand, have not been recovered from humans. A seventh proposed species, *B. rangiferi tarandi*, has been isolated exclusively from reindeer in Russia and from caribou in Alaska.

Table 11:1. Differential Characteristics of the Four Important Clinically Encountered Species of the Genus *Brucella*

Species	Reservoir	Co^2 (5%) Requirement	Urease Activity	H^2S Production	Growth Thionine A	Growth Thionine B	Growth Thionine C	Basic Fuchsin B	Basic Fuchsin C
B. melitensis 1-3	Goats, Sheep	–	v	– (4 Days)	+	+	+	+	+
B. abortus 1-9	Cattle	±	1-2 Hours	+ (2 Days)*	–	±	±	+†	+†
B. suis 1-4	Swine	–	0-30 minutes	– (4 Days)‡	±	+	+	–§	–§
B. canis	Dogs	–	0-30 minutes	–	+	+	+	–	–

v—Variable
* Biotype 6,7 variable
Biotype 5 negative
† Biotype 2 negative
‡ Biotype 1 positive
§ Biotype 3,4 positive

Slow growth occurs on agar media with colonies first appearing at 48 hours. *Brucella* grow best at 5-10% CO_2. No growth occurs under strictly anaerobic conditions. The addition of 1.5-2.5% glucose appears to favor growth, as does the addition of natural animal protein or erythritol. Thiamine, niocin, biotin and pantothenic acid are required for growth. Some strains also require the addition of serum.

Colonial morphology varies depending on medium composition and incubation conditions. Recommended media formulations include serum potato infusion agar, trypticase soy and tryptose agar, serum dextrose agar and 5% sheep blood agar.[9] Colonies after 5 days are nonhemolytic, nonpigmented, moist, slightly opalescent and glistening on the surface. A bluish-white tinge may be observed in reflected light. Optimal temperature for growth is 37°C with a range of 10-40°C. The optimal pH range is 6.6-7.4.

Brucella are catalase-positive, oxidase-positive and urease-variable. Production of hydrogen sulfide, urea hydrolysis and oxidative metabolism studies are necessary for species and biotype identification (Table 11:1). *Brucella melitensis* has 3 biotypes, *B. suis* has 4 and *B. abortus* has 9. If *Brucella* are exposed to conditions of extreme heat (60°C for 10 min), direct sunlight (hours) or 1% phenol (15 min), they are killed. They may survive in a moist, shaded environment for months, however, and have survived for days in sterile milk or tap water (57 days at 8°C and 10 days at 25°C). Further, they are relatively resistant to desiccation in either exudative materials or products of abortion.

CLINICAL MANIFESTATIONS

There are several clinical forms of brucellosis. The most common is acute illness which occurs in approximately 75% of individuals. The acute illness need not be severe or life-threatening. Seventy-five percent of individuals will recover within three months of the onset of disease, even if untreated. The incubation period is variable but usually is between one and three weeks. After the incubation period, several months may elapse before the onset of clinical manifestations. Symptoms of the acute illness are nonspecific and include chills, fever, sweating and headache.

In a study from Egypt, where all cases were due to *B. melitensis*, the acute illness occurred in 201 of 228 patients and lasted three months or less.[39] In the Egyptian series, fever was seen in 98% of patients, musculoskeletal pain was seen in 72%. Anorexia was seen much less frequently, i.e., 22%. Musculoskeletal pain was usually confined to the knees, ankles, shoulders, wrists, elbows and hips. True objective signs of joint disease as evidenced by erythema, warmth and effusion were uncommon. Hepatomegaly was seen in 62% of patients and splenomegaly in 70%. Combined enlargement of the liver and spleen was encountered in 52% of patients.

The age distribution was the 3rd to 5th decades in life, with 57% of cases occurring between 21 and 40 years of age.

In a large outbreak of brucellosis in U.S. abattoir-workers with 160 infected patients, 95% had malaise or chills, 93% had weakness or sweats, 68% had body aches, 52% had anorexia, 50% had weight loss and 44% had headache. Ninety-five percent of individuals had fever, but only 14% experienced lymphadenitis or lymphadenopathy and 10% experienced splenomegaly.

Another common presentation for brucellosis is subacute or chronic, insidious disease, reflected by the gradual onset of low-grade fever, sweating, weakness, headache and mental depression. Individuals may demonstrate intermittent fever over months with remittent symptoms. This symptom complex may be difficult to diagnose as brucellosis. Localized brucellosis occurs most often with the subacute presentation, although it may also be seen in the more chronic form. The joints, long bones and spinal column are frequently affected. Spondylitis and vertebral osteomyelitis have occurred in the cervical, thoracic and lumbosacral spine.[20,48] Sacroilitis has also been described.[34] The sternoclavicular joint has been involved[30] as have other joints, usually as monoarticular arthritis[25] or osteomyelitis.[14] Infectious bursitis has been reported.[23] Other sites of involvement have included the epididymis, kidney, testes, liver (non-caseating granulomas)[50] and spleen (target calcifications).[15] Infection of the central nervous system also occurs.[2] Cutaneous involvement[3,22] and pancytopenia[32] occur infrequently, although hematologic abnormalities, manifesting as lymphocytosis and leukopenia, are not uncommon.[11] Endocarditis is relatively rare but potentially devastating and management depends on the use of surgery and antimicrobics. Early recognition, coupled with valve replacement, can result in cure.[26,38,41] Brucellosis should be considered in any patient with fever of unknown origin.

THERAPY

Because *Brucella* are intracellular bacteria, antimicrobics which are both bactericidal and penetrate into cells are theoretically the most desirable agents. In vitro, the organisms are susceptible to all aminoglycosides, the tetracyclines, erythromycin, rifampin, chloramphenicol and trimethoprim-sulfamethoxazole.[24,25] Ampicillin is the only penicillin with in vitro activity.[43] First and second generation cephalosporins lack activity but moxalactam and some other third generation cephalosporins have been shown to be effective.

In vivo, the standard therapy has been tetracycline. Tetracycline may be used alone; however, relapse does occur and in some series has been reported to be as high as 80%. The usual dose is 500 mg 4 times daily for

21 days. When streptomycin is used in combination with tetracycline, relapse rates can be reduced to 10%. Streptomycin is usually given in a dose of 500 mg twice daily or once daily for 14 days. In addition, trimethoprim-sulfamethoxazole appears to have clinical efficacy as does rifampin.[10,12,29]

In localized disease of long bones and bursae, drainage procedures and antimicrobics (tetracycline and streptomycin) have been effective. Recurrences may occur; retreatment may be curative but osteomyelitis may be refractory despite multiple debridements and antimicrobics. Infection of the spine is usually amenable to antimicrobics alone. Joint disease may be refractory and synovectomy may be required. Soft tissue infections such as lymphadenitis are usually cured by excisional biopsy. Epidural abscesses respond to antimicrobics alone or antimicrobics combined with surgical drainage. In the absence of large, focal abscesses, hepatic, genitourinary and pulmonary brucellosis usually respond to antimicrobial therapy alone. Endocarditis due to *Brucella* is rare but very destructive to heart valves. Valve replacement has been done in all patients who have survived.

EPIDEMIOLOGY

Brucellosis has been found in virtually every country in the world.[6] Actual cases probably greatly exceed the numbers reported due to difficulties in diagnosis, particularly in lesser developed countries. The microorganism is enzootic in several animals, producing abortion and bacteremia. Milk is often infected due to localization of organism in the mammary glands. Countries reporting greater than 1,000 cases per year include Argentina, Peru, Mexico, Spain, Greece, Iran and Italy. Several countries (including Norway, Sweden, Switzerland, Czechoslovakia and Romania) have eradicated brucellosis through intensive control measures. Brucellosis is unknown in Iceland and the Virgin Islands. In the United States, there has been a steady decline in human brucellosis since 1945, which parallels the decline in prevalence of brucellosis in cattle as detected by surveillance serology testing. The decline in cases of bovine and human brucellosis began when public health laws, passed in 1934, were finally enforced in 1945. Reported cases of human brucellosis in the United States fell from 6,321 cases in 1945 to 175 in 1973.[3] For reasons that are unclear, brucellosis was reported more frequently in 1975 through 1977, with 328 cases in 1975. In 1983 there were only 185 cases.

Human cases of brucellosis are more common during the spring and summer months when the greatest outdoor activity and contact with animals occur.[21] Working-age males are at greatest risk as evidenced by the fact that between 1965-74, 74% of all cases of brucellosis occurred in men between the ages of 20 and 60.[21]

Currently, the largest percentage of human cases of brucellosis in the United States occur in abattoir-workers.[8,20] Others at risk include laboratory workers,[28,35] veterinarians and livestock handlers,[4] and individuals who ingest contaminated or improperly processed dairy products such as goat cheese and unpasteurized milk.[51,52] Brucellosis has also occurred in hunters who have butchered feral swine, elk, moose and bison in the United States and in persons ingesting raw meat, bone marrow or liver of reindeer, moose and caribou in Alaska. In the most recent published analysis from the Centers for Disease Control describing 2,047 cases of human brucellosis, 17% were secondary to cattle exposure, 39% from swine, 0.9% from sheep or goats, 10% from wild animals, 3.1% from domestic unpasteurized dairy products and 6.2% from imported cheese.

Humans become infected through direct contact with infected materials via penetration of skin or mucosal abrasions. Inhalation of organisms is felt to be a probable but uncommon mode of acquisition.[17] Direct human-to-human transmission is not known to occur.

Between 1965 and 1971, 77% of brucella infections in the United States were due to *B. suis*.[6] This represents a significant change since, during the early 20th century, 87% of human cases of brucellosis were due to *B. abortus*. One explanation for this change is the efficacy of public health control measures that have been directed almost exclusively against bovine brucellosis.

PUBLIC HEALTH SIGNIFICANCE, PREVENTION AND CONTROL

Brucellosis is a disease with major public health implications. Great strides have been made in the western world and developed countries toward reduction in exposure to these organisms. Disease in these countries is rare today.

Control measures aimed at eradicating brucellosis in animals is the key to elimination of this infection in the human host.[1] Renewed and continued vigilance in the testing and slaughtering of infected animals and the use of vaccines have been shown to reduce the incidence of brucellosis in humans. Regulation of the pasteurization of milk, cheese and other dairy products will prevent acquisition of brucellosis by the oral route. Education of the public and private sector is needed to caution against the ingestion of uncooked or unpasteurized meat and dairy products while traveling.

Cooperation is needed by livestock ranchers who face economic hardships if *Brucella* enters their herds. Quarantine and slaughter of herds have made ranchers wary of reporting suspected brucellosis. Currently, no uniform requirements exist for the utilization of *Brucella* vaccines in livestock and it is used only sporadically. Laboratory workers should use class III biohazard hoods and maintain meticulous care when handling *Brucella*.

Brucellosis is a zoonosis with a rich and storied medical heritage but one that is possible to eradicate with intensive preventive efforts.

DIAGNOSTIC PROCEDURES

The diagnosis of brucellosis depends upon help from the laboratory. Only the isolation of the microorganism from blood, tissue or body fluids definitely proves infection. *Brucella* are fastidious and successful cultivation is not always possible. Serologic tests provide useful adjunctive information and in many cases are the sole means for making the diagnosis.

Specimen Collection and Transport

The optimum specimen for culture is blood. Multiple blood cultures from peripheral or central veins should be performed when brucellosis is suspected. Collection of other specimens such as cerebrospinal fluid, synovial fluid and exudative material should be predicated on disease manifestations. Bone marrow specimens often increase the yield from patients without an evident focus of infection. Material for culture should be processed as soon as possible or should be refrigerated if delays in culture are anticipated.

Rapid Methods

Gram-stain microscopy is useful for determining morphology and staining characteristics. *Brucella* are gram-negative; however, counter stain is taken up poorly so counter staining should be performed for 1-3 min instead of the usual 30 s. A direct fluorescent antibody technique is a useful means for rapidly demonstrating *Brucella* directly in clinical specimens. Reagents, however, are not presently commercially available.

Primary Isolation And Culture

Several different media formulations have been recommended for isolation of *Brucella* including 5% sheep blood agar, brucella agar with 5% serum and serum dextrose agar.[9] A selective medium which has been used for the successful propagation of *Brucella* (i.e., Farrell's medium) contains bacitracin, polymixin B, nalidixic acid, vancomycin, cycloheximide and nystatin. Plates are incubated in an atmosphere of 5-10% CO_2 at 35-37°C for 10 days. Blood cultures may be performed using Castaneda bottles which utilize a biphasic medium consisting of solid agar and liquid broth.[9] The solid phase is prepared by adding 2.5% agar (final concentration) to trypticase soy, tryptose or brucella base broth. Subcultures of these bottles should be

FIGURE 11:1
Stages of Antibody Response in Brucellosis

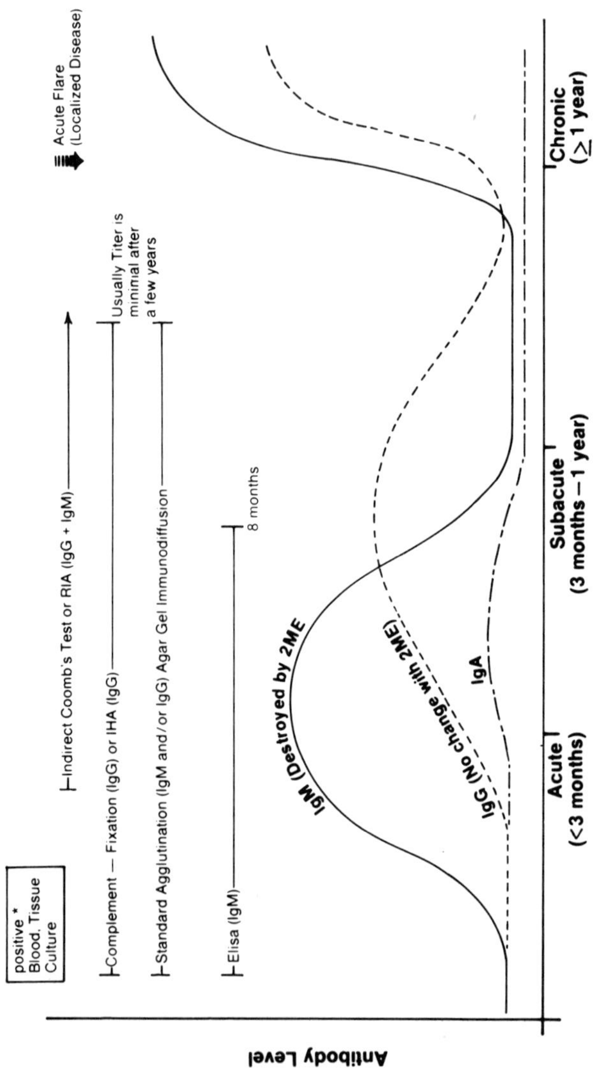

* culture positivity is variable

Total Agglutinating Antibody Peaks (IgM + IgG) in initial months
2 ME resistant IgG antibody demonstrable primarily in first year

performed every 4-5 days. Blood culture bottles should be vented and incubated at 35-37°C and examined for a total of 30 days.

Radiometric and lysis-centrifugation blood culture techniques may increase the yield and shorten the length of time to recovery of *Brucella*.[18] Subcultures may not be necessary with these methods. Furthermore, cultures do not need to be held longer than 7 days, as virtually all cultures will be positive within this time period.

Methods For Identification

Organisms suspected of being *Brucella* (i.e., oxidase-positive, catalase-positive, aerobic, nonmotile, nonhemolytic colonies of gram-negative coccobacilli that fail to ferment glucose and lactose) may be identified with a slide agglutination procedure using anti-smooth *Brucella* serum (Difco Laboratories). Among the four species of *Brucella* that are of concern as causes of human disease, *B. abortus, B. melitensis, B. suis* and *B. canis*, only the first three will yield an agglutination reaction with this antiserum. Identification of *B. canis* requires use of *B. canis* - specific antiserum which, at the present time, is not commercially available.

Definitive species identification of *Brucella* and determination of biotype require use of techniques and procedures not commonly employed in routine diagnostic microbiology laboratories (Table 11:1). As a result, isolates should be submitted to suitable reference laboratories for performance of these analyses.

Serodiagnosis

A variety of agglutination procedures have been developed for detecting serum antibody reactive with killed whole cells of *Brucella abortus*. A graphic representation of the antibody response in the human host is shown in Figure 11:1. All of the pathogenic *Brucella* species except *B. canis* crossreact with *B. abortus*. A specific agglutination test for *B. canis* is necessary for its diagnosis.[5,40,44] Agglutination tests can be performed either macroscopically in a tube[9] or on a card,[36,46] microscopically in a microtiter tray, or using the rose bengal plate method. A single titer of 1:160 or greater with a compatible illness or a 4-fold rise in titer is considered diagnostic.

The presence of blocking antibodies of the IgM class or the prozone effect can render the agglutination test falsely negative.[42] Crossreacting agglutinating antibodies have been noted after infection with *Francisella tularensis, Yersinia enterocolitica, Vibrio cholerae, Brucella* or *V. cholerae* vaccinations, and after skin testing with the *Brucella* skin test antigen, brucellergen.

Treatment of test serum with 2 mercaptoethanol (2ME) at a final concentration of 0.05 M serves to inactivate blocking IgM antibodies by disruption of disulfide bonds. As a result, agglutination tests utilizing 2ME-treated patient serum are generally more sensitive than the standard test, in particular when attempting to diagnose chronic infection and response to therapy.[7] In addition, the prozone effect may be eliminated from 2ME-treated serum. Using this procedure, a titer equal to or greater than 1:100 is considered consistent with *Brucella* infection.

Complement fixation (CF) and indirect hemagglutination (IHA) tests, when performed according to standardized techniques, are complementary to the performance of the agglutination procedure. [19,33,49] The CF and IHA tests permit better discrimination of IgG and IgA antibodies directed against *Brucella* antigens in active disease. A CF titer of 1:64 or more and an IHA titer of 1:100 or greater are considered consistent with *Brucella* infection. Crossreactions to *Yersinia* somatic antigen have been eliminated by the IHA procedure.

Several immunofluorescent tests have also been developed for the serodiagnosis of brucellosis.[16,27] They suffer from the necessity for considerable interpretive skill and appear to have no advantage over other procedures. They are not recommended for routine testing.

A radioimmunoassay (RIA) has been developed to detect IgA, IgM and IgG antibodies directed against *B. abortus*.[37] When RIA results were compared to the results of agglutination and complement-fixation tests, the RIA appeared to be more sensitive than tube agglutination in some instances and avoided the problems associated with blocking antibodies.

Perhaps most promising, is the use of enzyme immunoassays (EIA) for the serodiagnosis of brucellosis. EIA's have been developed for the detection of *Brucella*-specific IgG, IgM and total antibody.[13,47] Using these procedures, it appears to be possible to differentiate acute from chronic disease and to assess therapeutic efficacy. Because of the sensitivity of EIA, it may also be possible to differentiate active infection from subclinical background exposure.

REFERENCES

1. Barclay WR. Brucellosis control. JAMA 1980;244:2315.
2. Bashir R, Al-Kawi MZ, Harder EJ, Jinkins J. Nervous system brucellosis. diagnosis and treatment. Neurology 1985;35:1576-81.
3. Berger T, Guill MA, Goette DK. Cutaneous lesions in brucellosis. Arch Dermatol 1981;117:40-2.
4. Bigler WJ, Hoff GL, Hemmert WH, Tomas JA, Janowski HT. Trends of brucellosis in Florida. Am J Epidemiol 1977;105:245-51.
5. Blankenship RM, Sandord JP. *Brucella canis*. A cause of undulant fever. Am J Med 1975;59:424-6.
6. Brucellosis - Medical Staff Conference. West J Med 1975;122:232-7.
7. Buchanan TM, Faber LC. 2-Mercaptoethanol *Brucella* agglutination test: usefulness for predicting recovery from brucellosis. J Clin Microbiol 1980;11:691-3.

8. Buchanan TM, Hendricks SL, Patton CM, Feldman RA. Brucellosis in the United States, 1960-1972, Part I - III. An abattoir associated disease. Medicine 1974;53:403-13,415-25,427-39.
9. Castaneda MR. Laboratory diagnosis of brucellosis in man. Bull WHO 1961;24:73-84.
10. Conti R, Parenti F. Rifampin therapy for brucellosis, *Flavobacterium* meningitis, and cutaneous leishmaniasis. Rev Infect Dis 1983;5:5600-6.
11. Crosby E, Llosa L, Miro Quesada MM, Carillo C, Gotuzzo E. Hematologic changes in brucellosis. J Infect Dis 1984;150:419-24.
12. Daikos GK, Papapolyzos N, Marketos N, Mochlas S, Kastanakis S, Papasteriadis E. Trimethoprim-sulfamethoxazole in brucellosis. J Infect Dis 1973;128:5731-3.
13. DeKlerk E, Anderson R. Comparative evaluation of the enzyme-linked immunosorbent assay in the laboratory diagnosis of brucellosis. J Clin Microbiol 1985;21:381-6.
14. Del Rio DeLos AM. *Brucella* osteomyelitis. Pediatr Infect Dis 1983;2:50-2.
15. Demetropoulos KC, Lindenauer SM, Rapp R, Robins J. Target calcifications of the spleen in chronic brucellosis. J Can Assoc Radiol 1974;25:161-3.
16. Edwards JMB, Tannahill A, Bradstreet P. Comparison of the indirect fluorescent antibody test with agglutination, complement-fixation and Coombs Tests for *Brucella* antibody. J Clin Pathol 1970;23:161-5.
17. Elberg SS, Henderson DW. Respiratory pathogenicity of *Brucella*. J Infect Dis 1948;82:302-6.
18. Etemadi H, Raissadat A, Pickett MJ, Zafari Y, Vahedifar P. Isolation of *Brucella* spp. from clinical specimens. J Clin Microbiol 1984;20:586-9.
19. Farrell ID, Hinchcliffe PM, Robertson L. The use of the conglutinating complement fixation test in the diagnosis of human brucellosis. J Hyg (Camb) 1975;74:29-33.
20. Filstein MR, Potter ME, Payne R. Outbreak of brucellosis in upstate New York. NY State J Med 1980;80:1081-4.
21. Fox MD, Kaufman AF. Brucellosis in the United States, 1965-1974. J Infect Dis 1977;136:312-16.
22. Gee-Lew BM, Nicholas EA, Hirose FM, Yoshimori RN, Keller MA. Unusual skin manifestation of brucellosis. Arch Dermatol 1983;119:56-8.
23. Gotuzzo E, Alarcon GS, Bocanegra TS, et al. Articular involvement in human brucellosis. A retrospective analysis of 304 cases. Semin Arthritis Rheum 1982;12:245-55.
24. Hall WH, Manion RE. In vitro susceptibility of *Brucella* to various antibiotics. Appl Microbiol 1970;20:600-4.
25. Handel G, Le Compte M. Brucellosis. A treatable cause of monoarthritis. Clin Orthop Related Res 1982;168:211-13.
26. Heilig J, Beall AC Jr., Myers R, Harder E, Feteik N. *Brucella* aortic endocarditis corrected by prosthetic valve replacement. Am Heart J 1983;106:594-6.
27. Henderson RJ, Hill DM, Vickers AA, Edwards JM, Tillett H. Correlation between serological and immunofluorescence results in the investigation of brucellosis in veterinary surgeons. J Clin Pathol 1976;29:35-8.
28. Howe C, Miller ES, Kelly EH, Bookwalter HL, Ellingson HV. Acute brucellosis among laboratory workers. N Engl J Med 1947;236:741-3.
29. Kontoyannis PA, Papapoulos SE, Mortoglou AA. Co-trimoxazole in chronic brucellosis: A two-year follow-up study. Br Med J 1975;1:480-1.
30. Lam K, Silverstein LM, Carlisle RJ, Bayer AS. Disseminated brucellosis initially seen as sternoclavicular arthropathy. Arch Intern Med 1982;142:1193-4.
31. Lerro SJ. Human brucellosis in Texas. Texas Med 1971;67:60-6.
32. Martin-Moreno S, Soto-Guzman O, Bernaldo-de-Quiros J, Reverte-Cejudo D, Bascones-Casas C. Pancytopenia due to hemophagocytosis in patients with brucellosis: A report of four cases. J Infect Dis 1983;147:445-9.
33. Mittal KR, Ricciardi ID, Tizard JR. Indirect hemagglutination employing enterobacterial common antigen and *Yersinia* somatic antigen: a technique to differentiate brucellosis from infections involving crossreacting *Yersinia enterocolitica*. J Clin Microbiol 1980;11:149-52.

34. Neinstein LS, Goldenring J. *Brucella* sacroiliitis. Clin Pediatr 1983;22:645-8.
35. Nelson KE, Ruben FL, Andersen B. An unusual outbreak of brucellosis. Arch Intern Med 1975;135:691-5.
36. Nicoletti P, Fadai-Ghotbi MM. A comparison of the tube agglutination and card tests for the diagnosis of *Brucella melitensis* infection in humans. Can J Public Health 1971;62:442-5.
37. Parratt D, Nielson KH, White RG, Payne DJH. Radioimmunoassay of IgM, IgG, and IgA *Brucella* antibodies. Lancet 1977;1:1075-8.
38. Pazderka E, Jones JW. *Brucella abortus* endocarditis. Arch Intern Med 1982;142:1567-9.
39. Pfischner WCE, Ishak KG, Neptune EM Jr., et al. Brucellosis in Egypt. Am J Med 1957;23:915-29.
40. Polt SS, Schaefer J. A microagglutination test for human *Brucella canis* antibodies. Am J Clin Pathol 1982;77:,740-4.
41. Pratt DS, Tenney JH, Bjork CM, Reller LB. Successful treatment of *Brucella melitensis* endocarditis. Am J Med 1978;64:897-900.
42. Reddin JL, Anderson RK, Jenness R, Spink WW. Significance of 7S and macroglobulin *Brucella* agglutinins in human brucellosis. N Engl J Med 1965;272:1263-8.
43. Renner ED. Brucellosis. Clin Microbiol Newsletter 1979;1:1-4.
44. Rifkin GD, Supena RB, Axelson JA. *Brucella canis* bacteremia: A case with negative *B. canis* agglutinins. Am J Med Sci 1978;276:113-15.
45. Robertson L, Farrell ID, Hinchcliffe PM. The sensitivity of *Brucella abortus* to chemotherapeutic agents. J Med Microbiol 1973;6:549-57.
46. Russell AO, Patton CM, Kaufman AF. Evaluation of the card test for the diagnosis of human brucellosis. J Clin Microbiol 1978;7:454-8.
47. Sippel JE, Avad El-Masry N, Farid Z. Diagnosis of human brucellosis with ELISA. Lancet 1982;2:19-21.
48. Torres-Rojas J, Taddonio RF, Sanders CV. Spondylitis caused by *Brucella abortus*. South Med J 1979;72:1166-9.
49. Versilova PA, Cernyseva MI, Aslanjan RG, Knjazeva EN. Diagnosis of human and animal brucellosis by the indirect hemagglutination test. Bull WHO 1974;51:191-7.
50. Willaims RK, Crossley K. Acute and chronic hepatic involvement of brucellosis. Gastroenterology 1982;83:455-8.
51. Young EJ. Human brucellosis. Rev Infect Dis 1983;5:821-42.
52. Young EJ, Suvannoparrat U. Brucellosis outbreak attributed to ingestion of unpasteurized goat cheese. Arch Intern Med 1975;135:240-3.

CHAPTER 12

CAMPYLOBACTER INFECTIONS

Martin J. Blaser, M.D. and Wen-lan L. Wang, Ph.D.

INTRODUCTION

Although they were originally considered to be members of the genus *Vibrio* and primarily animal pathogens, it has become clear in recent years that campylobacters are distinct,[71] that they are common pathogens of humans and that new species are now being recognized with regularity. Human infections, first reported in 1947,[72] were systemic, occurred mostly in debilitated hosts and were largely due to *Campylobacter fetus* subsp. *fetus*. In 1957, Elizabeth King recognized a second group of bacteremic organisms associated with diarrheal illnesses.[40,41] These organisms are now known as *C. jejuni* and other closely related species, but it was not until the 1970s that techniques for isolating these organisms by stool culture became widely available.[20,61] Thus, only in the last decade has *C. jejuni* been recognized around the world as one of the most common bacterial pathogens of humans.[2,18,54] In 1984, first reports were published of a newly recognized organism now called *C. pylori* which was isolated from gastric contents of persons with peptic disease.[48] *C. fetus, C. jejuni, C. pylori* and several closely related organisms are of most clinical interest.

The nomenclature of the campylobacters has changed several times and continues to evolve as new organisms are recognized. Nevertheless, the classification now shown in the 9th edition of "Bergey's Manual of Systematic Bacteriology,"[63] (which is in agreement with the "Approved List of Bacterial Names,"[60]) is widely used.

CAUSATIVE ORGANISMS

Among the campylobacters, *C. jejuni* and *C. coli* are recognized as common causative agents of diarrhea in humans and have been isolated frequently from stool specimens; *C. laridis* is less common. *C. cinaedi* and *C. fennelliae* have been isolated from rectal swabs[22] and *C. cinaedi* from blood of homosexual men.[69] *C. fetus* subsp. *fetus* predominently causes systemic disease in patients with underlying disease.[29] *C. hyointestinalis* has been isolated from swine[23] and from humans. *C. pylori* has been isolated from biopsy specimens of humans with gastritis and peptic ulcer of the stomach and duodenum.[52] *C. concisus* has been isolated from the gingival crevices of humans with peridontal disease but its role in this disease is unknown.[75]

The other campylobacters have rarely been associated with human diseases. *Campylobacter sputorum* subsp. *sputorum* has been isolated as a commensal from the oral cavity of humans.[62] *C. sputorum* subsp. *bubulus* has been isolated from uterine and genital sites of cattle and sheep.[45] *C. sputorum* subsp. *mucosalis* has been associated with intestinal disease in pigs.[43] "*Campylobacter fecalis*" has been found in feces of healthy sheep and in cattle with enteric disease; it now is considered to be a biovar of *C. sputorum*.[56] *C. fetus* subsp. *venerealis* causes abortion and infertility in cattle and is generally not associated with human disease.[62,63] Nevertheless, new *Campylobacter* species[39] are being recognized in animals with regularity and it is likely that at least some will be associated with human disease.

CLINICAL MANIFESTATIONS

Three clinical forms of campylobacter infection are of major concern, i.e., enteric, bacteremic or disseminated and gastric infections. The organisms responsible for these manifestations and their relative significance is shown in descending order in Table 12:1.

Enteric Infection

The symptoms and signs of enteric campylobacter infection are not so distinctive that the physician can differentiate it from illness caused by

Table 12:1. Etiologic Agents Associated with Different Clinical Manifestations of *Campylobacter* Infection

	Disease Symptoms		
	Enteric	Disseminated	Gastric
Major pathogen	*C. jejuni*	*C. fetus*	*C. pylori*
Minor pathogens	*C. coli*	*C. jejuni*	GCLO–2
	C. laridis	*C. coli*	
	C. fetus	*C. laridis*	
	C. fennelliae	*C. fennelliae*	
	C. cineadi	*C. cineadi*	
	C. upsaliensis	*C. upsaliensis*	

many other enteric pathogens. At the mild end of the spectrum, symptoms may last for only 24 hours and can be indistinguishable from those seen in viral gastroenteritis. In contrast, *C. jejuni* also may cause fulminent or relapsing colitis that mimics ulerative colitis or Crohn's disease.[6]

Our knowledge of the clinical features of campylobacter infection is based largely on studies of patients whose symptoms were sufficiently severe to prompt their physicians to obtain a fecal culture.[46] The predominant symptoms of such affected persons are diarrhea, abdominal pain, fever, nausea, vomiting and constitutional problems. A prodrome of constitutional problems, chiefly fever, may be more prominent than the enteric symptoms. A history of grossly bloody stools is common and many patients have at least one day with eight or more bowel movements.[2] Fever has been noted in up to 80% of these patients and abdominal pain has been severe enough to mimic acute appendicitis. True rigors have occasionally been noted. Generalized abdominal tenderness is common, but peritoneal signs are rare. Fecal leukocytes are usually present. On occasion, a cholera-like illness with massive watery diarrhea may occur.

Most patients recover in less than a week, but 10%-20% have a relapse or a prolonged or severe illness. Although most infections are self-limited and the prognosis is generally good, hospitalization due to campylobacter enteritis is not rare and fatalities can occur.[64] Some patients with persistently high fevers and frequent bloody stools have been suspected of having an acute episode of inflammatory bowel disease before campylobacter infection has been diagnosed. Colonoscopic and radiographic examinations have provided evidence of inflammation throughout the colon. Cases of toxic megacolon, pseudomembranous colitis, and a massive lower gastrointestinal hemorrhage also have been described. Mesenteric adenitis and appendicitis have been reported in children and young adults. *C. jejuni* and closely related organisms have been shown to cause infectious proctitis in homosexual men.

Among populations in developing countries, infection by *C. jejuni* is associated with much milder illness, without bloody diarrhea, fever or fecal leukocytes.[1,4,16,24,54] Asymptomatic infection occurs much more commonly than in the developed countries, especially in older children and adults.[25] However, when travelers from developed countries acquire *C. jejuni* infections, they usually have symptoms associated with inflammatory illness.[65]

Disseminated Infection

This appears to be much less common than enteric infection but is probably significantly underreported, since organisms may be difficult to isolate and identify, and once identified are usually not reported to appropriate health authorities. Most disseminated infections occur in compromised hosts. Predisposing disorders include hepatic disease, malignancies, diabetes mellitus, generalized atherosclerosis, acute and chronic alcoholism, renal failure, immunosuppression and malnutrition.[13] Most patients are males and are at the extremes of age.[11] Three syndromes have been recognized.

Transient Bacteremia:

This is frequently associated with intestinal symptoms and usually is due to *C. jejuni*.[7] Systemic symptoms resolve spontaneously and the positive blood cultures are of little clinical significance. This usually occurs in a previously normal host.

Sepsis:

This is the most frequent manifestation of disseminated campylobacteriosis, usually occurs in debilitated hosts and is mostly due to *C. fetus*.[11,13,29] Intestinal symptoms may or may not be present. Clinically, the illness manifests as acute gram-negative sepsis and if untreated, mortality is high. In some hosts, onset of illness is gradual. The only sign of infection may be temperature elevation in a patient with known underlying disease. Untreated infection in these hosts may wax and wane but generally worsens. Thrombophlebitis of an extremity is a common complication.

Localized Infection:

Organisms may seed any organ but the most common syndromes are acute pyogenic meningitis or meningoencephalitis, subacute endocarditis, spontaneous peritonitis, septic arthritis and septic abortion.[8] Most of these infections are due to *C. fetus* but on occasion serum-resistant strains of *C. jejuni* may be the cause.[7] Drainage of abscesses or loculated fluid is essential for cure, but because of underlying poor host status prognosis is poor.

Gastric Infection:

C. pylori is now commonly isolated from gastritis or gastric ulcers in the lesser curvature of the stomach and sometimes from duodenal ulcers, but uncommonly from patients without peptic ulcer disease. Infected persons develop serum antibody responses to *C. pylori* cellular antigens.[36] The major question that must be resolved is whether these organisms cause peptic gastritis or a related syndrome, whether peptic disease predisposes to colonization with otherwise harmless bacteria, or whether after an initial peptic insult, continued colonization causes ongoing damage.

ANTIMICROBIAL SUSCEPTIBILITY AND TREATMENT

A large number of *C. jejuni, C. coli* and *C. fetus* isolates have been tested in vitro for susceptibility to antimicrobial agents.[70,73,76] Virtually all organisms are susceptible to clinically achievable concentrations of aminoglycosides, chloramphenicol, furazolidone and carbenicillin. *C. coli* strains are often resistant to erythromycin, clindamycin and tetracycline whereas *C. jejuni* and *C. fetus* strains are usually susceptible.[76] Trimethoprim-sulfamethoxazole and ampicillin should not be used for empiric treatment since many strains are resistant.

The cornerstone of treatment of acute diarrheal illness is replacement of fecal volume loss. Treatment with antimotility agents appears to worsen the course of illness and is contraindicated in patients with bloody diarrhea or with other signs of an inflammatory process such as fever or the presence of fecal leukocytes. Five to seven days of antibiotic therapy is indicated for patients who are acutely ill with enteritis, with persistant fever, bloody diarrhea, more than 8 bowel movements per day or significant volume loss, or in patients with persistence of symptoms for more than 1 week. Bacteremia and other systemic infections also should be treated with antibiotics. *C. fetus* infections should be treated for 2-3 weeks as relapses may occur, whereas systemic *C. jejuni* infections should be treated for 10 days. Occasionally, patients are acutely ill and septic-appearing, but spontaneously recover. Blood cultures may only be recognized as positive after the patient has recovered. In most such cases, antimicrobial therapy is not needed but physicians should individualize management of this problem.

When antimicrobial therapy of acute *Campylobacter* enteritis is indicated, erythromycin is the treatment of choice.[8] Alternative agents include the tetracyclines, clindamycin or furazolidone. For systemic *C. fetus* or *C. jejuni* infections, an aminoglycoside or chloramphenicol has been recommended but erythromycin also may be sufficient. The necessity for treating *C. pylori* infections is uncertain at present.

EPIDEMIOLOGY

In developed countries, *C. jejuni* is an important cause of diarrhea in both children and adults.[10,18] Highest age-specific attack rates occur in children under one year old, with a gradual and progressive lowering through childhood. A second peak in attack rate is seen in older children and young adults.[61] Although these infections occur throughout the year, summertime peaks are typical. Asymptomatic infection has been noted during outbreaks of *Campylobacter* enteritis, but culture surveys of healthy children in non-outbreak settings show that the prevalence of infection is low, usually less than 1%.[10] The ultimate reservoir for *C. jejuni* is the intestinal tracts of most domesticated and many wild animal species, including the animals used for food production (cattle, sheep, poultry, swine and goats). Transmission from these sources accounts for most human infections. For example, more than 50% of poultry sold on supermarket shelves is contaminated with *C.*

jejuni. Pets, including dogs, cats, birds and rodents, also may transmit infection to humans. Excreta from wild animals may contaminate water supplies. Therefore, transmission of *C. jejuni* infection to humans may be food- or waterborne, via direct contact with infected animals or person-to-person.

In developing countries, isolation of *C. jejuni* from both healthy children and those with diarrhea is common. In studies in Bangladesh and India, *Campylobacter* isolation rates in children who were ill or well were not significantly different[24,54] and as many as 40% of healthy children under 2 years old may be found by a single culture to excrete *C. jejuni*. However, among infants under 9 months in Soweto, South Africa, *Campylobacter* isolation was significantly associated with illness.[14] A striking epidemiologic characteristic of *Campylobacter* infection in developing countries is its age relationship; isolation rates vary inversely with age. In children with diarrheal illness from whom *C. jejuni* is the only pathogen isolated, clinical features are different from those in children in developed countries. Fever and bloody stools are less common, and diarrheal illness generally is less severe and briefer.[14,24,25] Similarly, duration of convalescent excretion is briefer among infected children in developing than in developed countries. Little is known about transmission of *Campylobacter* infection in developing countries.

The reservoir for *C. fetus* also includes domesticated animals but appears much more restricted than for *C. jejuni*; cattle and sheep predominate. Animal contact or ingestion of foods of animal origin, including raw milk, are known causes of transmission to humans. Previously normal hosts generally develop acute gastrointestinal illness whereas in debilitated hosts systemic illness predominates. Although the actual incidence of *C. fetus* infections is not known and is certainly underreported, it nevertheless appears to be much less common than *C. jejuni* infection.

The sources of *C. pylori* are not known and the epidemiology of infection appears to parallel that of idiopathic gastritis.

PUBLIC HEALTH SIGNIFICANCE AND PREVENTION

Much that has been learned about *C. jejuni, C. coli* and *C. fetus* is similar to that which is known about the salmonellae. As with salmonellae, the major identified reservoirs are animals and products obtained from animals. Although raw milk and untreated water[68] most frequently have been shown to be vehicles for epidemic *Campylobacter* infection, poultry, poultry products and meats are most important for sporadic cases. Although dogs, cats and birds have been shown to harbor salmonellae, they are not commonly recognized vectors for human infection. Similarly, although *Campylobacter* from puppies and kittens may infect some humans, pets are not the major vector for *Campylobacter*. Campylobacters have been found frequently in the developing world, while salmonellae are less frequently found. This phenomenon deserves exploration, since it suggests differences beween reservoirs or transmission patterns not yet identified. In the developed countries, *Campylobacter* infection is a very common cause of acute diarrheal illness. Although deaths occur, they appear to be uncommon. In contrast, the prevalence of *Campylobacter* infection in young children in developing countries suggests that it is probably a leading cause of morbidity and mortality in the first 2 years of life.

Control of *C. jejuni, C. coli* and *C. fetus* infections will ultimately be based on a better understanding of the reservoirs, epidemiology and pathophysiology of the infection. Since available evidence shows that farm and household animals constitute a major reservoir for these organisms, interruption of transmission to humans from these sources should have a high priority. Awareness of the necessity for handwashing after contact with animals or animal products and the importance of proper cooking and storage of foods of animal origin are probably as important for preventing *C. jejuni* infections as they are for preventing *Salmonella* infections. Pasteurization of milk, chlorination of water supplies[9] and thorough cooking of meat all readily kill *C. jejuni*. The public health significance of *C. pylori* is currently unknown. At the least, its presence is a marker for peptic ulcer disease and it could be involved in the pathogenesis of this disorder.

DIAGNOSTIC PROCEDURES

Rapid Methodology

Rapid specific diagnosis of *C. jejuni* or *C. fetus* infections using immunologic methods is not presently available. However, definition of group antigens makes it likely that such methodologies will be used in the future. Rapid diagnosis of *C. pylori* infection can be done. Gastric biopsy specimens may be crushed and introduced into Christensen's urea broth; the strong urease production by *C. pylori* will turn the tube positive within several hours and is a highly sensitive and specific test.[47,51]

Microscopic Methods:

It is possible to make a presumptive diagnosis of *Campylobacter* enteritis by direct examination of a fecal specimen. A wet preparation of stool in saline or broth may be observed for motility of the organisms by darkfield or phase-contrast microscopy.[52] Campylobacters in stool usually appear to be corkscrew or comma-shaped motile rods with darting motility. The organisms are so active that frequently they appear to jump from the slide preparation toward the observer. Distilled water inhibits motility and should not be used for preparation of mounts.[19] The wet mount is used only for presumptive diagnosis since occasional *Pseudomonas* strains can exhibit a similar motility pattern. A direct fecal smear may be Gram stained using carbolfuchsin as counterstain and examined by light microscopy. Many small gram-negative organisms with comma, "S", or seagull-shaped morphology constitute a presumptive diagnosis.

Primary Isolation

Important factors in cultivation of the campylobacters are transport of specimens, incubation temperature and selection of atmosphere and media.[74]

Transport of Specimens:

The majority of *C. jejuni, C. coli* and *C. laridis* are cultured from stool specimens, while most *C. fetus* subsp. *fetus* are isolated from blood and/or body fluids. These organisms survive well in blood culture media during transport, but they perish easily in unrefrigerated stool specimens. If immediate culturing of fecal specimens is not possible, a small portion should be kept in a preservative medium such as thioglycolate broth with pH 8.5 or alkaline peptone water with reducing agents (0.05 sodium thioglycolate with 0.025% cysteine).[77] Specimens with or without preservative should be kept at 4°C to prevent early death of the organisms.

Incubation Conditions:

Campylobacters and most campylobacter-like organisms grow well at 37°C, but *C. jejuni, C. coli* and *C. laridis* grow best at 42-43°C. Ideally, inoculated plates should be incubated at both 37°C and 42-43°C to facilitate the growth of different pathogenic campylobacters. As campylobacters are microaerophilic, a general method to achieve an appropriate atmosphere is to evacuate 75% of the air from an anaerobic jar and replace it with a gas mixture of 10% carbon dioxide and 90% nitrogen or completely evacuate the jar and fill with 5% oxygen, 10% carbon dioxide and 85% nitrogen. Other methods are listed in Table 12:2.

Filtration and Nonselective Media:

Membrane filtration has been used for the isolation of campylobacters in stool,[28,49,66] since campylobacters with a diameter of 0.2-0.5 μm will pass through a membrane with 0.65 μm pore size whereas other enteric bacteria will not. Filtrates then may be cultured on nonselective media. In one method, a low speed centrifugation (650-800 X g) precedes sequential 2-chamber filtration. The first stage of filtration uses a 8.0 μm and a 1.2 μm

Table 12:2. Methods for Achieving Appropriate Atmosphere Conditions for Incubation of *C. jejuni* and Related Organisms

Method	*Comment*	*Reference*
Evacuation-replacement	Impermeable polyethylene bags may be used instead of anaerobic jars	37
Disposable gas envelopes	Jars should have not more than 6 to 8 plates	75
Candle jar	Incubation at 42°C is usually necessary	74
Fortner principle	Requires a second plate with a facultative organism	38

non-sterile membrane and a lower chamber with a sterile 0.65 μm filter. Several drops of the filtrate are inoculated onto a nonselective medium and incubated.[28] One advantage of the filtration method is that nonselective media, such as chocolate and blood agar plates, are readily available in all clinical microbiology laboratories. Under appropriate incubation conditions, campylobacters will grow on these media if not subjected to the competition of the more common enteric bacteria. The disadvantages are the special effort required to prepare the 2-chamber filters and the 100-fold reduction of organisms during filtration. As human cases of *Campylobacter* enteritis usually contain 10^6 to 10^9 colony-forming units (CFU) of *C. jejuni* per gram of feces, the loss of 1-2 logs of organisms through filtration may not be significant. This technique has been simplified recently by placing a 0.65 μm filter directly on the nonselective medium and applying liquid stool or a fecal suspension to the filter. The filter may be removed after 1 h incubation at 37°C and the plate reincubated for 48 h.[66] This technique may be used to identify campylobacters susceptible to antibiotic agents present in selective media.[49]

Selective Media:

Selective media are much more widely used to isolate campylobacters from fecal specimens. Enrichment with 5%-10% sheep or horse blood is usual; however, bloodless media have been developed.[16] Various basal media are suitable, such as Brucella agar, Oxoid blood agar base No. 2, Columbia agar and tryptose agar (Difco Laboratories). The most commonly used selective media are: (1) Skirrow's medium[61] containing vancomycin, polymyxin B and trimethoprim as selective agents and requiring 7% lysed horse blood in order to neutralize trimethoprim antagonists such as thymidine; however, blood from other animals may be used as well; (2) Butzler's medium Oxoid using colistin, cefazolin, bacitracin, novobiocin and cycloheximide as selective agents;[18] (3) Butzler's medium Virion using cefaperazone, rifampin, colistin and amphotericin B as selective agents[27] to improve inhibition of *Pseudomonas* and *Proteus*; (4) Campy-BAP having the same

Table 12:3. Differential Characteristics of *Campylobacter* Species Related to Human Disease

	Growth							Susceptibility to 30 μg disk		
	25°C	37°C	42°C	Nirate reduction	TSI	H_2S in lead acetate paper	Hippurate hydrolysis	Cephalothin	Nalidixic acid	C-19 fatty acid production
C. jejuni	–	+	+	+	–	+	+	R*	S*	+
C. coli	–	+	+	+	–	+	–	R	S	+
C. laridis	–	+	+	+	–	+	–	R	R	–
C. fetus subsp. *fetus*	+	+	d*	+	–	d	–	S	R	–
C. hyointestinalis	d	+	d	+	+	+	–	S	R	–
C. cineadi	–	+	–	+	–	+	–	S	S	–
C. fennelliae	–	+	–	–	–	+	–	S	S	–
C. pylori	–	+	–	–		+	–	R	R	+
C. upsaliensis†	–	+	+	+	–	+	–	S	S	–

* R = resistant; S = susceptible; d = variable; † = catalase negative or weak

selective agents as Skirrow's medium plus cephalothin to inhibit spreading *Proteus* and amphotericin B to inhibit yeasts; and Brucella agar with 5% sheep blood as the basal medium; and (5) Preston medium using rifampin, polymyxin, trimethoprim and cycloheximide as selective agents.[16] Media with cephalosporins generally are most selective but may inhibit the non-*jejuni Campylobacter* species.

Several enrichment and/or selective media also have been described including: (1) Liquid enrichment medium[32] which has the same selective agents as Skirrow's medium with nutrient broth No. 2 (Oxoid) as base and 7% lysed horse blood; (2) Preston medium with FBP supplement;[16] (3) Waterman's enrichment broth with vancomycin, polymyxin, trimethoprim and cycloheximide as selective agents;[78] (4) Campy-thio which was originally designed to preserve and transport specimens, has served as an apparent enrichment broth;[57] and (5) Doyle's medium[21] which is especially useful for isolations from foods. Nevertheless, selective enrichment media for campylobacters are less efficient than those enrichment broths employed for isolation of salmonellae; consequently none are widely used.

Methods for Identification

Inoculated plates should be examined 24, 48 and 72 h after incubation. If only one reading is practical, then 48 h is the optimum time. *C. jejuni* and related organisms show two types of colonies in stool cultures. One is wet, mucoid, spreading and flat, with irregular borders. These are gray and nonhemolytic, but sometimes may be pink-tinged, depending on the type of medium used. Frequently, the growth is very flat resembling water condensation marks. The other colonial type is also nonhemolytic, discrete (1-2 μm in diameter), convex, entire and glistening. The experienced observer can distinguish *Campylobacter* colonies without difficulty. Suspect colonies should be Gram stained. *C. jejuni* are small, slender, curved to spiral gram-negative rods. In cultures older than 72 hours, *C. jejuni* cells become coccal, which may be confusing. Coccal forms are not readily subculturable; thus, if growth is beginning to show coccal forms, immediate subculturing is necessary.

Catalase and oxidase tests should be made on the primary growth. Virtually all the pathogenic campylobacters are catalase- and oxidase-positive; occasional strains may have weak or negative catalase reactions.[59] Suspend colonies of suspected campylobacters in a drop of saline or broth for assessment of motility. Use darkfield or phase-contrast microscopy to show typical darting motility. Since other bacteria also show this type of motility, confirmatory tests are necessary. Motility media such as motility-indole-ornithine (MIO) or sulfide-indole-motility (SIM) are not recommended because growth of *Campylobacter* in these media is difficult to interpret.

Table 12:3 shows the results of confirmatory tests. For study of growth temperature characteristics, three tubes of Brucella broth are inoculated with a suspension of bacterial growth, the optical density is standardized (MacFarland 1), 2 drops of the suspension are inoculated into each of the tubes, and one each is incubated at 25°C, 37°C or 42°C in the appropriate atmosphere. Alternatively, a plate medium such as 5% sheep blood agar may also be used for testing and several strains may be inoculated onto one plate. Tubes of TSI or Kliglers should be inoculated by stabbing the butt and streaking the slant as for cultures of *Enterobacteriaceae*, and a lead acetate paper strip should be suspended over the slanted medium. Incubate for 48 h and observe the blackening of the lead acetate paper (H_2S positive). Negatives may be reincubated for 7 days for further examination. Most campylobacters are nitrate-positive but *Campylobacter*-like organisms groups 2 and 3 are negative. *C. jejuni, C. coli* and *C. pylori* contain C-19 cyclopropane in their cell walls, whereas other *Campylobacter* species do not.[5,26] Although this characteristic appears to be definitive, analysis requires gas-liquid chromatography which is not routinely used in clinical microbiology laboratories.

A rapid method for testing hippurate hydrolysis is most useful for differentiating *C. coli* from *C. jejuni*.[30,31] A tube of hippurate testing medium should be heavily inoculated and then incubated in a waterbath for 2 h. Ninhydrin solution (0.2 mL of 3.5% ninhydrin in a mixture of acetone and butanol) should be added down the side of the tube to form an overlay. After a 10 min incubation at 37°C, the overlay should be examined for color change. Deep purple is considered a positive test. A weak color reaction is considered negative. Newly isolated strains of *C. jejuni* usually give strong positive reactions but frozen stock strains and occasional fresh isolates may show a weak or negative reaction. The clinical infections caused by *C. jejuni* and *C. coli* appear identical, and hippurate testing is recommended only for epidemiologic or research purposes.

Antimicrobial susceptibility tests also are used for identification of campylobacters. A blood agar plate is inoculated with the suspension of organisms prepared for temperature studies and 30 μg nalidixic acid and cephalothin disks are placed on its surface. Also add a 30 μg erythromycin disc for confirmation of susceptibility since this antibiotic is widely used to treat human infections. Plates with the 3 disks should be incubated at 35-37°C overnight for 24-48 h. The 48 h reading is taken only if no growth appears at 24 h. *C. fetus* subsp. *fetus* is resistant to nalidixic acid but is usually inhibited by the cephalothin disk. *C. jejuni* is sensitive to nalidixic acid but not to cephalothin.

A group of organisms resembling *C. jejuni* phenotypically but genetically different have been isolated from homosexual men with enteritis, proctitis and proctocolitis.[22] They grow slowly, unlike *C. jejuni* or *C. fetus*, and usually take more than 5 days to show visible growth. They do not grow at 25°C but grow well at 37°C. Growth at 42°C is variable. These campylobacter-like organisms (which now include *C. cineadi* and *C. fennelliae*) neither grow anaerobically nor at the level of oxygen (17%) in candle jars. Most of the results of the biochemical tests commonly used to identify these campylobacter-like organisms are similar to those for the other campylobacters. In contrast to *C. jejuni*, campylobacter-like organisms are hippurate-negative and some are nitrate-negative.[22,69]

Another group of organisms, currently called *C. pylori* have a morphology similar to that of *C. jejuni*, and their G + C content, 36 mol%, is in the range for the genus *Campylobacter*. They grow readily in an atmosphere of 5% oxygen, 10% carbon dioxide, 10% hydrogen and 75% nitrogen at 37°C in 3-5 days, and are nalidixic acid and cephalothin resistant. These organisms develop coccal forms after 2-4 days and appear to be very sensitive to air. Hippurate-positive strains have been reported and some strains are weakly catalase-positive. Most are strongly urease-positive.[47,51] Whether or not these organisms cause peptic ulceration, their presence is associated with, and may be a marker for, certain of these lesions.

Markers for Epidemiology

Serotyping of *C. jejuni* and *C. coli* is useful for understanding the epidemiology of these infections. Currently, two major methods are available. One is the Penner method,[53] which is an indirect hemagglutination technique using soluble heat-stable antigens, and the other is the Lior method which is a slide agglutination technique based on heat-labile antigens.[44] Absorbed antisera are not needed for the Penner method, making it easier to apply but more difficult to interpret. The Lior method requires absorbed antisera, but is simpler to perform. Crossreactions of cultures are encountered with the Penner method but are not frequent with the Lior method. Most routine laboratories will have little reason to serotype strains. Bacteriophages specific for several *Campylobacter* species have been described,[17] but none are routinely used in clinical microbiology laboratories.

Toxigenicity Tests

The pathogenesis of *C. jejuni* infection is uncertain. The finding of cellular infiltration in colonic biopsy specimens and the occasional presence of bacteremia suggest that these organisms may be invasive. Toxin production also has been demonstrated including an enterotoxin similar to cholera toxin[42,58] and several cytotoxins.[33,79] Toxigenicity studies have been done using tissue culture and other in vitro assays and various animal models but are not used in routine laboratories.

Serology

Most patients infected with *C. jejuni* show seroconversion to *C. jejuni* group cellular antigens[3,34,35] by two weeks postinfection. Antibodies to *C. fetus* can be measured using an indirect hemagglutination assay.[12]

EVALUATION OF LABORATORY FINDINGS

Isolation of any *Campylobacter* organism from a normally sterile site such as the bloodstream must be considered clinically significant. Isolation of campylobacters from stools is usually clinically significant; however, patients with asymptomatic or mild infections do not require specific treatment. Convalescent intestinal excretion persisting more than six months is distinctly unusual if it exists at all. Recurrent asymptomatic infection may occur in older children and adults in developing areas where levels of hygiene are poor and constant re-exposure is the rule. Although *C. pylori* is clearly associated with peptic disease, its etiologic significance is uncertain at present.

REFERENCES

1. Billingham JD. *Campylobacter* enteritis in the Gambia. Trans Roy Soc Trop Med Hyg 1981;75:641-4.
2. Blaser MJ, Berkowitz ID, LaForce FM, Cravena J, Reller LB, Wang WLL. *Campylobacter* enteritis: clinical and epidemiologic features. Ann Intern Med 1979;91:179-85.
3. Blaser MJ, Duncan DJ. Human serum antibody response to *Campylobacter jejuni* as measured in an enzyme-linked immunosorbent assay. Infect Immun 1984;44:292-8.
4. Blaser MJ, Glass RI, Huq MI, Stoll B, Kibriya GM, Alim ARMA. Isolation of *Campylobacter fetus* subsp. *jejuni* from Bangladeshi children. J Clin Microbiol 1980;12:744-7.
5. Blaser MJ, Moss CM, Weaver RE. Cellular fatty acid composition of *Campylobacter fetus*. J Clin Microbiol 1980;11:448-51.
6. Blaser JM, Parsons RB, Wang WLL. Acute colitis caused by *Campylobacter fetus* ss. *jejuni*. Gastroenterology 1980;78:448-53.
7. Blaser MJ, Perez GP, Smith PF, Patton C, Lastovica AJ, Wang WLL. Extraintestinal *Campylobacter jejuni* and *Campylobacter coli* infections: host factors and strain characteristics. J Infect Dis 1986;153:552-9.
8. Blaser MJ, Reller LB. *Campylobacter* enteritis. New Engl J Med 1981;305:1444-52.
9. Blaser MJ, Smith PF, Wang WLL, Hoff JC. Inactivation of *Campylobacter jejuni* by chlorine and monochloramine. Appl Environ Microbiol 1986;51:307-11.
10. Blaser MJ, Taylor DN, Feldman RA. Epidemiology of *Campylobacter jejuni* infections. Epidemiol Rev 1983;5:157-76.
11. Bokkenheuser V. *Vibrio fetus* infection in man. I. Ten new cases and some epidemiological observations. Am J Epidemiol 1970;91:400-9.
12. Bokkenheuser V. *Vibrio fetus* infection in man: a serological test. Infect Immun 1972;5:222-6.
13. Bokkenheuser V. *Vibrio fetus* infection in man. Occurrence, clinical picture, serology and source of infection. In: von Graevenitz A, Sall T, eds. Microorganisms and infectious disease. New York: Marcel Dekker, 1975;1:25-32.
14. Bokkenheuser VD, Richardson NJ, Bryner JH, et al. Detection of enteric campylobacteriosis in children. J Clin Microbiol 1979;9:227-32.
15. Bolton FJ, Coates D. Development of a blood-free *Campylobacter* medium; screening tests on basal media and supplements, and the ability of selected supplements to facilitate aerotolerance. J Appl Bacteriol 1983;54:125-30.
16. Bolton FJ, Robertson L. A selective medium for isolating *Campylobacter jejuni/coli*. J Clin Pathol 1982;35:462-7.

17. Bryner JH, Ritchie AE, Booth GD, Foley JW. Lytic activity of *Vibrio* phages on strains of *Vibrio fetus* isolated from man and animals. Appl Microbiol 1973;26:404-9.
18. Butzler JP, Skirrow MB. *Campylobacter* enteritis. Clin Gastroenterol 1979;8:737-65.
19. Chester B, Poulos G. Rapid presumptive identification of vibrios by immobilization in distilled water. J Clin Microbiol 1980;11:537-9.
20. Dekeyser P, Gossuin-Detrain M, Butzler JP, Sternon J. Acute enteritis due to related vibrio: first positive stool cultures. J Infect Dis 1972;125:390-2.
21. Doyle MP, Koidis P. Procedure for increased recovery of *Campylobacter jejuni* from inoculated unpasteurized milk. Appl Environ Microbiol 1984;47:455-60.
22. Fennell CL, Totten PA, Quinn TC, Patton DL, Holmes KK, Stamm WE. Characterization of campylobacter-like organisms isolated from homosexual men. J Infect Dis 1984;149:58-66.
23. Gebhart CJ, Edmonds P, Ward GE, Kurtz HJ, Brenner DJ. "*Campylobacter hypointestinalis*" sp. nov.: a new species of *Campylobacter* found in the intestines of pigs and other animals. J Clin Microbiol 1985;21:715-20.
24. Glass R, Stoll BJ, Huq MI, Struelens M, Blaser MJ, Kibriya AKMG. Epidemiological and clinical features of endemic *Campylobacter jejuni* infection in Bangladesh. J Infect Dis 1983;148:292-6.
25. Glass RI, Stoll BJ, Huq MI, Struelens M, Kibriya AKMG. Family studies of *Campylobacter jejuni* in Bangladesh: implications for pathogenesis and transmission. In: Pearson AD, ed. *Campylobacter* II. Proceedings of the second international workshop on campylobacter infections. London: Public Health Laboratory Systems, 1983:141-2.
26. Goodwin CS, McCulloch RK, Armstrong JA, Wee SH. Unusual cellular fatty acids and distinctive ultrastructure in a new spiral bacterium (*Campylobacter pyloridis*) from the human gastric mucosa. J Med Microbiol 1985;19:257-67.
27. Goossens H, DeBoeck M, Butzler JP. A new selective medium for the isolation of *Campylobacter jejuni* from human faeces. Eur J Clin Microbiol 1983;2:389-94.
28. Grant IH, Richardson NJ, Bokkenheuser VD. Broiler chickens as potential source of campylobacter infections in humans. J Clin Microbiol 1980;11:508-10.
29. Guerrant RL, Lajita RG, Winn WC Jr, Roberts RB. Campylobacteriosis in man: pathogenic mechanisms and review of 91 bloodstream infections. Am J Med 1978;65:584-92.
30. Harvey SM. Hippurate hydrolysis by *Campylobacter fetus*. J Clin Microbiol 1980;11:435-7.
31. Hebert GA, Hollis DG, Weaver RE, Lambert MA, Blaser MJ, Moss CW. Thirty years of campylobacters: their biochemical characteristics and a biotyping proposal for *C. jejuni*. J Clin Microbiol 1982;15:1065-73.
32. Hodge DS, Terro R. Comparative efficacy of liquid enrichment medium for isolation of *Campylobacter*. J Clin Microbiol 1984;19:434.
33. Johnson WM, Lior M. Toxins produced by *Campylobacter jejuni* and *Campylobacter coli*. Lancet 1984;1:229-30.
34. Jones DM, Eldridge J, Dale B. Serological response to *Campylobacter jejuni/coli* infection. J Clin Pathol 1980;33:767-9.
35. Kaldor J, Pritchard H. Serum antibodies in *Campylobacter* enteritis. J Clin Microbiol 1983;18:1-4.
36. Kaldor J, Tee W, McCarthy P, Watson J, Dwyer B. Immune response to *Campylobacter pyloridis* in patients with peptic ulceration. Lancet 1985;1:921.
37. Kaplan RL. *Campylobacter*. In: Lennette EH, Balows A, Hausler WJ Jr, Truant JP, eds. Manual of clinical microbiology. 3rd ed. Washington, DC: American Society for Microbiology, 1980:235-41.
38. Karmali MA, Fleming PC. Application of the Fortner principle to isolation of *Campylobacter* from stools. J Clin Microbiol 1979;10:245-7.
39. Karmali MA, Skirrow MB. Taxonomy of the genus *Campylobacter*. In: Butzler JP, ed. *Campylobacter* infection in man and animals. Boca Raton, FL: CRC Press, 1984:1-20.

40. King EO. Human infections with *Vibrio fetus* and a closely related *Vibrio*. J Infect Dis 1957;101:119-28.
41. King EO. The laboratory recognition of *Vibrio fetus* and a closely related *Vibrio* from cases of human vibriosis. Ann NY Acad Sci 1962;98:700-11.
42. Klipstein FA, Engert RF. Properties of crude *Campylobacter jejuni* heat-labile enterotoxin. Infect Immun 1984;45:314-19.
43. Lawson GHK, Leaver JL, Pettigrew GW, Rowland AC. Some features of *Campylobacter sputorum* subsp. *mucosalis* subsp. nov., nom. rev. and their taxonomic significance. Int J Syst Bacteriol 1981;31:385-91.
44. Lior H, Woodward DL, Edgar JA, LaRoche LJ. Serotyping by slide agglutination of *Campylobacter jejuni* and epidemiology. Lancet 1981;2:1103-4.
45. Loesche WJ, Gibbons RJ, Socransky SS. Biochemical characteristics of *Vibrio sputorum* and relationship to *Vibrio bubulus* and *Vibrio fetus*. J Bacteriol 1965;89:1109-16.
46. Mandal BK, De Mol P, Butzler JP. Clinical aspects of campylobacter infections in humans. In: Butzler JP, ed. *Campylobacter* infection in man and animals. Boca Raton, FL: CRC Press, 1984:21-30.
47. McNulty CAM, Wise R. Rapid diagnosis of *Campylobacter pyloridis* gastritis. Lancet 1986;1:387.
48. Marshall BJ, Warren JR. Unidentified curved bacilli in the stomach of patients with gastritis and peptic ulceration. Lancet 1984;1:1311-15.
49. Megraud F, Elharrif E. Isolation of *Campylobacter* species by filtration. Eur J Clin Microbiol 1985;4:437-8.
50. Morris GK, Patton CM. *Campylobacter*. In: Lennette EH, Balows A, Hausler WJ Jr, Shadomy HJ, eds. Manual of clinical microbiology. 4th ed. Washington, DC: American Society for Microbiology, 1985:302-8.
51. Owen RJ, Martin SR, Borman P. Rapid urea hydrolysis by gastric campylobacters. Lancet 1985;1:111.
52. Paisley JW, Mirrett S, Lauer BA, Roe M, Reller LB. Darkfield microscopy of human feces for presumptive diagnosis of *Campylobacter fetus* subsp. *jejuni* enteritis. J Clin Microbiol 1982;15:61-3.
53. Penner JL, Hennessey JN. Passive hemagglutination technique for serotyping *Campylobacter fetus* subsp. *jejuni* on the basis of soluble heat stable antigens. J Clin Microbiol 1980;12:732-7.
54. Rajan DP, Mathan VI. Prevalence of *Campylobacter fetus* subsp. *jejuni* in healthy populations in southern India. J Clin Microbiol 1982;15;749-51.
55. Riley LW, Finch MJ. Results of the first year of national surveillance of *Campylobacter* infections in the United States. J Infect Dis 1985;151:956-9.
56. Roop RM II, Smibert RM, Johnson JL, Krieg NR. DNA homology studies of the catalase-negative campylobacters and "*Campylobacter fecalis*," an emended description of *Campylobacter sputorum*, and proposal of the neotype strain of *Campylobacter sputorum*. Can J Microbiol 1985;31:823-31.
57. Rubin SJ, Woodard M. Enhanced isolation of *Campylobacter jejuni* by cold enrichment in Campy-thio broth. J Clin Microbiol 1983;18:1008-10.
58. Ruiz-Pallacios GM, Torres J, Torres NI, Escmilla E, Ruiz-Pallacios BR, Tamayo J. Cholera-like enterotoxin produced by *Campylobacter jejuni*. Lancet 1983;2:250-2.
59. Sandstedt K, Ursing J, Walder M. Thermotolerant *Campylobacter* with no or weak catalase activity isolated from dogs. Curr Microbiol 1983;8:209-13.
60. Skerman VBD, McGowen V, Sneath PHA. Approved lists of bacterial names. Int J Syst Bacteriol 1980;30:225-420.
61. Skirrow MB. *Campylobacter* enteritis: a "new" disease. Br Med J 1977;2:9-11.
62. Smibert RM. The genus *Campylobacter*. Ann Rev Microbiol 1978;32:674-709.

63. Smibert RM. Genus *Campylobacter* Sebald and Veron 1963, 907[AL]. In: Krieg NR, Hold JG, eds. Bergey's manual of systematic bacteriology; vol. 1. Baltimore: Williams and Wilkins, 1984:111-18.
64. Smith GS, Blaser MJ. Fatalities associated with *Campylobacter jejuni* infections. JAMA 1985;253:2873-5.
65. Speelman P, Struelens MJ. Detection of *Campylobacter jejuni* and other potential pathogens in travelers' diarrhea in Bangladesh. Scand J Gastroenterol 1983;18:19-25.
66. Steele TW, McDermott SN. The use of membrane filters applied directly to the surface of agar plates for the isolation of *Campylobacter jejuni* from feces. Pathology 1984;16:263-5.
67. Tanner ACR, Badges S, Lai CH, Listgarten MA, Visconti RA, Socransky SS. *Wolinella* gen. nov. *Wolinella succinogenes (Vibrio succinogenes*, Wolin et al). Comb. nov., and description of *Bacteroides gracilis* sp. nov., *Wolinella recta* sp. nov., *Campylobacter concisus* sp. nov., and *Eikenella corrodans* from humans with periodontal disease. Int J Syst Bacteriol 1981;31:432-45.
68. Taylor DN, McDermott KT, Little JR, Wells JG, Blaser MJ. *Campylobacter* enteritis from untreated water in the Rocky Mountains. Ann Intern Med 1983;99:38-40.
69. Totten PA, Fennell CL, Tenover FC, et al. *Campylobacter cinaedi* (sp. nov) and *Campylobacter fennelliae* (sp. nov): two new campylobacter species associated with enteric disease in homosexual men. J Infect Dis 1985;151:131-9.
70. Vanhoof R, Gordts B, Dierickx R, Coignau H, Butzler JP. Bacteriostatic and bactericidal activities of 24 animicrobial agents against *Campylobacter fetus* subsp. *jejuni*. Antimicrob Agents Chemother 1980;18:118-21.
71. Veron M, Chatelain R. Taxonomic study of the genus *Campylobacter* Sebald and Veron and designation of the neotype strain for the type species, *Campylobacter fetus* (Smith and Taylor) Sebald and Veron. Int J Syst Bacteriol 1973;23:122-34.
72. Vinzent R, Dumas J, Picard N. Septicemie grave au cours de la grossesse due a un vibrion: avortement consecutif. Bull Acad Natl Med (Paris) 1947;131:90-2.
73. Walder M. Susceptibility of *Campylobacter fetus* subsp. *jejuni* to twenty antimicrobial agents. Antimicrob Agents Chemother 1979;16:37-9.
74. Wang WLL, Luechtefeld NW, Blaser MJ, Reller LB. Effect of incubation atmosphere and temperature on isolation of *Campylobacter jejuni* from human stools. Can J Microbiol 1983;29:468-70.
75. Wang WLL, Luechtefeld NW, Blaser MJ, Reller LB. Comparison of CampyPak II with standard 5% oxygen and candle jar for growth of *Campylobacter jejuni* from human feces. J Clin Microbiol 1982;16:291-4.
76. Wang WLL, Reller LB, Blaser MJ. Comparison of antimicrobial susceptibility patterns between *Campylobacter jejuni* and *Campylobacter coli*. Antimicrob Agents Chemother 1984;26:351-3.
77. Wang WLL, Reller LB, Smallwood B, Luechtefeld NW, Blaser MJ. Evaluation of transport media for *Campylobacter jejuni* in human fecal specimens. J Clin Microbiol 1983;18:803-7.
78. Waterman SC, Park RWA, Bramley AJ. A search for the source of *Campylobacter jejuni* in milk. J Hyg 1984;93:333-8.
79. Yeen WD, Puthucheary SD, Pang T. Demonstration of a cytotoxin from *Campylobacter jejuni*. J Clin Pathol 1983;36:1237-40.

CHAPTER 13

CORYNEBACTERIAL INFECTIONS

Jill E. Clarridge, Ph.D. and Alice S. Weissfeld, Ph.D.

INTRODUCTION

The history of the corynebacteria, particularly *C. diphtheriae*, is a discussion of the very roots of clinical microbiology and infectious disease.[28] The term "diphtherite" was coined by Pierre Bretonneau in 1826, from the Greek root for skin or hide; this word was chosen because of the resemblance of the pharyngeal membrane in diphtheria to a piece of leather. Friedrich Loeffler published the definitive proof that a bacillus was the etiologic agent responsible for diphtheria in 1885, and Emil von Behring received the first Nobel Prize in medicine in 1901 for his suggestion that diphtheria antitoxin be used to treat patients with diphtheria.

In 1896, Lehmann and Neumann proposed that bacteria morphologically resembling the diphtheria bacillus be incorporated into the genus *Corynebacterium*. Corynebacteria other than *C. diphtheriae* are generally referred to as diphtheroids or coryneforms. Although immunization has virtually eliminated diphtheria from developed countries today, other coryneforms have been recognized as human pathogens.

CAUSATIVE ORGANISMS

C. diphtheriae, the type species of the genus, is a gram-positive, pleomorphic, nonsporulating, nonmotile, nonacidfast bacillus. It shares with other coryneform organisms the tendency to form palisading groups of bacteria ("Chinese letters") and for some rods to be thicker on one end than on the other (i.e., clubshaped; *coryne* means club in Greek). *C. diphtheriae* differs from some other *Corynebacterium* spp. in containing metachromatic granules and having an overall morphology that is more beaded, delicate, slender and difficult to stain (See color plate Fig. 13:1). It is facultatively anaerobic and grows well on common laboratory media. Its optimum temperature range is 34-37°C. This organism is the etiologic agent of diphtheria and causes natural infection only in humans.

The taxonomy of the other *Corynebacterium* spp. and coryneforms is complex and not fully delineated at this time, although considerable progress has been made by study of the cell wall, fatty acid, menaquinones and mycolic acid composition of these organisms. The genus *Corynebacterium* should be confined to coryneform bacteria which contain meso-diaminopimelic acid (meso DAP), arabinose and galatose in the cell wall.[17] The organisms are catalase-positive, generally facultatively anaerobic, have a DNA composition in the range of 51-63 mol% guanine + cytosine (G+C) and have short-chain mycolic acids (range 22-36 carbon atoms). They are not acidfast and do not form spores. Genera which resemble the corynebacteria, were formerly classified as *Corynebacterium*, or could because of their morphology be confused in a clinical microbiology laboratory with corynebacteria, include *Actinomyces, Arachnia, Arcanobacterium, Bacterionema, Mycobacterium, Nocardia, Oerskovia, Propionibacterium, Rhodococcus* and *Rothia*. There are reports of isolates from each of these groups being associated with human disease.[7,9,14,25,30,37,51,68,69,80,82] Except for those caused by *Mycobacterium* and *Nocardia*, the infections are usually opportunistic and of low virulence. *Brevibacterium* can be isolated from humans as well as from cheese, but have been reported only as normal flora.[65] Genera of gram-positive rods which are more easily distinguished from the corynebacteria and which contain major human pathogens include *Bacillus, Erysipelothrix* and *Listeria*. Differential characteristics of these genera are listed in Table 13:1. Some important cell wall and morphological data as well as biochemical tests are described. Other coryneform genera such as *Arthrobacter, Caseobacter, Cellulomonas, Curtobacterium* and *Microbacterium* have not been reported as isolated from humans. The taxonomy of the coryneform groups has been studied both by DNA homology and biochemical relatedness.[1,17,21,34,44,48,52,68,70,75] There are 16 *Corynebacterium* spp., including *C. diphtheriae*, described in "Bergey's Manual of Systematic Bacteriology."[17] The differential characteristics of the significant species are given in Table 13:2. The first eight species listed, *C. matruchotii*, the CDC groups and the unassigned groups have been isolated from humans. The other valid *Corynebacterium* spp. have not been associated with humans as either pathogens or normal flora. *C. flavescens* has been isolated from dairy products, *C. cystitidis, C. pilosum* and *C. renale* are associated with cystitis in cattle, *C. kutscheri* is associated with healthy and diseased rodents and *C. vitarumen, C. glutamicum* and *C. callunae* have been isolated from healthy plants or animals.[17] Some biochemical characteristics of *C. cystitidis, C. pilosum, C. renale* and *C. kutscheri* are included in Table 13:2 because their animal hosts are closely associated with humans.

The Centers for Disease Control (CDC) has tried to group the biochemically related coryneform organisms which have been isolated from humans.[79]

Although some are not valid species and a few are probably not even in the genus *Corynebacterium* (e.g., the motile organisms in CDC groups A-3, A-4 and A-5), there are reports of isolation of these organisms in association with human disease; therefore, descriptive and biochemical data on pertinent groups of these organisms are also included in Tables 13:2 and 13:3.

CORYNEBACTERIA DIPHTHERIAE

VIRULENCE

The virulence of *C. diphtheriae* is due almost entirely to the production of toxin. The toxin is a protein of 58,342 daltons molecular weight, coded for by the *tox* gene.[1,63] The *tox* gene is part of the DNA of the lysogenic phage which belongs to the β family of corynephage. The corynebacteria become virulent because the prophage enters the host cell (usually *C. diphtheriae*, but *C. ulcerans* and *C. pseudotuberculosis* can also be infected) and integrates its DNA into the chromosome of the host, forming a lysogenic bacterium, or lysogen.

Evidently, the occurrence of the *tox* gene or its expression varies in the types of *C. diphtheriae*. Usually, over 99% of the *gravis* and *intermedius* strains produce toxin, but only 60-85% of the *mitis* strains do.[82] Some of the naturally occurring *C. ulcerans* strains carry the phage or produce the toxin. Toxin production occurs only under iron-limiting conditions. Just as a β phage can convert a nontoxigenic strain to toxigenicity, the phage DNA can be lost from toxigenic strains, rendering them unable to produce toxin. This happens in nature and during subculture in the laboratory. Since there are also reports of toxigenic and nontoxigenic strains being isolated from the same patient[12], it is important to test more than one isolate for toxin production. In vitro loss of the *tox* gene might explain some reports of true diphtheria being caused by nontoxigenic strains.

Diphtheria toxin consists of two portions. Fragment A (21,500 daltons) catalyzes the transfer of adenosine diphosphoribose from nicotine adeninenucleotide (NAD) to elongation factor (EF), making EF nonfunctional. Since EF is needed for the translocation step of protein synthesis, this effectively inhibits protein synthesis. Fragment B (37,200 daltons) is responsible for the entry of Fragment A into the eukaryotic cell cytosol. It is interesting, with evolutionary implications, that portions of Fragment B show extensive homologies with apolipoprotein A1, the human protein that facilitates entry of lipids into cells.[61] It has been proposed that diphtheria was not known to the ancient Greeks and is, in fact, a more recent disease.[63] One can imagine that the DNA that encodes for at least part of the toxin was originally from the human genome, but became incorporated via a plasmid into the *C. diphtheriae* genome.[35]

Table 13:1. Preliminary Distinction of Some Groups of Gram Positive Rods Modified from reference 14, based on data in reference 44.

Name	Morphology	Catalase	Grows Better Anaerobically	Motility	Nitrate Reduction	Urease	Esculin	Hemolysis	Peptido-glycan in cell wall	Mycolic[a] acid	Comment
Bacillus	Med-lg, reg spore-forming	+	–	+	d	d	+	B, A NH	–	–	
Listeria monocytogenes	Sm-med, CB, R	+	–	+	–	–	+	B	–	–	Umbrella motility
Oerskovia	Br, fil, R	d	–	+[e]	d	–	+	NH, A	L-lysine	–	Yellow pig., isol. from soil, environ.
Rothia dentocariosa	Diph, sl br, pleo	+	–	–	+	–	+	NH	–	–	Normal mouth flora
Mycobacterium fortuitum complex	Sm-med R some sl curve	+	–	–	+	+	ND	NH	Meso-DAP	60–90	Acidfast
Rhodococcus equi	R, CB cycle	+	–	–	V	+	–	NH	Meso-DAP	30–38	Pink-coral pigment, sometimes acidfast
Nocardia	Br, fil, sometimes R	+	–	–	+[e]	+[e]	+	NH	Meso-DAP	46–60	Weak acidfast

Corynebacterium	Diph	+	–	–	V	d	–	NH, A	Meso-DAP	22–36	
Brevibacterium	Diph, R-coccus cycle	+	–	–	ND	–	ND	–	Meso-DAP	–	Isol. from cheese and human skin
Arcanobacterium	Small, sl br, sl curve, pleo	–	–[b]	–	+[e]	–	–	B	L-lysine	–	One species: *A. haemolyticum*
Actinomyces	Diph, pleo, sl br, fil	–[e]	+	–	d	d	d	NH	L-lysine	–	10 species, human and mammal isolates
Arachnia	Diph, Br, Fil, Pleo	–	+	–	+	–	–	NH	LL-DAP	–	Formerly *Actinomyces* normal mouth flora
Lactobacillus	Med R, Fil, Reg	–	+	–	–	–	+[e]	NH, A	–	–	Most grow on tomato juice agar
Erysipelothrix	Two forms: fil and CB	–	–	–	–	–	–	NH, A	–	–	Forms H_2S on TSI media
Propionibacterium	Diph, sl br	+[e]	+	–[e]	–	–	d	B, A NH	Meso-/ LL-DAP	–	Some species grow aerobically with CO_2.

Abbreviations: Br = branched rod; Diph = diphtheroid; Fil = filamentous; Reg = regular; Pleo = pleomorphic; + = 90% or more positive; – = 10% or less positive; d = 11–89% of strains are positive; e = some species are exceptions; V = variable; ND = no data; sm = small; lg = large; med = medium; CB = coccobacillus; R = rod; sl = slight; B = beta; A = alpha; NH = No hemolysis; a = number of carbon atoms in the mycolic acid, if present; b = Growth enhanced by CO_2; Meso-DAP = meso-diamino-pimelic acid.

Table 13:2. Some Characteristics of *Corynebacteria* spp. and Groups Isolated from Humans and Mammals

	Nitrate Reduction	Carbohydrate Utilization				Pyrazinamidase	Comments
		Urease Hydrolysis	Glucose	Maltose	Sucrose		
C. diphtheriae	+*	−*	+	+	−	−	Phospholipase D−; Halo on Tinsdale
C. pseudotuberculosis	V*	+	+	+	V	−	Phospholipase D+; Starch & Glycogen−; Halo on Tinsdale
"*C. ulcerans*"	−	+	+	+	−	−	Phospholipase D+; Starch & Glycogen+; Halo on Tinsdale
C. xerosis	+	−	+	−	+	+	
C. pseudodiphtheriticum	+	+	−	−	−	+	
C. kutscheri	+	+	+	+	+	+	Associated with rats. Hydrolyzes esculin.
C. minutissimum	−	−	+	+	V	+	
C. striatum	−	−	+	+	−	ND	CDC charts give Maltose negative, Sucrose positive.
C. renale	−	+	+	ND*	−	+	
C. cystitidis	−	+	+	+	−	+	

C. pilosum	+	+	+	+	–	+	
C. mycetoides	–	–	+	–	ND	ND	
C. matruchotii	+	V	+	V	V	+	Nitrate and urease differ from CDC. "Whip with handle" shape.
CDC groups:							
Group JK	–	–	+	V	–		Small grey colony
Group D2	–	+	–	–	–		Also called *C. urealyticum*. Small grey colony
Group G1	+	–	+	V	+		
Group G2	–	–	+	V	+		
Group F1	V	+	+	V	+		
Group F2	V	+	+	+	–		
Group I	+	–	+	V	–		No halo on Tinsdale
Unassigned groups:							
C. aquaticum	V	–	+	+	+		Yellow, motile, esculin V
C. bovis	–	–	+	–	–		
CDC Group A	V	–	+	+	+		Motile, esculin positive, pigment V

* + = positive; – = negative; V = variable; ND = Not Done.

Table 13:3. Nomenclature Changes and Partial Description for Some Coryneform Bacteria.

Old Name	New Name	Comments
C. equi	*Rhodococcus equi*	Causes pneumonia in foals. Salmon colored colonies; mucoid.
C. pyogenes	*Actinomyes pyogenes*[18]	
C. haemolyticum	*Arcanobacterium haemolyticum*[19]	
C. genitalium	Probably the same as CDC group JK[29]	
C. ulcerans	*C. diphtheriae* group but not a separate species.	Biochemicals listed in Table 13:2.
C. aquaticum	Unassigned	Motile, yellow pigment.
C. bovis	Unassigned	Similar to rhodococci, causes bovine mastitis.
CDC Groups A 3, 4, 5	Unassigned	Motile, hydrolyze esculin, utilize glucose, maltose, sucrose.
C. ovis	*C. pseudotuberculosis*	
C. hofmanni	*C. pseudodiphtheriticum*	
Bacterionema matruchotti	*C. matruchotii*[20]	
CDC Group D-2	*C. urealyticum*	

CLINICAL MANIFESTATIONS

The classic form of diphtheria is characterized by a local pseudomembranous lesion covering the tonsils, pharynx, larynx or nose. The pseudomembrane can extend into the trachea and completely obstruct the air passages; patients may die of suffocation. Diphtheria toxin produced in the local lesion may be absorbed systemically and damage distant organs and tissues, such as the heart, liver, kidneys and peripheral nerves. This damage, particularly to the heart, is often cited as the immediate cause of death from diphtheria.

C. diphtheriae can also produce cutaneous infections.[50,64] Although a sharply demarcated lesion with a pseudomembranous base often is seen, the appearance may not be distinctive, and the infection can only be confirmed by culture. Usually, other bacterial species (staphylococci and streptococci) can be isolated from the abscess, so coryneforms should never be discarded as skin contaminants until *C. diphtheriae* is ruled out.

Primary infection can also affect the ear, conjunctiva, umbilicus and vagina. The organism is rarely found in the blood or internal organs, but has been reported as a cause of endocarditis.[54,55]

THERAPY

Diphtheria antitoxin is the most important specific therapy. Daily doses range from 20,000-100,000 units administered intravenously, depending upon the extent of membrane formation. Initiation of therapy to neutralize toxin should be started immediately, based on clinical symptoms and should NEVER await laboratory confirmation. Diphtheria antitoxin is produced in horses and intradermal testing for immediate hypersensitivity should precede its administration.

Adjunctive therapy includes intravenous penicillin or erythromycin, given to eradicate the infecting organism. Nontoxigenic strains of *C. diphtheriae* have been shown to be erythromycin-resistant.[24] Therefore, susceptibility testing of all isolates should be performed on Mueller-Hinton agar supplemented with 5% sheep blood or in brain heart infusion broth supplemented with 10% fetal calf serum or Tween 80.

Antibiotics are also used to treat asymptomatic carriers. Treatment of these individuals reduces their risk of having an active infection and limits the degree to which they can spread the organism. Identifying and treating *C. diphtheriae* carriers during outbreaks is thus an important control measure.[16]

EPIDEMIOLOGY

Diphtheria remains endemic in many devloping countries, where less than 10% of infants are fully immunized and approximately one million deaths occur each year. In contrast, the incidence of diphtheria in the Unites States has declined steadily since the 1920s. A large cutaneous diphtheria outbreak in Seattle, Washington, occurred during the 1970s[64] in a "Skid Row" population. These cases represented 50% of all cases reported in this country during that period. However, the diphtheria case incidence in the U.S. declined dramatically after 1975[13] and reached its lowest recorded level in 1980, i.e., two patients (0.01 cases per million). During 1959-70, South Dakota was the state with the highest average annual incidence (12.4 cases per million), followed by New Mexico, Alaska, Washington, Arizona and Montana.[8] The highest average annual incidence between 1971-81 occurred in the West (1.4 cases per million) instead of the South (0.3 case per million). Diphtheria continued to be rare in the North (less than 0.1 case per million). A definite decline in diphtheria was observed during the warmer months of the year; the highest incidence occurred between January and March. Children less than 15 years old had the highest average annual incidence (0.8 case per million); white and black persons had similar average annual attack rates, but the incidence in American Indians was approximately 100-fold greater.

Studies on the molecular epidemiology of diphtheria using restriction enzyme analysis of bacterial DNA[62] have shown that toxigenic and nontoxigenic strains of *C. diphtheriae* isolated fom a single outbreak had almost identical DNA. Investigators postulated, therefore, that the variation in toxin production was probably due to lysogenic conversion, i.e., acquisition of the β-bacteriophage in situ. Current vaccination programs are designed merely to eliminate the toxigenic organisms and individuals who carry nontoxigenic strains run the risk of an imported β-bacteriophage converting these benign microorganisms into virulent, toxin-producing strains capable of causing diphtheria in nonimmunized hosts.

PUBLIC HEALTH SIGNIFICANCE, PREVENTION AND CONTROL

Although *C. diphtheriae* is most frequently disseminated by aerosol (respiratory) or direct contact (cutaneous), the organism may be spread by fomites or, rarely, by milk.[40] Diphtheria is a highly contagious disease, especially among crowded, nonimmunized individuals. Case fatality rates of 5-10% for respiratory diphtheria have remained constant for more than 50 years; the highest case fatality ratios were in the very young and the elderly.

Interruption of transmission is the major goal for preventing outbreaks; the use of diphtheria toxoid vaccine has been associated with marked decreases in the incidence of and mortality from diphtheria worldwide.[40] A primary series of 4 doses of diphtheria toxoid is recommended for children less than 7 years old by the Immunization Practices Advisory Committee.[11] Active protection should then be maintained by administering a single dose every 10 years thereafter.

Experience with diphtheria immunization indicates that an immunization level between 70-95% of the population is needed to prevent epidemic spread.[13] However, surveys of immunization records of children less than 14 years old in 1981 showed that 10% of white and 32% of nonwhite children were not fully immunized.

Since immunization does not protect against carriage of *C. diphtheriae*, the organism may persist in a population with little or no clinical diphtheria. Although carriage of the organism can be eliminated by antibiotic therapy, the cost of locating carriers makes this approach impractical except in outbreak situations.

Diphtheria is a reportable disease in most states and countries. Strict isolation is recommended for pharyngeal diphtheria and contact isolation for cutaneous cases.[4,50] Isolation may be discontinued after 14 days of appropriate antibiotic therapy.

CORYNEFORMS OTHER THAN *C. diphtheriae*

Clinical Manifestations

Corynebacterium species other than *C. diphtheriae* are some of the most common isolates in the clinical laboratory. *Corynebacterium* spp. and the morphologically similar *Propionibacterium* spp. comprise a significant portion of the normal flora of the skin. They are sometimes found as a predominant colonizing species in the respiratory tract after antibiotic therapy. Indwelling catheters in either blood lines or the urinary tract can become colonized by these organisms and subsequently cause contamination of a specimen during collection or provide a source of infection.

Infections caused by coryneform bacteria other than *C. diphtheriae* have been reviewed.[15,42,45,53,78] Some of the most commonly cited bacterial species in these reviews have subsequently been found not to be valid *Corynebacterium* spp. Such organisms, including *Propionibacterium acnes*, [78] *Rhodococcus equi*,[37] and *Arcanobacterium hemolyticum*,[51,80] have been associated primarily with wound infections, respiratory infections and infections mimicking Group A streptococcal disease, respectively.

Although *C. ulcerans* is no longer a valid species but is considered in the *C. diphtheriae* group, the clinical literature generally retains the name. This organism has been associated with mastitis in cattle and pharyngitis in humans.[17] Since it can be carried as a commensal in both humans and animals, true pathogenicity may be difficult to prove. Toxigenic strains of *C. ulcerans* can cause diphtheria.[57] *C. pseudotuberculosis*, previously called *C. ovis*, is rarely isolated from humans who have not been exposed to animals. In humans, it may cause lymphadenitis and pneumonia.[33,47,53,78] In sheep, goats, horses and other warm-blooded animals, it may cause ulcerative lymphangitis, abscesses and other chronic purulent infections.[17]

C. xerosis and *C. pseudodiphtheriticum* are normal skin and mucous membrane flora. Overgrowth by these organisms after antibiotic treatment is not uncommon. *C. pseudodiphtheriticum* has been isolated from patients with pneumonia[26] and from the urine. *C. xerosis* has also been associated with pneumonia.[66]

C. minutissimum can cause abscess formation[6] and possibly erythrasma of the skin. *C. mycetoides* has been associated with tropical ulcers; *C. (Bacterionema) matruchotii* with eye infections[82] and opportunistic infections.

Of the groups described by CDC, *Corynebacterium* CDC group D-2, renamed *C. urealyticum*, has been isolated from the urine of patients with cystitis,[72] although it can be found in the urine at other times.[15] It is often highly antibiotic-resistant and could be confused with CDC group JK. Endophthalmitis due to CDC group A-4 has been reported.[22,39] "*C. aquaticum*," which is not considered a *Corynebacterium* species, can be isolated from the environment and has been reported to have caused meningitis in a child.[3] Endocarditis, often in patients who have prosthetic heart valves, and infections of pacemakers or other prostheses are the most commonly reported diseases caused by nondiphtheria corynebacteria or coryneform groups.[42,49,53,54,77,78] Etiologic agents which are often part of the normal flora include *C. xerosis, C. pseudodiphtheriticum*, group JK and the ill-defined "skin" bacteria. Similarly, bacteremia, usually in immunocompromised hosts, can be caused by these organisms, particularly group JK.[38,67,84]

Virulence, Therapy, Epidemiology, Public Health Significance, Prevention and Control

The virulence of *Corynebacterium* spp. other than *C. diphtheriae* or corynebacteria carrying the *tox* gene is generally very low. Toxins have been described for *C. pseudodiphtheriticum*.[43] Many of these infections are in compromised hosts and, in most part, the source of the organism seems to be the host himself. However, the organisms can be spread by hands and objects. Nosocomial spread of group JK has been documented.[84]

The susceptibility pattern for the *Corynebacterium* spp. is not predictable.[46] Organisms involved in hospital-acquired infections, such as group JK or D-2, are often highly antibiotic-resistant but highly sensitive in vitro to vancomycin. This is not, however, a reliable characteristic for identification. Agents, such as ciprofloxacin and the lipopolypeptide antibiotics may have useful activity. Most corynebacteria that have caused endocarditis were susceptible to vancomycin, teichoplanin (a polypeptide antibiotic), ciprofloxacin and rifampin; but there was strain variability to erythromycin, imipenem and the aminoglycosides. Penicillins and cephalosporins are generally not effective.[73]

DIAGNOSTIC PROCEDURES

Primary Isolation and Culture

C. diphtheriae Isolation: Media containing potassium tellurite at a final concentration of 0.03-0.04% is inhibitory to many organisms but allows the growth of *C. diphtheriae*. Cystine-tellurite blood agar (CTA), chocolate-blood-tellurite agar, modified Tinsdale (MTM) and Hoyles media all contain tellurite and have proved satisfactory.[32] The CDC found that CTA yielded more isolates from mixed cultures than MTM, although all strains grew on MTM.[81] Because *C. diphtheriae* (as well as *C. ulcerans* and *C. pseudotuberculosis*) colonies form a halo on MTM, it may be easier for inexperienced workers to recognize the organism on MTM plates.[59] CTA may be preferred by some laboratories because it has a longer shelf life than MTM.

Swabs or exudative material from the infected site, usually the nasopharynx or skin, are inoculated to a blood plate, an agar medium containing tellurite and a Loeffler's slant. Both nasopharynx and throat of suspected cases of diphtheria should be sampled. Growth on the Loeffler's agar can be examined by Gram stain as soon as 8 h and up to 24 h, looking for typical beaded gram-positive rods. Since this medium allows not only rapid growth of *C. diphtheriae* but of other coryneforms as well, the results of Gram stains are only presumptive. An egg-based media developed by Pai gives similar results. A flow chart for the initial isolation and workup is shown in Figure 13:2. It is well to emphasize that *C. diphtheriae* grows well on many ordinary laboratory media which support gram-positive cell growth. On plates such as trypticase soy agar with 5% sheep blood (SBA), Columbia agar with or without added colistin and nalidixic acid (CNA) and blood agars made with horse or rabbit blood, small to medium sized colonies can be seen at 24 hours. The problem with these agars is that they are not selective or differential so that many bacteria, including essentially all *Corynebacterium* spp. will grow. Since coryneforms are a significant part

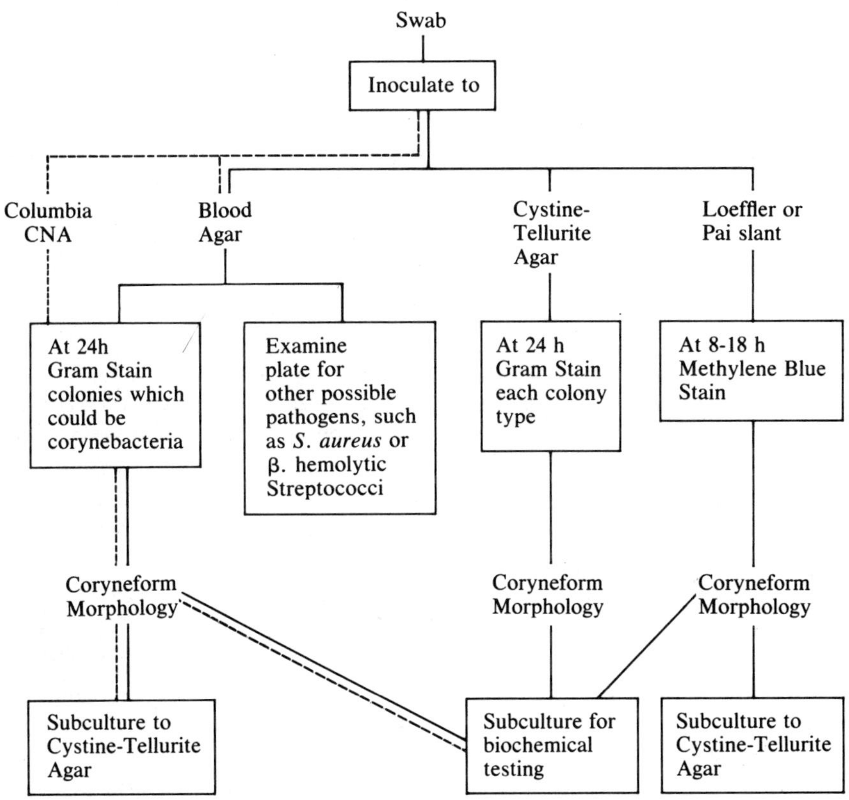

FIGURE 13:2. Scheme for the isolation of corynebacteria: (_____) *C. diphtheriae* under ideal conditions; (------) *C. diphtheriae* under less than ideal conditions and other corynebacteria.

of the normal flora in sites such as the skin and pharynx, distinguishing *C. diphtheriae* from these groups would be difficult without selective or differential media. However, because diphtheria is so rare in developed countries, many clinical laboratories do not stock fresh tellurite or Loeffler's media. When there is clinical suspicion of skin or pharyngeal diphtheria but specialized media are not available, specimens may be plated on several blood-containing media. All coryneforms that grow on these media should be isolated and identified to the point where it is clear whether they are or are not *C. diphtheriae*.

Other *Corynebacterium* spp.: All corynebacterial species grow well on ordinary laboratory media, so essentially all would grow on SBA and CNA. However, colonies of some strains are extremely small (less than 0.5 mm at 24 h) and some strains require serum for growth.

Methods for Identification

Identification of *C. diphtheriae:* The distinctive characteristics of *C. diphtheriae* and other *Corynebacterium* spp. are shown in Table 13:2. All strains of *C. diphtheriae* are nitrate-positive (except *C. diphtheriae* subsp. *mitis* var *belfanti*), urease-negative and produce a halo on Tinsdale medium. *C. ulcerans* and *C. pseudotuberculosis*, which are considered in the *C. diphtheriae* group, not only produce this halo which is the result of production of ferric sulfide by sulfhydrolase or cystinase, but also are negative in the pyrazinamidase test.[74] *C. diphtheriae* usually ferments glucose and maltose but not xylose, mannitol, lactose or sucrose. Three different types of *C. diphtheriae*, called *gravis, intermedius* and *mitis*, which differ in colonial morphology, Gram stain, a few biochemical reactions and severity of associated disease, have been described. The cause and significance of these differences is not clear. The colonial morphology of each of these strains is described here primarily for historical interest, as morphology is not invariably associated with certain biochemical types nor is it expected that laboratories which rarely isolate *C. diphtheriae* would have the experience to distinguish the strains on this basis.

On tellurite blood agar, the *gravis* type produces the largest colonies (1-2 mm at 24 h); they are circular, convex, friable, grey and sometimes hemolytic. The *intermedius* type colonies are small (less than 1 mm at 24 h), greyish-black and nonhemolytic, with a smooth or granular surface. The *mitis* colonies are usually 1-1.5 mm in size, emulsifiable, butryous and slightly hemolytic. The *gravis* type ferments starch and glycogen whereas the other two types do not.[83]

There are several methods to test the ability to produce toxin of a strain of *C. diphtheriae* (and *C. ulcerans or C. pseudotuberculosis*). The classic method described by Elek[5,27] involves streaking the strain to be tested on an iron-deficient medium so that toxin-producing capacity is expressed. A paper strip containing antitoxin is placed perpendicularly to the streak. As the toxin diffuses from the line of bacterial growth and the antitoxin diffuses from the paper strip, a line of precipitation forms at a 45° angle between the two.

A method using tissue culture cells to detect toxin has been described.[60,71] Tissue culture cells are inoculated with test supernatants in a manner similar to that for the test for *Clostridium difficile* toxin. Cytotoxic effects are shown if diphtheria toxin is present. In one assay,[60] the presence of the toxin prevents Chinese hamster ovary cell cultures from growing and producing sufficient acid to change a pH indicator. Screening is therefore rapid and macroscopic.

The in vivo test for toxigenicity involves inoculating a 48 h broth culture of the test organism into each of two guinea pigs. One receives an injection of diphtheria antitoxin and the other does not. Toxigenicity is presumed if the guinea pig without the protective antitoxin dies.[81]

Since all of these methods require stringent controls, the materials are often not easily available and the interpretations are difficult, a definitive test for toxigenicity is best done in laboratories with proper facilities and experience.

Fluorescent antibody techniques for the detection of *C. diphtheriae* have been described[58] and are used in some parts of the world now.[31]

Identification of *C. ulcerans* and *C. pseudotuberculosis:* These two strains, which have been previously called *C. ovis*, resemble *C. diphtheriae* in the production of a halo on Tinsdale medium and in the potential to produce diphtheria toxin. In one study, about 31% of the *C. ulcerans* strains and 3% of the *C. pseudotuberculosis* strains produced toxin.[56] Although the *tox* gene portion of the DNA is homologous in these strains, the lesser degree of homology in the rest of the genome indicates that *C. ulcerans* and *C. pseudotuberculosis* are distinct though related species.[36] As shown in Table 13:2, both *C. ulcerans* and *C. pseudotuberculosis* differ from *C. diphtheriae* in producing urease, hydrolyzing gelatin (after prolonged incubation at lower temperatures) and producing phospholipase D.[2] The two species can be biochemically distinguished because *C. ulcerans* generally ferments starch and glycogen whereas *C. pseudotuberculosis* does not.

Identification of Other *Corynebacterium* species: Table 13:2 lists the major differential biochemical reactions of the *Corynebacterium* spp. or groups which have been associated with humans or animals. It is readily apparent that this does not provide unique identification of all species. A study of well known identification schemes[17,23,29] reveals significant differences in the published reactions. We have chosen to list those in "Bergey's Manual of Systematic Bacteriology"[17] but have noted under "Comments" misleading differences. Because of ambiguities in taxonomy, it is important to publish the observed biochemical reactions as well as the name of the organism when trying to associate an organism with a disease. The observation of the halo on Tinsdale medium and the absence of pyrazinamidase activity[74] are important in distinguishing the *C. diphtheriae* group from the rest of the corynebacteria.

Clinical laboratories should be expected to distinguish *C. diphtheriae* from other *Corynebacterium* spp., using the tests listed in Table 13:2. However, speciating the other corynebacteria is difficult even after performing the extensive testing described elsewhere.[17,23,79] Some standard tests require up to 2 weeks for a definitive result (the carbohydrate utilization tests), some organisms grow poorly in standard media and require serum (e.g., Group JK, Group G) and there are some clinical isolates that do not fit published patterns.[15]

Rapid tests which will help identify the majority of clinically important isolates would be useful. The commercially available API 20S[46] and the API zym[48] strips have been tested with coryneform organisms, but the results, though interesting, are not promising. Modifications that do not require growth (and therefore are more rapid) of methods using standard biochemicals seem the most useful.[41,76]

CLINICAL SIGNIFICANCE OF LABORATORY FINDINGS

The isolation of a toxinogenic strain of *C. diphtheriae* is always significant, since it is either the agent of disease in a particular patient or an agent capable of producing disease in non-immunized individuals. The isolation of a nontoxinogenic strain of *C. diphtheriae* has less significance, because the organism must first be converted to virulence by the addition of the β-bacteriophage before causing disease. Treatment, however, should be initiated on the basis of clinical symptoms and not await laboratory results.

Non-diphtheria *Corynebacterium* spp. are very frequent isolates in the laboratory and are rarely clinically significant. However, as delineated in "Clinical Manifestations", many species have the capability of producing disease, especially in compromised patients. In determining relevance, one should examine specimens in which coryneforms are the predominant or only isolate and identify these isolates at least to genera. It is possible that some species of highly virulent genera such as *Nocardia, Mycobacterium, Listeria* or *Erysipelothrix* may be confused with *Corynebacterium* spp. In addition, organisms in the coryneform genera *Arcanobacteria, Propionibacterium, Actinomyces* and *Rhodococcus* can be clinically significant. However, due to the scarcity of data, distinguishing among the species within the genus *Corynebacterium* (except for *C. diphtheriae*) will give few clues to the treatment or severity of disease. Also, because of difficulties in *Corynebacterium* spp. identification, the information is generally too delayed to be clinically useful.

Performing antibiotic susceptibility testing is important, as the results are not predictable. It is probable that high resistance in strains of *Corynebacterium* CDC group JK and *Corynebacterium urealyticum* is a virulence factor and contributes to their clinical significance.

REFERENCES

1. Barksdale L. The genus *Corynebacterium*. In: Starr MP, Stolp H, Truper HG, Balows A, Schlegel HG, eds. The prokaryotes: a handbook on habitats, isolation and identification of bacteria. Berlin: Springer Verlag, 1981:1827-37.
2. Barksdale L, Linder I, Sulea T, Pollice M. Phospholipase D activity of *Corynebacterium pseudotuberculosis, (Corynebacterium ovis)* and *Corynebacterium ulcerans*, a distinctive marker within the genus *Corynebacterium*. J Clin Microbiol 1981;13:335-43.
3. Beckwith DG, Jahre JA, Haggerty S. Isolation of *Corynebacterium aquaticum* from spinal fluid of an infant with meningitis. J Clin Microbiol 1986;23:375-6.
4. Benenson AS, ed. Control of communicable diseases in man. 14th ed. Washington, DC: American Public Health Association, 1985:116-20.
5. Bickham ST, Jones WL. Problems in the use of the in vitro toxigenicity test for *Corynebacterium diphtheriae*. Am J Clin Pathol 1972;57:244-6.
6. Berger SA, Gorea A, Stadler J, Dan M, Zilberman M. Recurrent breast abscesses caused by *Corynebacterium minutissium*. J Clin Microbiol 1984;20:1219-20.
7. Broeren SA, Peel MM. Endocarditis caused by *Rothia dentocariosa*. J Clin Pathol 1984;37:1298-1300.
8. Brooks GF, Bennett JV, Feldman RA. Diphtheria in the United States, 1959-70. J. Infect Dis 1974;129:172-8.
9. Broughton RA, Wilson HD, Goodman NL, Hendrick JA. Septic arthritis and osteomyelitis caused by an organism of the genus *Rhodococcus*. J Clin Microbiol 1981;13:209-11.
10. Centers for Disease Control. Fatal diphtheria, Wisconsin. Morbid Mortal Weekly Rep 1982;31:553-5.
11. Centers for Disease Control. Immunization Practices Advisory Committee. Diphtheria, tetanus and pertussis: guidelines for vaccine prophylaxis and other preventive measures. Ann Intern Med 1985;103:896-905.
12. Chang DN, Laughren GS, Chalvardjian NE. Three variants of *Corynebacterium diphtheriae* subsp. *mitis (belfanti)* isolated from a throat specimen. J Clin Microbiol 1978;8:767-8.
13. Chen RT, Broome CV, Weinstein RA, Weaver R, Tsai TF. Diphtheria in the United States, 1971-81. Am J Public Health 1985;75:1393-7.
14. Clarridge, JE, Weissfeld AS. Aerobic asporogenous gram-positive bacilli. Clin Microbiol Newsletter 1984;6:115-18.
15. Clarridge JE. When, why and how far should coryneforms be identified? Clin Microbiol Newsletter 1986;8:32-4.
16. Collins CH, Dulake C. Diphtheria: the logistics of mass swabbing. J Infect 1983;6:227-30.
17. Collins MD, Cummins CS. Genus *Corynebacterium* Lehmann and Neumann. In: Sneath PHA, Mair NS, Sharpe ME, Holt JG, eds. Bergey's manual of systematic bacteriology; vol 2. Baltimore: Williams and Wilkins, 1986:1266-76.
18. Collins MD, Jones D. Reclassification of *Corynebacterium pyogenes* (Glage) in the genus *Actinomyces*, as *Actinomyces pyogenes* comb. nov. J Gen Microbiol 1982;128:901-3.
19. Collins MD, Jones D, Schofield GM. Reclassification of *"Corynebacterium haemolyticum"* (MacLean, Liebow and Rosenberg) in the genus nov. as *Arcanobacterium haemolyticum* nom. rev. comb. nov. J Gen Microbiol 1982;128:1279-81.

20. Collins MD. Reclassification of *Bacterionema matruchotii* (Gilmour, Howell and Bibby) in the genus *Corynebacterium* as *Corynebacterium matruchotii* comb. nov. Zentral Bakteriol Mikrobiol Hyg I Abt Orig C 1982;3:364-7.
21. Corino DL, Sesardic D. Profile analysis of total mycolic acids from skin corynebacteria and from named *Corynebacterium* strains by gas-liquid chromatography and spectrometry. J Gen Microbiol 1980;116:61-8.
22. Coudron PE, Harris RC, Vaughn MG, Dalton HP. Two similar but atypical strains of coryneform Group A-4 isolated from patients with endophthalmitis. J Clin Microbiol 1985;22:475-7.
23. Coyle MB, Hollis DG, Groman NB. *Corynebacterium* spp. and other coryneforms. In: Lennette EH, Balows A, Hausler WJ Jr, Shadomy HJ, eds. Manual of clinical microbiology. 4th ed. Washington, DC: American Society for Microbiology 1985:193-204.
24. Coyle MB, Minshew BH, Bland JA, Hsu PC. Erythromycin and clindamycin resistance in *Corynebacterium diphtheriae* from skin lesions. Antimicrob Agents Chemother 1979;16:525-7.
25. Crickshank JG, Gawler AH, Shaldon C. *Oerskovia* species: rare opportunistic pathogens. J Med Microbiol 1979;12:513-17.
26. Donaghy M, Cohen J. Pulmonary infection with *Corynebacterium hofmannii* complicating systemic lupus erythematosus. J Infect Dis 1983;147:962.
27. Elek SD. The plate virulence test for diphtheria. J Clin Pathol 1949;2:250-8.
28. English PC. Diphtheria and theories of infectious disease: centennial appreciation of the critical role of diphtheria in the history of medicine. Pediatrics 1985;76:1-9.
29. Evangelista AT, Coppola KM, Furness G. Relationship between group JK corynebacteria and the biotypes of *Corynebacterium genitalium* and *Corynebacterium pseudogenitalium*. Can J Microbiol 1984;30:1052-7.
30. Fell HWK, Nagington J, Naylor GRE. *Corynebacterium haemolyticum* infections in Cambridgeshire. J Hyg (Camb) 1977;79:269-74.
31. Formiga LCD. New possibilities for the laboratory diagnosis of diphtheria. Brazilian J Med Res 1985;18:401-2.
32. Frobisher M, Lankford EI, Yates E, Gay KF. A comparative study of tellurite plating media for *Corynebacterium diphtheriae*. Am J Hyg 1948;48:1-5.
33. Goldberger AC, Lipsky BA, Plorde JJ. Suppurative granulomatous lymphadenitis caused by *Corynebacterium ovis (pseudotuberculosis)*. Am J Clin Pathol 1981;76:486-90.
34. Goodfellow M, Weaver CR, Minnikin DE. Numerical classification of some rhodococci, corynebacteria and related organisms. J Gen Microbiol 1982;128:731-45.
35. Groman NB. Conversion by corynephages and its role in the natural history of diphtheria. J Hyg (Camb) 1984;93:405-17.
36. Groman N, Schiller J, Russell J. *Corynebacterium ulcerans* and *Corynebacterium pseudotuberculosis*: responses to DNA probes derived from Corynephage β and *Corynebacterium diphtheriae*. Infect Immun 1984;45:511-17.
37. Habinchak DR, Jeffrey B, Higbee JW, Everett ED. Infections caused by *Rhodochrous*. Amer J Med 1978;65:298-302.
38. Hande KR, Witebsky FG, Brown MS, et al. Sepsis with a new species of *Corynebacterium*. Ann Intern Med 1976;85:423-6.
39. Hanscom T, Maxwell WA. *Corynebacterium* endophthalmitis: laboratory studies and report of a case treated by vitrectomy. Arch Ophthalmol 1979;97:500-2.
40. Hewlett EL. Selective primary health care: strategies for control of disease in the developing world. XVIII. Pertussis and diphtheria. Rev Infect Dis 1985;7:426-33.
41. Hollis DG, Sottnek FO, Brown MJ, Weaver RE. Use of the rapid fermentation test in determining carbohydrate reactions of fastidious bacteria in clinical laboratories. J Clin Microbiol 1980;12:620-3.
42. Johnson WD and Kaye D. Serious infections caused by diphtheroids. Ann NY Acad Sci 1970;174:568-76.

43. Jolly RD. The pathogenic action of the exotoxin of *Corynebacterium ovis*. J Comp Pathol 1965;75:417-31.
44. Jones D, Collins MD. Irregular nonsporing gram-positive rods. In: Sneath PHA, Mair NS, Sharpe ME, Holt JG, eds. Bergey's manual of systematic bacteriology; vol 2. Baltimore: Williams and Wilkins, 1986:1261-6.
45. Kaplan K, Weinstein L. Diphtheroid infections of man. Ann Intern Med 1969;70:919-29.
46. Kelly MC, Smith ID, Anstey RJ, Thornley JH, Rennie RP. Rapid identification of antibiotic-resistant corynebacteria with the API 20S system. J Clin Microbiol 1984;19:245-7.
47. Keslin MH, McCoy EL, McCuskey JJ, Lutch JS. *Corynebacterium pseudotuberculosis*: a new cause of infections and eosinophilic pneumonia. Amer J Med 1979;67:228-31.
48. Kilian M. Rapid identification of *Actinomycetacea* and related bacteria. J Clin Microbiol 1978;8:127-33.
49. Klima M, Clarridge J, Chapman A, Young E. Pacemaker associated infection due to a *Corynebacterium* species. Texas Heart Institute J 1985;12:177-82.
50. Koopman JS, Campbell J. The role of cutaneous diphtheria infections in a diphtheria epidemic. J Infect Dis 1975;131:239-44.
51. Kovatch AL, Schuit KE, Michaels RH. *Corynebacterium haemolyticum* peritonsillar abscess mimicking diphtheria. JAMA 1983;249:1757-8.
52. Lechevalier HA. Nocardioforms. In: Sneath PHA, Mair NS, Sharpe ME, Holt JG, eds. Bergey's manual of systematic bacteriology; vol 2. Baltimore: Williams and Wilkins, 1986:1458-85.
53. Lipsky BA, Goldberger AC, Tompkins LS, Plorde JJ. Infections caused by nondiphtheria corynebacteria. Rev Infect Dis 1982;4:1220-35.
54. Love JW, Medina D, Anderson S, Braniff B. Infective endocarditis due to *Corynebacterium diphtheriae*: report of a case and review of the literature. Johns Hopkin Med J 1981;148:41-2.
55. Marcus JC, Spector I, Chin WWN, Levin SE. Infective endocarditis due to non-toxigenic *Corynebacterium diphtheriae* in a child. South African Med J 1983;63:285-7.
56. Maximescu P, Oprisan A, Pop A, Potorac E. Further studies on *Corynebacterium* species capable of producing diphtheria toxin (*C. diphtheriae, C. ulcerans, C. ovis*). J Gen Microbiol 1974;82:49-56.
57. Meers PD. A case of classical diphtheria and other infections due to *Corynebacterium ulcerans*. J Infect 1979;1:139-42.
58. Moody MD, Jones WL. Identification of *Corynebacterium diphtheriae* with fluorescent antibacterial reagents. J Bacteriol 1963;86:285-93.
59. Moore MS, Parsons EI. A study of a modified Tinsdale's medium for the primary isolation of *Corynebacterium diphtheriae*. J Infect Dis 1958;102:88-93.
60. Murphy JR, Bacha P, Teng M. Determination of *Corynebacterium diphtheriae* toxigenicity by a colorimetric tissue culture assay. J Clin Microbiol 1978;7:91-6.
61. Neville DM Jr, Hudson TH. Transmembrane transport of diphtheria toxin, related toxins and colicins. Ann Rev Biochem 1986;55:195-224.
62. Pappenheimer AM Jr, Murphy JR. Studies on the molecular epidemiology of diphtheria. Lancet 1983;2:923-6.
63. Pappenheimer AM Jr. The diphtheria bacillus and its toxin: A model system. J Hyg Camb 1984;93:397-404.
64. Pedersen AHB, Spearman J, Tronca E, Bader M, Harnisch J. Diphtheria on skid row, Seattle, Washington, 1972-75. Public Health Rep 1977;92:336-42.
65. Pitcher G, Malnick H. Identification of *Brevibacterium* from clinical sources. J Clin Pathol 1984;37:1395-8.
66. Porschen RK, Goodman Z, Rafai B. Isolation of *Corynebacterium xerosis* from clinical specimens. Am J Clin Pathol 1977;68:290-3.
67. Riley PS, Hollis DG, Utter GB, Weaver RE, Baker CN. Characterization and identification of 95 diphtheroid (group JK) cultures isolated from clinical specimens. J Clin Microbiol 1979;9:418-24.

68. Schaal KP, Pulverer G. The genera *Actinomyces, Agromyces, Arachnia, Bacterionemia* and *Rothia*. In: Starr MP, Stolp H, Truper HG, Balows A, Schlegel HG, eds. The prokaryotes: a handbook on habitats, isolation and identification of bacteria. Berlin: Springer Verlag, 1981:1923-50
69. Schafer FJ, Wing EJ, Norden CW. Infectious endocarditis caused by *Rothia dentocariosa*. Ann Intern Med 1979;91:747-8.
70. Schofield GM, Schaal KP. A numerical taxonomic study of members of the *Actinomycetaceae* and related taxa. J Gen Microbiol 1981;127:237-59.
71. Schubert JH, Bickham ST, Wiggins GL. Tissue culture method for toxigenicity testing of *Corynebacterium diphtheriae*. Appl Microbiol 1968;16:1748-52.
72. Soriario F, Ponte C, Santamaria M, Castilla C, Roblas RF. In vitro and in vivo study of stone formation by *Corynebacterium* Group D2 (*Corynebacterium urealyticum*). J Clin Microbiol 1986;23:691-4.
73. Spitzer PG, Eliopoulos GM, Karchmer AW, Moellering RC. Activity of newer polypeptide antibiotic compared with other agents against pathogenic *Corynebacterium* species [Abstract]. Interscience Conference on Antimicrobiol Agents and Chemotherapy. Washington, DC: American Society for Microbiology, 1986:263.
74. Sulea IT, Pollice MC, Barksdale L. Pyrazine carboxylamidase activity in *Corynebacterium*. Int J Syst Bacteriol 1980;30:466-72.
75. Suzuki K, Kaneko T, Komagata K. Deoxyribonucleic acid homologies among coryneform bacteria. Int J Syst Bacteriol 1981;31:131-8.
76. Thompson JS, Gates-Davis DR, Yong DCT. Rapid microbiological identification of *Corynebacterium diphtheriae* and other medically important corynebacteria. J Clin Microbiol 1983;18:926-9.
77. Van Scoy RE, Cohen SN, Geraci JE, Washington JA II. Coryneform bacterial endocarditis. Mayo Clinic Proc 1977;52:216-19.
78. Washington JA II. Bacteriology, clinical spectrum of disease and therapeutic aspects of coryneform bacterial infection. In: Remington JS, Swartz MN, eds. Current clinical topics in infectious diseases; vol 2. New York: McGraw Hill, 1981:196-219
79. Weaver RE, Hollis DB. Gram-positive organisms: a guide to presumptive identification. Atlanta: Center for Disease Control, 1983.
80. Wickremeinghe RSB. *Corynebacterium haemolyticum* infections in Sri Lanka. J Hyg (Camb) 1981;87:271-6.
81. Wiggins GL, Sottnek FO, Hermann GJ. Diphtheria and other corynebacterial infections. In: Balows A, Hausler WJ Jr, eds. Diagnostic procedures for bacterial, mycotic and parasitic infections. 6th ed. Washington, DC: American Public Health Association, 1981:317-33.
82. Wilhelmus KR, Robinson NM, Jones DB. *Bacterionema matruchotii* ocular infections. Am J Ophthalmol 1979;87:143-7.
83. Wilson G. *Corynebacterium* and other coryneform organisms. In: Wilson G, Miles A, Parka MT, eds. Topley and Wilson's principles of bacteriology, virology and immunity; vol 2. 7th ed. London: Edward Arnold, 1983:94-113.
84. Young VM, Meyers WF, Moody MR, Schimpff SC. The emergence of coryneform bacteria as a cause of nosocomial infections in compromised hosts. Am J Med 1981;70:646-50.

CHAPTER 14

ENTEROBACTERIACEAE INFECTIONS

J.J. Farmer, III, Ph.D., Joy G. Wells, M.S., Patricia M. Griffin, M.D.,

and I. Kaye Wachsmuth, Ph.D.

It is difficult to treat the *Enterobacteriaceae* as a single group because their ecology, epidemiology and pathogenicity have evolved quite differently.[26,27,42] Thus, this chapter is divided into five major sections. The first section covers procedures used with the *Enterobacteriaceae* as a group and with the "opportunistic pathogens." The next four sections deal individually with *Escherichia coli, Shigella, Salmonella* and *Yersinia enterocolitica*. For more detailed treatment of the *Enterobacteriaceae*, consult references 26, 28, 40, 42, 45 and 78. Space limitations have prevented citation of numerous other primary references of importance, but many of these may be found in the reviews cited.

ENTEROBACTERIACEAE

INTRODUCTION

The family *Enterobacteriaceae* is a large group of diverse bacteria with certain common properties. Members are found in almost all environments including soil, water, plants and the normal flora of animals. They also cause diseases in plants and animals. Some species occupy a very limited ecological niche. *Salmonella typhi* is found only in man and causes typhoid fever. In contrast, strains of *Klebsiella pneumoniae* are widely distributed in the environment and contribute to biochemical and geochemical processes. However, *K. pneumoniae* can also cause human diseases ranging from asymptomatic colonization of the intestinal, urinary or respiratory tract to fatal septicemia. In this chapter we concentrate on the species which cause human disease, with much of the emphasis on infections in the United

States, which are often quite different from those in other parts of the world, particularly developing nations.

The species which comprise the family *Enterobacteriaceae* have the following properties in common: appear as gram-negative rods; are motile by peritrichous flagella or nonmotile; do not form spores; grow on peptone or meat extract media without additional supplements; grow well on MacConkey agar; grow both aerobically and anaerobically; ferment (rather than oxidize) D-glucose, often with gas production; are catalase-positive; are oxidase-negative; reduce nitrate to nitrite; and have a 39-59% range of guanine plus cytosine (G+C) content of deoxyribonucleic acid (DNA). Although most strains have these properties, occasionally exceptions occur which can be explained by mutation or other genetic mechanisms.

The classification of *Enterobacteriaceae* has changed as more scientific data have become available. In this chapter we use the nomenclature and classification used by the Enteric Bacteriology Laboratories at the Centers for Disease Control (CDC) which may differ from that used by other authors. The reader interested in the development of this classification should consult the recent review of the family.[28] Table 14:1 is a list of genera and species added to the family *Enterobacteriaceae* since the 6th edition of this manual. The section on *Salmonella* discusses nomenclatural changes in this group of organisms.[29]

CAUSATIVE ORGANISMS

Many of the species of *Enterobacteriaceae* have been incriminated in human disease and occur in clinical specimens.[26,28,42,47] In the last 30 years many of the species have been implicated as causes of "opportunistic infections". *Escherichia, Proteus, Morganella, Providencia, Citrobacter, Klebsiella, Enterobacter, Hafnia* and *Serratia* are leading causes of nosocomial infections (infections acquired during hospitalization), and many laboratories now identify all *Enterobacteriaceae* to the species level.

CLINICAL MANIFESTATIONS, EPIDEMIOLOGY AND PUBLIC HEALTH SIGNIFICANCE

Although certain types of infections, such as those of the lower respiratory tract caused by *K. pneumoniae*, have been recognized for many years, the fact that many species of *Enterobacteriaceae* are nosocomial pathogens has been appreciated only in the last few decades. Before antimicrobial therapy was available, most life-threatening infections were acquired outside hospitals. Most nosocomial infections in the preantibiotic era were caused by *Staphylococcus* or *Streptococcus*. During the 1950s, there was a shift in both the place where serious infections were acquired and the types of

Table 14:1. New Organisms in the Family *Enterobacteriaceae* Isolated from Clinical Specimens*

Organism	Clinical significance in extraintestinal human infections
Budvicia aquatica	−†
Cedecea davisae	+
Cedecea lapagei	(−)
Cedecea neteri	+
Cedecea species 3	(−)
Cedecea species 5	(−)
Citrobacter amalonaticus biogroup 1	+
Edwardsiella hoshinae	−
Enterobacter asburiae	(+)
Enterobacter amnigenus biogroup 1	−
Enterobacter taylorae	(+)
Escherichia fergusonii	(−)
Escherichia hermannii	(−)
Escherichia vulneris	(−)
Ewingella americana	+
Klebsiella planticola	(−)
Klebsiella group 47, indole$^+$ ornithine$^+$	+
Kluyvera ascorbata	+
Kluyvera cryocrescens	(−)
Moellerella wisconsensis	(−)
Morganella morganii biogroup 1	(+)
Proteus penneri	+
Providencia rustigianii	(−)
Rahnella aquatilis	(−)
Serratia ficaria	(−)
Serratia fonticola	(−)
Serratia marcescens biogroup 1	+ +
Serratia odorifera biogroup 1	(−)
Serratia odorifera biogroup 2	(+)
Serratia plymuthica	(−)
Tatumella ptyseos	(+)
Yersinia frederiksenii	(+)
Yersinia intermedia	(+)
Yersinia kristensenii	(+)
Yersinia ruckeri	(−)
Enteric Group 41	(−)
Enteric Group 45	(−)
Enteric Group 57	(−)
Enteric Group 58	(−)
Enteric Group 59	(−)
Enteric Group 60	(−)
Enteric Group 68	(−)

* The organisms in this table have been described since the 1981 edition of this book. See reference 28 for a more detailed description of these organisms and their role in human disease.

† Definitions for clinical significance: + + + +, + + +, and + + = definitely clinically significant; + = reported to be clinically significant at least at some sites, but may not be significant at other sites; (+) = clinical significance at least suggested in the literature, but more data are needed; (−) = no data at present to suggest significance, but significance can not be totally excluded because of occurrence in extraintestinal clinical specimens; − = no evidence for significance, but may occur in feces.

organisms isolated.[67] With effective antimicrobial therapy available for many community-acquired infections such as those caused by gram-positive cocci and *Mycobacterium tuberculosis*, relatively fewer patients entered the hospital with a serious infection. In contrast, proportionately more patients developed nosocomial infections, and instead of *Staphylococcus aureus* causing most of these infections, hospitalized patients frequently were infected by *Enterobacteriaceae* and *Pseudomonas aeruginosa*. Some *Enterobacteriaceae*, such as *Serratia marcescens*, previously thought to be benign saprophytes, were actually causing serious disease.

This shift in the place where serious infections were acquired and in the agents known to cause nosocomial infections was primarily the result of the interplay of advances in medical therapy during the 1950s. Increasing antibiotic usage which led to the development of antibiotic-resistant strains of *Enterobacteriaceae* was probably instrumental in an evolutionary process which continues today. Simultaneous progress in other forms of treatment was also a factor because it gave rise to a population of patients within hospitals who were frequently more susceptible to infection than patients in general had been in the past. Therapy for serious illnesses such as leukemia, diabetes, pulmonary and renal diseases resulted in a population of patients who were often debilitated by the effects of chronic disorders or by their treatment and were thus susceptible to a superimposed infection. Medications such as corticosteroids, immunosuppressive therapy and antineoplastic drugs which suppress host defenses were introduced during this period. Treatment with these agents tends to facilitate colonization and subsequent infection, often with gram-negative organisms from the patient's own bacterial flora. Invasive procedures, such as bladder catheterization, assisted ventilation and intravascular catheterization were also used more often in routine supportive care. These procedures disrupt local epithelial barriers and provide access for invading microorganisms.

Although these changes in medical therapy led to decreased resistance to infection in the patient, the *Enterobacteriaceae* were intrinsically well adapted to become nosocomial pathogens. They are ubiquitous organisms which have numerous potential reservoirs within hospitals. As part of the animate environment (patients and personnel), the *Enterobacteriaceae* normally inhabit the large bowel and less often the vagina and pharynx. They are sometimes part of the transient flora of normal skin and can frequently be cultured from the hands of hospital personnel. Another reservoir which is sometimes overlooked in hospital outbreaks is the colonized or infected patient.

In the inanimate environment, strains of *Enterobacteriaceae* can survive and some can even multiply in aqueous solutions. They can contaminate[27] intravenous fluids (especially those containing glucose), parenteral medications, irrigating solutions and even some antiseptic solutions containing hexachlorophene. In fact, gram-negative bacteria can spread so readily in the hospital environment that it may be difficult to determine whether an inanimate reservoir is a primary source of infectious organisms or has become secondarily contaminated, as is often the case with countertops or sink drains in patient care areas. Routine cultures of the animate or inanimate environment in the absence of a specific disease problem are unlikely to provide meaningful information and are generally considered to be a waste of infection control resources.

The number of nosocomial infections caused by *Enterobacteriaceae* can only be estimated. Approximately 7% of hospitalized patients develop nosocomial infections, with published rates ranging from 3.5-15%. However, no standardized "acceptable" level of nosocomial infections has been set. Nosocomial infection rates vary with the type and size of the hospital, the characteristics of the patient population, the number of acute care beds, the number and type of surgical procedures performed, the definitions used to distinguish infection from colonization and particularly, nosocomial from community-acquired infections, the scope and activity of the surveillance program in each institution and other factors. Through a consistent ongoing program of surveillance, each hospital should establish its own baseline nosocomial infection rate.

Nosocomial infections are most often acquired by those patients who are least able to tolerate them, the very old, the very young and the very ill. It has been estimated that each nosocomial infection increases the duration of hospital stay for that patient by an average of 7 days. Besides the increased morbidity and mortality associated with nosocomial infections, the yearly monetary costs associated with them in the United States are in the billions of dollars.

Almost half of all nosocomial infections are caused by *Enterobacteriaceae*. Table 14:2 shows the percentage of nosocomial infections caused by individual pathogens at various sites of infection. These data were obtained in the National Nosocomial Infection Study (NNIS), an ongoing nationwide surveillance program in over 50 American hospitals. In 1984 the overall nosocomial infection rate reported by these hospitals was 3.4 infections per 100 patient discharges, which may underestimate the true infection rate by as much as 30%. *Enterobacteriaceae* were associated with about 40% of all infections in which a pathogen was identified.

The urinary tract is the most common site of nosocomial infection, accounting for about 41% of all such infections (Table 14:2). Most nosocomial urinary tract infections are caused by the *Enterobacteriaceae*, particularly *E. coli*. Of the hospitalized patients who develop a urinary tract infection, 75% have had some type of prior urologic instrumentation. Bladder catheterization is most frequently involved, although other forms of manipulation such as cystoscopy are important as well. An indwelling catheter is more likely to lead to a urinary tract infection than is a single, short-term catheterization. However, the risk of infection with an indwelling catheter

Table 14:2. Important Causes of Nosocomial Infections in the United States*

Pathogen	Proportion (%) of infections caused by each pathogen at site: Urin. tract†	Surg. wound	Lower resp.	Prim. bact.	Cutan.	Other	Total isolates	%
E. coli	30.7	11.5	6.4	10.1	7.0	7.4	5,266	17.8
P. aeruginosa	12.7	8.9	16.9	7.6	9.2	6.7	3,366	11.4
Enterococcus	14.7	12.1	1.5	7.1	8.8	7.0	3,063	10.4
S. aureus	1.6	18.6	12.9	12.3	28.9	14.6	3,059	10.3
Klebsiella spp.	8.0	5.2	11.6	7.8	3.8	4.6	2,193	7.4
Coagulase-negative staphylococcus	3.4	8.3	1.5	14.9	11.5	11.6	1,868	6.3
Enterobacter spp.	4.8	7.0	9.4	6.3	4.5	3.9	1,748	5.9
Candida spp.	5.4	1.7	4.0	5.6	5.8	14.1	1,620	5.5
Proteus spp.	7.4	5.2	4.2	0.8	3.3	2.1	1,522	5.1
Serratia spp.	1.2	2.1	5.8	3.0	2.2	1.5	691	2.3
Other fungi	2.2	0.4	1.4	1.3	0.9	2.8	496	1.7
Citrobacter spp.	1.8	1.4	1.4	0.7	0.7	0.9	414	1.4
Bacteroides spp.	0.0	3.7	0.2	3.4	1.2	1.4	355	1.2
Streptococcus, Gp. B	0.9	1.3	0.7	2.3	1.1	1.9	348	1.2
Other anaerobes	0.0	1.7	0.1	1.8	0.8	4.4	300	1.0
All others‡	5.2	10.9	22.0	15.0	10.3	15.1	3,253	11.1
Number of isolates	12,218	5,500	4,567	2,264	1,690	3,323	29,562	100.0

* Based on nosocomial infection surveillance for the United States in 1984.

† Abbreviations: Urin. tract = urinary tract infections; Surg. wound = Surgical wound infections; Lower resp. = Lower respiratory tract infections; Prim. bact. = Primary bacteremia; Cutan. = Cutaneous infections; spp. = species

‡ Other pathogens were combined since none accounted for more than 3% of the isolates at any site.

can be substantially reduced by maintaining a continuously closed sterile drainage system, rather than having an open system or one which is frequently opened and irrigated.

A substantial proportion of community-acquired and nosocomial urinary tract infections caused by *E. coli* are caused by O-antigen groups O4, O6 and O75.[18] Strains of these serogroups colonize the large bowel and often cause infection in the patient. There is a higher prevalence of these serogroups in stools of hospitalized patients than in stools of individuals in the community. Hospital personnel have a colonization rate similar to that of patients. A similar situation exists with urinary tract infections caused by *K. pneumoniae* in which the patient's intestinal tract is an important intermediate reservoir. In this instance, infection is often acquired endogenously. *Klebsiella* which cause urinary tract infection apparently colonize the gastrointestinal tract only after a period of hospitalization. The prevalence of *Klebsiella* colonization in hospital personnel is generally low and the organism is probably transmitted to patients on the hands of personnel. Antibiotic therapy is a definite factor predisposing to the development of *Klebsiella* intestinal colonization and subsequent urinary tract infection.

In contrast, urinary tract infections with *Serratia* and *Providencia* almost never result from organisms in the patient's own intestine. In outbreaks caused by these bacteria, the major reservoirs are patients whose urinary tract is colonized or patients with unrecognized infection. Infection is acquired extrinsically through passive transmission of organisms from patient to patient on the hands of hospital personnel. Broad spectrum antimicrobial therapy and catheterization are associated with infection. Measures for controlling outbreaks of urinary tract infections caused by the *Enterobacteriaceae* are aimed at diminishing or eradicating the reservoir, interrupting the mode of spread and modifying the factors placing the patients at risk.[72]

After surgical wound and other cutaneous infections, the next most frequent nosocomial infection site is the lower respiratory tract, which accounts for 15% of nosocomial infections in NNIS hospitals (Table 14:2). Over half of these infections are caused by *Enterobacteriaceae* or *Pseudomonas*. The mortality rate associated with lower respiratory tract infections caused by gram-negative bacteria is high, ranging from 30-60%. Most lower respiratory tract infections are probably caused by microorganisms from the pharynx that are spread to the bronchial tree and lungs by inapparent aspiration of oral secretions. However, this mechanism has not been demonstrated conclusively.[62] Hospitalized patients are more likely than nonhospitalized persons to have pharyngeal colonization with gram-negative bacteria. Chronic or severe illness predisposes to pharyngeal colonization and subsequent lower respiratory tract infections, presumably because of impaired clearance mechanisms. Antibiotic therapy is also a predisposing factor. Gram-negative bacteria that colonize the pharynx may come from other patients or from the individual's own gastrointestinal tract.

Although pharyngeal colonization may be the cause of nosocomial lower respiratory tract infection with gram-negative bacilli, hospitalized patients are frequently exposed to other potential sources of infectious microorganisms. Contaminated respiratory therapy equipment allows potential pathogens to be inhaled directly. Inspired gas mixtures used in respiratory therapy must be saturated with water vapor to keep the respiratory tract mucosa from drying. This saturation can be achieved by either nebulizers or humidifiers. Of the two reservoirs, nebulizers are the more risky because the aerosolized water droplets in which bacteria may be suspended are small enough to be deposited directly in the alveoli. In one hospital, the prevalence of necrotizing pneumonia caused by gram-negative bacteria and seen at autopsy increased 4-fold over a 5-year period after such equipment was introduced and widely used. The rate subsequently returned to baseline levels when a routine program of nebulizer decontamination was instituted. Common-source outbreaks of respiratory tract infection have been caused by contaminated medications and by contaminated water in reservoirs. Multiple-dose vials of medications should not be used and reservoirs should be emptied and refilled every 8-12 h. Reusable respiratory therapy equipment should be sterilized before it is used and breathing circuits should be changed every 24 hours. Many strains of *Klebsiella, Enterobacter* and *Serratia* can multiply in high quality distilled water, which explains some of the problems with moist environments.

The gram-negative bacteria are also the most common etiologic organisms in nosocomial bacteremias. Although bacteremia in hospitalized patients is less common than nosocomial infections at other sites, invasion of the bloodstream by gram-negative organisms often has a poor prognosis. Mortality from nosocomial bacteremia may approach 90% in certain groups of patients. Outcome is largely dependent on the age of the patient (newborns and the elderly are most likely to have fatal infections) and the severity of the underlying disease. A particularly high mortality rate is associated with septic shock.

Most cases of nosocomial bacteremia are secondary infections. The organism is transmitted from an identifiable primary infection at another site. The urinary tract is the most common primary site of infection resulting in bacteremia, with less frequent sites being the respiratory tract, gastrointestinal tract and surgical wounds. With some clinical conditions such as severe burns, secondary bacteremia is almost inevitable. The frequency with which the *Enterobacteriaceae* cause secondary bacteremia reflects their involvement in primary infections at other sites.

In approximately 20-30% of nosocomial bacteremias, there is no readily identifiable focus. These bacteremias are termed primary and have special epidemiologic importance. In some instances, particularly in immunosuppressed or otherwise debilitated patients, organisms enter from an occult portal in the gastrointestinal tract or pharynx. Alternatively, the bloodstream may be seeded during a surgical procedure involving the urinary tract, gastrointestinal tract or biliary system, or during cystoscopy or colonoscopy. Primary bacteremias may also result from contaminated fluids or other materials being introduced into the vascular system. This was the situation in the United States when intravenous fluids contaminated with *Enterobacter agglomerans* and *E. cloacae* caused a nationwide outbreak of primary bacteremia. Bacteremia associated with intravenous fluid therapy is more likely to result from extrinsic contamination with microorganisms which gain access to the delivery system during the process of preparation and infusion. Outbreaks of primary bacteremias have also been caused by parenteral injection of contaminated medications from multiple-dose vials, contamination of infused blood products, particularly platelets, and contamination of intravascular pressure monitoring systems.

Markers for Epidemiology

Marker systems are most useful in differentiating common species, including *E. coli, Proteus mirabilis, Morganella morganii, Providencia rettgeri, Klebsiella, Enterobacter* and *Serratia*.[45] Marker systems are usually not needed for the rare species of opportunistic *Enterobacteriaceae*. A cluster of cases caused by one of these rare pathogens suggests an infection problem which should be investigated.

Specialized or reference methods are very useful in epidemiologic studies, but most laboratories should not attempt to do them unless they can allocate the necessary personnel. Setting up typing methods is time-consuming and the laboratory staff must do them often to maintain adequate skill. It is best to refer isolates for typing to a laboratory with necessary reagents and expertise.

Serological Typing

Many serologic schemes have been proposed for typing the *Enterobacteriaceae*. Those used for *E. coli, Shigella, Salmonella* and *Klebsiella* are standardized by international agreement, but others are poorly standardized. Some of the sera are commercially available. Laboratories should not routinely type the opportunistic *Enterobacteriaceae*, except as part of carefully planned studies or when epidemiologic questions must be answered. When antisera are not available commercially, few laboratories should attempt to produce them. When sera are available commercially, they can be used as the specific circumstances dictate. Several reviews contain many details on serotyping.[26]

DIAGNOSTIC PROCEDURES

Collection and Processing of Specimens

This subject must be considered in relation to other microorganisms likely to be present in specimens. Fortunately, almost all procedures designed for isolating bacterial pathogens from extraintestinal specimens are designed to isolate fastidious pathogens,[42,47] insuring that *Enterobacteriaceae* will also be isolated since they survive well and grow on normal plating media. Tables 14:1 and 14:3 list some of the species which can occur in extraintestinal specimens. These tables can be used as a guide to the possible clinical relevance and relative frequency at different sites. The stool culture is an

Table 14:3. Distribution of *Enterobacteriaceae* and Other Organisms in Significant Blood Cultures and in Meningitis*

Organism	Blood	Spinal Fluid
Family *Enterobacteriaceae*		
Escherichia coli	4019 (559)†	65 (17)
Klebsiella pneumoniae	768 (152)	12 (2)
Proteus mirabilis	610 (96)	5 (1)
Enterobacter cloacae	218 (39)	2
Salmonella (subgroup 1)	222 (31)	1
Klebsiella oxytoca	141 (23)	4
Salmonella typhi	133 (1)	—
Citrobacter freundii	82 (13)	1
Morganella morganii	77 (13)	1 (1)
Serratia marcescens	65 (13)	5 (2)
Proteus vulgaris	40 (7)	1
Serratia liquefaciens group	34 (4)	—
Enterobacter agglomerans group	34 (5)	1 (1)
Salmonella paratyphi A	31	—
Enterobacter aerogenes	28 (6)	3
Providencia stuartii	19 (2)	1 (1)
Citrobacter diversus	13 (1)	6 (3)
Hafnia alvei	9 (1)	—
Yersinia enterocolitica	6 (2)	—
Other Organisms (for comparison)		
Aeromonas hydrophila	50 (14)	—
Pseudomonas aeruginosa	514 (203)	12 (6)
Staphylococcus aureus	2459 (371)	40 (9)
Haemophilus influenzae	408 (18)	461 (22)
Streptococcus pneumoniae	1638 (328)	286 (70)
Streptococcus—group B	290 (45)	73 (16)
Neisseria meningitidis	102 (18)	395 (25)

* Data for bacteremia and meningitis are from the latest surveillance report from England, Wales and Ireland for one year. These are not reportable diseases in the United States.

† The first number gives the number of cases and the number in parentheses gives the number of these which were fatal: — indicates that none were reported.

exception and is discussed in more detail because the procedure is designed primarily to isolate enteric pathogens such as *Salmonella, Shigella*, pathogenic strains of *E. coli* and *Y. enterocolitica*.

Stool Culture

Stool cultures are usually submitted with a request to isolate and identify the cause of diarrhea. The groups of *Enterobacteriaceae* usually associated with diarrhea in the United States are *Salmonella, Shigella*, certain pathogenic strains of *E. coli* and *Y. enterocolitica*. Occasionally other *Enterobacteriaceae* have been implicated as causing diarrhea. This list includes such groups as *Citrobacter, Proteus, Klebsiella, Enterobacter* and *Serratia*. Enterotoxin-producing strains of *Enterobacteriaceae* other than *E. coli* have been isolated from people with diarrhea,[85] but their etiologic role is not well established. Currently, there is no evidence that these enterotoxin-producing strains are important causes of diarrhea in the United States.

Stool cultures should be plated as soon as possible after they are collected in order to recover fastidious pathogens such as *Shigella*. If rapid processing is not possible, a small portion of the stool (0.2-0.5 g) or a swab coated with feces should be placed in a transport medium and held refrigerated until it can be examined in the laboratory. Commonly used transport media include Stuart's, Amies, Cary-Blair and buffered-glycerol saline. Cary-Blair is probably the best overall transport medium for diarrheal stools.

There are many different procedures for processing stool specimens.[47] Many laboratories are content to isolate *Salmonella* and *Shigella*, but isolation procedures for stools can be designed to include all the possible pathogens. In cases of chronic or severe diarrhea, rare pathogens should be considered. Specific points about the isolation and identification of *Salmonella, Shigella, E. coli* and *Y. enterocolitica* will be considered in subsequent sections.

Microscopic Examinations

Many specimens are Gram stained and then examined microscopically. Any gram-negative rod found on microscopic examination may be an *Enterobacteriaceae*, but microscopic examination cannot exclude rod-shaped species in other families.

Stool specimens should be examined macroscopically for the presence of blood and/or mucus. They can also be examined microscopically for leukocytes.[61] Small flecks of mucus or stool are mixed with 0.1 mL of Loeffler's methylene blue stain on a glass microscopy slide. A cover slip is added and the suspension is examined microscopically for leukocytes. Pickering et al[61] found leukocytes more frequently in stools which were positive for *Shigella* (24 of 36 or 69% contained leukocytes) than from stools

Table 14:4. Biochemical Reactions of the *Enterobacteriaceae* that Cause the Most Important Human Infections or are Frequently Isolated from Clinical Specimens*

Species	Indole production	Methyl red	Voges-Proskauer	Citrate (Simmons')	Hydrogen sulfide (TSI)	Urea hydrolysis	Phenylalanine deaminase	Lysine decarboxylase	Arginine dihydrolase	Ornithine decarboxylase	Motility (36°C)	Gelatin hydrolysis (22°C)	D-Glucose, gas	Lactose fermentation	Sucrose fermentation	D-Mannitol fermentation	Dulcitol fermentation	Adonitol fermentation	D-Sorbitol fermentation	L-Arabinose fermentation	Raffinose fermentation	L-Rhamnose fermentation	D-Xylose fermentation	Melibiose fermentation	DNase, 25°C	ONPG†
Escherichia coli	98	99	0	1	1	1	0	90	17	65	95	0	95	95	50	98	60	5	94	99	50	80	95	75	0	95
Shigella serogroups A, B, and C	50	100	0	0	0	0	0	0	5	1	0	0	2	0	0	93	2	0	30	60	50	5	2	50	0	2
Shigella sonnei	0	100	0	0	0	0	0	0	2	98	0	0	0	2	1	99	0	0	2	95	3	75	2	25	0	90
Salmonella, most serotypes	1	100	0	95	95	1	0	98	70	97	95	0	96	1	1	100	96	0	95	99	2	95	97	95	2	2
Salmonella typhi	0	100	0	0	97	0	0	98	3	0	97	0	0	1	0	100	0	0	99	2	0	0	82	100	0	0
Salmonella paratyphi A	0	100	0	0	10	0	0	0	15	95	95	0	99	0	0	100	90	0	95	100	0	100	0	95	0	0
Citrobacter freundii	5	100	0	95	80	70	0	0	65	20	95	0	95	50	30	99	55	0	98	100	30	99	99	50	0	95
Citrobacter diversus	99	100	0	99	0	75	0	0	65	99	95	0	98	35	45	100	50	98	99	100	0	100	100	0	0	96
Klebsiella pneumoniae	0	10	98	98	0	95	0	98	0	0	0	0	97	98	99	99	30	90	99	99	99	99	99	99	0	99
Klebsiella oxytoca	99	20	95	95	0	90	1	99	0	0	0	0	97	100	100	99	55	99	99	98	100	100	100	99	0	100
Enterobacter aerogenes	0	5	98	95	0	2	0	98	0	98	97	0	100	95	100	100	5	98	100	100	96	99	100	99	0	100
Enterobacter cloacae	0	5	100	100	0	65	0	0	97	96	95	0	100	93	97	100	15	25	95	100	97	92	99	90	0	99
Hafnia alvei	0	40	85	10	0	4	0	100	6	98	85	0	98	5	10	99	0	0	0	95	2	97	98	0	0	90
Serratia marcescens	1	20	98	98	0	15	0	99	0	99	97	90	55	2	99	99	0	40	99	0	2	0	7	0	98	95
Proteus mirabilis	2	97	50	65	98	98	98	0	0	99	95	90	96	2	15	0	0	0	0	0	1	1	98	0	50	0
Proteus vulgaris	98	95	0	15	95	95	99	0	0	0	95	91	85	2	97	0	0	0	0	0	1	5	95	0	80	1
Providencia rettgeri	99	93	0	95	0	98	98	0	0	0	94	0	10	5	15	100	0	100	1	0	5	70	10	5	0	5
Providencia stuartii	98	100	0	93	0	30	95	0	0	0	85	0	0	2	50	10	0	5	1	1	7	0	7	0	10	10
Providencia alcalifaciens	99	99	0	98	0	0	98	0	0	1	96	0	85	0	15	2	0	98	1	1	1	0	1	0	0	1
Morganella morganii	98	97	0	0	5	98	95	0	0	98	95	0	90	1	0	0	0	0	0	0	0	0	0	0	0	5
Yersinia enterocolitica	50	97	2	0	0	75	0	0	0	95	2	0	5	5	95	98	0	0	99	98	5	1	70	1	5	95
Yersinia pestis	0	80	0	0	0	5	0	0	0	0	0	0	0	0	0	97	0	0	50	100	0	1	90	20	0	50
Yersinia pseudotuberculosis	0	100	0	0	0	95	0	0	0	0	0	0	0	0	0	100	0	0	0	50	15	70	100	70	0	70

* Each number gives the percentage of positive reactions after 2 days of incubation at 36°C. The vast majority of these positive reactions occur within 24 h. Reactions that become positive after 2 days are not considered.

† ONPG = *o*-Nitrophenyl-β-D-galactopyranoside.

which yielded other pathogens (14%) or no pathogen (17%). This procedure is seldom used in clinical laboratories and should not be used as a substitute for culture.

Definitive identification of *Enterobacteriaceae* is almost always based on biochemical reactions on pure cultures rather than on microscopic examination. Although identification by fluorescent antibody staining is theoretically possible for all species, in practice it has been limited to *Salmonella* and to certain serogroups of *E. coli*, and has not been used routinely. Serological crossreactions with other species of *Enterobacteriaceae* have limited this approach.

Inoculation of Primary Plates

Specimens, except stools, are processed for isolation of any pathogen with no particular emphasis on the *Enterobacteriaceae*.[42,47] Culture materials such as urine, sputum or wound specimens will be plated onto a nonselective medium such as blood agar which supports growth of most bacteria, and onto a medium such as MacConkey agar (interchangeable throughout this chapter with eosine methylene blue agar (EMB)) which permits growth and some differentiation of *Enterobacteriaceae* and other nonfastidious gram-negative rods. With a few exceptions, *Enterobacteriaceae* will grow on most plating media and form colonies 1-3 mm in diameter within 18-24 h.

Identification

There are many different approaches to identifying *Enterobacteriaceae*. Twenty years ago this topic was less complicated than today because the basic question was "Which, and how many, conventional biochemical tests are needed for identification?" Today many more methods are available.[28,42,47].

Conventional Biochemical Tests in Tubes: This approach was once used by all clinical and public health microbiology laboratories. Biochemical test media are prepared, dispensed into glass tubes and sterilized. Although many laboratories prepare their own, most media are also available commercially. Growth from one colony is inoculated into each of the tubes. The tubes are incubated and the reactions are read at 24 h and usually also at 48 h (and kept longer by reference laboratories). Unfortunately, the media and the tests are not well standardized and few laboratories use the same tests. Even with so many variables, this approach usually results in correct identification of the more common species of *Enterobacteriaceae*. Table 14:4 gives the results obtained with the commonly used biochemical tests for the species of *Enterobacteriaceae* most often isolated from clinical specimens. A more detailed biochemical identification chart (over 100 species and biogroups and 45 tests) for all species of *Enterobacteriaceae* is available.[28]

The question has been asked "How many tests are needed to identify *Enterobacteriaceae* correctly?" There is no single answer to this question. Before it can be answered, another question must be asked and answered—"What is the acceptable percentage of incorrect identifications?" Because reference centers must strive for 100% accuracy in identification, 25-50 biochemical tests are done on each culture. Other helpful information can be obtained from staining reactions, growth on different media, genus- or species-specific tests, antimicrobial susceptibility patterns, serological typing and computer analysis. Reference laboratories are not required to obtain results as rapidly as are primary laboratories and can work for 100% accuracy with essentially no time or cost restraints. This is a luxury a busy hospital microbiology laboratory cannot afford. Most laboratories have developed their own flow charts or abbreviated differentiation charts for identification.[42] Since a few species of *Enterobacteriaceae* represent 95-98% of all those found, such shortcuts usually yield acceptable results. Misidentifications do occur when these schemes are used due to the biochemical similarity of some species. Table 14:4 can be used as the first stage in identifying an isolate of *Enterobacteriaceae*. Tables 14:5-18 give the differential reactions of most of the commonly isolated genera and species in the family.

"Kits" for Identifying *Enterobacteriaceae:* A "kit" is defined as a series of miniaturized or standardized tests available commercially. A single colony

Table 14:5. Differentiation of *Buttiauxella, Kluyvera* and Two Related Enteric Groups

Test	*Buttiauxella agrestis*	Enteric Group 63	Enteric Group 64	*Kluyvera ascorbata*	*Kluyvera cryocrescens*
Sucrose fermentation	−*(60)†	−	−	+	(+)
Ascorbate test (7 day)	−	+	−	+	−
D-Arabitol fermentation	−	−	+	−	−
Melibiose fermentation	+	−(67)	−	+	+
Raffinose fermentation	+	−	−	+	+
α-Methyl-D-glucoside fermentation	−	v(100)	−(100)	+	+
Citrate utilization (Simmons')	+	−(67)	v(100)	+	(+)
Lysine decarboxylase	−	+	−	+	(−)
Lactose fermentation	+	−	+	+	+

* Symbols (all data are for reaction within 2 days at 36°C unless otherwise specified): + = 90–100% positive; (+) = 75–89.9% positive; v = 25.1 to 74.9% positive; (−) = 10.1 to 25% positive; − = 0–10% positive.

† If delayed reactions are useful for differentiation, the % positive within the time period 3 to 7 days is given in parentheses; otherwise no delayed reactions are given.

Table 14:6. Differentiation Within the Genus *Cedecea*

Test	*C. davisae*	*C. lapagei*	*C. neteri*	*C. species 3*	*C. species 5*
Ornithine decarboxylase (Moellers)	+*	−	−	−	v
Fermentation of:					
Sucrose	+	−	+	v	+
D-Sorbitol	−	−	+	−	+
Raffinose	−	−	−	+	+
D-Xylose	+	−	+	+	+
Melibiose	−	−	−	+	+
Malonate utilization	+	+	+	−	−

* Symbols, same as Table 14:5.

Table 14:7. Differentiation Within the Genus *Citrobacter*

Test	*C. amalonaticus*	*C. freundii*	*C. diversus*
BIOCHEMICAL TESTS			
Indole production	+*	−	+
H_2S production (TSI)	−	+	−
Malonate utilization	−	(−)	+
KCN, growth in	+	+	−
Tyrosine-clearing	−	−	+
Adonitol fermentation	−	−	+
ANTIBIOGRAM—ZONE SIZES			
Cephalothin (30 μg)†	18.0(2.0)‡	10.9(2.9)	23.5(1.2)
Ampicillin (10 μg)	8.7(2.4)	14.3(3.1)	7.1(1.2)
Carbenicillin (100 μg)	16.5(2.4)	24.1(0.9)	12.6(1.6)

* Symbols same as Table 14:5.
† The number in parentheses is the amount of the antibiotic in the disc.
‡ The first number is the mean, the number in parentheses is the standard deviation of the zones of inhibition.[8] Data are based on 10 strains of each species. One strain was found to have multiple antibiotic resistance. It was excluded and replaced with a sensitive strain.

is picked (in some kits additional processing is required) and inoculated into the test system. This approach is similar to the "conventional tube" method, with the main differences being in the miniaturization, the number of tests available and the method of analyzing results. Kits are now used by most United States laboratories. An excellent review of the kits describes their routine use.[47]

Markers for Epidemiology

Sometimes an isolate must be typed to aid in an epidemiologic study. Serotyping is often used because it has several advantages. However,

Table 14:8. Differentiation Within the Genus *Edwardsiella*

Test or Property	*E. tarda* Most strains	*E. tarda* Biogroup 1	*E. hoshinae*	*E. ictaluri*
Indole production	+*	+	(−)	−
H_2S production (TSI)	+	−	−	−
Motility	+	+	+	−
Malonate utilization	−	−	+	−
Fermentation of:				
D-Mannitol	−	+	+	−
Sucrose	−	+	+	−
Trehalose	−	−	+	−
L-Arabinose	−	+	(−)	−
Tetrathionate reduction	+	−	+	
Present in human clinical specimens	+	−	rare	−

* Symbols same as Table 14:5.

serotyping is not always the method of choice. For example, *Shigella sonnei* cannot be divided into further serologic types. In this and similar instances, other typing methods may be used.

Biotyping: Simple phenotypic properties are determined, such as fermentation of D-xylose, production of indole and growth at 45°C. The procedures can be done in conventional test tubes or with one of the commercial kit systems.

Bacteriophage Typing: A standard set of bacteriophages is applied to the isolates to determine similarities or differences in their lysis patterns.[47]

Bacteriocin Production or Bacteriocin Sensitivity: Bacteriocins are inhibitory substances produced by one strain which kill or inhibit other strains of the same species. Typing by bacteriocin sensitivity is comparable to bacteriophage typing except that a standard set of bacteriocins is used. When bacteriocin production is used for typing, a strain is grown under conditions that allow it to produce bacteriocins, which are then assayed against a standard set of indicator strains.

Plasmid Profile Analysis: Strains of the same species often differ in their plasmid content. Cultures are lysed; plasmid DNA is extracted and applied to agarose gels to separate plasmids by size. Strains can then be compared by the number and size of their plasmids. For example, a strain of *Salmonella* typhimurium with 4 plasmids 70, 39, 34 and 28 megadaltons in size, would be quite different from a strain with a single 73 megadalton plasmid.

Table 14:9. Differentiation Within the Genus *Enterobacter*

Test or Property	*E. aerogenes*	*E. agglomerans*	*E. amnigenus* biogroup 1	*E. amnigenus* biogroup 2	*E. cloacae*	*E. gergoviae*	*E. intermedium*	*E. sakazakii*	*E. taylorae*
Lysine decarboxylase	+*	−	−	−	−	+	−	−	−
Arginine dihydrolase	−	−	−	v	+	−	−	+	+
Ornithine decarboxylase	+	−	v	+	+	+	(+)	+	+
KCN—growth in	+	v	+	+	+	−	v	+	+
Fermentation of:									
Sucrose	+	(+)	+	−	+	+	v	+	−
Dulcitol	−	(−)	−	−	(−)	−	+	−	−
Adonitol	+	−	−	−	(−)	−	−	−	−
D-Sorbitol	+	v	−	+	+	−	+	−	−
Raffinose	+	v	+	−	+	+	+	+	−
α-methyl-D-glucoside	+	−	v	+	(+)	−	+	+	v
D-Arabitol	+	v	−	−	(−)	+	−	−	−
Yellow pigment	−	(+)	−	−	−	−	−	+	−
Present in human clinical specimens	+	+	−	−	+	+	−	+	+

* Symbols same as Table 14:5.

Table 14:10. Differentiation Within *Escherichia-Shigella*

	Shigella serogroups A, B, and C	*Shigella sonnei*	*E. coli* "Inactive"	*E. coli* "Normal"	*E. blattae*	*E. fergusonii*	*E. hermannii*	*E. vulneris*
Indole production	v*	–	(+)	+	–	+	+	–
Lysine decarboxylase	–	–	v	+	+	+	–	(+)
Ornithine decarboxylase	–	+	–	v	+	+	+	–
Motility	–	–	–	+	–	+	+	+
Gas produced during fermentation	–	–	–	+	+	+	+	+
Acetate utilization	–	–	v	+	–	+	(+)	v
Mucate fermentation	–	–	v	+	v	–	+	(+)
Lactose fermentation	–	–	(–)	+	–	–	v	(–)
KCN-Growth in	–	–	–	–	–	–	+	(–)
Yellow pigment	–	–	–	–	–	–	+	v
D-Mannitol fermentation	(+)	+	+	+	–	+	+	+
Adonitol fermentation	–	–	–	–	–	+	–	–
D-Sorbitol fermentation	v	–	(+)	+	–	–	–	–
Cellobiose fermentation	–	–	–	–	–	+	+	+
D-Arabitol fermentation	–	–	–	–	–	+	–	–
Present in human clinical specimens	+	+	+	+	–	+	+	+
Isolated from cockroaches	–	–	–	–	+	–	–	–

* Symbols same as Table 14.5.

Table 14:11. Differentiation Within the Genus *Klebsiella*

Test	*K. pneumoniae*	*K. oxytoca*	*K. terri gena*	*K. planticola**	*K.* Group 47 indole$^+$, ornithine$^+$
Indole production†	−‡	+‖	−	(−)	+
Ornithine decarboxylase†	−	−	−	−	+
Growth and D-glucose fermentation at:‡					
5°C	−	−	+	+	+
10°C	−	+	+	+	+
41°C	+	+	+	−	−
44.5°C§	+	−	−	−	−

* The reactions of *Klebsiella trevisanii* (*Klebsiella* Group K) are the same as *K. planticola*.
† Based on CDC data.
‡ Based on limited CDC data; compiled from the literature.
§ 44.5°C is the temperature setting of water baths used for the "fecal coliform" test.
‖ Symbols same as Table 14:5.

Table 14:12. Differentiation Within the Genus *Kluyvera*

Test	*K. ascorbata*	*K. cryocrescens*
Ascorbate test	+*	−
D-glucose fermentation at 5°C (21 days)	−	+
Zone sizes for cephalothin and carbenicillin	small†	large†

* Symbols same as Table 14:5.
† *K. ascorbata* has zone size of 17mm or less around cephalothin; *K. cryocaescens* usually has larger zones.

Table 14:13. Differentiation of the Three Genera in the *Proteus* Group

Test or Property	*Proteus*	*Providencia*	*Morganella*
Citrate utilization	v*	+	−
H_2S production (TSI)	+	−	−
Ornithine decarboxylase	v	−	+
Gelatin liquefaction	+	−	−
Lipase (corn oil)	+	−	−
D-Mannose fermentation	−	+	+
Swarming†	+	−	−

* Symbols same as Table 14:5.
† On sheep blood agar or trypticase soy agar.

The series of books "Methods in Microbiology" review typing methods for most of the species of *Enterobacteriaceae*.

Problem Strains

Most strains of *Enterobacteriaceae* grow readily on plating media, but there are exceptions. Some strains grow poorly on blood agar but grow much better on chocolate agar incubated in a candle jar. This fact suggests a possible nutritional requirement or a mutation involved with respiration. There are slow-growing strains of *E. coli, K. pneumoniae* and *Serratia*, but this kind of metabolic change presumably could occur in any species. Biochemical reactions usually require several days of additional incubation before a typical pattern is obtained and a correct identification is possible. A second type of "sluggish" organism is sometimes found in specimens from patients who have been given antimicrobial agents. Li et al[50] described such "pleiotropic" mutants in *S. marcescens* and *Salmonella*. These strains react atypically in many of the standard biochemical tests and are difficult to identify.

Laboratories often isolate strains which grow rapidly but whose biochemical reactions do not fit any of the described species of *Enterobacteriaceae*. At present these cultures can only be reported as "unidentified." In time, these organisms will probably be named as new species which can then be routinely identified.[28] Most newly identified species will probably be rare in clinical specimens.

Susceptibility To Antimicrobial Agents

When antibiotics were first introduced, there was only slight resistance among the *Enterobacteriaceae*. However, today many strains of *Enterobacteriaceae* isolated from human disease are antibiotic-resistant.

Intrinsic Resistance: Intrinsic resistance is a genetic property of most strains of a species and evolved long before antibiotic usage by man. Intrinsic resistance can best be shown by studying strains that were isolated and stored in a culture collection before the "antibiotic era" or by studying strains from nature that have not been exposed (presumably) to antibiotics. A third way is to collect a large number of strains from a wide variety of sources and study those that have the most sensitive patterns. For example, all strains of *S. marcescens* apparently have intrinsic resistance to penicillin G, colistin and cephalothin.[27] Table 14:19 lists other species of *Enterobacteriaceae* and their resistance patterns.

Non-intrinsic Resistance: Much antibiotic resistance is due to the selective pressure of antibiotic usage in the hospital. Many strains of *Enterobacteri-*

Table 14:14. Differentation Within the Genus *Proteus*

Test or Property	*P. mirabilis*	*P. myxofaciens*	*P. penneri*	*P. vulgaris* biogroup 2	*P. vulgaris* biogroup 3
Indole production	–*	–	–	+	+
Ornithine decarboxylase	+	–	–	–	–
Maltose fermentation	–	+	+	+	+
D-Xylose fermentation	+	–	+	+	+
Salicin fermentation	–	–	–	+	–
Esculin hydrolysis	–	–	–	+	–
Chloramphenicol susceptibility	S	S	R	V	S
Present in human clinical specimens	+	–	+	+	+
Occurs as a pathogen of gypsy moth larvae	–	+	–	–	–

* Symbols same as Table 14:5: S = susceptible; R = resistant; V = variable.

Table 14:15. Differentiation Within the Genus *Providencia*

Test	*P. alcalifaciens*	*P. rustigianii*	*P. stuartii*	*P. rettgeri*
Urea hydrolysis	–*	–	v	+
Myo-Inositol fermentation	–	–	+†	+
Adonitol fermentation	+	–	–†	+
D-Arabitol fermentation	–	–	–	+
Trehalose fermentation	–	–	+	–
D-Galactose fermentation	–	+	+	+

* Symbols same as Table 14:5.
† *Providencia stuartii* biogroup 4 strains are inositol negative and biogroup 6 strains are adonitol positive; these two biogroups are rare.

aceae that cause disease have become highly antibiotic-resistant through the evolutionary selective pressure of antibiotic usage by man. Genetic studies have shown that this type of antibiotic resistance is often plasmid-mediated.

The Antibiogram as a Marker in Epidemiologic Studies: Antibiotic susceptibility testing is usually done on isolates which are clinically significant, providing an "antibiogram" which can be useful in comparing isolates in epidemiological studies. When the selective ecological pressure of antibiotics is changed, the resistance pattern of epidemic (or endemic) strains may also change. These changes have been documented in outbreaks which have lasted for several months or longer. Even with these limitations in genetic stability, the antibiogram is one of the most useful laboratory markers in investigating infection problems.

Table 14:16. Properties of the Six Subgroups Within the Genus *Salmonella* (“the Salmonella-Arizona Group”)*

	Designation:					
	Salmonella subgroup 1	*Salmonella* subgroup 2	*Salmonella* subgroup 3a	*Salmonella* subgroup 3b	*Salmonella* subgroup 4	*Salmonella* subgroup 5
DNA-hybridization group of Crosa et al.	1	2	3	4	5	Not Studied
Salmonella subgenus names formerly used	I	II	III	III	IV	V
Genus according to Ewing	*Salmonella*	*Salmonella*	*Arizona*	*Arizona*	*Salmonella*	*Salmonella*
Subspecies according to Le Minor et al.	*choleraesuis*	*salamae*	*arizonae*	*diarizonae*	*houtenae*	*bongori*
Usually Monophasic (Mono) or Diphasic (Di) flagella	Di	Di	Mono	Di	Mono	Mono
Usually isolated from humans and warm-blooded animals	+	–	–	–	–	–
Usually isolated from cold-blooded animals and the environment	–	+	+	+	+	+
Pathogenic for humans	+ + + +	+	+	+	+	+ ?
TESTS TO DIFFERENTIATE THE SUBGROUPS						
Dulcitol fermentation	96†	90	0	1	0	100
Lactose fermentation	1	1	15	85	0	0
ONPG Test	2	15	100	100	0	100
Malonate utilization	1	95	95	95	0	0
Growth in KCN medium	1	1	1	1	95	100
Mucate fermentation	90	96	90	30	0	100
Gelatin hydrolysis‡	–	+	+	+	+	–
D-Galacturonate fermentation‡	–	+	–	+	+	+
Lysis by 01 bacteriophage‡	+	+	–	+	–	V

* Adapted from Farmer et al. [28, 29]

† The numbers give the % positive for the tests after 2 days incubation at 36° C; the results for the first six tests are based on CDC data. The vast majority of the positive tests occur within 24 hours; reactions positive after 2 days are not considered.

‡ Based on the data of Le Minor et al. + = 90% or more positive, – = 10% or less positive. The test for gelatin hydrolysis is the rapid “film” method at 36°C (almost all strains are negative by the tube method at 22°C within 2 days).

Table 14:17. Differentiation Within the Genus *Serratia*

Biochemical test	*S. ficaria*	*S. liquefaciens*	*S. marcescens*	*S. odorifera*	*S. plymuthica*	*S. rubidaea*	"*Serratia*" *fonticola*
Deoxyribonuclease (25°C)	+*	(+)	+	+	+	+	−
Lipase (corn oil)	(+)	(+)	+	V	V	+	−
Gelatinase (22°C)	+	+	+	+	V	(+)	−
Lysine decarboxylase	−	+	+	+	−	V	+
Ornithine decarboxylase	−	+	+	V	−	−	+
Odor of *S. odorifera*	+	−	−	+	−	(−)	−
Red, pink or orange pigment	−	−	V	−	V	V	−
Fermentation of:							
L-Arabinose	+	+	−	+	+	+	+
D-Arabitol	+	−	−	−	−	(+)	+
D-Sorbitol	+	+	+	+	V	−	+
Adonitol	−	−	V	V	−	+	+
Dulcitol	−	−	−	−	−	−	+

* Symbols same as Table 14:5.

Table 14:18. Differentiation of the Five Species in the *Yersinia enterocolitica* Group*

	Y. enterocolitica	*Y. kristensenii*	*Y. intermedia*	*Y. frederiksenii*	*Y. aldovae*
Sucrose fermentation	+†	−	+	+	v
Raffinose fermentation	−	−	+	−	−
Rhamnose (L-) fermentation	−	−	+	+	+
Cellobiose fermentation	+	+	+	+	−
α-Methyl-D-glucoside fermentation	−	−	+	−	−
Melibiose fermentation	−	−	+	−	−

* These characteristic fermentation patterns usually occur within 1 to 4 days at 25°C, but are often delayed at 36°C.
† Symbols same as Table 14:5.

ESCHERICHIA COLI

INTRODUCTION

Escherichia coli may present one of the most challenging problems in bacterial pathogenesis. The organism is a common inhabitant of the human (and animal) intestine and, based on routine laboratory tests, saprophytic strains are virtually indistinguishable from inherently pathogenic strains. As pathogenicity mechanisms and markers have been identified, we are beginning to understand the complicated etiology of *E. coli* infections. There are apparently 4 distinct groups now recognized within this species: (1)Normal flora *E. coli* which may cause opportunistic infections such as wound or lower urinary tract infections and various manifestations in the immunocompromised host; (2) *E. coli* causing septicemia or meningitis in neonates; (3) *E. coli* causing upper urinary tract infections or pylonephritis; and (4) *E. coli* causing diarrhea, dysentery, hemorrhagic colitis and hemolytic uremic syndrome.

Isolation of any organism from spinal fluid, blood or kidney suggests a causal role for that organism in infection. Isolation of *E. coli* from these sites does not require selection or differentiation at the clinical level but has generated considerable debate as to their opportunistic versus pathogenic nature. In the past decade, fimbriae adherent for urinary epithelial cells (antigenic designations F7-F12), a hemolysin associated with cytolysis and release of host iron, aerobactin and enterochelin iron sequestering systems, K-1 capsular antigen and colicin V have been identified as virulence markers in these extraintestinal pathogens.[58] The diarrheogenic *E. coli* pose a special problem and will be reviewed in detail, following a general discussion of the methods of primary isolation, identification and determination of epidemic strain markers which are similar for all pathogenic *E. coli*.

Table 14:19. Intrinsic Antibiotic Resistance in *Enterobacteriaceae**

Organisms	Most strains resistant to:
Citrobacter amalonaticus	ampicillin
Citrobacter freundii	cephalothin
Citrobacter diversus	ampicillin, carbenicillin
Edwardsiella tarda	colistin
Enterobacter cloacae	
Enterobacter aerogenes	cephalothin
Enterobacter, other	
Hafnia alvei	
Klebsiella	ampicillin, carbenicillin
Proteus mirabilis	polymyxins, tetracycline, nitrofurantoin
Proteus vulgaris	polymyxins, ampicillin, cephalothin, nitrofurantoin
Morganella morganii	polymyxins, ampicillin, cephalothin
Providencia rettgeri	polymyxins, cephalothin, nitrofurantoin, tetracycline
Providencia, other	polymyxins, nitrofurantoin†
Serratia marcescens	polymyxins, cephalothin‡
LESS COMMON GENERA AND SPECIES	
Buttiauxella	cephalothin
Cedecea	polymyxins, ampicillin, cephalothin
Escherichia hermannii	ampicillin, carbenicillin
Ewingella americana	cephalothin
Kluyvera ascorbata	ampicillin, cephalothin
Kluyvera cryocrescens	ampicillin
Serratia fonticola	ampicillin, carbenicillin, cephalothin
Serratia, other	polymyxins,§ cephalothin

* Adapted from references 17, 25, 26, 45 and from the original papers describing new genera and species.
† Most strains of *Providencia stuartii* are also resistant to cephalothin and tetracycline.
‡ *Serratia marcescens* can also have intrinsic resistance to ampicillin, carbenicillin, streptomycin and tetracycline.
§ Resistance to polymyxins is common, but many strains have zones of 12mm or more.

DIAGNOSTIC PROCEDURES

Primary Isolation

Fecal specimens should be plated directly on a nonselective plating medium such as blood agar and on a differential medium of low selectivity such as MacConkey agar. Media of low selectivity which use lactose as the differentiating sugar are best because the proportion of lactose (lac)$^+$ and lac$^-$ colonies can be determined (gram-positive organisms do not form colonies) on this medium. The disadvantage of the sugar-containing media, however, is that organisms are more likely to be rough (autoagglutinable) in serological tests if they are grown on a medium which contains sugar. MacConkey agar appears to be preferable, since lac$^+$ and lac$^-$ colonies can

Table 14:20. Biochemical Tests Helpful in Differentiating *Escherichia coli* from *Shigella*

Test	*E. coli* "normal"	*E. coli* inactive	*S. dysenteriae*	*S. flexneri* groups 1–5	*S. flexneri* group 6	*S. boydii*	*S. sonnei*
Motility	85*	0	0	0	0	0	0
Gas from D-Glucose	91	0	0	0	18	0	0
Lactose	90	0	0	0	0	1	2
Indole	99	90	44	62	0	29	0
Mucate	94	25	0	0	0	0	16
Acetate	84	59	0	0	0	0	0
Christensen's (Citrate)	24	NA†	0	0	0	0	0
Lysine	88	43	0	0	0	0	0
Arginine	17	2	1.5	0	49	18	1
Ornithine	63	18	0	0	0	3	99
Sucrose	51	11	0	2	0	0	0.1
Salicin	37	3	0	0	0	0	0

* Gives the % positive for the test after 48 h of incubation.
† NA = data not available.

be selected without additional testing. *E. coli* isolates can be correctly selected with a reasonable degree of accuracy directly from the plating media. Since some *E. coli* strains ferment lactose slowly or are lac$^-$, both lac$^+$ and lac$^-$ colonies should be selected from plating media for additional testing, but most should be lac$^+$. For reference procedures it is generally recommended that 10 colonies be selected, but laboratory resources will dictate how many isolates can be reasonably handled (five colonies is suggested as the minimum number). Specimens may be examined for *E. coli* O157:H7 by utilizing sorbitol fermentation as a strain marker. *E. coli* O157:H7 is sorbitol-negative (or delayed positive) while 93% of *E. coli* strains are sorbitol-positive. Specimens can be plated on MacConkey-sorbitol agar if the laboratory resources permit use of a separate plating medium. MacConkey-sorbitol agar is prepared by adding 1% D-sorbitol to MacConkey agar base without lactose (available commercially). If MacConkey-sorbitol agar is not used, then lactose-positive colonies selected from MacConkey agar may be screened for sorbitol fermentation. Isolates that do not ferment sorbitol within 24 h should be screened with commercial *E. coli* O157 antiserum. If examining a large number of specimens, a laboratory may find it useful to use media which combines sorbitol fermentation and immobilization with *E. coli* H7 antiserum prior to serotyping.

Once the *E. coli* colonies have been isolated, there are two basic laboratory approaches to implicate them as the cause of diarrhea: assaying for virulence mechanisms and serotyping. For serological typing, colonies should be transferred to a nonselective medium such as blood agar, blood agar base or infusion agar. They should not be inoculated to a sugar-containing media such as triple sugar iron (TSI) agar which could cause the isolate to become rough.

Biochemical Identification

This topic is included because many cultures identified as *Shigella* by clinical or even reference laboratories are actually *E. coli*. Lactose$^+$, motile, gas-producing strains of *E. coli* are easily identified, but some *E. coli* strains are negative in these tests. The biochemical properties of this group are given in Table 14:20 under "*E. coli* inactive." Misidentification often results because *E. coli* strains crossreact serologically with *Shigella*, and identification is based on agglutination in one of the *Shigella* antisera. A complete set of biochemical reactions would have shown that the organism was *E. coli* rather than *Shigella*. Unlike *Shigella*, these strains are not inherent causes of dysentery in man; however, certain strains have been implicated in some cases of dysentery.

Differentiation from Shigella: This process can pose one of the most difficult problems for a laboratory and may reflect the fact that *E. coli* and *Shigella* should be placed in the same species on the basis of their close DNA relatedness. The best approach is to do a complete set of biochemical reactions and compare the pattern to that of *E. coli* and to those of all the *Shigella* groups (Tables 14:10, 14:20). The following generalizations are suggested as guidelines:

(1) *Shigella* cultures are always nonmotile and lysine negative.

(2) With the exception of some *Shigella flexneri* 6, *Shigella* do not produce gas during carbohydrate fermentation (there have been reports of gas production by a few strains of *S. boydii* 13 and 14 and *S. dysenteriae*.

(3) Cultures which ferment mucate or give an alkaline reaction on acetate or Christensen's citrate are much more likely to be *E. coli* than *Shigella*.

(4) *Shigella boydii* and *S. dysenteriae* are very rare in the United States. Cultures which have been presumptively identified as one of these two species should be carefully checked before any report is made.

It is obvious from this discussion that no definitive rules can be made. Most *Shigella* agglutinate in one of the polyvalent *Shigella* sera and in an individual typing serum. Although this fact can be very helpful in deciding that a culture is *Shigella, E. coli* cultures frequently crossreact in these sera. Because it is very important to differentiate *E. coli* from *Shigella*, complete biochemical and serological typing should be done in each instance.

Marker Systems

Serotyping is probably the most effective marker system for *E. coli*.[59] There are 171 recognized O somatic antigens, 80 K acidic polysaccharide antigens, 12 F or proteinaceous fimbrial antigens and 56 H protein flagellar antigens. There are rare reports of phase variation and several F antigens are plasmid-mediated, but the serotype is generally a very stable marker. An example of one strain designation is O6:K2:H1:F7.[58] Lack of availability of the many necessary reagents and subsequently, the small number of laboratories which can serotype is a primary limitation of serotyping. Another, more recently recognized limitation, is the mounting evidence that there is significant genetic diversity within a serogroup and even within the same O-H group (serotype).[14] This realization may be important in redefining pathogenic strains within groups such as O18:K1 and O2:K1.[14]

Techniques other than serotyping have also been used to type or subdivide groups of *E. coli*. Biotyping can be a useful marker since *E. coli* strains vary in their biochemical reactions (Table 14:10). It is important to note that many biochemical reactions occur after 18-24 h, and most reactions are held in reference laboratories for at least 7 days. Otherwise strains may appear to be one biotype at 24 h and a different biotype at 3 days. Certain biotype markers have been most useful within serotypes. The sorbitol-negative reaction of O157:H7 strains of *E. coli* has made this an excellent screening assay prior to serotyping. Bacteriophage typing, colicin typing and antimicrobial susceptibility patterns can be useful in epidemiological studies,[18] but phage and colicin techniques are not widely used, and resistance characters are frequently on plasmids which are transmissible or easily lost. These methods should be reserved for outbreak investigations or for special studies.

Plasmid profile analysis has provided an effective epidemiologic marker in several outbreaks of *E. coli* diarrheal disease. This methodology has become more widespread as reagents and equipment have become commercially available. Plasmid profiles in conjunction with restriction endonuclease digests have proven to be sensitive clonal and epidemic markers, especially within one serotype.[86]

There are several new techniques which may prove to be even more sensitive and specific markers than any of the above. Outer membrane protein (OMP) patterns, lipopolysaccharide (LPS) patterns and multilocus enzyme electrophoresis have provided evidence that there is genetic diversity within serogroups and serotypes of *E. coli*.[14] These techniques presently are limited to research and reference laboratories and require relatively complex procedures, reagents and equipment.

DIARRHEOGENIC *E. COLI*

Because *E. coli* strains are common inhabitants of the human gastrointestinal tract, virulent strains were not recognized as intestinal pathogens until the 1940s. At that time, certain strains were identified as the cause of outbreaks of explosive, severe (often fatal) gastrointestinal illness in infants. Our knowledge about diarrheogenic *E. coli* has expanded greatly since that time, especially in the past 10 years. There are now four recognized classes of *E. coli* that cause diarrhea: (1) enteropathogenic, EPEC; (2) enterotoxigenic, ETEC; (3) enteroinvasive, EIEC; and (4) enterohemorrhagic, EHEC. Each class is composed of various, and often unique, O:H serotypes and possesses virulence properties characteristic of that class. The serotypes which seem to be "inherent" pathogens are listed within this classification in Table 14:21.

Enteropathogenic *E. coli*

Causative Organism: This is the subject of much controversy today, and to understand the problem, it is necessary to understand how certain strains of *E. coli* were incriminated as the cause of diarrhea in infants.[26,41]

Between 1945 and 1950, *E. coli* was implicated as a cause of epidemics of infantile diarrhea, but there was evidence that other microorganisms were also important causes. The classical study which incriminated *E. coli* as an important cause of infantile diarrhea was done by Kauffmann and DuPont.[41]

Table 14:21. Serotypes of *Escherichia coli* Associated with Human Diarrheal Diseases

Enterotoxigenic (ETEC)		Enteropathogenic (EPEC)		Enteroinvasive (EIEC)	Enterohemorrhagic (EHEC)
O6:H16	O85:H7	O26:NM	O114:H2	O28ac:NM	O157:H7
O8:NM	O114:H21	O26:H11	O119:H6	O29:NM	
O8:H9	O115:H21	O55:NM	O125ac:H21	O112ac:NM	
O11:H27	O115:H40	O55:H6	O127:NM	O115:NM	
O15:H11	O126:H9	O55:H7	O127:H6	O124:NM	
O20:NM	O128ac:H7	O86:NM	O127:H9	O124:H7	
O25:NM	O128ac:H12	O86:H2	O127:H21	O124:H30	
O25:H42	O128ac:H21	O86:H34	O128ab:H2	O135:NM	
O27:H7	O148:H28	O111ab:NM	O142:H6	O136:NM	
O27:H20	O149:H4	O111ab:H2	O158:H23	O143:NM	
O63:H12	O159:H4	O111ab:H12		O144:NM	
O78:H11	O159:H20	O111ab:H21		O152:NM	
O78:H12	O166:H27			O164:NM	
	O167:H5			O167:NM	

They showed that *E. coli* strains from outbreaks in several countries belonged to the following O-K-H antigen groups: O55:K59:H6, O111:K58:H2, O111:K58:H12 and O111:K58:NM (NM = nonmotile). These O-K-H combinations had not been observed in the feces of healthy infants or adults. It must be emphasized that they did not say that all *E. coli* strains with O antigen 55 or 111 are enteropathogenic. Most recently, Orskov and Orskov have reported that these K antigens are not true acidic polysaccharides and that antigenic designation has been dropped.[59]

In the early 1950s, microbiologists all over the world began to look for the Kauffmann-DuPont strains in epidemics of infantile diarrhea and often found them. The evidence suggested that these strains were distributed worldwide and were important causes of diarrhea, particularly in nursery outbreaks. Sometimes these specific strains were not found in outbreaks, but other strains of *E. coli* were. Soon it became apparent that other strains of *E. coli* could cause outbreaks of infant diarrhea. The list of EPEC serotypes increased until specific mechanisms of pathogenicity were discovered for ETEC and EIEC strains. As certain "one-time EPEC" serotype strains were found to produce enterotoxin or invade the epithelium, these strains were dropped from the EPEC classification.[49]

Pathogenicity: We do not yet understand the precise mechanism by which EPEC serotype strains cause diarrhea, but we do know that some strains within this group adhere to intestinal epithelial tissue and that some produce Shiga-like Vero toxin(s).[49,53] As mechanisms of pathogenicity are determined, the EPEC serotypes in Table 14:21 may be split into new categories. At present, many EPEC strains seem to be enteroadherent as defined by adherence to HeLa cells in culture or by DNA probes which detect the presence of genes coding for HeLa adherence. Other EPEC serotype strains produce a cytopathogenic effect on Vero or HeLa tissue culture cells.[53] The pathogenicity of many of these strains has been confirmed on several occasions in the ultimate infection model, the human volunteer.[49]

Antisera directed against the O group antigens are the only commercially available diagnostic tools. These reagents and methods are described and discussed in detail in the *Enterobacteriaceae* chapter of the previous edition of this book. Data from several field studies indicate that less than 50% of the EPEC serogroup strains are actually EPEC serotypes. This means that presumptive EPEC strains, as determined by serogroup and clinical manifestations, should be sent to reference laboratories for further characterization (stool specimens or cultures from suspect outbreaks of diarrhea may be sent to the CDC for serotyping and pathogenicity assays, but isolates from suspect sporadic cases should preferably be sent to Dr. Richard Wilson, Director of the *E. coli* Reference Center, 115 William L. Henning Building, Pennsylvania State University, University Park, PA 16802, Telephone (814) 863-2630).

One recent report describing the use of commercial diagnostic antisera was rather discouraging. None of 118 *E. coli* that agglutinated in the commercial sera were identified as EPEC serotypes by the reference laboratory (approximately 30% were confirmed as EPEC serogroups). The investigators also tested 105 of these strains with the adhesiveness DNA probe and found that none hybridized. It is important therefore to use caution when interpreting serotype results and to use these reagents only when there are well-documented and compelling clinical reasons.[24,49]

Clinical Manifestations and Therapy: EPEC produce moderate to severe, watery, dehydrating diarrhea which may be associated with fever (60%), respiratory symptoms (50%) and abdominal distension (10%).[20] Although the average duration of illness is about one week, many patients have exacerbations. In addition, EPEC is one of the few known causes of chronic diarrhea in infants.[49] Outbreaks of EPEC diarrhea in the 1940s and 1950s were associated with case fatality rates as high as 70%. Although the case fatality rate is much lower now, the disease is often more severe than that due to *Shigella*, enterotoxigenic *E. coli* or nonbacterial pathogens. Risk factors for death include young age and virulence of the associated EPEC strain. Strains of serogroup O111 have been associated with a striking clinical illness and a high mortality rate.[20]

The role of antibiotics in the treatment of EPEC infections is not clear; most studies have failed to show any benefit. In one study, patients treated with methicillin or trimethoprim-sulfamethoxazole recovered more quickly than controls.[84] However, drug resistance among EPEC is high both in developed and developing areas.

Epidemiology: The section on causative organisms details the epidemiologic studies by which EPEC were first recognized as a cause of diarrhea in infant nurseries. Case-control studies confirmed that EPEC are also pathogens in sporadic infant diarrhea in the community. After the 1950s, reports of outbreaks of EPEC diarrhea in industrialized countries became rare and many hospitals stopped serotyping *E. coli*. However, EPEC have remained an important cause of infant diarrhea in the developing world. Nearly all episodes of EPEC diarrhea occur in children under 2 years of age. Illness is uncommon in older children and adults even though they often carry the organism.[20] Many investigations have suggested that the transition from breast-feeding to bottle-feeding or weaning foods in areas with high environmental contamination is a frequent antecedent to the development of EPEC diarrhea.[84] It is likely that age-specific variations in peak attack rates for EPEC diarrhea in different areas are related partly to age at weaning. EPEC can cause large outbreaks of diarrhea in infant care institutions and affected infants can represent a means of spread of this organism into the community.[20]

Volunteer studies have demonstrated that ingestion of 10^7 to 10^9 organisms will cause disease in adults and infants.[49] The early EPEC outbreaks in industrialized countries occurred in summer months, but by the 1960s, the seasonality appeared to have shifted to the cooler months. In developing countries today, diarrhea due to EPEC is found must frequently in the warm season.[49]

EPEC are an important cause of infant morbidity and mortality worldwide; up to 30% of acute sporadic infant diarrhea in Brazil and South Africa is attributed to these organisms. Even in industrialized countries, both outbreaks and sporadic cases continue to be reported.

Public Health: Efforts most likely to be effective in preventing EPEC diarrhea are encouragement of breast-feeding, assurance of clean baby bottles and safe weaning foods, and good hygiene in homes and hospitals.

Enterotoxigenic *E. coli*

Causative Organisms: Certain strains of *E. coli* can colonize the human small intestine and cause an influx of secretions mediated by the action of heat-labile and/or heat-stable enterotoxins (LT and/or ST). The properties of both toxins are summarized in Table 14:22. As seen in this table, the genetic determinants for LT and ST are located on plasmid DNA,[23] and these plasmids appear to be stable in the serotypes listed in Table 14:21. These ETEC serotype strains usually produce both toxins and specific colonization factors. Other serotypes have been reported as producers of LT and/or ST, but there is some indication that many of these strains are

Table 14:22. Enterotoxins of *Escherichia*

Property	Heat-labile enterotoxin	Heat-stable enterotoxin
Heat sensitive	+	–
Trypsin sensitive	+	–
Acid sensitive	+	–
Molecular weight	87,000	1500–5000
Gene(s) location	plasmid	transposon (plasmid)
Stimulation of adenylcyclase	+	–
Stimulation of guanylcyclase	–	+
Immunogenic	+	–
Neutralized by anti-CT	+ (⅓)	–
Neutralized by GM	+	–

Table 14:23. Assays for Enterotoxins of *Escherichia coli*

Assay	Heat-labile enterotoxin	Heat-stable enterotoxin
Rabbit ileal loop		
6–7 h	+*	+
18 h	+	+ or –
Infant mouse (4 h)	–	+
Infant rabbit	+	+
Rabbit skin	+	–
Y1 mouse adrenal cells	+	–
Chinese hamster ovary cells	+	–
Enzyme-linked immunoassay	+	+
Radioimmune assay	+	+
Agglutination	+	–
Staphyloccocal coagglutination		
Latex particle agglutination		
Reverse passive latex agglutination		
Genetic probe	+	+

*+ = positive result in assay, – = negative result, (+ or –) = variable result. Refer to article reviewing enterotoxin methodology.[85]

unstable producers (reflecting spontaneous plasmid loss) and are often isolated from asymptomatic individuals.

Colonization factors may be a requirement in the pathogenesis of ETEC infections. There may be as many as five distinct fimbrial antigens associated with human ETEC isolates, most of which can be detected by the mannose-resistance agglutination of red blood cells. Orskov and Orskov have proposed to include these and other fimbrial antigens, such as those associated with colonization of urinary epithelial cells, in the F antigenic schema.[59]

Pathogenicity: Table 14:23 describes some of the available toxin assays for LT and/or ST. In general, the biological assays measure intestinal fluid influx (rabbit loop, infant mouse, infant rabbit) or tissue culture response to adenylcyclase activation. The application of these assays to diagnosis of ETEC infections is limited by inherent problems and the expense involved in acquiring and maintaining animal or tissue culture systems. The detailed methods, sensitivities and requirements for most of the assays listed in Table 14:23 are reviewed elsewhere.[85] Agglutination assays for LT and several enzyme-linked immunosorbent assays (ELISA) for ST have been published more recently and offer procedures potentially more adaptable to the diagnostic microbiology laboratory.[30,51] Reagents for the latex agglutination and reverse passive agglutination assays for LT are commercially available in the United States.

Since ETEC are not a major cause of diarrhea in the United States and the disease is generally self-limited, we do not recommend that the routine clinical laboratory conduct enterotoxin assays. Specimens or isolates from clusters of illness or epidemics can be sent to CDC for toxin testing.

Clinical Manifestations and Therapy: Illness due to ETEC consists of watery, nonbloody diarrhea, abdominal cramps and little or no fever. It usually lasts for 4 or 5 days.[21] Illness is mild in the vast majority of patients but a dehydrating cholera-like picture may occur. Controlled trials in adults have demonstrated that tetracycline or trimethoprim-sulfamethoxazole (TMP-SMX) shorten the duration of both the diarrhea and the excretion of the organism.[65] Similar studies in children have not been performed. However, since disease is self-limited in most patients, replacement of fluid and electrolytes is usually the only therapy required.

Chemoprophylaxis of travelers' diarrhea, which is often due to ETEC, has been well studied. Bismuth subsalicylate (trade name Pepto-Bismol) can prevent or decrease the severity of diarrhea. Enterovioform and related drugs are not helpful in preventing travelers' diarrhea and may have serious neurological side effects. Deoxycycline and trimethoprim-sulfamethoxazole (TMP-SMX) are effective in reducing the incidence of diarrhea but their risks must be considered; both drugs can cause serious side effects and may cause alterations in the colonic and vaginal flora which may favor infection by pathogenic organisms. In addition, laboratory studies suggest that antibiotic pressure on ETEC may promote the acquisition of both antibiotic resistance and enterotoxin production. Most travelers do not develop diarrhea, and, since diarrhea, when it does occur, responds well to either fluids alone or to antibiotic therapy, the risks of prophylactic antimicrobials are not warranted for most travelers.[1]

Epidemiology: Although diarrhea due to ETEC occurs in the United States, it is a common problem only in developing areas, where it occurs primarily in young children and in visitors.

In developing countries, the incidence of ETEC diarrhea appears to be highest in the first two years of life and to decrease progressively with age. In a study in Bangladesh, children under five had an average of one to two episodes of ETEC diarrhea each year.[8] In Mexico, children show a progressive increase in antibodies to heat-labile enterotoxin over the first few years of life.[20] Illness due to ETEC in children in developed countries appears to be rare, although outbreaks in nurseries have been reported.

ETEC are the major etiologic agents of travelers' diarrhea. The illness is common among groups traveling from low-risk areas (e.g., U.S., northwestern Europe, Canada and Japan) to high-risk areas (e.g., Latin America, Asia and Africa).[20] Immunity to infection develops with increasing time in an endemic area. In a study of students attending school in Mexico, the attack rate for diarrhea was inversely proportional to the amount of time spent in the country. In endemic areas, ETEC may frequently be cultured from stools of asymptomatic adults.[20]

A relatively large inoculum, $>10^8$ viable cells, is necessary to produce disease in adults.[20] Disease is usually transmitted through contaminated food or water and is common during the warm season.[65] Outbreaks of ETEC diarrhea in adults in the United States have been traced to sewage-contaminated water, restaurant food and imported cheese.

Public Health: Assurance of safe food and water is the best protection against diarrhea due to ETEC. Health officials should prevent fecal contamination of water and should enforce food hygiene in eating establishments. Persons traveling in developing areas should select hot foods, hot or carbonated beverages and fruits which can be peeled. Leafy green vegtables and tapwater should be avoided.[20]

Enteroinvasive *E. coli*

Causative Organisms: There are certain strains of *E. coli* which cause an illness indistinguishable from shigellosis. The enteroinvasive strains listed in Table 14:21 may be similar to (and occasionally indistinguishable from) shigellae. The first description of an EIEC (isolated from diarrheal cases in Italy in 1944 and 1945) identified the organism as a paracolon bacillus.[26] The organism was later identified as an *E. coli* O124:H30. This same serogroup has been implicated in diarrheal disease outbreaks in the United States as recently as 1981. In a study which examined several serotypes within the O124 serogroup, investigators were able to show that only certain H types and nonmotile strains were enteroinvasive.[33]

Most EIEC strains are lysine decarboxylase-negative while *E. coli* in general are positive (about 85%). Although most enteroinvasive O124 strains appear unable to ferment lactose, this does not apply to many of the other

EIEC serotypes. Many of the EIEC strains fall within the previously discussed category of "inactive *E. coli*" and can be distinguished from *Shigella* by the characteristics described in Table 14:20. There are, however, more fermentatively active EIEC which are not clearly *E. coli* or *Shigella*. The antigenic relatedness of EIEC and *Shigella* reflects the close DNA relatedness and certain EIEC serotypes have O antigens identical to *Shigella* O antigens. As an example, the *E. coli* O124 antigen is identical to the O antigen of *Shigella dysenteriae* 3.[17]

Pathogenicity: This class of diarrheogenic *E. coli* may be the most difficult to diagnose. Like ETEC strains, they are identified by their pathogenic mechanism, which has been extremely difficult to demonstrate in vitro. The pathogenicity of EIEC is similar, or identical, to that of shigellae and is similarly mediated by a large-molecular-weight plasmid.[44] These characteristics and assays are described in detail in the *Shigella* Section of this chapter.

In general, EIEC has been identified by invasiveness of the guinea pig or rabbit conjunctiva (Sereny Test). This means that 10 guinea pigs or rabbits would be required to test 10 *E. coli* colonies from a primary isolation plate of one patient's stool culture. With the advent and use of an ELISA[60] and gene probe for enteroinvasiveness, investigators learned that in acute illness there may be only 1 or 2 enteroinvasive colonies out of 20 colonies tested per patient.[81] It is apparent that these newer and more sensitive assays could provide much-needed epidemiologic information on EIEC strains and infections. However, these assays are not commercially available or in general use.

Clinical Manifestations and Therapy: Information about illness due to EIEC has been obtained from volunteer studies[21] and from outbreak investigations.[33,52] In one large outbreak, diarrhea was the most common symptom, occurring in 88% of patients. Fever occurred in 72%, nausea in 71% and cramps in 66%.[52] The diarrhea is usually watery; bloody stools occur in fewer than 10% of patients. The presence of mucus and polymorphonuclear leukocytes in the stool is probably typical.[21] Illness is usually self-limited, lasting for 2-3 days;[52] illness severe enough to require hospitalization is uncommon.[21,52] Deaths have not been reported.

Epidemiology and Public Health Significance: For unknown reasons (other than the potential limitations of laboratory identification), illness due to EIEC appears to be rare both in developed and developing areas. Only three outbreaks of disease have been reported in the United States. One affected at least 387 persons who ate imported cheese.[52] Another occurred among passengers on a cruise ship and the third affected children and adults in an institution for the mentally retarded. Outbreaks of EIEC have not been reported from day-care centers or infant nurseries.

A relatively high dose (10^8 cells) or pretreatment with sodium bicarbonate is necessary to produce disease in healthy volunteers.[21] Foodborne spread appears to be the usual mode of transmission. Person-to-person spread has also been reported.[33] The median incubation period in one outbreak was 18 hours (range 2-48 hours).[52] Due to the rarity of reported illness due to EIEC, little epidemiologic and public health information is available.

Enterohemorrhagic *E. coli*

Causative Organism: Hemorrhagic colitis was recognized as a disease entity in 1982 when two outbreaks of illness occurred in the United States and *E. coli* serotype O157:H7 was isolated from ill people.[66] These two outbreaks provided information on a "new illness" and a "new pathogen." Review of the CDC culture collection revealed that serotype O157:H7 had been isolated from a patient with a similar illness in 1975. All isolates fermented sorbitol slowly or not at all. Plasmid profile data indicated that all of these isolates were closely related, if not clonal. Profiles appeared to be identical, but there was a slight difference in Hind III restriction endonuclease digests of plasmid DNA. Oregon isolates contained one additional digest fragment, indicating that there was not one immediate source of both outbreaks. Other H types of O157 were found in the culture collection; these were sorbitol-positive and had a variety of plasmid profiles completely unlike the outbreak strains.

Pathogenicity: Much like EPEC, O157:H7 strains were defined as pathogens on the basis of epidemiologic data.[66] These strains possessed none of the traditional *E. coli* virulence properties. Among several laboratory animals initially tested, they produced diarrhea only in the infant rabbit. However, the infection did not mimic human illness. The most recently-described infection model is the gnotobiotic piglet. Piglets develop some striking symptoms and pathology, but not bloody diarrhea.[32]

All wild type O157:H7 strains appear to produce large quantities of a Shiga-like toxin, referred to as Vero toxin (VT), which is cytotoxic for HeLa or Vero cell culture. Although we do not know the exact role of toxin in pathogenesis, toxin does seem to play some role in hemorrhagic colitis and hemolytic uremic syndrome.[38,39,53] We know now that there are at least two immunologically distinct Vero toxins; they appear to be mediated by phage DNA and they share the neurotoxic, enterotoxic and cytotoxic properties of the Shiga toxin.[25,39,59,73]

All isolates of O157:H7 examined to date have contained a plasmid of approximately 60 Mdal. These strains are generally susceptible to antibiotics, and the function of this plasmid is unknown.

Several O157:NM strains have been isolated from patients with hemorrhagic colitis; they produce large quantities of VT, are generally sorbitol-negative and possess the 60 Mdal plasmid. These strains appear to be EHEC, probably variants of the O157:H7. There may be other EHEC serotypes, but without appropriate epidemiologic data, these must be defined by the existing assays, i.e., the infant rabbit or gnotobiotic piglet.

Clinical Manifestations and Therapy: Uncomplicated illness due to *E. coli* O157:H7 is characterized by bloody diarrhea (76%), abdominal pain which may be severe (76%) and vomiting (56%). Few patients with uncomplicated infection develop fever.[66] The proportion of patients requiring hospitalization has ranged from 16-80% in different studies. In most patients, illness lasts 4-8 days, although patients with more severe symptoms may be ill for 13 days or more.[66,77]

In patients with bloody diarrhea, barium enemas show a striking "thumb-printing" pattern in the right colon, indicative of submucosal edema.[66] The clinical picture may suggest acute ulcerative or ischemic colitis. Laparatomy performed on one patient revealed severe colonic inflammation, most marked at the hepatic flexure. Deaths due to *E. coli* O157:H7 infection have been reported only in elderly patients and in patients who develop the hemolytic uremic syndrome (HUS). In three nursing home outbreaks, mortality was 3%, 14% and 36% respectively.[69]

HUS, recognized by the findings of acute renal failure, microangiopathic hemolytic anemia and thrombocytopenia, is an important complication of infection with *E. coli* O157:H7. In outbreak settings, O to 8% of patients have developed HUS.[77] Risk factors for disease which progresses to HUS have not been determined. A prospective study of 40 patients with HUS found that 30 (75%) had evidence of infection with VT-producing *E. coli.* Six different O serogroups of verotoxin-producing *E. coli* were isolated from stools of 12 of these patients; 3 of the isolates were serogroups O157:H7.[38] Infection with *E. coli* O157:H7 may also precede thrombotic thrombocytopenic purpura (TTP), an illness which shares many features with HUS.[16]

Although *E. coli* O157:H7 is usually sensitive to all antimicrobials, antimicrobial therapy did not shorten the duration of illness.[66] Randomized treatment studies have not been reported.

Epidemiology: The 6 reported outbreaks of hemorrhagic colitis due to *E. coli* O157:H7 in which detailed information is available have together involved almost all age groups. In 2 community-wide outbreaks the median ages were 17 and 28, respectively.[66] Three outbreaks occurred in nursing homes,[69] and one in a day-care center. In 3 outbreaks, infection was linked to ingestion of contaminated hamburger and the organism was isolated once from a suspected lot of beef.[66] The incubation period was estimated to be 4 days in 2 outbreaks and 8 days in another.

Laboratory studies have indicated that *E. coli* O157:H7 is an important pathogen. It was isolated from the stools of 15% of patients with sporadic bloody diarrhea in two reports.[64] In another study of 1,425 stool specimens, *E. coli* O157:H7 was isolated more frequently than *Salmonella*.

Public Health Significance: Proper cooking of hamburger and other meat, avoidance of cross-contamination of foods in the kitchen and attention to personal hygiene may prevent cases of hemorrhagic colitis. More directed public health efforts will require new information about the reservoirs of this organism and its means of entrance into the food chain.

SHIGELLA

CAUSATIVE ORGANISMS

Organisms of the genus *Shigella* are the most common causes of bacillary dysentery, a disease entity recognized since the time of Hippocrates and Galen. Before the age of bacteriology, dysentery was regarded as a single, well-defined disease, but between 1875 and 1901 it became apparent that at least two classes of microorganisms were involved; one protozoan and the other bacterial. From 1898 to 1901, Shiga in Japan, Kruse in Germany and Flexner in the Philippines, showed that bacillary dysentery was caused by a bacillus that somewhat resembled the agent causing typhoid fever. Since that time, a number of *Shigella* "species" and serological types that cause dysentery have been described.

Today the four named groups of *Shigella* are *S. dysenteriae* (Group A), *S. flexneri* (Group B), *S. boydii* (Group C) and *S. sonnei* (Group D). Strains are also isolated from dysentery that appear biochemically to be *Shigella* but cannot be serotyped. The latter groups of *Shigella* are given the status of "Provisional" and each may be added to the *Shigella* schema as a new O group in one of the species. These strains are best called "*Shigella* spp." until they can be further defined. Although the four major groups are given different species names, they are very close genetically and could be considered one species.[12]

PATHOGENICITY

The genus *Shigella* is host-adapted to man and higher primates and is rarely isolated from other animal species. Pathology studies of both humans and monkeys have shown that the primary site of infection for *Shigella* is the terminal ilium and the colon.[48] Shigellae penetrate the epithelium and multiply within the cells, less often penetrating the deeper crypt cells or lamina propria and rarely causing bacteremia. Although limited to the mucosal layer, the inflammatory response can be dramatic; the surface epithelium becomes necrotic, possibly due to toxin activity. Polymorphonuclear leucocytes are stimulated and infiltrate areas of the infected intestine. Necrotic areas become ulcerated, and red blood cells and serum proteins infiltrate the lumen, resulting in the dysenteric stool characterized by blood and mucous; milder forms of diarrheal disease also result from *Shigella* infections.[48]

One prerequisite for virulence in *Shigella* seems to be a smooth lipopolysaccharide (LPS), which protects the organism from host defense mechanisms. When shigellae reach the terminal ileum and colon, they cause disruption of the microvilli, are internalized by epithelial cells and eventually multiply freely in the cytoplasm. The intracellular organisms soon invade neighboring epithelial cells, leading to inflammation and cell death, and causing necrotic ulcerations. The genetic determinants for LPS, penetration, multiplication and other steps in the invasiveness process are discussed in detail elsewhere.[44]

There is also evidence for the role of enterotoxin in the pathogenicity of shigellae. Initial observations were made using a laboratory animal model,[43] but the natural primate disease process may also reflect enterotoxic activity. Human volunteers infected with *S. flexneri* were reported to have diarrhea preceding dysentery by several days.[22] When monkeys were fed live shigellae, they also experienced fluid influx in the jejunum which was not detected when shigellae were inoculated directly into the cecum. Both routes of inoculation induced dysentery. Toxin is apparently formed in natural infection and antitoxin titers are demonstrable in patients who have had shigellosis.[43]

The role of enterotoxin in shigellosis is unclear. One study in monkeys reported that toxigenic, noninvasive *S. dysenteriae* 1 strains did not cause illness. Invasive, nontoxigenic shigellae have not been available for study. Additionally, there is new evidence that the toxin(s) produced by shigellae are similar to those produced by other bacterial species, including nonpathogenic organisms. The toxin may be more important in the destruction of epithelial cells by intracellular shigellae than in enterotoxic activity during shigellosis. Perhaps it is this intracellular presentation of toxin which would make it a virulence factor for shigellae and not for normal flora *E. coli*. It is thought that the one protein has enterotoxic, cytotoxic and neurotoxic activity.[25]

CLINICAL MANIFESTATIONS AND THERAPY

Shigellosis, or bacillary dysentery, has an incubation period that varies from less than 12 hours to 4 days. It often begins with fever, abdominal pain and watery diarrhea, and at this stage is clinically difficult to distinguish from diarrhea due to other agents. With invasion of the colonic mucosa, frequent, scant stools containing blood, mucus and pus, and accompanied by abdominal cramps, become characteristic.[43] The more virulent the organism (*S. dysenteriae* 1 > *S. flexneri* > *S. sonnei*), the more likely and the more rapid is the appearance of dysentery.[43] In well-nourished subjects, the illness is usually limited to 7-10 days without treatment. In the malnourished, it may cause chronic relapsing disease for months.[43]

Prolonged carriage of *Shigella* is rare in healthy persons in developed countries. However, in poor or institutionalized patients, symptomatic infections or asymptomatic carriage may last weeks or months.[43]

In controlled trials, antibiotics appear to be effective at reducing both the clinical symptoms and the duration of excretion of the organism. Treatment may be withheld in mild cases but is definitely indicated in severe cases or when the risk of transmission is high.[65] Ampicillin (not amoxicillin), trimethoprim-sulfamethoxazole (TMP-SMX) and tetracycline are effective for sensitive strains.[43,65] Ampicillin resistance in *Shigella* strains is high in many areas and has led to the use of TMP-SMX as the empiric drug of choice. Resistance to TMP-SMX, however, is occurring in some areas.

EPIDEMIOLOGY

A small number of viable *Shigella* (10 to 200 organisms) is sufficient to initiate an infection. As a result, the majority of cases of shigellosis are spread by person-to-person transmission. Outbreaks due to contaminated food or water occur, but less frequently. In homosexual men,[43] anal-oral sexual transmission is important.

S. sonnei and *S. flexneri* are the most commonly isolated serogroups in the United States (Table 14:24, Table 14:25).[15] Changes in the predominant serotypes in the United States in the past decades are similar to those of other developed countries.[68] *S. dysenteriae* has almost completely disappeared and is usually found only in travelers to underdeveloped areas. Before 1966, *S. flexneri* was responsible for over 50% of isolates in the United States. Since then, *S. sonnei* has emerged as the predominant species.

In the United States, the highest reported attack rates are in children 1-4 years of age, with the peak rate in 2-year olds. In the past, the reported isolation rates by sex were similar except for a female predominance in the age groups 10-29 and 60-79, possibly reflecting exposure to young children. In the early 1970s, a shift in the age and serotype distribution of *Shigella* cases was noted in urban areas. For example, in San Francisco, the male to female ratio of *Shigella* cases in the 20-39 year old age group rose to 7:1 in 1975. In San Francisco, cases of *Shigella* in men ages 20-39 represented 65% of all reported cases and the predominant serotype was *S. flexneri*.[19]

Table 14:24. *Shigella* and *Salmonella* Isolates Reported in the United States for 1984

Organism	Number of isolates
Shigella sonnei	7,847
Shigella flexneri	3,765
Shigella boydii	388
Shigella dysenteriae	179
Shigella, serotype not reported	611
Salmonella typhimurium	12,670
Salmonella enteritidis	3,685
Salmonella heidelberg	3,562
Salmonella newport	1,605
Salmonella infantis	1,226
Salmonella agona	937
Salmonella saintpaul	650
Salmonella montevideo	635
Salmonella muenchen	523
Salmonella oranienburg	499
Salmonella typhi	443
Salmonella, other serotypes	7,200
Salmonella, serotype not reported	2,227

Groups with an increased risk of shigellosis are those in which inadequate hygiene, crowding or sexual behavior make person-to-person transmission likely. These include children in day-care centers, American Indians, travelers, male homosexuals, persons in some custodial institutions and those in homes with inadequate water for handwashing.

S. dysenteriae has been responsible for recent epidemics in Central America, Bangladesh and Central Africa.[65] These epidemics tend to be associated with multiply-resistant strains and high mortality rates.

PUBLIC HEALTH SIGNIFICANCE

Control of bacillary dysentery can be achieved by measures within the household and the local community. *Shigella* infections can be prevented by attention to handwashing to minimize person-to-person transmission and by protection of the water supply from human fecal contamination. Live oral vaccines for several *Shigella* serotypes have been prepared and some have been effective in experimental studies.[43] However, an effective commercially available vaccine is still some years in the future.

DIAGNOSTIC PROCEDURES

Primary Isolation

Although the preferred method for maximal recovery of *Shigella* from fecal specimens is direct plating on agar media,[60] enrichment of fecal

Table 14:25. Serotypes of *Shigella* Isolated in the United States in 1984

Organism	O-group	Number	Percentage
S. dysenteriae	unsp*	131	1.0
S. dysenteriae	1	8	0.1
S. dysenteriae	2	18	0.1
S. dysenteriae	3	12	0.1
S. dysenteriae	4	4	0.0
S. dysenteriae	7	3	0.0
S. dysenteriae	9	3	0.0
S. boydii	unsp	285	2.2
S. boydii	1	5	0.0
S. boydii	2	64	0.5
S. boydii	3	2	0.0
S. boydii	4	12	0.1
S. boydii	5	4	0.0
S. boydii	8	3	0.0
S. boydii	9	2	0.0
S. boydii	10	5	0.0
S. boydii	14	5	0.0
S. boydii	18	1	0.0
S. flexneri	unsp	2,296	18.0
S. flexneri	1unsp†	219	1.7
S. flexneri	1a	99	0.8
S. flexneri	1b	18	0.1
S. flexneri	2unsp	336	2.6
S. flexneri	2a	197	1.5
S. flexneri	2b	23	0.2
S. flexneri	3unsp	156	1.2
S. flexneri	3a	170	1.3
S. flexneri	3b	22	0.2
S. flexneri	3c	2	0.0
S. flexneri	4unsp	58	0.5
S. flexneri	4a	59	0.5
S. flexneri	4b	1	0.0
S. flexneri	5	16	0.1
S. flexneri	6	93	0.7
S. sonnei		7,847	61.4
Shigella, not serotyped		611	4.8
TOTAL		12,790	

* unsp = unspecified (not further subdivided).
† Some laboratories did not subdivide serotypes of *S. flexneri*, but others did. Those not subdivided are listed as unspecified.

specimens in gram-negative (GN) broth[83] has been reported effective. Selenite broth may also be used in isolating *S. sonnei*. It is advisable to use plating media of at least 2 and possibly 3 levels of selectivity for isolation. Xylose lysine deoxycholate (XLD) agar (intermediate selectivity) is excellent for isolating *Shigella*[55,82] and should be included. It contains D-xylose as a differentiating agent, and since most *Shigella* strains do not ferment xylose, they appear as colorless colonies on the plate. However, *Shigella* isolates which ferment xylose rapidly can be missed on this medium. Therefore, additional plating media containing lactose as a differentiating agent should be used in conjunction with XLD agar. A lactose-containing medium of low selectivity such as Tergitol 7, MacConkey or EMB agar should be included as the second medium. A medium of low selectivity is needed to isolate certain fastidious strains of *Shigella* (such as *S. dysenteriae* 1) which grow poorly on the more inhibitory media. If laboratory resources permit use of a third plating medium, a more selective agar which contains lactose such as SS, Hektoen enteric (HE) or deoxycholate citrate agar may also be used. Occasional strains of *Shigella* may not grow on some of the more selective media. *S. sonnei* is suppressed more than other species by SS[55] and deoxycholate citrate agars. *S. dysenteriae* 1 is inhibited on SS agar,[63] slightly suppressed by XLD agar and is best isolated with media of low selectivity, such as Tergitol 7 or MacConkey agar.

At least two colonies typical of *Shigella* should be transferred from each selective agar plate to triple sugar iron (TSI) and Kliger iron (KI) agar slants. Only the center of the desired colony should be touched, since organisms which are inhibited may still be viable. These contaminants will grow on differential agar stabs and interfere with identification of *Shigella*. Isolates whose TSI or KI reaction is alkaline/acid with no H_2S or gas should be screened serologically with antisera to *Shigella* O groups A, B, C and D and inoculated to urea agar and motility medium. Urea-positive or motile cultures can then be discarded. Isolates that are nonmotile, anaerogenic and react serologically may be considered presumptive *Shigella* spp. Presumptive positives as well as suspicious cultures which are serologically negative should be tested further biochemically. A suspension of biochemically typical *Shigella* isolates which agglutinate poorly or not at all should be heated in a water bath at 100°C for 15-30 min, cooled and retested for agglutination.

Marker Systems

The species designation and O antigen group are the most useful markers for epidemiologic analysis. The World Health Organization International Collaborating Center for *Shigella* in Atlanta, Georgia, now recognizes 38 serotypes of *Shigella: S. dysenteriae* consists of 13 serotypes; *S. flexneri* consists of 6 serotypes (actually 13 including subfactors); *S. boydii* consists of 18 serotypes and *S. sonnei* consists of smooth (form I) and rough (form II) variants of a single serotype. Unfortunately, many absorbed antisera must be used to differentiate some of the serological groups, such as those in *S. flexneri*. Also, the phenotypic differentiation of shigellae is a prerequisite for serotyping because most serotypes share common or crossreacting O antigens with *E. coli*. For serotypes which are isolated infrequently, the serotype alone may provide an effective epidemiologic marker.

Antimicrobial susceptibility pattern (antibiogram), biochemical reactions (biotype), susceptibility to chemical substances (resistotype), production and/or susceptibility to bacteriocins (colicin type), susceptibility to a set of bacteriophages (phage type), electrophoretic mobility of plasmid DNA (plasmid profile) and R plasmid characterization have all been used to discriminate individual (epidemic) strains or clones of *S. sonnei*. All of these techniques demand rigorous standardization. Some methods are overly sensitive and others are influenced by the loss or acquisition of plasmid DNA, especially when those plasmids possess resistance or colicin determinants. Shigellae seem to readily acquire R-plasmids under the selective pressures of antibiotic therapy,[79] apparently changing "types" in the course of an epidemic.

Plasmid profiles have been used in conjunction with antibiograms and have been effective in identifying epidemic strains during outbreaks and in assessing control measures. A more detailed analysis of R plasmids was effective in defining apparently similar *S. sonnei* strains and in identifying apparently identical plasmids in different strains.[54]

Pathogenicity Assays

Although man and higher primates are the only known hosts for *Shigella* species, several animal models of disease have been established. The monkey, a natural host, is probably the best studied model, mimicking the human illness. The availability, cost and maintenance requirements of monkeys have limited the use and value of such a model. The rabbit ileal model measures invasiveness and fluid accumulation, but has the disadvantage of being a whole animal assay, requiring surgical procedures to establish an infection. The guinea pig has also been used but requires pretreatment with opiates to slow intestinal motility. The most widely used infection model is the Sereny test[74] originally described as keratoconjunctivitis in the rabbit following inoculation of shigellae into the conjunctival sac. Guinea pigs and mice have also been used successfully.

Invasiveness can also be measured in HeLa and Henle tissue culture assays. One recent modification of these assays measures invasiveness and intracellular multiplication. A positive assay is read as plaque formation or the killing of cells rather than the internalization of shigellae. This distinction could prove to be important in identifying the actively pathogenic strains. Toxic activity is also measured in the HeLa cell assay and is read as destruction of the monolayer by culture supernatants or lysates.

A new and promising assay for *Shigella* species and enteroinvasive *E. coli* was described by Pal et al.[60] An enzyme-linked immunosorbent assay was developed, based on antisera to an invasive strain of *E. coli* absorbed with an avirulent derivative. This would appear to be a simple, inexpensive diagnostic assay for invasive organisms and could be used as a screening assay to be confirmed by the Sereny test or some other biological assay.

One DNA probe derived from the large invasiveness plasmid of *S. flexneri* was used effectively in at least one field study and was applied directly to diarrheal stools.[81] Shigellae are not always the predominant enteric organisms on plating media and direct assay of the stool may identify more cases of shigellosis. DNA probes should prove to be sensitive and specific tools for screening large numbers of organisms or specimens and for increasing understanding of the epidemiology of dysentery.

SALMONELLA

CAUSATIVE ORGANISMS

Salmonella is a very important genus in human disease and public health. This point was reemphasized by the recent outbreak in Chicago where there were an estimated 150,000-300,000 cases of diarrhea due to *Salmonella typhimurium*.

Because the evolution of strains in this group represents a continuum, it is not surprising that *Salmonella* nomenclature and classification have been confused over the years. Since the last edition of this book, there have been some changes in the nomenclature, classification and reporting of the *Salmonella-Arizona* group of bacteria.[29] Several independent studies have shown that most strains of the group are highly related in an evolutionary sense and, in one recent classification, all strains are considered as belonging in a single species. However, there are 6 subgroups within the *Salmonella* group. The differences among these 6 subgroups are summarized in Table 14:16. One proposal has been to use subspecies names for the 6 subgroups. However, there is almost universal agreement that a more simplified nomenclature is preferable for routine use. For this reason it is convenient to artificially treat all the named serotypes of *Salmonella* as if they were species. Thus, *Salmonella* serotype typhimurium is conveniently written as *Salmonella typhimurium*. This simple notation is universally accepted and understood and will be used in this chapter. As indicated in Table 14:16, most *Salmonella* serotypes associated with human diseases belong to subgroup 1, but strains in subgroups 3a and 3b (''Arizona'') are occasionally isolated (see review[88]). Strains of *Salmonella* subgroups 2, 4 and 5 are much rarer.

Serotyping of *Salmonella* is done in almost all laboratories, but to a different extent. Clinical laboratories do ''grouping'' in commercial antisera. This simple procedure determines the ''O'' antigen and provides information to quickly issue reports such as ''*Salmonella* serogroup B'' or ''*Salmonella* serogroup C1.''

In contrast, many reference laboratories, such as state and territorial laboratories in the United States, do complete antigenic analysis of both ''O'' and ''H'' antigens and report serotype name such as ''*Salmonella* serotype typhimurium" or "*Salmonella* serotype newport." This complete serotyping is time consuming and requires a complex set of *Salmonella* typing sera.

Serotypes of *Salmonella* are defined on the basis of their antigenic structure and occasionally by an additional biochemical reaction(s). In antigenic formulas, major antigens are separated by colons, and the components of an antigen are separated by commas. The formula "1,4,5,12:i:1,2" means the strain has O antigen components "1,4,5,12" (Group B antigens), flagella phase one antigen "i" and flagella phase two antigen "1,2" (if flagella antigens in one of the phases had been missing, it would have been designated by a "-"). Names were given for most of the important *Salmonella* serotypes to avoid having to remember complex antigenic formulas. Thus, if laboratory test results show that a strain has the antigenic formula 1,4,5,12:i:1,2, "*Salmonella* serotype typhimurium" or "*S. typhimurium*" is reported. Although over 2000 serotypes of *Salmonella* have been described, most of them are rarely isolated from human infection.

CLINICAL MANIFESTATIONS

Human infections with *Salmonella* have various clinical symptoms and involve both intestinal and extraintestinal sites.[6,7,9,35,71] Patients may have intestinal and extraintestinal infections concurrently.

The most common syndrome is that of uncomplicated enterocolitis. After an incubation period of 8-48 hours, the typical patient experiences nausea, vomiting, cramps, diarrhea and fever. Symptoms generally resolve in 2-14 days. Severe diarrhea may occur, but death occurs primarily among neonates, the elderly and patients with underlying diseases. Following recovery, some patients may continue to excrete organisms for weeks or months.

The incidence of the chronic carrier state after infection with *S. typhi* (typhoid fever) is 1-3%. The chronic carrier state after nontyphoidal *Salmonella* infection is less common. Chronic enteric carriers have a higher incidence of bilary tract disease than the general population.

The syndrome of enteric fever includes fever, headache and prostration, which may last days to weeks. The syndrome has been classically associated with *S. typhi* (typhoid fever) and with the "paratyphoid" bacilli *S. paratyphi* A, *S. paratyphi* B (synonym = *S. schottmuelleri*) and *S. paratyphi* C (synonym = *S. hirschfeldii*), but it may be caused by other *Salmonella* serotypes. Enteric fever due to *S. typhi* is called typhoid fever and is more prolonged, has a higher case fatality ratio and may be complicated by gastrointestinal perforation, bleeding, hemorrhage or focal infections.

Salmonella can produce bacteremia in patients with or without enterocolitis or enteric fever. Bacteremia is especially common in infections with

S. choleraesuis. Invasive infections have been reported in patients with abnormalities in host defenses. These include infants, the elderly, patients with neoplastic disease, (particularly lymphoreticular malignancies), uremia, recent surgery, hemolytic disease and the acquired immunodeficiency syndrome (AIDS).[57] Localized infections following *Salmonella* bacteremia can affect almost any site. Common associations include meningitis in infants, pneumonia in the elderly and osteomyelitis in patients with sickle cell disease.

The treatment of *Salmonella* infections depends upon the site of the infection and the condition of the patient. Fluid and electrolyte replacement is the treatment of choice for patients with uncomplicated enterocolitis. Antidiarrheal drugs containing components which reduce gut motility may worsen salmonellosis; therefore, these agents should be avoided. Antibiotic therapy is not indicated in uncomplicated intestinal infection in normal hosts because it prolongs excretion of the organism and does not alter the clinical course of the illness.[2] However, antibiotic therapy of intestinal infection should be considered for patients with abnormalities in host defenses. Antibiotics are indicated for patients with enteric fever, bacteremia and focal infections.

Antibiotic resistance among *Salmonella* strains isolated from humans has increased over the years. The percentage of resistant strains will depend on many different factors and varies markedly by serotype.[80] Foods of animal origin constitute the major source of most human nontyphoidal *Salmonella*, including antibiotic-resistant organisms. One interstate outbreak of human illness due to tetracycline-resistant *Salmonella* was traced to farms where cattle were fed chlortetracycline for growth promotion.[36]

Antibiotic-resistant strains of *Salmonella* are of concern for several reasons. First, treatment of those *Salmonella* infections which require antibiotics can be ineffective if the organism is resistant to the antibiotics used. Second, the case-fatality rate for infections due to resistant *Salmonella* is higher than that for infections due to antibiotic-sensitive *Salmonella*. And third, exposure to an antibiotic for other reasons increases the risk of symptomatic infection with an antibiotic-resistant *Salmonella*.[80]

EPIDEMIOLOGY

Humans usually acquire *Salmonella* by ingestion of contaminated food or water. Person-to-person and animal-to-person (such as from pet turtles) transmission occurs less frequently.

Since humans are the only known reservoir of *S. typhi*, infection with this organism indicates exposure to human feces. The major reservoir of nontyphoidal *Salmonella* is domestic food animals and this fact is key to understanding the epidemiology of *Salmonella* infections. Animal feeds containing *Salmonella* are major sources of animal infection; carcasses of infected animals may contaminate previously uninfected meat during processing. Poultry and meat products are the most common vehicles of transmission. Foodborne transmission occurs through either the inadequate preparation of contaminated food or the cross-contamination of other food. Person-to-person spread has been a serious problem in hospitals and institutions, primarily among neonates and in patients with underlying diseases.[2,3]

Over 2000 *Salmonella* serotypes have been described, but 10 serotypes account for over 75% of human isolates (Table 14:24). Although, in general, *Salmonella* infections occur with greatest frequency during the warm season and in children under 5 years old, individual serotypes vary widely in seasonality and age-specificity, presumably reflecting differences in their sources. Thus, serotyping is a very important marker in epidemiologic studies.

PUBLIC HEALTH SIGNIFICANCE

In contrast to *S. typhi*, the incidence of illness due to nontyphoid *Salmonella* has increased steadily over the past 20 years. Approximately 37,000 *Salmonella* isolations are reported annually in the United States (Table 14:24), with the highest rates in children 2-4 months old. Since these isolates are estimated to represent approximately 1% of those clinically ill with salmonellosis, the true number of cases of salmonellosis may approach 4 million annually.[9,80]

Efforts to prevent human salmonellosis have centered on reducing the contamination of food products, educating consumers to prevent food handling errors and eliminating sources of high risk (such as banning the interstate shipment of pet turtles). Efforts by industry and government to pasteurize egg products have been associated with a decrease in salmonellosis associated with eggs. On the other hand, outbreaks associated with meat and poultry still occur. The incidence of salmonellosis will only be reduced if the reservoir among food animals is reduced, thus resulting in less overall contamination of food with *Salmonella*.

DIAGNOSTIC PROCEDURES

Primary Isolation

Salmonella colonies are usually found on primary plates inoculated with feces from persons who are acutely ill with diarrhea. However, an enrichment broth is also recommended for use in clinical laboratories to increase the isolation rate of *Salmonella* from stool specimens. Most enrichment broths for *Salmonella* are highly selective. They allow the growth of *Salmonella* and inhibit growth of other bacteria. The three selective enrichment media most widely used to isolate *Salmonella* from fecal specimens are: tetrathionate broth, tetrathionate broth with brilliant green and selenite F broth. Tetrathionate brilliant green broth is an excellent medium for recovering most *Salmonella*, but it inhibits *S. typhi*. Many prefer to use either selenite or tetrathionate without the brilliant green dye because neither inhibits *S. typhi*, and both are equally good for recovering most other *Salmonella*. However, both selenite and tetrathionate enrichment broths inhibit certain serotypes of *Salmonella*. Smith found that direct plating of intestinal contents on a selective or differential agar was superior to both selenite and tetrathionate enrichments for isolating *S. choleraesuis* and *S. abortusovis*, and recommended brilliant green MacConkey broth for isolating *S. choleraesuis*.[75] Leifson[46] also noted the high toxicity of selenite broth for *S. choleraesuis* when he first described the medium. Similarly, tetrathionate inhibits the growth of *S. paratyphi* A.[4]

Numerous selective plating media have been used to isolate *Salmonella* from fecal specimens. These media are differential and vary from slightly selective to highly selective. The media of low selectivity include MacConkey, EMB and deoxycholate agar. Media of intermediate selectivity such as XLD, deoxycholate citrate, SS and HE agar are widely used by laboratories that screen for both *Salmonella* and *Shigella* because they support the growth of both. If laboratory resources permit the use of an additional plate just for *Salmonella*, one of the highly selective media such as brilliant green (BG) or bismuth sulfite agar (BS) is superior to the less selective media. Although media of low and intermediate selectivity suppress growth of some gram-negative bacteria, they are not as selective as brilliant green or bismuth sulfite and allow growth of contaminants which cannot be differentiated from *Salmonella* without further testing. The combination of brilliant green agar and tetrathionate brilliant green broth is particularly good for isolating *Salmonella* other than *S. typhi*. Some workers have reported overgrowth or spreading of *Proteus* on brilliant green agar. This problem may result from improper sterilization, a critical factor in the preparation of the medium. It should be sterilized for exactly 15 min at 121°C because a longer period decreases its selectivity, and less time results in inhibition of *Salmonella*.

Bismuth sulfite agar is the preferred medium for isolating *S. typhi* and is very useful for detecting strains of *Salmonella* which ferment lactose. Bismuth sulfite has been reported to inhibit *Salmonella* serotypes other than *S. typhi* unless it is refrigerated at 4°C for at least 24 h before use. For isolating *S. typhi*, however, pour plates are preferable although streak plates can be substituted if they are prepared immediately before use. If pour plates are used, subsurface colonies should be restreaked on MacConkey or EMB agar before biochemical tests are done. This step eliminates mixed cultures.

"Suspicious *Salmonella* colonies" should be selected from the plating medium and transferred to either triple sugar iron (TSI) or Kliger's iron (KI) agar. At least two representatives of each type of suspicious colony should be selected from each plate. Another medium, lysine iron agar (LIA), indicates the decarboxylation or deamination of lysine and the production of hydrogen sulfide. LIA used in conjunction with TSI agar is particularly helpful in the presumptive identification of *Salmonella*. Both of these media can be inoculated from one colony by first inoculating the TSI in the usual manner and then inoculating the LSI by stabbing the butt of the medium twice and streaking the slant. If results are needed quickly, a trypticase soy tryptose (TST) broth for determining H antigens can also be inoculated from this colony. Otherwise, this broth can be inoculated from the TSI culture. If a culture appears contaminated on either TSI or LIA, it should be replated on MacConkey or EMB agar before proceeding. The usual reaction of *Salmonella* on TSI or KI will be alkaline/acid, gas and H_2S. Strains may occasionally occur which are lactose-positive, giving an acid slant, and that do not produce H_2S or gas. The usual reaction on LIA is alkaline/alkaline with H_2S. Occasionally lysine-negative (acid butt) and H_2S-negative strains occur. Isolates with typical *Samonella* reactions on either TSI or LIA should be kept for further analysis. If there is no need to know the serogroup or serotype of an organism, isolates can be screened for *Samonella* antigens by using a polyvalent O or H antiserum. A positive reaction in either the polyvalent H or O group antisera with typical TSI and LIA reactions indicate a presumptive *Salmonella*. If serotyping information is desired, colonies should be examined by slide agglutination with commercial polyvalent grouping antisera (*Samonella* O group antigens A,B,C_1,C_2,D,E and Vi). Those cultures positive in the O group antiserum can be screened for H antigens using Spicer-Edwards pooled antisera.[76] The Spicer-Edwards pools include 7 pools of antisera for determining 17 flagellar antigens. Additional absorbed antisera are required for final serotyping. If the serologic screening yields negative reactions, the following tests should be done: urea, indole, lysine decarboxylase, growth in KCN and motility. Typical *Salmonella* cultures are urea$^-$, indole$^-$, lysine$^+$, KCN$^-$ and motile. If these biochemical reactions are not characteristic, and *Salmonella* antigens are found, the cultures should be plated on MacConkey or EMB agar to obtain a pure culture, tested biochemically (complete set) or forwarded to a reference laboratory.

Markers for Epidemiology

Serotyping is the most important marker for *Salmonella* and is very useful in epidemiologic studies. In many countries, including the United States, most *Salmonella* are serotyped by reference laboratories. In the United States, *S. typhimurium* accounts for over 30% of all *Salmonella* infections (Table 14:24); thus additional typing of this serotype can be helpful in epidemiologic studies. The antibiogram can be useful because strains of *S. typhimurium* have many different resistance patterns. A biotyping scheme has been described and used in several countries, but it has not been evaluated in the United States. Bacteriophage typing has provided additional sensitivity for *S. typhimurium* and for some of the other common serotypes, but unfortunately, bacteriophage typing is a complicated procedure that requires careful standardization and should be attempted only by a laboratory that can devote considerable time to it. Plasmid profile analysis has been used recently and this technique appears very useful since it can be used for all serotypes. Typing (other than serotyping) should only be used in well-defined epidemiological investigations where specific questions can be answered with laboratory data. A carefully selected control group should be included.

Serodiagnosis

A method sometimes used in attempting to diagnose typhoid fever is based on a patient's antibody response to one of the antigens of *S. typhi*, a procedure historically known as the Widal reaction. This test measures agglutinating antibodies to O and H antigens of *S. typhi* and has been used when typhoid fever is in the differential diagnosis but *S. typhi* cannot be isolated. Many consider an antibody titer to the H antigen of little value because it is much less specific than the O titer, although concurrent rises in H and O titers are mutually supportive. To interpret febrile agglutination test results, it is necessary to examine acute and convalescent sera (1-2 weeks apart). A 4-fold or greater increase in titer to the O antigen is considered significant by some, but must be interpreted cautiously, since other serologically related (Group D) *Salmonella* could cause the antibody rise. Several points to consider in interpreting results of this test are: (1) the commercial antigens that are available are poorly standardized; (2) patient antibodies to other bacteria with common O and H antigens can crossreact, so diagnosis of typhoid fever should never be based on this test alone; (3) production of O and H agglutinins may be suppressed by early treatment with chloramphenicol; and (4) prior typhoid immunization may be responsible for the patient's antibody titers. An O titer of 1:50 or 1:100 on a single serum in the first 2 weeks of illness is considered significant by some, if it can be established that the patient has definitely not been vaccinated.

It has also been shown that typhoid carriers may have titers against the Vi antigen; however, the test is difficult to perform and false-negative as well as false-positive results may be obtained. Both favorable and unfavorable evaluations of this test have been reported. A standardized test with improved sensitivity and specificity has been described[58] but the antigen is not commercially available.

YERSINIA ENTEROCOLITICA

INTRODUCTION

The genus *Yersinia* is a recent addition to the family *Enterobacteriaceae*. It was formerly classified in the family *Pasteurellaceae*, but studies over the last few years have indicated that the genus more appropriately belongs in the family *Enterobacteriaceae*. Strains of *Yersinia* contain the enterobacterial common antigen and are related by DNA-DNA hybridization to *E. coli*. The genus is now a well-accepted member of the family.

CAUSATIVE ORGANISMS

The genus *Yersinia* has eight named species, all of which occur in clinical specimens. The most important species in human disease are *Y. pestis, Y. pseudotuberculosis* and *Y. enterocolitica*. *Y. pestis* causes plague[13] which historically has been one of the most important infectious diseases and a scourge through the ages. *Y. pseudotuberculosis* causes infections which have a broad clinical picture that closely resembles that of *Y. enterocolitica*. Both *Y. pestis* and *Y. pseudotuberculosis* are covered in Chapter 25, "Plague," and discussion here will be limited to the other species, the most important being *Y. enterocolitica*. This organism causes infections of the intestinal tract and extraintestinal infections. Until the early 1970s, *Y. enterocolitica* was thought to be a single species with considerable variation in all its properties. However, a number of studies have clarified the classification of the "atypical strains" of this species, now classified as four additional species: *Y. aldovae, Y. frederiksenii, Y. intermedia* and *Y. kristensenii*. These four organisms are included in the "*Y. enterocolitica* group" but do not cause intestinal infections. They occasionally cause extraintestinal infections and can easily be confused with *Y. enterocolitica* in routine identifications. Unless otherwise indicated, the remainder of this section is limited to *Y. enterocolitica*.

CLINICAL MANIFESTATIONS

Y. enterocolitica can cause many different clinical syndromes.[10,11,13,31] Enteritis, mesenteric adenitis, arthritis and erythema nodosum are frequently reported. Less frequently recognized manifestations include septicemia, pharyngitis, iritis, myocarditis, liver abscess, osteomyelitis and meningitis. An excellent review and summary has been published.[13]

Enteritis, with symptoms of diarrhea and abdominal pain, is the most common clinical syndrome. It is seen mainly in infants and young children. Diarrhea may vary from a few loose stools per day to fulminant enterocolitis. Fever is generally low grade but may be spiking or absent. Nausea and vomiting occur but are usually not prominent. Disease generally resolves within 2 or 3 weeks without treatment, but can be protracted.[10,13]

Patients with mesenteric adenitis have right lower quadrant pain, fever and leukocytosis, and often undergo laparotomy for suspected appendicitis. In most patients, inflammation of the appendix is absent and the surgeon finds an inflamed terminal ileum and enlarged mesenteric lymph nodes. This syndrome is seen primarily in older children and adolescents.

A reactive migratory polyarthritis, mainly affecting adults, is the most common extraintestinal manifestation associated with *Y. enterocolitica* infection. It occurs in about 30% of infected patients in Finland, but appears to be less common in the Unites States. Arthritis may develop during or after enteric infection and usually lasts 1-3 months. White cell counts in synovial fluid are elevated but cultures of the fluid are sterile. Patients with histocompatibility antigen HLA-B27 have an increased risk of developing arthritis. Reiter's syndrome has also been reported following infection with *Y. enterocolitica*.

Erythema nodosum may also develop after infection and occurs more commonly in women than in men. Tender nodules appear on the anterior part of the legs and other areas within 2-20 days after onset of enteritis. It usually resolves within a month.

Septicemia is uncommon and is most often reported in the elderly and in patients with diabetes mellitus, cirrhosis, hemochromatosis and malignancy. Diarrhea may be absent. Patients with sepsis may develop osteomyelitis, meningitis and hepatic or splenic abscesses. Sepsis can carry a high mortality rate, correlating in general with the severity of the underlying condition.

THERAPY

There is no data on the value of antimicrobial therapy in patients with enteritis or mesenteric adenitis, and most such infections are self-limited. Patients with bacteremia or with infection at a site that is normally sterile should receive antibiotic therapy. The drug of choice has not yet been identified, so current infectious disease literature will be needed for guidance.

EPIDEMIOLOGY AND PUBLIC HEALTH SIGNIFICANCE

Y. enterocolitica has been isolated from many animals, but most serotypes found in animals have not been demonstrated to cause human disease.[10,13]

However, isolates from swine are often similar to those causing human infection.[13] In the Unites States, milk and tofu have caused outbreaks of *Yersinia* infection. Drinking water and sick animals have also been suspected as sources.

The reported incidence of human *Y. enterocolitica* infections has increased dramatically in the last decade, probably due to improved bacteriologic techniques for isolation. The incidence is highest in Scandinavia and Europe, where serogroups O3 and O9 are predominant. Many isolates from the United States have been serogroup O8.[13] There seems to be an association between *Y. enterocolitica* infection and a cold climate. The organism seems to be rarely found in warmer climates.

DIAGNOSTIC PROCEDURES

Primary Isolation

Most authors agree that *Y. enterocolitica* differs from other enteric bacteria in that it is best isolated at 22-26°C rather than at 35-37°C. Incubating selective media at 25°C may allow *Y. enterocolitica* to compete better with other organisms. *Y. enterocolitica* incubated at 25°C for 24 h will appear as pinpoint to 0.1 mm, transparent to translucent, smooth colonies that can best be visualized with a dissecting microscope using oblique lighting. The colonies become larger (0.5-2 mm) after an additional 24 h incubation. Although *Y. enterocolitica* grows on most plating media commonly used for recovery of enteric pathogens, several serogroups are inhibited on SS and Hektoen agars.[10] A medium designed specifically for recovery of *Y. enterocolitica*, cefsulodin-irgasan-novobiocin (CIN) agar, appears to be the most effective among selective plating media.[34] It should be included as a routine plating medium for stool specimens if laboratory resources permit. CIN agar may be incubated at 32°C for 24 h or at 22-25°C for 48 h. MacConkey agar would be a good second choice in place of CIN agar or in addition to CIN. Many laboratories screen for *Y. enterocolitica* by incubating enteric plating media an additional 24 h at 25°C after initial incubation at 37°C for 24 h (when they look for *Salmonella* and *Shigella*). Although this technique has proven successful in recovering *Y. enterocolitica*, it has never been compared with incubation at 25°C for 48 h, so its sensitivity is not known. Incubation at 37°C may cause the *Yersinia* virulence plasmid[10,13,37] to be lost.

Cold enrichment enhances recovery of *Y. enterocolitica* from fecal specimens. *Y. enterocolitica* grows at 4°C, in contrast to most other enteric organisms, which gradually die. Specimens can be inoculated into phosphate-buffered saline (PBS) pH 7.4-7.6 and held for 21 days at 4°C. Subculture may be done at 3, 7 and 14 days, but maximal recovery will be obtained at

21 days. Because of the long delay in obtaining results, cold enrichment is not popular in hospital microbiology laboratories. If initial direct plating of specimens yields *Y. enterocolitica* or other pathogens, the cold enrichment procedure could be omitted.

In picking from primary plates, lactose-negative colonies should be selected from MacConkey agar and mannitol-positive colonies from CIN agar. Occasional strains of *Y. enterocolitica* may be lactose-positive, so lactose-positive colonies that are typical of *Y. enterocolitica* in size and morphology should also be selected. At least two representatives of each type of suspicious colony should be picked from each plate to either TSI or KI agar, which is then incubated at 25°C for 24 h. The reaction of *Y. enterocolitica* on TSI will be acid/acid, with no gas and no H_2S. Strains which ferment sucrose rapidly may cause the slant to revert to alkaline. The reaction on KI agar is alkaline/acid, with no gas and no H_2S. Isolates typical of *Y. enterocolitica* on TSI or KI should be screened further by inoculation into urea and motility media, which are incubated at 25°C for 24 h. A second tube of motility agar is inoculated and incubated at 35-37°C for 24 h. Isolates that are urea-positive, motile at 25°C and nonmotile at 35-37°C should be considered presumptively positive. Occasionally, strains of *Y. enterocolitica* are weakly motile at 25°C and require additional incubation or passage through semisolid agar. All cultures that have screening reactions suspicious for *Y. enterocolitica* should be definitely identified (incubation at 25°C).

Methods for Identification

Identification of *Yersinia* cultures can be more difficult than for many other *Enterobacteriaceae*. Strains of the *Y. enterocolitica* group tend to grow more slowly at 35-37°C than other *Enterobacteriaceae*. Colonies are typically 1/2 to 1/3 the size of fast-growing species. *Yersinia* cultures are also less active in some biochemical tests at 35-37°C than at 22-26°C. Since most incubators in clinical microbiology laboratories are set at 35-37°C, initial biochemical testing of *Yersinia* cultures will almost never be done at the optimum temperature. A culture identified as a member of the *Y. enterocolitica* group should be retested with biochemical tests incubated at 25°C (Tables 14:4, 14:18). Strains are typically urea-positive, motile at 25°C, but nonmotile at 35-37°C. All 5 species in the *Y. enterocolitica* group are very similar, but can be differentiated by the tests listed in Table 14:18. Typical reaction patterns are usually observed within a few days at 25°C, but reactions are often delayed if incubation is at 35-37°C. Most strains of *Y. enterocolitica* do not ferment lactose or raffinose, but occasionally strains become lactose-and raffinose-positive through the acquisition of a metabolic plasmid. These strains can be confused with *Y. intermedia* which is also raffinose-positive (Table 14:18).

Markers for Epidemiology

More research has been devoted to differentiating virulent from avirulent strains than in subdividing strains below the level of species. However, several typing methods have been described.

Biotyping: The first step is to assign a strain of the *Y. enterocolitica* group to its correct species (Table 14:18). Strains of *Y. enterocolitica* can then be further differentiated into a number of biotypes, which vary in their biochemical reactions.[10] The two biotyping schemes most often used are those described by Nilehn, and by Wauters, which is a simplication of the former. Biotype 1 strains produce indole and lecithinase and rapidly ferment salicin and esculin. Biotype 2 strains are indole-positive, but are negative for lecithinase and for rapid fermentation of salicin and esculin. Biotypes 3-5 are negative on all 4 of the above tests. Strains of biotype 3 ferment D-xylose and lactose (in OF medium) which differentiates them from biogroup 4 strains which are negative for these two reactions. Biogroup 5 strains are very inactive biochemically and are negative for all the above tests. Biotyping has been used extensively by those with an active interest in *Yersinia*, but is not usually done in clinical microbiology laboratories.

Serotyping: Serotyping of *Y. enterocolitica* has been well studied, and there is an antigenic schema for both O and H antigens. Currently, there are at least 57 O antigens and 20 H antigens. The exact number of O and H antigens varies, depending on the author. There is no international standardization, which has caused confusion in the literature. Serotyping can often provide valuable information in relation to pathogenicity. In many countries, virulent strains of serogroup O3 predominate and strains of serogroup O9 make up the majority of the remaining isolates. In these countries, the use of only two antisera, O3 and O9, will allow serogrouping of the majority of clinical strains. In the United States, the situation is quite different because serogroups O3 and O9 do not predominate. The most common O groups are O3, O4, O8, O9, O13, O18, O2O and O21. It is not practical for most laboratories to do extensive serotyping and most reference laboratories will probably want to use only sera for the most important O groups. Only a very few *Yersinia* reference centers can maintain and use a complete set of O and H typing sera. Serotyping of the other species in the *Y. enterocolitica* group is not usually necessary because of their rarity. The current antigen schema for *Y. enterocolitica* still includes the other *Yersinia* species, but some workers have proposed their removal. This would leave an antigenic schema specific for *Y. enterocolitica*.

Bacteriophage Typing: Several phage typing schemes have been described for the *Y. enterocolitica* group, but their use has been limited to a few *Yersinia* reference centers.

Virulence Tests

Some, but not all, strains of *Y. enterocolitica* can cause human disease. This fact is well accepted, but the difficulty has been in the differentiation of the virulent strains from the nonvirulent ones. Strains known to be pathogenic have not been positive in all virulence assays. The pathogenic strains of serogroup 03 from Europe appear to be quite different from the pathogenic strains of serogroup 08 from America. Virulent strains of *Y. enterocolitica* contain a 70-kilobase virulence plasmid (45 megadaltons), and the loss of this plasmid is accompanied by a loss in the ability to invade tissue and cause disease. Table 14:26 lists many of the methods which have

Table 14:26. Methods Used to Define Virulence in Cultures of *Yersinia enterocolitica*

Method	Dependence on virulence plasmid
Simple Laboratory Methods	
Pyrazinamidase test	−
Biotyping	−
Calcium-dependent growth at 37°C on Congo red agar	+
Calcium-dependent growth at 37°C on magnesium oxylate agar	+
Congo red uptake	+
O antigen group (such as O3, O8, or O9)	−
Temperature-dependent colonial morphology on trypticase soy agar	+
Temperature-dependent autoagglutination in tissue culture or other broth media	+
Other Laboratory Methods	
Plasmid profile analysis	+
Serotyping, complete	−
Tissue culture, adherence to human epithelial cells such as HEp-2	
Tissue culture, invasion of human cell lines such as HeLa, Hep-2 and Henle	−
Tissue culture, cytotoxicity to human epithelial cells such as HEp-2	
Serum resistance (to normal human serum)	
Agglutination in "virulence specific" antiserum	
Electron microscopy—detection of fibril structures	+
DNA probes	
Other membrane protein profiles	
Hemagglutination (mannose-resistant) of guinea pig erythrocytes	
Phagocytosis of *Y. enterocolitica* cells	+
Growth within macrophages	+
Animal Models	
Sereny test (guinea pig eye)	+
Mouse lethality	+
Infant mouse intestine—accumulation of fluid	+

been used to measure virulence. The "simple" methods listed in the top part of the table have application in routine clinical microbiology because they are easy to do. The reference methods and animal models are more difficult and are usually done only in reference laboratories or in clinical laboratories where there is a special interest in *Yersinia*. Only the simple laboratory methods are considered in detail here.

Pyrazinamidase Test: This test measures the enzyme pyrazine-carboxylamidase (pyrazinamidase), and was originally used to characterize the mycobacteria and corynebacteria. In 1985, Kandolo and Wauters[37] used it to characterize 381 strains of *Yersinia*. They found an excellent correlation between virulence in *Yersinia* and a negative test for pyrazinamidase. *Y. pestis* and *Y. pseudotuberculosis* were pyrazinamidase-negative, as were strains of *Y. enterocolitica* which belonged to biogroups-serogroups usually associated with human disease. One interesting observation was that the pyrazinamidase test does not depend on the actual presence of the 70-kilobase virulence plasmid. Strains cured of this plasmid remained pyrazinamidase-negative. The advantage of the pyrazinamidase test is that it can detect strains that were originally virulent, but which have lost their virulence plasmid through laboratory manipulation such as the picking of single colonies and/or growth at 37°C. The present virulence of a strain can be determined by one of the assays that depends on the actual presence of the virulence plasmid (Table 14:26).

Calcium-dependent Growth at 37°C: A culture of *Y. enterocolitica* is grown on a medium such as magnesium oxylate agar (tryptic soy agar with added $MgCl_2$ and sodium oxalate). Strains that contain the virulence plasmid are Ca^{++} dependent at 37°C and thus fail to grow, or they produce small colonies compared to colonies on a control plate such as blood agar.

Congo Red Uptake: A culture of *Y. enterocolitica* is grown at 37°C on tryptic soy agar with added congo red dye. Strains which contain the virulence plasmid take up the dye and appear as red colonies.

Autoagglutination: A culture of *Y. enterocolitica* is inoculated into 2 tubes of tissue culture media (such as Eagle minimum essential medium plus Earle salts and L-glutamine). One tube is incubated at 37°C and the other at 22°C. Autoagglutination at 37°C, but not at 22°C, usually indicates a temperature-dependent Ca^{++} requirement associated with the virulence plasmid. Other broth media can also be used.

Serodiagnosis

As with most bacterial diseases, definitive diagnosis is based on the isolation and identification of *Y. enterocolitica* from appropriate clinical specimens taken when symptoms are present. Yersiniosis is sometimes considered in the differential diagnosis of a patient's illness in the absence of positive culture results.[10,13,31] Antibody levels to *Y. enterocolitica* are then ordered as a diagnostic aid (see review[31]).

Serodiagnosis of *Y. enterocolitica* infection is a complex subject. An infection due to *Y. enterocolitica* is usually accompanied by a rise in antibody titer to antigens of the infecting strains. The titer then drops after recovery and elimination of the infecting strain. Serodiagnosis has proved very useful in countries where only one or two O serogroups of *Y. enterocolitica* cause the majority of the infections. For example, in Europe, Japan and much of the world, most infections are caused by *Y. enterocolitica* serogroup O3. *Y. enterocolitica* serogroup O9 often comprises the majority of the remaining cases. In addition, strains of serogroup O3 and possibly O9 may cause a more disseminated illness, or at least an infection more likely to produce a good antibody response. Thus, serodiagnosis based on the antibody response to those two O antigens has a very good correlation with infection.

Unfortunately, serodiagnosis is much more complex in the United States. Many different O group of *Y. enterocolitica* are involved in enteric infections. Thus, sera must be tested against a wide variety of different O antigens to insure complete coverage. This difficulty, along with many documented serological crossreactions, has limited the availability and usefulness of serodiagnosis. However, there is still some demand for the test, enough so that at least one commercial company does testing on a "fee for services bases." Specialty Laboratories, 2122 Granville Ave., Los Angeles, CA 90025 has developed an "EIA Panel for antibodies to the *Y. enterocolitica* serotypes (O3, O4, O5 and O8) found to be most prevalent in the United States." In addition, Virion, 4 Upperfield Rd., Morristown, NJ 07969 offers complement fixation reagents for the serodiagnosis of *Y. enterocolitica* serotypes O3, O8 and O9.

The criteria for defining a positive and a negative test are poorly standardized in the serodiagnosis of *Y. enterocolitica* infections, particularly if the test is done on a single serum specimen.

REFERENCES

1. Anonymous. Travelers' diarrhea. National Institutes of Health consensus development conference statement; vol 5, No 8. Bethesda, MD: National Institutes of Health, 1985:1-20.
2. Aserkoff BA, Bennett JV. Effect of antibiotic therapy in acute salmonellosis on the fecal excretion of salmonellae. N Engl J Med 1969;281:636-40.
3. Baine WB, Gangarosa EJ, Bennett JV, Barker WH. Institutional salmonellosis. J Infect Dis 1973;128:357-60.
4. Banwart GJ, Ayres JC. Effect of various enrichment broths and selective agars upon the growth of several species of *Salmonella*. Appl Microbiol 1953;1:296-301.

5. Bartlett RC. Medical microbiology: How fast to go - how far to go. In: Lorian V, ed. Significance of medical microbiology in the care of patients. Baltimore: Williams and Wilkin, 1977:15-35.
6. Bennett IL, Hood EW. Infectious diseases (some aspects of salmonellosis). Ann Rev Med 1959;10:1-20.
7. Black PH, Kunz LJ, Swartz MN. Salmonellosis - A review of some unusual aspects. New Engl J Med 1960;262:813-17.
8. Black RE, Brown KH, Becker S, Abdul Alim ARM, Huq I. Longitudinal studies of infectious diseases and physical growth of children in rural Bangladesh. II. Incidence of diarrhea and association with known pathogens. Am J Epidemiol 1982;115:315-24.
9. Blake PA, Feldman RA. Salmonellosis. In: Last JM, ed. Maxey-Rosenau public health and preventive medicine. 12th ed. Norwalk, CT: Appleton-Century-Crofts, 1986:407-10.
10. Bottone EJ, ed. *Yersinia enterocolitica*. Boca Raton, FL: CRC Press, 1981.
11. Boyce JM. *Yersinia* species. In: Mandell GL, Douglas RG Jr, Bennett JE, eds. Principles and practice of infectious diseases. 2nd ed. New York: John Wiley, 1985:1296-1301.
12. Brenner DJ, Steigerwalt AG, Wathen HG, Gross RJ, Rowe B. Confirmation of aerogenic strains of *Shigella boydii* 13 and further study of *Shigella* serotypes by DNA relatedness. J Clin Microbiol 1982;16:432-6.
13. Butler T. Plague and other *Yersinia* infections. New York: Plenum Medical Book Co., 1983.
14. Caugant DA, Levin BR, Orskov I, et al. Genetic diversity in relation to serotype in *Escherichia coli*. Infect Immun 1985;49:407-13.
15. Centers for Disease Control. Shigellosis - United States, 1984. Morbid Mortal Weekly Rep 1985;34:600-2.
16. Centers for Disease Control. Thrombotic thrombocytopenic purpura associated with *Escherichia coli* O157:H7. Morbid Mortal Weekly Rep 1986;35:549-51.
17. Cheasty T, Rowe B. Antigenic relationships between the entero-invasive *Escherichia coli* O antigens O28ac, O112ac, O124, O136, O143, O144, O152 and O164 and *Shigella* O antigens. J Clin Microbiol 1983;17:681-4.
18. Cooke EM. *Escherichia coli* and man. London: Churchill Livingstone, 1973.
19. Dritz SK, Ainsworth TE, Back A, et al. Patterns of sexually transmitted enteric diseases in a city. Lancet 1977;2:3.
20. DuPont HL. *Escherichia coli* diarrhea. In: Evans AS, Feldman HA, eds. Bacterial infections of humans. New York: Plenum Medical Book Co., 1982.
21. DuPont HL, Formal SB, Hornick RB, et al. Pathogenesis of *Escherichia coli* diarrhea. N Engl J Med 1971;285:1-9.
22. DuPont HL, Hornick RB, Dawkins AT, Snyder MJ, Formal SB. The response of man to virulent *Shigella flexneri*. J Infect Dis 1969;119:296-9.
23. Echeverria P, Seriwatana J, Taylor DN, Tirapat C, Rowe B. *Escherichia coli* contains plasmids coding for heat-stable b, other enterotoxins and antibiotic resistance. Infect Immun 1985;48:843-6.
24. Echeverria P, Taylor DN, Leksomboon U, et al. Identification of enteric pathogens in the small and large intestine of children with diarrhea. Diagn Microbiol Infect Dis 1986;4:277-84.
25. Eiklid K, Olsnes S. Animal toxicity of *Shigella dysenteriae* cytotoxin: Evidence that the neurotoxic, enterotoxic and cytotoxic activities are due to one toxin. J Immunol 1983;130:38-84.
26. Ewing WH. Edwards and Ewing's identification of *Enterobacteriaceae*. 4th ed. New York: Elsevier Science, 1986.
27. Farmer JJ III, Davis BR, Hickman FW, et al. Detection of *Serratia* outbreaks in hospital. Lancet 1976;2:787-9.
28. Farmer JJ III, Davis BR, Hickman-Brenner FW, et al. Biochemical identification of new species and biogroups of *Enterobacteriaceae* isolated from clinical specimens. J Clin Microbiol 1985;21:46-76.

29. Farmer JJ III, McWhorter AC, Brenner DJ, Morris GK. The *Salmonella-Arizona* group of *Enterobacteriaceae*: Nomenclature, classification and reporting. Clin Microbiol Newsletter 1984;6:63-6.
30. Finkelstein RA, Yang Z. Rapid test for identification of heat-labile enterotoxin-producing *Escherichia coli* colonies. J Clin Microbiol 1983;18:23-8.
31. Fowler JM, Brubaker RR. Immunology of yersiniae. In: Rose NR, Friedman H, Fahey JL, eds. Manual of clinical laboratory immunology. 3rd ed. Washington, DC: American Society for Microbiology, 1985:371-4.
32. Francis DH, Collins JE, Duimstra JR. Infection of gnotobiotic pigs with an *Escherichia coli* O157:H7 strain associated with an outbreak of hemorrhagic colitis. Infect Immun 1986;51:953-6.
33. Harris JR, Mariano J, Wells JG, Payne BJ, Donnell HD, Cohen ML. Person-to-person transmission in an outbreak of enteroinvasive *Escherichia coli*. Am J Epidemiol 1985;122:245-52.
34. Head CB, Whitty DA, Ratnam S. Comparative study of selective media for recovery of *Yersinia enterocolitica*. J Clin Microbiol 1982;16:615-21.
35. Hook EW. *Salmonella* species (including typhoid fever). In: Mandell GL, Douglas RG Jr, Bennett JE, eds. Principles and practice of infectious diseases. 2nd ed. New York: John Wiley, 1985:1256-69.
36. Holmberg SD, Osterholm MT, Senger KH, Cohen ML. Drug resistant *Salmonella* from animals fed antimicrobials. N Engl J Med 1984;311:617-22.
37. Kandolo K, Wauters G. Pyrazinamidase activity in *Yersinia enterocolitica* and related organisms. J Clin Microbiol 1985;21:980-2.
38. Karmali MA, Petric M, Lim C, Fleming PC, Arbus GS, Lior H. The association between idiopathic hemolytic uremic syndrome and infection by verotoxin-producing *Escherichia coli*. J Infect Dis 1985;151:775-82.
39. Karmali MA, Petric M, Louie S, Cheung R. Antigenic heterogeneity of *Escherichia coli* verotoxins. Lancet 1986;1:164-5.
40. Kauffmann F. The bacteriology of *Enterobacteriaceae*. Baltimore: Williams and Wilkins, 1966.
41. Kauffman F, DuPont A. *Escherichia* strains from infantile gastroenteritis. Acta Pathol Microbiol Scand 1950;27:552-64.
42. Kelly MT, Brenner DJ, Farmer JJ III. *Enterobacteriaceae*. In: Lennette EH, Balows A, Hausler WJ Jr, Shadomy HJ, eds. Manual of clinical microbiology. 4th ed. Washington, DC: American Society for Microbiology, 1985:363-77.
43. Keusch GT. Shigellosis. In: Evans AS, Feldman HA, eds. Bacterial infections of humans - Epidemiology and control. New York: Plenum Medical Book Co., 1982:487-509.
44. Kopecko DJ, Baron LS, Buysse J. Genetic determinants of virulence in *Shigella* and dysenteric strains of *Escherichia coli*: their involvement in the pathogenesis of dysentery. Current topics in microbiology and immunology. Berlin: Springer-Verlag, 1985;118:71-95.
45. Krieg NR, ed. Bergey's manual of systematic bacteriology; vol 1. Baltimore: Williams and Wilkins, 1984.
46. Leifson E. New selenite enrichment media for the isolation of typhoid and paratyphoid (*Salmonella*) bacilli. Amer J Hyg 1936;24:423-32.
47. Lennette EH, Balows A, Hausler WJ Jr, Shadomy HG, eds. Manual of clinical microbiology. 4th ed. Washington, DC: American Society for Microbiology, 1985.
48. Levine MM, DuPont HL, Formal SB, et al. Pathogenesis of *Shigella dysenteriae* 1 (Shiga) dysentery. J Infect Dis 1973;127:261-70.
49. Levine MM, Edelman R. Enteropathogenic *Escherichia coli* of classic serotypes associated with infant diarrhea: Epidemiology and pathogenesis. Epidemiologic Rev 1984;6:31-51.
50. Li K, Farmer JJ III, Coppola A. A novel type of resistant bacteria induced by gentamicin. Trans NY Acad Sci 1974;36:369-96.

51. Lockwood DE, Robertson DC. Development of a competitive enzyme-linked immunosorbent assay (ELISA) for *Escherichia coli* heat-stable enterotoxin (ST_a). J Immunol Meth 1984;75:295-307.
52. Marier R, Wells JG, Swanson RC, Callahan W, Mehlman IJ. An outbreak of enteropathogenic *Escherichia coli* foodborne disease traced to imported French cheese. Lancet 1973;2:1376-8.
53. Marques LR, Moore MA, Wells JG, Wachsmuth IK, O'Brien AD. Production of Shiga-like toxin by *Escherichia coli.* J Infect Dis 1986;154:338-41.
54. Marranzano M, Giammanco G, d'Hauteville H, Sansonetti P. Epidemiological markers of *Shigella sonnei* infections: R-plasmid fingerprinting, phage-typing and biotyping. Ann Inst Pasteur 1985;136:339-45.
55. Morris GK, Koehler JA, Gangarosa EJ, Sharrar RG. Comparison of media for direct isolation and transport of shigellae from fecal specimens. Appl Microbiol 1970;19:434-7.
56. Nadelman RB, Mathur-Wagh U, Yancovitz SR, Mildvan D. *Salmonella* bacteremia associated with the acquired immunodeficiency syndrome (AIDS). Arch Intern Med 1985;145:1968-71.
57. Nolan CM, Feeley JC, White PC Jr, Hambie EA, Brown SL, Wong KH. Evaluation of a new assay for Vi antibody in chronic carriers of *Salmonella typhi.* J Clin Microbiol 1980;12:22-6.
58. O'Brien AD, LaVeck GD. Purification of a *Shigella dysenteriae* 1-like toxin produced by *Escherichia coli.* Infect Immun 1983;40:675-83.
59. Orskov F, Orskov I. Serotyping of *Escherichia coli.* In: Bergan T, ed. Methods in microbiology; vol 14. London: Academic Press, 1984:43-112.
60. Pal T, Pacsa AS, Emody L, Voros S, Selley E. Modified enzyme-linked immunosorbent assay for detecting enteroinvasive *Escherichia coli* and virulent *Shigella* strains. J Clin Microbiol 1985;21:415-18.
61. Pickering LK, DuPont HL, Olarte J, Conklin R, Ericsson C. Fecal leucocytes in enteric infections. Am J Clin Pathol 1977;68:562-5.
62. Pierce AK, Sanford JP. Aerobic gram-negative bacillary pneumonias. Ann Rev Respir Dis 1974;110:647-58.
63. Rahaman MM, Huq I, Dey CR. Superiority of MacConkey's agar over Salmonella-Shigella agar for isolation of *Shigella dysenteriae* Type 1. J Infect Dis 1975;131:700-3.
64. Ratnam S, March SB. Sporadic occurrence of hemorrhagic colitis associated with *Escherichia coli* 0157:H7 in Newfoundland. Can Med Assoc J 1986;134:43-6.
65. Rennels MB, Levine MM. Classical bacterial diarrhea; perspectives and update - *Salmonella, Shigella, Escherichia coli, Aeromonas* and *Plesiomonas*. Pediatr Infect Dis 1986;5:91-9.
66. Riley LW, Remis RS, Helgerson SD, et al. Hemorrhagic colitis associated with a rare *Escherichia coli* serotype. N Engl J Med 1983;308:681-5.
67. Rodgers DE. The changing patterns of life-threatening microbial disease. New Engl J Med 1959;261:677-83.
68. Rosenberg ML, Weissman JB, Gangarosa EJ, Reller LB, Beasley RP. Shigellosis in the United States: Ten-year review of nationwide surveillance, 1964-1973. Am J Epidemiol 1976;104:543-51.
69. Ryan CA, Tauxe RV, Hosek GW, et al. *Escherichia coli* O157:H7 diarrhea in a nursing home: clinical, epidemiological and pathological findings. J Infect Dis 1986;154:631-8.
70. Sack RB. Serologic tests for the diagnosis of enterobacterial infections. In: Rose WR, Freeman H, Fahet JL, eds. Manual of clinical laboratory immunology. 3rd ed. Washington, DC: American Society for Microbiology, 1986:359-62.
71. Saphra I, Winter JW. Clinical manifestations of salmonellosis in man. N Engl J Med 1957;256:1128-34.
72. Schaberg DR, Alford RH, Anderson R, Farmer JJ III, Melly MA, Schaffner W. An outbreak of nosocomial infection due to multiply resistant *Serratia marcescens*: Evidence of interhospital spread. J Infect Dis 1976;134:181-8.

73. Scotland SM, Smith HR, Willshaw GA, Rowe B. Vero cytotoxin production in strains of *Escherichia coli* is determined by genes carried on bacteriophage. Lancet 1983;2:216.
74. Sereny B. Experimental *Shigella* keratoconjunctivitis. Acta Microbiol Acad Sci Hung 1955;2:293-6.
75. Smith HW. The isolation of salmonellae from the mesenteric lymph nodes and faeces of pigs, cattle, sheep, dogs and cats and from other organs of poultry. J Hyg 1959;57:266-73.
76. Spicer CC. A quick method for identifying *Salmonella* "H" antigens. J Clin Pathol 1956;9:378-9.
77. Spika JS, Parsons JE, Nordenberg D, Wells JG, Gunn RA, Blake PA. Hemolytic uremic syndrome and diarrhea associated with *Escherichia coli* O157:H7 in a day care center. J Pediatr 1986;109:287-91.
78. Starr MP, Stolp H, Truper HG, Balows A, Schlegal HC, eds. The prokaryotes. Berlin: Springer Verlag, 1981.
79. Tanaka T, Hashimoto H, Mitsuhashi S. Conjugal transferability of multiple resistance in *Shigella* strains. Microbiol Immunol 1983;27:479-84.
80. Tauxe RV. Antimicrobial resistance in human salmonellosis in the United States. J Animal Sci 1983;62(Suppl 3):65-73.
81. Taylor DN, Echeverria P, Pal T, et al. The role of *Shigella* spp., enteroinvasive *Escherichia coli* and other enteropathogens as causes of childhood dysentery in Thailand. J Infect Dis 1986;153:1132-8.
82. Taylor WI, Harris B. Isolation of shigellae: II. Comparison of plating media and enrichment broths. J Clin Pathol 1965;44:476-9.
83. Taylor WI, Schelhart D. Isolation of shigellae. V. Comparison of enrichment broths with stools. Appl Microbiol 1968;16:1383-6.
84. Thorén A. The role of enteropathogenic *E. coli* in infantile diarrhea: aspects on bacteriology, epidemiology and therapy. Scand J Infect Dis 1983;37(Suppl):1-51.
85. Wachsmuth K. Laboratory detection of entertoxins. In: Ellner PD, ed. Infectious diarrheal diseases: Current concepts and laboratory procedures. New York: Marcel Dekker, 1984:93-115.
86. Wachsmuth K. Molecular epidemiology of bacterial infections: Examples of methodology and of investigations of outbreaks. Rev Infect Dis 1986;8:682-92.
87. Wadstrom T, Aust-Kettis A, Habte D, et al. Enterotoxin-producing bacteria and parasites in stools of Ethiopian children with diarrhoeal disease. Arch Dis Childhood 1976;51:865-70.
88. Weiss SH, Blaser MJ, Paleologo FP, et al. Occurrence and distribution of serotypes of the Arizona subgroup of *Salmonella* strains in the United States from 1967 to 1976. J Clin Microbiol 1986;23:1056-64.

CHAPTER 15

ERYSIPELOID

Judy A. Daly, Ph.D.

INTRODUCTION

Erysipelothrix rhusiopathiae (Erysipelothrix insidiosa) was first isolated from mice by Koch in 1880, then from pig blood vessels in 1882 by Loeffler and described as the etiologic agent for the cutaneous lesion of erysipeloid by Rosenbach in 1884.

CLINICAL MANIFESTATIONS

E. rhusiopathiae causes a slowly spreading, purplish-red, cellulitis-like lesion called erysipeloid.[2,4] Symptoms usually include burning, throbbing and itching; fever and other systemic aspects occur in only 10 percent of the cases. The differential diagnosis includes streptococcal and staphylococcal infections, cutaneous diphtheria, anthrax and erythema multiforme. These infections differ from erysipeloid by the absence of suppuration and pitting.

Erysipeloid may disseminate to cause septicemia with arthritis or endocarditis.[1,5,7] Among the 30 reported cases of septicemia, the incidence of endocarditis is high. Persons at risk include those working in occupations known to predispose to *Erysipelothrix* infection, and those with a history of a prior debilitating disease.

Penicillin is the therapeutic agent of choice for *Erysipelothrix* infections. Uncomplicated infections are treated with oral medication. In vitro, *E. rhusiopathiae* is susceptible to erythromycin, lincomycin, cephalosporins, tetracyclines and chloramphenicol. Complicated infections, such as endocarditis, require administration of 12 million units/day of penicillin, with or without an aminoglycoside, for 4 weeks.

EPIDEMIOLOGY

E. rhusiopathiae is primarily a pathogen of animals (both wild and domestic), fish and birds. Clinical disease, (e.g., sepsis, endocarditis and arthritis) has been documented in swine and also occurs in sheep, rabbits, cattle, birds, turkeys and rats. Transmission of disease to humans occurs from contact with infected meat or animal-contaminated soil, food and water. Persons at greatest risk of *Erysipelothrix* infections include fish handlers, butchers, meat processing workers, poultry workers, farmers, veterinarians, abattoir workers and housewives. Outbreaks of infection have been described among workers who produce buttons from bone.

PUBLIC HEALTH SIGNIFICANCE, PREVENTION AND CONTROL

Erysipeloid is an occupational risk for veterinarians, laboratory workers, abattoir workers, fish handlers, poultry workers, farmers and housewives. Gloves and frequent handwashing are advised for protection from this infection.

LABORATORY DIAGNOSIS

Collection

Erysipeloid lesions can be sampled by biopsy[6] or aspiration. After cleansing, inject 1% procaine or saline into the edge of the lesion and either excise a full-thickness portion of skin or aspirate. Routine blood cultures can be used to isolate *E. rhusiopathiae* from patients with sepsis or endocarditis.

Culture And Isolation

Biopsy specimens and tissue aspirates should be cultured in an infusion broth containing 1% glucose, incubated at 35-37°C in 5% CO_2 or air, and subcultured to a blood agar plate at 24 h intervals. Blood can be cultured with routine blood culture media.

Identification

A 24-hour colony of *E. rhusiopathiae* on trypticase soy agar with 5% sheep blood appears smooth or rough, convex, circular and transparent with a 0.1 to 0.5 mm diameter. Often alpha hemolysis is noted. *E. rhusiopathiae*, a small (0.2-0.4 μm by 0.5-2.5 μm), slender, pleomorphic gram-positive rod, is catalase- and oxidase-negative. Triple sugar iron (TSI) agar reactions include an acidic slant and butt and sufficient H_2S to cause a blackened butt. The H_2S reaction by a gram-positive rod is usually diagnostic for *E. rhusiopathiae*. Rapid carbohydrate reactions can be used to determine the fermentation patterns of this organism.[3] *E. rhusiopathiae* ferments glucose and lactose within 48 hours but not xylose, mannitol or sucrose. No serological techniques are available for clinical laboratory use. *Actinomyces (Corynebacterium) pyogenes*, *Arcanobacterium (Corynebacterium) haemolyticum* and *Listeria monocytogenes* are other gram-positive rods which are differentiated from *E. rhusiopathiae* by hemolysis on blood agar, H_2S production in TSI agar, catalase and motility (Table 15:1).

Table 15:1. Differential characteristics of *Erysipelothrix*, *Listeria*, *Actinomyces* and *Arcanobacterium*

Test	*Erysipelothrix rhusiopathiae*	*Actinomyces (Corynebacterium) pyogenes*	*Arcanobacterium (Corynebacterium) haemolyticum*	*Listeria monocytogenes*
Hemolysis	alpha	beta	beta	beta
H_2S production (TSI)	+	−	−	−
Catalase	−	−	−	+
Motility	−	−	−	+

REFERENCES

1. Borchardt K, Sullivan R, Blumberg H, et al. *Erysipelothrix rhusiopathiae* endocarditis. South Med J 1982;75:892-5.
2. Grieco M, Sheldon C. *Erysipelothrix rhusiopathiae*. Ann NY Acad Sci 1970;174:523-5.
3. Hollis DG, Sottnek FO, Brown WJ, Weaver RE. Use of the rapid fermentation test in determining carbohydrate reactions of fastidious bacteria in clinical laboratories. J Clin Microbiol 1980;12:620-3.
4. Nelson E. Five hundred cases of erysipeloid. Rocky Mt Med J 1955;52:40-3.
5. Park C, Poretz D, Goldenberg R. *Erysipelothrix* endocarditis with cutaneous lesion. South Med J 1976;69:1101-2.
6. Price JEL, Bennett WEJ. The erysipeloid of Rosenbach. Br Med J 1951;2:1060-2.
7. Townshend RH, Jephcott AE, Yekta MH. *Erysipelothrix* septicaemia without endocarditis. Br Med J 1973;1:464-7.

CHAPTER 16

HAEMOPHILUS INFECTIONS

Paul M. Mendelman, M.D.

INTRODUCTION

The first associations of *Haemophilus* with human disease were made in 1883 by Koch for *H. aegyptius* (Koch-Weeks bacillus) with contagious conjunctivitis, in 1889 by Ducrey for *H. ducreyi* with chancroid or soft chancre, and in 1892 by Pfeiffer for *H. influenzae* with pandemic influenza. The latter etiologic association was disproved nearly 40 years later when the first influenza virus was isolated. However, the role of *H. influenzae* as a secondary invader following influenza appears to be substantiated by serologic data from the 1918 epidemic.[51] This species name has persisted and it is clearly the predominant human pathogen in the genus *Haemophilus*.

In the 1930's, Pittman described encapsulated and nonencapsulated *H. influenzae*.[41] Six capsular types (a through f) were recognized and capsule production was correlated with invasive disease. Strains which expressed the type b capsule were identified as the most invasive of the serotypes. Despite advances in our understanding of the significant factors in *H. influenzae* pathogenesis, the organism remains one of the most important agents of childhood disease.

CAUSATIVE ORGANISMS

The genus *Haemophilus* currently consists of 19 species. All are obligate parasites of humans (10 species) or other animals (9 species) (Table 16:1). The genus belongs to the family *Pasteurellaceae* and its members are aerobic or facultatively anaerobic, nonmotile, pleomorphic, gram-negative rods which require complex media for growth. Specific factors required for growth include the heat stable X (haemin) factor and the heat labile V (NAD, nicotinamide adenine dinucleotide) factor. These requirements and

Table 16:1. *Haemophilus* Speciation*

Human Isolates	Animal Isolates (Animal Host)
1. *H. influenzae*	11. *H. haemoglobinophilus* (dogs)
2. *H. aegyptius*	12. *H. pleuropneumoniae* (swine)
3. *H. ducreyi*	13. *H. paracuniculus* (rabbits)
4. *H. parainfluenzae*	14. *H. parasuis* (swine)
5. *H. parahaemolyticus*	15. *H. paragallinarum* (chicken)
6. *H. paraphrohaemolyticus*	16. *H. avium* (poultry)
7. *H. aphrophilus*	17. *H. somnus* (cattle)
8. *H. paraphrophilus*	18. *H. agni* (sheep)
9. *H. segnis*	19. *H. equigenitalis* (mares)
10. *H. haemolyticus*	

* Nineteen species are currently listed within the genus *Haemophilus*[20]

other differentiating characteristics of *Haemophilus* species isolated from humans are listed in Table 16:2.

CLINICAL MANIFESTATIONS

The 10 *Haemophilus* species isolated from humans may be part of the normal flora of the respiratory tract, the genitourinary tract or the oral cavity of healthy humans; all have been associated with certain clinical diseases (Table 16:3). All encapsulated *H. influenzae* may cause invasive disease (meningitis and other bloodborne infections); however, serovar b is responsible for over 95% of illness. Nonencapsulated *H. influenzae* are also important respiratory pathogens causing otitis media and sinusitis in children, sepsis in newborn infants, pneumonia in children in developing countries and both community-acquired and nosocomial pneumonia in adults.[33,49] Nontypable *H. influenzae* are also associated with acute exacerbations of chronic bronchitis in patients with chronic obstructive pulmonary disease. Of the *Haemophilis* species, *H. influenzae, followed by H. parainfluenzae, H. aphrophilus* and *H. paraphrophilus* are the species most commonly associated with bacteremic infections, primarily endocarditis. Although comparative data are limited, 3% of invasive disease was due to non-influenza *Haemophilus* in two Swedish communities.[60]

THERAPY

The pathogenesis of invasive disease involves bacteremia, and occult invasion of the central nervous system must always be considered. The choice of specific antibiotic therapy must take into account current regional antibiotic susceptibility patterns. Resistance to ampicillin, chloramphenicol, trimethoprim/sulfamethoxazole (TMP/SMZ), rifampin, and relative resist-

Table 16:2. Certain Differential Characteristics of *Haemophilus* Species Isolated from Humans*

	Requirement for:†						Acid from:					
	X	V	Indole	Urease	Hemolysis	Ornithine decarboxylase	D-xylose	D-ribose	D-mannose	D-fructose	Sucrose	Lactose
H. influenzae												
Biovar I	+	+	+	+	–	+	+	+	–	–	–	–
Bivoar II	+	+	+	+	–	–	+	+	–	–	–	–
Biovar III	+	+	–	+	–	–	+	+	–	–	–	–
Biovar IV	+	+	–	+	–	+	+	+	–	–	–	–
Biovar V	+	+	+	–	–	+	+	+	–	–	–	–
Biovar VI	+	+	–	–	–	+	+	+	–	–	–	–
Biovar VII	+	+	+	–	–	–						
Biovar VIII	+	+	–	–	–	–						
H. haemolyticus	+	+	V	+	+	–	V	+	–	w	–	–
H. ducreyi	+	–	–	–	D	–	–	–	–	–	–	–
H. parainfluenzae												
Biovar I	–	+	–	–	–	+	–	–	+	+	+	–
Biovar II	–	+	–	+	–	+	–	–	+	+	+	–
Biovar III	–	+	–	+	–	–	–	–	+	+	+	–
Biovar IV	–	+	+	+	–	+	–	u	+	+	+	–
Biovar V	–	+	+	+	–	+	u	u	v	+	+	–
Biovar VI	–	+	+	–	–	+	–	–	u	u	+	–
Biovar VII	–	+	+	+	–	–	–	–	u	u	+	–
H. paraphrophilus	–	+	–	–	–	–	–	+	+	+	+	+
H. aphrophilus	–	–	–	–	–	–	–	+	+	+	+	+
H. segnis	–	+	–	–	–	–	–	–	–	w	w	–
H. aegyptius	+	+	–	+	–	+	–	D	–	–	–	–
H. parahaemolyticus	–	+	–	+	+	V	–	–	–	+	+	–
H. paraphrohaemolyticus	–	+	–	+	+	–	–	–	–	+	+	–

* adapted from references 20 and 52 or references cited therein;
\+ indicates that 90 percent or more of the strains are positive
– indicates that 10 percent or less of the strains are positive
V indicates that the majority of strains are positive
v indicates that the majority of strains are negative
D indicates that the majority of strains give a delayed positive reaction
w indicates a weakly positive reaction
u indicates unknown
† x and v factors are haemin and nicotinamide adenine dinucleotide, respectively.

Table 16:3. Clinical Manifestations of *Haemophilus* in Humans*

H. influenzae
- **Encapsulated** (primarily serovar b organisms)
  - Meningitis, Bacteremia, Pneumonia
  - Epiglottitis, Cellulitis
  - Septic Arthritis, Osteomyelitis
  - Preseptal and Orbital Cellulitis
  - Pericarditis
  - Epididymitis
  - Urinary Tract Infection
  - Cerebrospinal Fluid Shunt Infection
  - Neonatal Sepsis
  - Abscess Formation: soft tissue, peritonsillar, periappendiceal, brain, lung and liver
  - Endocarditis
  - Endophthalmitis
  - Peritonitis
- **Unencapsulated**
  - Otitis Media, Sinusitis
  - Conjunctivitis
  - Chronic Bronchitis, Bronchiectasis
  - Pneumonia, Tracheobronchitis, Lung Abscess, Empyema
  - Meningitis, Bacteremia
  - Vaginitis, Urethritis
  - Chorioamnionitis

H. parainfluenzae
- Endocarditis,
- Chronic Bronchitis, Pneumonia, Empyema
- Meningitis, Brain Abscess, Bacteremia
- Septic Arthritis
- Urinary Tract Infection
- Urethritis, Myositis
- Liver Abscess, Chorioamnionitis
- Neonatal Sepsis, Puerperal Bacteremia
- Conjunctivitis, Chronic Prostatitis
- Epiglottitis
- Corneal Ulcer/Endophthalmitis
- Otitis Media
- Chronic gingivitis

H. aphrophilus
- Endocarditis
- Meningitis/Bacteremia, Brain Abscess
- Pneumonia, Lung Abscess, Sinusitis
- Cholecystitis
- Soft Tissue Infection
- Vertebral Osteomyelitis
- Septicemia
- Necrotizing Fasciitis

H. paraphrophilus
- Endocarditis
- Meningitis, Brain Abscess
- Epiglottitis
- Mouth Abscess
- Osteomylitis of the Jaw
- Urinary Tract Infection
- Appendicitis
- Paronychia
- Pneumonia

H. paraphrohaemolyticus
- Liver Abscess
- Urethritis

H. haemolyticus
- Endocarditis
- Chronic Bronchitis
- Conjunctivitis

H. parahaemolyticus
- Endocarditis
- Purulent Oral Infections
- Chronic Bronchitis
- Empyema of the gall bladder
- Periorbital cellulitis

H. segnis
- Pancreatic Abscess
- Appendicitis

H. aegyptius
- Conjunctivitis
- Bacteremia
- Endocarditis (single report)

H. ducreyi
- Chancroid
- Conjunctivitis (single report)
- Oropharyngeal Infection (symptomatic and asymptomatic)

* Tabulated from published reports.

ance to certain second and third generation cephalosporins has been observed.[4,32,62]

Due to the high incidence of beta-lactamase producing strains, ampicillin should never be used alone for initial therapy of invasive disease. Ampicillin in combination with chloramphenicol remains the therapy of choice for invasive disease in the United States. Ampicillin, amoxicillin, cefaclor, erythromycin-sulfamethoxazole, TMP/SMZ or augmentin may be used for oral therapy of noninvasive diseases of the respiratory tract. With the exception of ampicillin and amoxicillin, the remaining antibiotics would be acceptable for the treatment of infection due to a beta-lactamase producing, ampicillin-resistant strain. Unfortunately, ampicillin-resistant, non-beta-lactamase producing isolates have been reported with increasing frequency. These isolates are primarily nontypable and isolated from the respiratory tract. Augmentin, which will successfully inhibit beta-lactamase-producing strains due to the inclusion of a beta-lactamase inhibitor along with amoxicillin, would have no inhibitory effect. In addition, other beta-lactams would have reduced efficacy presumably due to altered penicillin-binding proteins in these strains.[30,31]

H. ducreyi antibiotic susceptibility patterns exhibit marked geographic variation. Many isolates produce beta-lactamase and thus are resistant to the penicillins. Increasing resistance to sulfonamides and tetracycline has also been noted. At present, the treatment of choice is a 10-day course of TMP/SMZ or erythromycin. Augmentin, ceftriaxone, rosaramicin and rifampin have also proved effective.[43,47,55]

EPIDEMIOLOGY

Members of the genus *Haemophilus* may colonize the human host without causing injury or harm. *H. parainfluenzae, H. haemolyticus, H. parahaemolyticus, H. paraphophilus* and *H. segnis* are routinely isolated from the nasopharynx, pharynx and the oral cavity. In addition, *H. influenzae, H. parainfluenzae* and *H. paraphrophilus* have been cultured from the vagina of mature women. *H. paraphrohaemolyticus, H. aphrophilus* and *H. segnis* have been isolated from dental plaque, and *H. ducreyi* has been associated with asymptomatic carriage in the genitourinary tract and the oropharynx.[22] Nonencapsulated *H. influenzae* may be isolated from the respiratory tract (nose or throat) of children at a frequency of 60 to 90% depending upon age.[24] In contrast, the colonization rate with serovar b organisms averages less than 5%, and there is no correlation between carriage rate, socioeconomic status, sex or race.

Serovar b organisms cause over 95% of invasive *H. influenzae* disease in children, while the other five capsular types have rarely been reported to cause disease. Due to ease of case definition and high frequency of occurrence, most studies have examined meningitis. In fact, the most common agent of bacterial meningitis in children is *H. influenzae* serovar b, causing 8,000 to 10,000 cases each year in the United States with 400 to 500 deaths.[48] The yearly incidence of other invasive disease due to this organism has been estimated to be equal to that of meningitis. *H. influenzae* serovar b (Hib) meningitis is a disease of infancy. Approximately 80% of children with Hib meningitis are less than 2 years of age and almost two thirds are less than one year. Most population-based studies have shown an equal occurrence of Hib meningitis in boys and girls. In contrast, epiglottitis and pneumonia cases have revealed a 1.5:1 and a 2:1 male to female ratio, respectively. Hib meningitis has a bimodal seasonal incidence with a peak in the fall and spring. The overall risk of secondary household spread has been well described. Certain patients have an increased incidence of Hib disease. These include low-birth weight infants, patients with leukemia or other malignancy undergoing chemotherapy or in remission, those with cerebrospinal fluid (CSF) shunts, skull defects, splenectomy, congenital asplenia, sickle cell disease, disorders of immunoglobulin synthesis (hereditary deficiency of IgG or IgG2 and IgG4) and disorders of complement (C_2, C_3, C_{3b} inactivator deficiency). Genetic predisposition also appears to play a role; Caucasian children without the MNSs erythrocyte antigen, black children without the Km (1) immunoglobulin allotype, as well as Navajo and Eskimo children are at increased risk of developing disease.[8,33]

H. ducreyi, the etiologic agent of chancroid, is sexually transmitted. Military personnel and prostitutes are important in transmission of disease.[3,42,44] The incidence of chancroid is probably intermediate between that of gonorrhea and of syphilis. In the United States the annual incidence is $<$1 case per 100,000 population with $<$1000 cases reported annually between 1966-1985. A tripling of cases occurred in the United States in 1986, (2994 cases), which has been attributed to prostitution. Due to importation, clusters of disease are usually observed.[3] A higher incidence has been associated with noncaucasian populations (primarily uncircumcised males) of lower socioeconomic status in tropical, third world countries, where the disease may be endemic.

H. ducreyi has been isolated from asymptomatic carriers and may be transmitted without active disease. More recently, *H. ducreyi* has been observed as a secondary pathogen in genital ulcers due to herpes simplex virus. These data place in question the traditional view of *H. ducreyi* as the most common cause of genital ulcer disease.[21] Future studies should include isolation for herpes simplex virus.

H. aegyptius causes acute contagious conjunctivitis of endemic or epidemic proportions primarily in tropical climates. Epidemiologically and clinically, *H. aegyptius* is distinct from *H. influenzae* biotype III. However, these species are closely related by DNA homology studies.[26] Recently, bacteremia due to *H. aegyptius* has been reported in association with Brazilian Purpuric Fever.[7] The clinical presentation is similar to meningococcemia and case fatality rates have varied from 44-100%.

PUBLIC HEALTH SIGNIFICANCE, PREVENTION AND CONTROL

As noted previously, *H. influenzae* serovar b is the most common cause of bacterial meningitis in children. Although the mortality rate for Hib meningitis is only 5%, the neurologic sequelae in survivors has been reported to be nearly 50%, with significant neurologic deficits in 30%.[48]

In April 1985, the first Hib vaccine was licensed in the United States for use in children from 2-5 years of age.[39,40] The vaccinogen is the polysaccharide capsule, polyribose-ribitol-phosphate (PRP). Unfortunately, the PRP vaccine is ineffective in children less than 24 months of age. Currently, three additional vaccines (PRP covalently linked to diphtheria toxoid, PRP linked to a diphtheria protein and PRP linked to a meningococcal outer membrane protein) have undergone limited clinical study in young infants. After repeated doses they appear safe and immunogenic.[1,12,13] However, clinical efficacy data are not yet available and these vaccines are not licensed.

Rifampin chemoprophylaxis will eradicate the carrier state of *H. influenzae* serovar b;[33] however, little information is available on the efficacy of disease prevention. Rifampin prophylaxis has been advocated for all household contacts of the index case (including adults) if another child less than 48 months of age resides in the home.[40] The index case may receive rifampin during or at completion of his course of parenteral therapy. A requirement for rifampin prophylaxis for daycare center attendees whenever a single case has occurred remains controversial. However, if two cases of invasive disease occur in the same daycare center within 60 days, all attendees and caregivers should receive prophylaxis. Because 54% of secondary cases will occur within 7 days of the index case, parents should be notified promptly and instructed to seek medical attention if their child becomes febrile or ill.

CHANCROID

The incidence of chancroid is unknown; however, it is common in Southeast Asia, Africa and Central America, where it is more prevalent than syphilis. In developed countries, sporadic outbreaks of disease continue to occur due to importation.

Prevention of chancroid has not been well studied. Circumcision may reduce the susceptibility of males to infection, and careful washing of the genitalia with soap and water immediately following intercourse is effective.[44] Condoms have been thought to be less effective in protecting against chancroid than against syphilis or gonorrhea. Efficacy of topical antibiotic prophylaxis and prospective treatment of prostitutes has not been reported. Nevertheless, antimicrobial treatment of index cases and their sexual contacts should interrupt disease transmission.[3]

DIAGNOSTIC PROCEDURES

Selection and Processing of Specimens

Speciation should be performed on all significant isolates. These include (a) any strain associated with invasive disease (cerebrospinal fluid or blood isolate), (b) any strain isolated from a sterile site and (c) any relatively pure or abundant isolate from a respiratory site when associated with clinical disease. Any transport system used should be quality controlled to be sure that it maintains viability. Cultures should be processed promptly and incubated upon media containing both X and V factors and under conditions (increased CO_2) that would support the growth of all members of the genus. Selective media may be used initially but only in addition to the nonselective media for primary isolation. The necessity to obtain follow-up cultures should be dictated only by the clinical response of the patient; routine follow-up cultures are not required to assess standard antimicrobial therapy.

SPECIFIC PROCEDURES

Microscopy and Other Rapid Methodology

Haemophilus species are small gram-negative organisms which exhibit pleomorphism in vivo; predominant filamentous forms interspersed with coccobacillary forms are observed in Gram stained smears of CSF specimens, whereas coccobacilli predominate on primary isolation. *H. aegyptius* and *H. ducreyi* appear as slender rods, the latter in pairs or chains. Pleomorphism in vitro occurs more commonly when cultures are stressed nutritionally or in the presence of sublethal concentrations of cell wall-active antibiotics. Upon subculture, most strains will become uniformly coccobacillary.

Meningitis due to *H. influenzae* serovar b can be diagnosed by direct Gram stain examination of cerebrospinal fluid, by using specific antiserum to demonstrate capsular swelling (Quellung reaction), or by fluorescence microscopy using specific antiserum linked to a fluorescent stain. Disk susceptibility tests should be done immediately on any CSF specimen with a positive direct examination. In the case of culture-negative disease due to prior treatment with oral antibiotics, an acridine orange stain of the cerebrospinal fluid may yield positive morphology when the Gram stain examination is negative.[23]

Antigen-detection assays are available, but they should not supplant culture and Gram stain of infected material. Detection of the type b capsular antigen in body fluids may be of diagnostic value in confirming etiology for a patient whose cultures are sterile due to prior antibiotic therapy or prior to the time bacterial growth occurs. These assays are discussed under Serologic Tests.

The clinical diagnosis of chancroid is not always reliable and ability to culture *H. ducreyi* remains problematic. Indirect immunofluorescence assays using recently developed monoclonal antibodies have been observed to stain organisms in smears of lesion material from patients and experimental animals, and such rapid diagnostic techniques may be quite useful in the future.[16,46]

Primary Isolation and Culture

Media used for primary isolation should support the growth of all ten *Haemophilus* species isolated from humans. Complex media containing X and V factors will support the growth of *Haemophilus* better than nutritionally limited or chemically defined media with similar supplementation. Chocolate agar with added X and V factors (enriched chocolate agar) should be used for primary isolation. Other media which will support the growth of *Haemophilus* include brain heart infusion (BHI) agar supplemented with X and V factors, Fildes enrichment agar, supplemented Levinthal agar and chocolate agar with 1% vitamin supplements. All media should be quality controlled for ability to support growth of test organisms as X and V factor concentrations vary over time and from lot to lot. Sheep blood agar alone will not support the growth of XV or V factor-requiring *Haemophilus* species. Cross-streaking with *Staphylococcus aureus* after inoculation provides V factor and *Haemophilus* colonies will surround the staphylococcal colonies as satellites. *Haemophilus* species may also satellite around other organisms, such as *Neisseria* spp., diphtheroids, etc. To avoid confusion, CSF specimens should be cultured on supportive media without the need for cross-streaking. *H. influenzae* will grow on rabbit blood agar, presumably because the V factor is more available. A disk containing 10 units of bacitracin may be used to select *Haemophilus* spp. from sputum specimens.

Although many blood culture media have been shown to support the growth of *H. influenzae*, these media should also be evaluated with test organisms as part of a quality control program. Hypertonic blood culture medium has been shown to yield earlier growth than standard aerobic media.[9] A recent comparison of standard trypticase soy broth with a new blood culture system which involves lysis of blood cells and direct plating suggests that the contents of the new system are toxic to *H. influenzae* serovar b in the presence of human blood,[45] emphasizing the need for parallel testing of new systems, including automated ones.

H. ducreyi can be isolated on chocolate agar with 1% supplements although recovery rates are generally poor. Addition of 3 μg of vancomycin per mL to enriched chocolate agar medium provides a selective medium for the isolation of the organism from chancroid lesions, which usually contain mixed flora. Other supportive media for *H. ducreyi* have been described[37,50,54] and more than a single medium and a single culture has been recommended.[11,14] Incorporation of vancomycin and/or bacitracin (and/or clindamycin) into enriched media can also be used to select for other species of *Haemophilus* from specimens harboring mixed microbial flora.

Although not an absolute requirement, increased ambient CO_2 enhances the growth of 4 of the 10 *Haemophilus* species isolated from humans -- *H. aphrophilus, H. paraphrophilus, H. paraphrohaemolyticus* and *H. ducreyi*.[20,37] The other 6 species, including *H. influenzae* , do not require increased CO_2 for growth. *Haemophilus* species do not require X factor when grown under anaerobic conditions.

Except for *H. ducreyi*, which grows better at a lower temperature (33°C), all *Haemophilus* species grow best at 35-37°C, and most can be detected after 18 to 24 hours of incubation. *H. aegyptius* may require 2 to 4 days and *H. ducreyi* up to 9 days for isolation. A moist environment (such as sterile, wet paper towels in a candle jar) will aid the isolation of *H. ducreyi*.

Encapsulated *H. influenzae* colonies are mucoid and irridescent on translucent media whereas unencapsulated strains are smaller and smooth but nonrefractile to light. Identification of serovar b organisms may be performed by incorporating type specific antiserum into the agar medium; a precipitating ''halo'' surrounds capsule-producing colonies.[34] Placement at 4°C for several hours and observation in tangential light will enhance detection of the halo. The amount of antiserum required is large, which represents a limitation to this procedure.

Methods for Identification

Members of the genus *Haemophilus* are most easily speciated on the basis of their requirement for X and/or V factors (Table 16:2). The media used for testing must be devoid of one or both of these factors, but otherwise support the growth of *Haemophilus* species. Complex media lacking both factors are difficult to obtain; thus testing with appropriate control strains prior to their use is imperative. Chemically defined media which support the growth of *Haemophilus* and lack one or both factors have been described,[6] and may be considered as an alternative to complex media.

After inoculation onto a medium minus X and V factor, separate paper disks containing X, V or X and V factors are placed on the surface and the cultures incubated. Growth around the disk containing both X and V factors but not the other two is evidence of a requirement for both factors, whereas growth around an individual X or V disk plus the X and V disk is evidence of a single factor requirement. Confluent growth on the entire plate is most often evidence of contamination, but may also suggest the presence of *H. aphrophilus*, which requires neither factor (Table 16:2).

There are several sources of error in the paper disk approach, which include the spurious transfer of growth factors from the primary culture and placement of the V factor disk too close to the X factor disk. The latter can usually be recognized by the appearance of growth around only one side of the X factor disk. V-independence should not be assumed for hemolytic *Haemophilus* species growing on sheep blood agar plates as hemolysis will release V factor.

Determination of the X factor requirement is complicated by the fact that the X factor is heat-stable and thus cannot be selectively destroyed as can the V factor. It is thought that X factor is present in many of the complex media which support the growth of *Haemophilus* species and it has been proposed that the overlap in the clinical manifestations between encapsulated *H. influenzae* (X-dependent) and *H. parainfluenzae* (X-independent) is due to misidentification.[56] However, misidentification of *H. parainfluenzae* can be reduced by confirming strain identity with biochemical tests and fermentation reactions (Table 16:2).

The porphyrin test[20] is an accurate, rapid, visual non-medium-dependent method to determine the X-factor requirement, and this assay is now commercially available. X-independent *Haemophilus* synthesize heme when supplied with delta-aminolevulinic acid. Porphobilinogen and porphyrins are intermediates in the pathway and can be detected by exposure of the cell suspension to ultraviolet light. Red fluorescence indicates a positive test. X-requiring *Haemophilus* species do not have the capacity to synthesize heme, do not excrete these intermediates and thus have a negative test (no red fluorescence). Quality control using known control strains is mandatory.

Table 16:2 lists other differentiating tests for the 10 *Haemophilus* species isolated from humans. For example, fermentation reactions may differentiate *H. influenzae* biovar III from *H. aegyptius* and can easily differentiate *H. influenzae* from *H. parainfluenzae*. These latter two species may also be subdivided into 8 and 7 biovars, respectively, based on production of indole, presence of urease and presence of ornithine decarboxylase activity.[33,52] Commercial biotyping and fermentation assays are available.[27]

MARKERS FOR EPIDEMIOLOGY

Although biotyping is easy to perform, it is not a useful epidemiologic tool for invasive disease due to serovar b organisms. Over 80% of organisms isolated from patients with meningitis are biovar I and biovar I represents greater than 80% of all serovar b isolates studied from all sources. Epidemiologic markers for *H. influenzae* which have been used in addition to biotyping include outer membrane protein (OMP) profiles, lipopolysaccharide (LPS) patterns and electrophoretic enzyme isotypes (ETs).

The outer membrane of *H. influenzae* contains 2-3 dozen proteins, but there are only 4-6 major proteins. Twenty-one distinctive subtypes based on relative mobility of OMPs have been identified among strains isolated from the United States.[48] Of these, 3 account for 75% of isolates and 6 are responsible for 89% of the patterns observed. Temporal shifts in OMPs have been observed when *H. influenzae* serovar b isolates separated by 3-5 decades were compared.[2] Comparison of OMP subtypes of strains isolated from healthy children and strains from those with disease revealed no significant difference in the frequencies of the most common subtypes.[15]

The OMP profiles of nontypable strains of *H. influenzae* are distinct from those of serovar b strains, and exhibit marked variability. Nontypable strains isolated from the blood of newborns with sepsis have been shown to have a unique OMP profile. OMP analyses have revealed that *H. aegyptius* and *H. influenzae* biovar III appear distinct, in spite of significant DNA homology, although no markers have been shown to unequivocally differentiate these two species.[5,26]

Heterogeneity of the OMPs of *H. ducreyi* has also been observed and the profiles appear to be species-specific.[38] At least seven different subtypes have been described and identical OMP patterns have been used to define a common-source outbreak.

Electrophoretic profiles of lipopolysaccharide (LPS) have been used to classify *H. influenzae* serovar b into 11 subtypes.[17] LPS subtyping has revealed differences between isolates with identical OMP profiles.[17,18] However, a recent report suggests that the LPS profile may not be a stable characteristic and thus may not be useful as an epidemiologic marker.[59]

More recently, a population genetic framework for *H. influenzae* using the electrophoretic mobilities of multiple metabolic enzymes or electrophoretic types for an analysis of variance has been developed.[35,36] Fifty-five distinctive combinations of ET, OMP and biovar have been described for *H. influenzae* serovar b. ET analysis demonstrated extensive genetic diversity among unencapsulated isolates and confirmed that unencapsulated strains are genetically distinct from encapsulated serovar b organisms.

Use of enzyme activities for 28 different substrates in evaluating isolates of *H. ducreyi* has proved contradictory and, to date, has not been useful epidemiologically.[53]

Serologic Tests (Antigen Detection)

Serotyping (antigen detection) is commercially available only for encapsulated *H. influenzae*. Six capsular types (a through f) can be identified by specific antisera. Commercial assays have been directed primarily at detection of the type b capsular antigen, PRP. Key to detecting the type b capsular antigen is specific, high-titered antiserum. This, in part, may contribute to the variability among commercial kits. Levels of PRP are significantly higher at the focus of infection (CSF, pleural fluid, joint fluid, etc.) compared to serum and urine. The three most commonly used techniques for antigen detection are countercurrent immunoelectrophoresis (CIE), latex particle agglutination (LPA) and coagglutination (CoA).[19,28,29] Enzyme linked immunoassays (ELISA) for PRP detection have been developed[57] and may offer an advantage over LPA in detection of antigen in urine and sputum.[10] However, the level of antigen detected is similar, and although technically simple, ELISA assays take longer to perform and are more difficult than LPA assays. Furthermore, a blocking test is required to rule out false-positive reactions.[19,61]

Natural crossreactions may occur with pneumococci, meningococci, *E. coli* and *Staphylococcus aureus*. False-positive reactions have been rare with CSF, but more common when testing serum and urine.[19,58] This problem has been resolved to some extent by heating, treating with dithiothreitol or by dilution.[25] In addition, false-negative reactions can occur with antigen excess. Although direct detection methods may be useful in some circumstances (e.g., partially treated meningitis), it should be noted that the Gram stained smear has equivalent sensitivity to most of the serologic procedures.

REFERENCES

1. Anderson P, Pichichero ME, Insel RA. Immunization of 2-month-old infants with protein-coupled oligosaccharides derived from the capsule of *Haemophilus influenzae* type b. J Pediatr 1985;107:346-51.
2. Barenkamp SJ, Granoff DM, Pittman M. Outer membrane protein subtypes and biotypes of *Haemophilus influenzae* type b: relation between strains isolated in 1934-1954 and 1977-1980. J Infect Dis 1983;148:1127.
3. Blackmore GA, Limpakarnjanarat K, Rigau-Perez JG, Albritton WL, Greenwood JR. An outbreak of chancroid in Orange County, California: Descriptive epidemiology and disease-control measures. J Infect Dis 1985;151:840-4.
4. Campos J, Garcia-Tornel J, Sanfeliv I. Susceptibility studies of multiply resistant *Haemophilus influenzae* isolated from pediatric patients and contacts. Antimicrob Agents Chemother 1984;25:706-9.
5. Carlone GM, Sottnek FO, Plikaytes BD. Comparison of outer membrane protein and biochemical profiles of *Haemophilus aegyptius* and *Haemophilus influenzae* biotype III. J Clin Microbiol 1985;22:708-13.
6. Catlin BW. Nutritional profiles of *Neisseria gonorrhoeae, Neisseria meningitidis* and *Neisseria lactamica* in chemically defined media and the use of growth requirements for gonococcal typing. J Infect Dis 1973;128:178-94.
7. Centers for Disease Control. Brazilian purpuric fever: *Haemophilus aegyptius* bacteremia complicating purulent conjunctivitis. Mortal Morbid Weekly Rep 1986;35:553-4.
8. Coulehan JL, Michaels RH, Hollowell C, Schults R, Welty TK, Kuo JS. Epidemiology of *Haemophilus influenzae* type b disease among Navajo Indians. Public Health Rep 1984:99:404-9.
9. Crist AE, Amsterdam D, Neter E. Superiority of hypertonic culture medium for detection of *Haemophilus influenzae* by the Bactec Procedure. J Clin Microbiol 1982;15:528-30.
10. Drow DL, Manning DD. Comparison of coagglutination, latex agglutination and enzyme-linked immunosorbent assay for detection of *Haemophilus influenzae* type b infection. Diagn Microbiol Infect Dis 1983;1:317-22.
11. Dylewski J, Nsanze H, Maitha G, Ronald A. Laboratory diagnosis of *Haemophilus ducreyi*: sensitivity of culture media. Diagn Microbiol Infect Dis 1986;4:241-5.
12. Einhorn M, Weinberg GA, Anderson EL, Granoff PD, Granoff DM. Immunogenicity in infants of *Haemophilus influenzae* type b polysaccharide in a conjugate vaccine with *Neisseria meningitidis* outer-membrane protein. Lancet 1986;2:299-302.
13. Eskola J, Kayhty H, Peltola H, et al. Antibody levels achieved in infants by course of *Haemophilus influenzae* type b polysaccharide/diphtheria toxoid conjugate vaccine. Lancet 1985;1:1184-6.

14. Hafiz S, McEntegart MG, Kinghorn GR. Sheffield medium for cultivation of *Haemophilus ducreyi*. Br J Vener Dis 1984;60;196-8.
15. Hampton CM, Barenkamp SJ, Granoff DM. Comparison of outer membrane protein subtypes of *Haemophilus influenzae* type b isolates from healthy children in the general population and from diseased patients. J Clin Microbiol 1983;18:596-600.
16. Hansen EJ, Loftus TA. Monoclonal antibodies reactive with all strains of *Haemophilus ducreyi*. Infect Immun 1984;44:196-8.
17. Inzana TJ. Electrophoretic heterogeneity and interstrain variation of the lipopolysaccharide of *Haemophilus influenzae*. J Infect Dis 1983;148:492-9.
18. Inzana TJ, Pichichero ME. Lipopolysaccharide subtypes of *Haemophilus influenzae* type b from an outbreak of invasive disease. J Clin Microbiol 1984;20:145-50.
19. Kaplan SL. Antigen detection in cerebrospinal fluid - pros and cons. Am J Med 1983;75:109-18.
20. Kilian M, Biberstein EL. *Haemophilus*. In: Krieg NR, Holt JG, eds. Bergey's manual of systematic bacteriology; vol 1. Baltimore: Williams and Wilkins, 1984:558-69.
21. Kinghorn GR, Hafiz S, McEntegart MG. Pathogenic microbial flora of genital ulcers in Sheffield with particular reference to herpes simplex virus and *Haemophilus ducreyi*. Br J Vener Dis 1982;58:377-80.
22. Kinghorn GR, Hafiz S, McEntegart MG. Oropharyngeal *Haemophilus ducreyi* infection. Br Med J 1983;287:650.
23. Kleiman MB, Reynolds JK, Watts NH, Schreiner RL, Smith JW. Superiority of acridine orange stain versus gram-stain in partially treated bacterial meningitis. J Pediatr 1984;104:401-4.
24. Kulinska D, Kilian M. Relative proportions of *Haemophilus* species in the throat of healthy children and adults. Eur J Clin Microbiol 1984;3:249-52.
25. Marcon MJ, Hamoudi AC, Cannon HJ. Comparative laboratory evaluation of three antigen detection methods for diagnosis of *Haemophilus influenzae* type b disease. J Clin Microbiol 1984;19:333-7.
26. Martel AY, Sottnek FO, Thomas ML, Albritton WL. Susceptibility of *Haemophilus aegyptius* to trooleandomycin: lack of taxonomic value. Can J Microbiol 1986;32:289-93.
27. Matthews JS, Reynolds JA, Weesner DE, Perry JL, Jenkins AL. Rapid species identification and biotyping of respiratory isolates of *Haemophilus* spp. J Clin Microbiol 1983;18:472-5.
28. McGraw TP, Bruckner DA. Sensitivity of commercial agglutination and countercurrent immunoelectrophoresis methods for the detection of *Haemophilus influenzae* type b capsular polysaccharide. Am J Clin Pathol 1983;80:703-6.
29. McGraw TP, Bruckner DA. Evaluation of the Directigen and Phadebact agglutination tests. Am J Clin Pathol 1984;82:97-9.
30. Mendelman PM, Chaffin DO, Clausen C, et al. Failure to detect ampicillin-resistant, non-β-lactamase-producing *Haemophilus influenzae* by standard disk susceptibility testing. Antimicrob Agents Chemother 1986;30:274-80.
31. Mendelman PM, Chaffin DO, Stull TL, Rubens CE, Mack KD, Smith AL. Characterization of non-β-lactamase-mediated ampicillin resistance in *Haemophilus influenzae*. Antimicrob Agents Chemother 1984;26:235-44.
32. Mendelman PM, Doroshow CA, Gandy SL, Syriopoulou V, Weigen CP, Smith AL. Plasmid-mediated resistance in multiply resistant *Haemophilus influenzae* type b causing meningitis: Molecular characterization of one strain and review of the literature. J Infect Dis 1984;150:30-9.
33. Mendelman PM, Smith AL. *Haemophilus influenzae*. In: Feigin RD, Cherry JD, eds. Textbook of pediatric infectious diseases. 2nd ed. Philadelphia: WB Saunders, 1987:1142-63.
34. Michaels RH, Stonebraker FE, Robbins JB. Use of antiserum agar for detection of *Haemophilus influenzae* type b in the pharynx. Pediatr Res 1975;9:513-16.
35. Musser JM, Barenkamp SJ, Granoff DM, Selander RK. Genetic relationships of serologically nontypable and serotype b strains of *Haemophilus influenzae*. Infect Immun 1986;52:183-91.

36. Musser JM, Granoff DM, Pattison PE, Selander RK. A population genetic framework for the study of invasive diseases caused by serotype b strains of *Haemophilus influenzae*. Proc Natl Acad Sci 1985;82:5078-82.
37. Oberhofer TR, Back AE. Isolation and cultivation of *Haemophilus ducreyi*. J Clin Microbiol 1982;15:625-9.
38. Odumeru JA, Ronald AR, Albritton WL. Characterization of cell proteins of *Haemophilus ducreyi* by polyacrylamide gel electrophoresis. J Infect Dis 1983;148:710-14.
39. Peltola H, Kayhty H, Virtanen M, Makela PH. Prevention of *Haemophilus influenzae* type b bacteremic infections with the capsular polysaccharide vaccine. N Engl J Med 1984;310:1561-6.
40. Peter G, Giebink GS, Hall CB, Plotkin SA, eds. Report of the Committee on Infectious Diseases. *Haemophilus influenzae* infections. 20th ed. Elk Grove Village, IL: American Academy of Pediatrics, 1986;3:169-74.
41. Pittman M. Variation and type specificity in the bacterial species *Haemophilus influenzae*. J Exp Med 1931;53:471-95.
42. Plummer FA, D'Costa LJ, Nsanze H, Dylewski J, Karasira P, Ronald AR. Epidemiology of chancroid and *Haemophilus ducreyi* in Nairobi, Kenya. Lancet 1983;2:1293-5.
43. Plummer FA, Nsanze H, D'Costa LJ, et al. Short course and single-dose antimicrobial therapy for chancroid in Kenya: studies with rifampin alone and in combination with trimethoprim. Rev Infect Dis 1983;5(S3):565-72.
44. Ronald AR, Albritton WL. Chancroid and *Haemophilus ducreyi*. In: Holmes KK, Mardh P-A, Sparling PF, Wiesner PJ, eds. Sexually transmitted diseases. New York: McGraw-Hill, 1984:385-93.
45. Rubin LG, Baranowski J. Comparison of the DuPont isolator 1.5 microbial tube and trypticase soy broth for the recovery of *Haemophilus influenzae* type b in experimental bacteremia. J Clin Microbiol 1985;22:815-18.
46. Schalla WD, Sanders LL, Schmid GP, Tam MR, Morse SA. Use of dot-immunobinding and immunofluorescence assays to investigate clinically suspected cases of chancroid. J Infect Dis 1986;153:879-87.
47. Schmid GP. The treatment of chancroid. JAMA 1986;255:1757-62.
48. Sell S, Wright PF, eds. *Haemophilus influenzae*: epidemiology, immunology and prevention of disease. Amsterdam: Elsevier Biomedical, 1982:1-321.
49. Shann F, Germer S, Hazlett D, Gratten M, Linnemann V, Payne R. Aetiology of pneumonia in children in Goroka Hospital, Papua, New Guinea. Lancet 1984;2:537-41.
50. Sottnek FO, Biddle JW, Kraus SJ, Weaver RE, Stewart JA. Isolation and identification of *Haemophilus ducreyi* in a clinical study. J Clin Microbiol 1980;12:170-4.
51. Stevens KM. The pathophysiology of influenzal pneumonia in 1918. Perspec Biol Med 1981;25:115-23.
52. Sturm AW. Isolation of *Haemophilus influenzae* and *Haemophilus parainfluenzae* from genital-tract specimens with a selective culture medium. J Med Microbiol 1986;21:349-52.
53. Sturm AW, Zanen HC. Enzymic activity of *Haemophilus ducreyi*. J Med Microbiol 1984;18:181-7.
54. Sturm AW, Zanen HC. Characteristics of *Haemophilus ducreyi* in culture. J Clin Microbiol 1984;19:672-4.
55. Taylor DN, Pitarangsi C, Echeverria P, Panikabutra K, Suvongse C. Comparative study of ceftriaxone and trimethoprim-sulfamethoxazole for the treatment of chancroid in Thailand. J Infect Dis 1985;152:1002-6.
56. Tebbutt GM. Evaluation of some methods for the laboratory identification of *Haemophilus influenzae*. J Clin Pathol 1983;36:991-5.
57. Tiller PW, Diener E. *Haemophilus influenzae* type b capsular polysaccharide detection and measurement by an enzyme-linked immunosorbent assay (ELISA). Zentral Bakt Hyg 1981;248:488-93.

58. Tilton RC, Dias F, Ryan RW. Comparative evaluation of three commercial products and counter-immunoelectrophoresis for the detection of antigens in cerebrospinal fluid. J Clin Microbiol 1984;20:231-4.
59. Tolan RW, Muson RS, Granoff DM. Lipopolysaccharide gel profiles of *Haemophilus influenzae* type B are not stable epidemiologic markers. J Clin Microbiol 1986;24:223-7.
60. Trollfors B, Brorson J-E, Claesson B, Sandberg T. Invasive infections caused by Haemophilus species other than *Haemophilus influenzae*. Infection 1985;13:12-14.
61. Wetherall BL, Hallsworth PG, McDonald PJ. Enzyme-linked immunosorbent assay for detection of *Haemophilus influenzae* type b antigen. J Clin Microbiol 1980;11:573-8.
62. Yogev R, Moxon ER. Elaboration of type b capsule by *Haemophilus influenzae* as a determinant of pathogenicity and impaired killing by trimethoprim-sulfamethoxazole. J Clin Invest 1982;69:658-65.

CHAPTER 17

LEGIONELLOSIS

Washington C. Winn, Jr., M.D.

INTRODUCTION

The genus *Legionella* was recognized as an important cause of human disease only after public and scientific attention was focused on an epidemic of pneumonia at the Pennsylvania American Legion convention in 1976.[34] The etiology of the pneumonia was established the following year, when investigators at the Centers for Disease Control isolated a bacterium from lung tissue and documented a serologic response among Legionnaires who had survived.[57] This Legionnaires' disease bacillus was unrelated by phenotypic and genetic analysis to any previously described families of bacteria. The bacterium was, therefore, placed in a new family, *Legionellaceae*, as a new genus and species, *Legionella pneumophila*.[8] Subsequently, it became apparent that neither the bacterium nor the disease was new. Members of the genus had been isolated from human blood in the 1940s and 1950s by inoculation of guinea pigs, but these individual isolates were not associated with outbreaks at the time.[41] Several epidemics of *Legionella* infection which occurred between 1957-1974 have been documented by retrospective seroepidemiology.[37,63,72]

CAUSATIVE ORGANISMS

Recognition of the diversity of the genus *Legionella* has increased steadily in the past decade. There is every reason to believe that the complexity will continue to increase.

Twenty-three species, several of which contain multiple serogroups, have been established (Table 17:1). Many of these species have been isolated only from environmental sites. Alternative taxonomic proposals have been made for some species,[35] but not widely accepted. *L. pneumophila* was

Table 17:1. Identification of *Legionella* species

Species	Number of serogroups	Browning of tyrosine medium	Gelatin lique—faction	Hippurate hydrolysis	Oxidase	Beta lactamase	Fluorescence Wood's lamp
L. pneumophila	11	+	+	+	+, +/−	+	−
L. feeleii	1	w	−	+/−	−	−	−
L. spiritensis	1	+	+	w	+	+	−
L. longbeachae	2	+	+	−	+	+/−	−
L. jordanis	1	+	+	−	+	+	−
L. oakridgensis	1	+	+	−	−	w	−
L. wadsworthii	1	−	+	−	−	+	−
L. sainthelensi	1	+	+	−	+	+	−
L. hackeliae	2	+	+	−	+	+	−
L. maceachernii	1	+	+	−	+	−	−
L. jamestowniensis	1	+	+	−	−	+	−
L. santicrucis	1	+	+	−	+	+	−
L. micdadei	1	−	−	−	+	−	−
L. israelensis	1	−	w	−	−	+	−
L. bozemanii	2	+	+	−	+/−	+/−	BW
L. dumoffii	1	+*	+	−	−	+	BW
L. gormanii	1	+	+	−	−	+	BW
L. anisa	1	+	+	−	+	+	BW*
L. cherrii	1	+	+	−	−	+	BW
L. steigerwaltii	1	+	+	−	−	+	BW
L. parisiensis	1	+	+	−	+	+	BW
L. rubrilucens	1	+	+	−	−	+	R
L. erythra	1	+	+	−	+	+	R

All species are gram negative, require 1-cysteine for primary isolation, and contain catalase or peroxidase. They do not grow on sheep blood agar, reduce nitrate to nitrite, produce urease, or produce acid from D-glucose. With the single exception of *L. oakridgenis,* they are motile by means of polar flagella and require 1-cysteine for continued growth after subculture.

+ = positive; − = negative; +/− = variable; w = weak reaction; * = rare exceptions reported.

Autofluorescence under long wavelength UV light (Wood's lamp): BW = blue-white; R = red.

Adapted from Reference 7.

known as the "Legionnaires' disease bacillus" and *L. micdadei* as the "Pittsburgh pneumonia agent" before the taxonomy of the genus was established. The most important human pathogens in the genus *Legionella* are *Legionella pneumophila* serogroups 1 and 6 and *L. micdadei*. Eighty-five percent of specimens identified by the Centers for Disease Control between 1980-1982 as containing *Legionella* spp. contained *L. pneumophila; L. micdadei* was detected in 6% of specimens. Sixty-one percent of the specimens containing *L. pneumophila* yielded serogroup 1 and 14% serogroup 6.[66] It is unclear whether the uneven distribution of species and serogroups in human infections reflects differences in virulence or in exposure to environmental bacteria.

Members of the *Legionella* genus are gram-negative, nonsporeforming bacilli. In clinical specimens, the bacilli measure 0.5-1.0 x 2-4 μm. After isolation, long filamentous forms may be observed (Figure 17:1). Carbohydrates are neither oxidized nor fermented. Amino acids provide the primary source of energy. L-cysteine is required for isolation of all species and is also necessary for continued subculture of all species except *L. oakridgensis*. All species except this latter organism are motile by means of polar flagella.

CLINICAL MANIFESTATIONS AND THERAPY

Legionella spp. may produce either acute pneumonia (Legionnaires' disease)[34] or a flu-like syndrome (Pontiac fever).[37] The two syndromes are

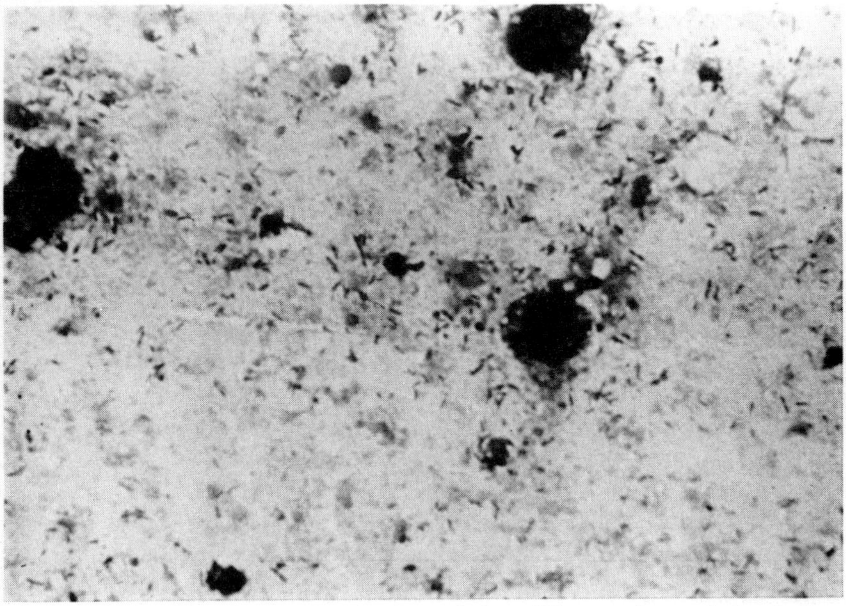

FIGURE 17:1a. Touch preparation from infected human lung. A few inflammatory cells and many small coccobacilli are present. *L. pneumophila* serogroup 1 was isolated from the lung. Gram stain. X 1000.

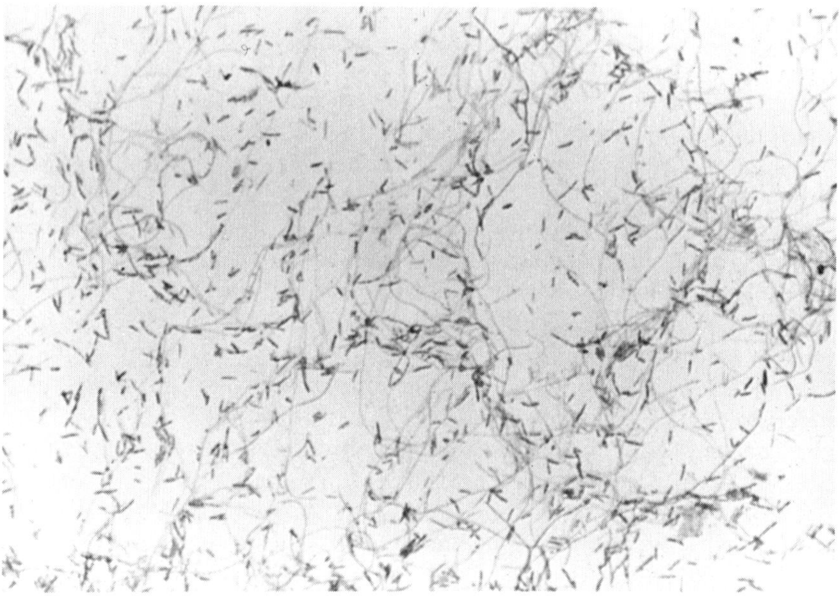

FIGURE 17:1b. Bacterial cells of the *L. pneumophila* strain isolated on supplemented Mueller-Hinton agar from the lung shown in Figure 1a. Long filamentous forms are present. Gram strain. X 1000.

differentiated on clinical and epidemiologic grounds.[10] Legionnaires' disease has a long incubation period (2-10 days), a low attack rate, radiographic evidence of pneumonia and a prolonged convalescence. Approximately half of the recognized species have been associated with this syndrome. In contrast, Pontiac fever has a short incubation period (5-6 hours), a high attack rate (up to 95%), absence of pneumonia on radiographs and a short course without residua. To date only *L. pneumophila* serogroups 1 and 6, and *L. feeleii* have been incriminated as causes of Pontiac fever.[37,43,53]

Some signs and symptoms are common to the two clinical presentations. Fever, chills, malaise, myalgias, nonproductive cough and leukocytosis are often present. Extrapulmonary manifestations are common in Legionnaires' disease. Changes in mental status, including confusion disproportionate to the height of the fever, depression, disorientation and lethargy, or gastrointestinal symptoms, such as nausea, vomiting, abdominal pain and diarrhea may suggest the diagnosis of *Legionella* infection, but are not pathognomonic.

Asymptomatic *Legionella* infections probably occur, even in immunosuppressed patients.[18] Nonpneumonic infection and severe pneumonia have been reported to occur after exposure to the same environmental site.[36] Pontiac fever is distinguished from nonpneumonic Legionnaires' disease by epidemiologic rather than clinical criteria.

The course of Legionnaires' disease is dominated by increasing respiratory distress.[47] Among patients who produce sputum, hemoptysis is common. Rales are the first sign of pulmonary disease. Radiographic infiltrates are usually unilateral and patchy initially,[47] progressing over several days to ipsilateral and contralateral lobes. A variety of radiographic patterns may be seen, including diffuse, patchy infiltrates and lobar consolidation.[30] A distinctive, although not pathognomonic pattern is the presence of poorly marginated, rounded, peripheral lesions. Cavitation has been observed infrequently in radiographs,[30] but small abscesses are common in pathological specimens.[86]

Biochemical abnormalities are frequent, but not diagnostic of *Legionella* infections.[47] Hyponatremia, hypophosphatemia, abnormalities in liver function tests and proteinuria are common. Myoglobinuria and renal failure have been reported.[65]

Dissemination of bacteria from the lung to other organs is common in fatal cases,[29] but is not usually associated with inflammatory disease. *L. pneumophila* has produced pyelonephritis,[16] pericarditis,[55] endocarditis,[56] perirectal abscess,[2] hepatic abscess[14] and hemodialysis fistula infections.[46] *L. micdadei* has been isolated from a cutaneous abscess in an immunocompromised patient.[1]

Convalescence from the pneumonia is often prolonged. Radiographic abnormalities may persist for months.[30] Abnormal pulmonary function tests have been documented as long as two years after a primary infection.[52]

Erythromycin is the antibiotic of choice for therapy of Legionnaires' disease. The efficacy of erythromycin was suggested by the analysis of data from the original Philadelphia epidemic[34] and confirmed in a subsequent epidemic in Vermont.[11] Rifampin may be considered as additional therapy in patients who have serious disease. Trimethoprim-sulfasoxazole has been shown to be effective in experimental animals.[64]

EPIDEMIOLOGY

Most species of *Legionella* have been isolated from aquatic environmental sources. *L. pneumophila* is ubiquitous.[32] The factors that promote the growth of *Legionella* in potable and surface water are incompletely known. Algal products can stimulate the growth of *L. pneumophila* in vitro[6] and a variety of free-living protozoa may be parasitized.[4] The nature of interactions in the environment is difficult to document. *L. pneumophila*, amoebae and two ciliates were isolated from a single cooling tower, after which in vitro infection of the protozoa by *Legionella* was documented.[4] The presence of other bacterial genera may also contribute to the growth of *Legionella* spp.[77]

Legionella spp., most commonly *L. pneumophila*, are frequently present in potable water.[5] Hot water systems in which the temperature is maintained below 65°C or in which the bacteria are protected by organic matter are particularly prone to colonization.[78] Freshly isolated strains of *L. pneumophila* which have been grown in tap water are more resistant to chlorine than are those subcultured on agar.[50]

Environmental sites are the most important and perhaps the only sources for human infection. Person-to-person transmission of infection has not been documented.[88] Epidemics of Pontiac fever have been associated with evaporative condensers from which the bacteria were aerosolized,[37] with a coolant in a manufacturing plant[43] and with whirlpools.[53]

Three epidemiologic patterns of Legionnaires' disease have been documented: explosive epidemics,[34] prolonged hyperendemic cases[40] and sporadic cases.[71] Cooling towers and evaporative condensers are important sources for epidemic Legionnaires' disease.[15,36] Potable water is the best documented source for epidemics and for hyperendemic foci not associated with cooling towers.[5,42,60,70]

Less is known about the source of sporadic cases. In several instances, epidemiological data suggest potable water.[3,45] The use of home airconditioners was associated with community-acquired disease in Burlington, Vermont, but this association was not proved to be an etiologic one.[11]

Both epidemic and sporadic Legionnaires' disease have a seasonal distribution, with cases occurring most frequently in the summer months. Many epidemics have been institutional, striking hospitals, hotels or resorts in a pattern that suggests a common source. Severe *Legionella* pneumonia may occur in otherwise healthy persons. A number of risk factors have been identified for the development of severe infection, particularly smoking,[34,71] immunosuppression[40] and chronic disease.[71] Underlying disease and exposure to an environmental source undoubtedly magnifies the risk of serious infection.[3]

The frequency of *Legionella* infection is difficult to determine. In some populations the frequency of seropositivity may be high.[11] A retrospective analysis of unselected sera from patients with acute respiratory disease suggested an incidence of 1%.[33] In some hospitals *L. pneumophila* has been identified as a common etiology of community-acquired[54] or nosocomial[58] pneumonia. Elsewhere, Legionnaires' disease has been documented infrequently in patients who should have been at high risk.[38] The geographic differences may reflect variations in colonization of local water systems or differences in virulence among environmental isolates.

PUBLIC HEALTH SIGNIFICANCE, PREVENTION AND CONTROL

In the ten years since the recognition of Legionnaires' disease, concerted efforts by scientists from many disciplines have been dramatically successful in reducing the frequency of this lethal infection in multiple locales.[5,42,70]

Prevention of infection can be accomplished best by minimizing exposure to environmental *Legionella*, especially for individuals who are at risk of developing serious disease. The development of vaccines for *Legionella* is unlikely until the immunology of the infection is better understood. Prophylactic administration of erythromycin to patients at high risk has been employed during epidemics,[75] but is not generally advised.

Elimination of *Legionella* spp. from surface waters is impossible and permanent decontamination of cooling towers is extremely difficult, if not also impossible. Standard methods for general maintenance of cooling towers should be followed carefully. The most effective biocides can suppress or eliminate *Legionella* temporarily, but do not produce permanent decontamination.[51] Continuous treatment with chlorine is an effective means by which to prevent recolonization of cooling towers, but is destructive to the equipment.

Chlorination and/or heat have proved effective at suppressing bacterial growth in potable water systems, but each has drawbacks. Elevated water temperature may produce scalding unless rigorous precautions are taken. As the level of chlorination increases, risk of accelerating the decay of plumbing systems is magnified. Treatment must be continuous or recurrent because recolonization of the system is likely. Devices that measure and adjust the chlorine concentration in potable water allow titration of chlorine to levels that minimize deterioration of the water pipes (Philip Mead, personal communication).

Prevention of *Legionella* infections should be addressed by surveillance of patients rather than of the environment. The high prevalence of *Legionella* in water, multiplicity of potential sources, likely recolonization of environmental sites and frequency of environmental bacteria in the absence of clinical disease should discourage routine environmental sampling. Microbiologic and serologic testing of patients with undiagnosed pneumonia should be available, either locally or in a reference laboratory. Hospital epidemiologists should include this genus in the differential diagnosis of clusters of pneumonia, even if cases have not been documented previously. If cases are detected, vigorous attempts should be made to assess the epidemiologic relationship of all potential sources to infected patients. Once a focus of disease has been defined, ongoing control measures should be instituted.

DIAGNOSTIC PROCEDURES

Selection and Processing of Specimens

Specimens from any respiratory site are acceptable for culture. Production of sputum from the lower respiratory tract should be encouraged, but a paucity of neutrophils cannot be used to exclude specimens. *Legionella* has been identified in expectorated sputum, tracheal aspirates, bronchial washings and brushings, lung aspirates and biopsies.[12,25,87] Isolates have been recovered from pleural fluid with less frequency. Induction of sputum by nebulization of saline has not been evaluated. *L. pneumophila* has been isolated from blood and extrapulmonary sites.[24,46] Culture of non-respiratory sites may be considered if clinical data suggest the possibility of disseminated infection.

No special transport media are required. *Legionella* spp. are relatively hardy bacteria, but their viability in clinical specimens has not been systematically evaluated.

Acute and convalescent serum samples should be collected for serological evaluation: convalescent sera should be obtained 3-6 weeks after onset of disease. Early morning urine specimens may be tested if immunoassays for *Legionella* antigen are available.

Microscopy and Other Rapid Methodology

If large numbers of bacteria are present, as in a lung biopsy, *Legionella* may be visualized by Gram stain. Addition of 0.05% carbolfuchsin to the safranin counterstain facilitates the visualization of faintly staining gram-negative bacilli. Other stains that contain carbolfuchsin, such as the Gimenez stain for rickettsia and *Chlamydia*, may also be employed.[19]

Immunofluorescence has been used most frequently to detect *Legionella* spp. directly in respiratory specimens. The sensitivity of the test is low, ranging from 25-50%.[12,25,87] The specificity is high, varying from approximately 90% for epidemic cases[25,87] to 99% for sporadic cases. The test must be performed with scrupulous attention to detail, a high quality fluorescence microscope must be available and observers must be skilled in fluorescent techniques. Immunologic crossreactions between *Legionella* spp. and other bacteria have been documented. Most false-positive results probably occur, however, when environmental *Legionella* contaminate reagents or slides that are used in the test.[87] Slides should be carefully cleaned and all aqueous reagents, including formalin, should be filter-sterilized. Positive results should be confirmed by retesting with species- or serogroup-specific reagents and substantiated by culture and/or serology.

Fluorescein-conjugated polyclonal sera, in which immunoglobulins against multiple species and serogroups have been pooled, are available commercially. A monoclonal reagent that recognizes all serogroups of *L. pneumophila* appears equivalent to the polyclonal reagents in sensitivity and specificity, but stains background less intensely.[22] Inclusion of a counterstain, such as Evan's blue or rhodamine, facilitates observation. Rhodamine-conjugated normal serum may be useful to block Fc-mediated attachment of staphylococci and streptococci to the specific antibodies.

The direct fluorescence test is useful to document *Legionella* infection when the frequency of disease is high. When the prevalence is low, even a very small number of false-positive results may become unacceptable and it is difficult to maintain proficiency of personnel.

Radioimmunoassay, enzyme immunoassay and latex agglutination have proved effective at detecting bacterial antigen in urine[68] in research laboratories, but the reagents are not commercially available. Antigens of *L. pneumophila* may be excreted for long periods after the acute infection has subsided.[49] The persistence of antigen facilitates diagnosis at a time when cultures may be negative, but this persistence must be taken into consideration when attempting to associate the antigen with an episode of pneumonia.

A DNA probe against bacterial cRNA has been used effectively for identification of isolates, but has not yet been tested for detection of bacteria in specimens.[21]

Primary Isolation and Culture

Recovery of *Legionella* in culture is the preferred means of diagnosis.[25,87,90] *Legionella* spp. have not been grown from respiratory secretions of healthy individuals.[9] The specificity of microbiologic diagnosis is therefore 100%. The sensitivity of culture is better than that of direct fluorescence and approximates that of serological diagnosis.

Legionella spp. are classified as Class II pathogens and do not present any special hazard to laboratory workers. Manipulations that may produce aerosols, such as the homogenization of tissues, are best performed in a biological safety cabinet. Other organisms that do represent significant biohazard, such as *Francisella tularensis*, may grow on *Legionella* media.[79]

The best media for primary isolation are those that contain charcoal, a buffer to stabilize the pH at the optimum (6.85-6.95) and alpha-ketoglutarate. The preferred basic isolation medium is buffered charcoal yeast extract agar with alpha-ketoglutarate (BCYEα).[19] The charcoal probably inactivates toxic superoxides and hydrogen peroxides in the media.[44] Addition of aniline dyes may provide some differentiation of colonies,[76] but has not been demonstrated to increase isolation.

Competing microbial flora may inhibit the growth of *Legionella*.[31] Antibiotics may be added to medium for examination of specimens from potentially contaminated sites. The addition of cefamandole, polymyxin B and anisomycin (BMPα medium) will provide moderate inhibition of competing flora.[19] Cefamandole may inhibit species other than *L. pneumophila*. Vancomycin may be substituted for cefamandole in BMPα medium or MWY (Modified Wadowsky Yee) medium containing glycine, vancomycin, polymyxin B and anisomycin may be used.[19,20] Acid treatment of potentially contaminated specimens, with or without the use of selective media, may additionally enhance recovery of *L. pneumophila*. A 1:10 dilution of the specimen is prepared in 0.2M KCl-HCl (pH 2.2), homogenized, incubated at room temperature and inoculated onto agar plates.[12]

Media for isolation of *Legionella* must be prepared with care. A final pH of 6.85-6.95 after autoclaving should be achieved with KOH, because NaOH is inhibitory. Quality control should be performed with a virulent *Legionella* strain, derived from a patient or from an experimental animal. Avirulent laboratory strains may grow well on media that do not support the growth of clinical isolates. *L. pneumophila* maintains virulence after multiple subcultures on BCYEα agar,[28] but other species may lose virulence after one or two subcultures. Commercially prepared plates and dehydrated media are available. Suppliers should be able to document the procedures and results of their quality control.

Inoculated plates should be incubated in air at 35-37°C for 2 weeks. Recovery of some species may be enhanced by low concentrations of CO_2, but the concentration should not exceed 5%. Macroscopic colonies appear after plates have been incubated for at least 2 days. Half of the isolates are detected after incubation for 72 h. The macroscopic appearance of young *Legionella* colonies is characteristic (Figure 17:2). Colonies are smooth, convex and entire. When viewed with a dissecting microscope, they have

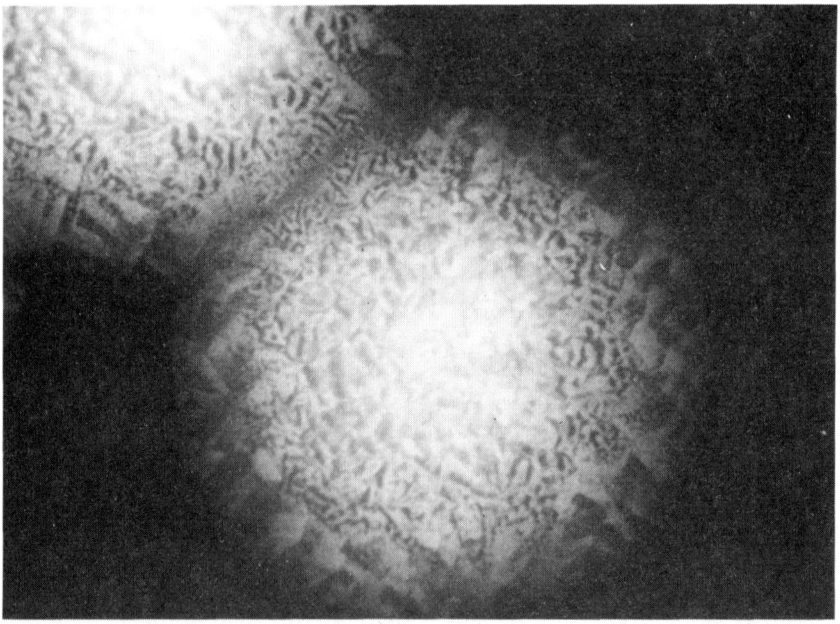

FIGURE 17:2. Dissecting microscopic appearance of colonies of *L. pneumophila,* serogroup 1, viewed with oblique light. Note the tracery of patterns, resembling cut-glass, in the colony. X 35.

a mottled appearance with shades of blue, pink, or green. A multi-faceted ("cut-glass") effect may be observed with oblique light, although the surface of the colony is regular. As the colony enlarges, the center and eventually the whole becomes opaque. It is useful, therefore, to observe plates daily, at least for the first 5-7 days. Colonies have a sticky consistency and cannot be removed cleanly from the plate. If a bacteriologic loop is removed slowly from a colony, a tenacious strand of bacteria may be demonstrated, resembling pulled taffy.

L. pneumophila was first recovered from blood in biphasic media.[24] The bacteria grow slowly, so incubation should be continued for one month. Isolates have also been recovered in conventional and radiometric blood culture systems. Blind subculture is required, because neither turbidity nor a positive growth index is achieved with regularity. The frequency of bacteremia is not known.[29,67] Lysis-centrifugation may also be useful for laboratories that use this methodology,[17] but clinical studies using this methodology have not been reported. Recovery of *Legionella* spp. from environmental sites may be difficult if large numbers of other bacteria are present. Samples are efficiently collected by swabbing inside surfaces of plumbing fixtures, such as faucets and shower heads, or collecting sediment from hot water tanks. Swabs may be placed in 1 mL of sterile distilled water for transport. Use of selective media and acid treatment are often needed to inhibit other bacteria. To culture water, large volumes should be concentrated by filtration or centrifugation.

Methods for Identification

Methods for identification of *Legionella* spp. may be categorized into two groups—those that are sufficient for reporting results in hospital laboratories and those that are necessary for definitive speciation in reference laboratories. As knowledge of the complexity of the genus has increased, it has become apparent that no single method can provide definitive identification of all isolates. The choice of diagnostic protocols will depend on the resources of the laboratory and the frequency with which *Legionella* spp. are isolated.

In most situations, a simple diagnostic scheme will provide sufficient information to identify clinical isolates with reasonable certainty. Suspect colonies should be subcultured to BCYEα and trypticase soy-sheep blood agar (TSA). Strains that grow on blood agar may be eliminated from consideration. Alternatively, subculture may be made in parallel to BCYEα agar with and without l-cysteine. *L. oakridgensis*, however, may replicate on media that do not contain l-cysteine when subcultured. Some non-*Legionella* species may grow on BCYEα agar only in the presence of this amino acid; in at least one instance the colonial morphology of such an isolate resembled that of *Legionella* spp.[73]

Isolates that do not grow on TSA may then be serogrouped, using commercially available immunofluorescence reagents. Simple protocols, using slide agglutination[74] or coagglutination[83] have also been described. Serological crossreactions do occur among the *Legionella* serogroups and species. These crossreactions do not obviate the routine use of serological confirmation, especially if antisera are used at the highest possible working dilution. *L. anisa*, however, may be indistinguishable serologically from *L. longbeachae* serotype 2.[39] It has been suggested that some strains, previously identified by biochemical and serologic criteria as *L. pneumophila* serogroup 1, actually belong to a new species, because the genes that code for bacterial enzymes diverge from the reference patterns.[26]

Isolates that do not react with grouping sera may represent a serogroup not included in the available panel of antisera, a new serogroup or an organism other than *Legionella*. *F. tularensis*, for instance, has been recovered on BCYEα agar;[79] this fastidious organism also requires l-cysteine for growth and will not be detected on TSA.

Biochemical characterization is not generally useful for differentiation among species of *Legionella* (Table 17:1), but may be helpful as additional presumptive evidence that the isolate belongs to the genus.[7] Most species liquefy gelatin,[7,62] produce browning on charcoal-treated yeast extract agar that contains tyrosine[7,62] and contain catalase or peroxidase. Close observation may be necessary to detect the catalase reaction. Nitrates are not reduced to nitrites, carbohydrates are not utilized and urease is not produced. Nine species produce a blue-white or red autofluorescence when the colonies are observed with a long wavelength ultraviolet light. All species, with the exception of *L. oakridgensis*, are motile by means of one or two polar flagella. Only *L. pneumophila* consistently produces strongly positive hippurate hydrolysis.[7,62]

Additional tests are required for definitive identification or for characterization of isolates that resemble *Legionella* spp. but do not react with specific antisera. All species, except *L. erythra*, contain prominent branched-chain fatty acids by gas-liquid chromatography.[7] Isoprenoid quinones with more than 10 isoprene units in the side chain may be detected by reverse-phase, high-performance liquid chromatography. The ultimate identification is provided by the determination of genetic relatedness, using DNA hybridization.[7] The commercial availability of molecular techniques for analysis of *Legionella* may bring this reference procedure into the realm of the clinical laboratory.[26]

Markers for Epidemiology

The multiplicity of environmental sources for human exposure and the predominance of *L. pneumophila* serogroup 1 among both environmental and clinical isolates diminish the effectiveness of simple serogrouping for epidemiologic investigations. Analysis of plasmid content,[61] comparison of reactivity of strains with a panel of monoclonal antibodies[45,60] and determination of allelic variation of the structural genes for bacterial enzymes[69] have been used to increase the discrimination of epidemiologic analysis. In several instances, these subtyping schemes have incriminated a single source for human disease among several that would have been candidates had serogrouping alone been available.[45,60] Characterization of genetic structure produces the largest number of subdivisions within *L. pneumophila* serogroup 1.[26] It is not yet clear whether any single method is superior for detecting meaningful epidemiologic associations.

Serologic Diagnosis

The diagnosis of *Legionella* pneumonia was facilitated by the development of reliable tests for serodiagnosis. Documentation of a serologic response to *Legionella* spp. was the primary diagnostic method before the advent of reliable media for recovery of the bacteria in culture.[34] Today, detection of antibodies remains a useful adjunct for diagnosis, especially for those patients who do not produce adequate sputum for culture.

Of the several serologic tests that have been applied to the diagnosis of *Legionella* infections, the indirect fluorescent antibody (IFA) test has been evaluated most extensively. Reagents for the IFA test are readily available from commercial sources. Various methods for preparation of bacterial antigen in the IFA test have been described. Heat-killed antigen appears comparable to a formalin-inactivated preparation if the diagnostic endpoints are adjusted.[80] Enzyme immunoassays have also been successfully used for serodiagnosis.[27] The sensitivity of the enzymatic method is greater than that of IFA, but the specificity is somewhat less.

Antibodies of IgG, IgM and IgA classes are produced.[82] Anti-immunoglobulin reagents must detect IgM, because a substantial minority of patients produce antibodies of this class alone, especially in the early weeks after infection.[59,89] Crossreactions among serogroups and species of *Legionellla* are extensive. The infecting organism cannot always be pinpointed by serologic analysis.[84]

The IFA test and a double-sandwich version of the enzyme immunoassay may be used to detect IgM antibodies. Although the presence of anti-*Legionella* IgM suggests recent infection, this class of immunoglobulin may persist for as long as a year in a few patients.[59]

Seroconversion, defined as at least a 4-fold increase in antibodies to a titer of 1:128 in the IFA technique with heat-killed antigen, is considered indicative of recent infection. Convalescent serum should be collected at least 3 weeks and, preferably, 6 weeks after the first specimen.[25] A single titer of 1:256 or more may suggest infection during an epidemic, but is difficult to interpret if the infection is sporadic. As the number of antigens tested increases, so does the need for rigorous diagnostic criteria.[85]

The sensitivity of the IFA test is approximately 75%, whether defined by positive culture[25] or by epidemiologic criteria.[81] The specificity is very high if strict positive criteria are enforced.[81] Crossreactions have been reported between *Legionella* spp. and several other bacterial genera,[13,23,48,85] but the importance of these observations has not been established.

CLINICAL SIGNIFICANCE OF LABORATORY FINDINGS

Recovery of *Legionella* spp. by culture of clinical specimens is diagnostic of current infection. Demonstration of antigen in clinical specimens or a seroconversion is presumptive evidence of a recent infection, but must be evaluated in light of clinical and epidemiologic data.

REFERENCES

1. Ampel NM, Ruben FL, Norden CW. Cutaneous abscess caused by *Legionella micdadei* in an immunosuppressed patient. Ann Intern Med 1985;102:630-2.
2. Arnow PM, Boyko EJ, Friedman EL. Perirectal abscess caused by *Legionella pneumophila* and mixed anaerobic bacteria. Ann Intern Med 1983;98:184-5.
3. Arnow PM, Chou T, Weil D, Shapiro EN, Kretzschmar C. Nosocomial Legionnaires' disease caused by aerosolized tap water from respiratory devices. J Infect Dis 1982;146:460-7.
4. Barbaree JM, Fields BS, Feeley JC, Gorman GW, Martin WT. Isolation of protozoa from water associated with a legionellosis out-break and demonstration of intracellular multiplication of *Legionella pneumophila*. Appl Environ Microbiol 1986;51:422-4.
5. Best M, Yu VL, Stout J, Goetz A, Muder RR, Taylor F. *Legionellaceae* in the hospital water-supply. Epidemiological link with disease and evaluation of a method for control of nosocomial Legionnaires' disease and Pittsburgh pneumonia. Lancet 1983;2:307-10.
6. Bohach GA, Snyder IS. Cyanobacterial stimulation of growth and oxygen uptake by *L. pneumophila*. Appl Environ Microbiol 1983;46:528-31.
7. Brenner DJ, Steigerwalt AG, Gorman GW, et al. Ten new species of *Legionella*. Int J Syst Bacteriol 1985;35:50-9.
8. Brenner DJ, Steigerwalt AG, McDade JE. Classification of the Legionnaires' disease bacterium: *Legionella pneumophila*, genus novum, species nova, of the family *Legionellaceae*, familia nova. Ann Intern Med 1979;90:656-8.
9. Bridge JA, Edelstein PH. Oropharyngeal colonization with *Legionella pneumophila*. J Clin Microbiol 1983;18:1108-12.
10. Broome CV, Fraser DW. Epidemiologic aspects of legionellosis. Epidemiol Rev 1979;1:1-16.
11. Broome CV, Goings SA, Thacker SB, Vogt RL, Beaty HN, Fraser DW. The Vermont epidemic of Legionnaires' disease. Ann Intern Med 1979;90:573-7.
12. Buesching WJ, Brust RA, Ayers LW. Enhanced primary isolation of *Legionella pneumophila* from clinical specimens by low-pH treatment. J Clin Microbiol 1983;17:1153-5.
13. Collins MT, McDonald J, Hiby N, Aalund O. Agglutinating antibody titers to members of the family *Legionellaceae* in cystic fibrosis patients as a result of cross-reacting antibodies to *Pseudomonas aeruginosa*. J Clin Microbiol 1984;19:757-62.

14. Cutz E, Thorner PS, Rao CP, Toma S, Gold R, Gelfand EW. Disseminated *Legionella pneumophila* infection in an infant with severe combined immunodeficiency. J Pediatr 1982;100:760-2.
15. Dondero TJ Jr, Rendtorff RC, Mallison GF, et al. An outbreak of Legionnaires' disease associated with a contaminated air-conditioning cooling tower. N Engl J Med 1980;302:365-70.
16. Dorman SA, Hardin NJ, Winn WC Jr. Pyelonephritis associated with *Legionella pneumophila*, serogroup 4. Ann Intern Med 1980;93:835-7.
17. Dorn GL, Barnes WR. Rapid isolation of *Legionella pneumophila* from seeded donor blood. J Clin Microbiol 1979;10:114-15.
18. Dowling JN, Pasculle AW, Frola FN, Zaphyr MK, Yee RB. Infections caused by *Legionella micdadei* and *Legionella pneumophila* among renal transplant recipients. J Infect Dis 1984;149:703-13.
19. Edelstein PH. *Legionella*. In: Lennette EH, Balows A, Hausler WJ Jr, Shadomy HJ, eds. Manual of clinical microbiology. 4th ed. Washington, DC: American Society for Microbiology, 1985:373-81.
20. Edelstein PH. Comparative study of selective media for isolation of *Legionella pneumophila* from potable water. J Clin Microbiol 1982;16:697-9.
21. Edelstein PH. Evaluation of the Gen-Probe DNA probe for the detection of legionellae in culture. J Clin Microbiol 1986;23:481-4.
22. Edelstein PH, Beer KB, Sturge JC, Watson AJ, Goldstein LC. Clinical utility of a monoclonal direct fluorescent reagent specific for *Legionella pneumophila*: comparative study with other reagents. J Clin Microbiol 1985;22:419-21.
23. Edelstein PH, McKinney RM, Meyer RD, Edelstein MA, Krause CJ, Finegold SM. Immunologic diagnosis of Legionnaires' disease: cross-reactions with anaerobic and microaerophilic organisms and infections caused by them. J Infect Dis 1980;141:652-5.
24. Edelstein PH, Meyer RD, Finegold SM. Isolation of *Legionella pneumophila* from blood. Lancet 1979;1:750-1.
25. Edelstein PH, Meyer RD, Finegold SM. Laboratory diagnosis of Legionnaires' disease. Am Rev Respir Dis 1980;121:317-27.
26. Edelstein PH, Nakahama C, Tobin JO, et al. Paleoepidemiologic investigation of Legionnaires' disease at Wadsworth Veterans Administration Hospital by using three typing methods for comparison of legionellae from clinical and environmental sources. J Clin Microbiol 1986;23:1121-6.
27. Elder EM, Brown A, Remington JS, Shonnard J, Naot Y. Microenzyme-linked immunosorbent assay for detection of immunoglobulin G and immunoglobulin M antibodies to *Legionella pneumophila*. J Clin Microbiol 1983;17:112-21.
28. Elliott JA, Johnson W. Virulence conversion of *Legionella pneumophila* serogroup 1 by passage in guinea pigs and embryonated eggs. Infect Immun 1982;35:943-6.
29. Evans CP, Winn WC Jr. Extrathoracic localization of *Legionella pneumophila* in Legionnaires' pneumonia. Am J Clin Pathol 1981;76:813-15.
30. Fairbank JT, Mamourian AC, Dietrich PA, Girod JC. The chest radiograph in Legionnaires' disease. Further observations. Radiology 1983;147:33-4.
31. Flesher AR, Kasper DL, Modern PA, Mason EO Jr. *Legionella pneumophila*: growth inhibition by human pharyngeal flora. J Infect Dis 1980;142:313-17.
32. Fliermans CB, Cherry WB, Orrison LH, Smith SJ, Tison DL, Pope DH. Ecological distribution of *Legionella pneumophila*. Appl Environ Microbiol 1981;41:9-16.
33. Foy HM, Broome CV, Hayes PS, Allan I, Cooney MK, Tobe R. Legionnaires' disease in a prepaid medical-care group in Seattle 1963--75. Lancet 1979;1:767-70.
34. Fraser DW, Tsai TR, Orenstein W, et al. Legionnaires' disease: description of an epidemic of pneumonia. N Engl J Med 1977;297:1189-97.
35. Garrity GM, Brown A, Vickers RM. *Tatlockia* and *Fluoribacter*: Two new genera of organisms resembling *Legionella pneumophila*. Int J Syst Bacteriol 1980;30:609-14.

36. Girod JC, Reichman RC, Winn WC Jr, Klaucke DN, Vogt RL, Dolin R. Pneumonic and nonpneumonic forms of legionellosis. The result of a common-source exposure to *L. pneumophila*. Arch Intern Med 1982;142:545-7.
37. Glick TH, Gregg MB, Berman B, Mallison G, Rhodes WW Jr, Kassanoff I. Pontiac fever. An epidemic of unknown etiology in a health department: I. Clinical and epidemiologic aspects. Am J Epidemiol 1978;107:149-60.
38. Goldstein JD, Keller JL, Winn WC Jr, Myerowitz RL. Sporadic *Legionellaceae* pneumonia in renal transplant recipients. A survey of 70 autopsies, 1964 to 1978. Arch Pathol Lab Med 1982;106:108-11.
39. Gorman GW, Feeley JC, Steigerwalt A, Edelstein PH, Moss CW, Brenner DJ. *Legionella anisa*: a new species of *Legionella* isolated from potable waters and a cooling tower. Appl Environ Microbiol 1985;49:305-9.
40. Haley CE, Cohen ML, Halter J, Meyer RD. Nosocomial Legionnaires' disease: a continuing common-source epidemic at Wadsworth Medical Center. Ann Intern Med 1979;90:583-6.
41. Hebert GA, Moss CW, McDougal LK, Bozeman FM, McKinney RM, Brenner DJ. The rickettsia-like organisms TATLOCK (1943) and HEBA (1959): bacteria phenotypically similar to but genetically distinct from *Legionella pneumophila* and the WIGA bacterium. Ann Intern Med 1980;92:45-52.
42. Helms CM, Massanari RM, Zeitler R, et al. Legionnaires' disease associated with a hospital water system: a cluster of 24 nosocomial cases. Ann Intern Med 1983;99:172-8.
43. Herwaldt LA, Gorman GW, McGrath T, et al. A new *Legionella* species, *Legionella feeleii* species nova, causes Pontiac fever in an automobile plant. Ann Intern Med 1984;100:333-8.
44. Hoffman PS, Pine L, Bell S. Production of superoxide and hydrogen peroxide in medium used to culture *Legionella pneumophila*: catalytic decomposition by charcoal. Appl Environ Microbiol 1983;45:784-91.
45. Joly JR, Winn WC. Correlation of subtypes of *Legionella pneumophila* defined by monoclonal antibodies with epidemiological classification of cases and environmental sources. J Infect Dis 1984;150:667-71.
46. Kalweit WH, Winn WC Jr, Rocco TA Jr, Girod JC. Hemodialysis fistula infections caused by *Legionella pneumophila*. Ann Intern Med 1982;96:173-5.
47. Kirby BD, Snyder KM, Meyer RD, Finegold SM. Legionnaires' disease: report of sixty-five nosocomially acquired cases and review of the literature. Medicine 1980;59:188-205.
48. Klein GC. Cross-reaction to *Legionella pneumophila* antigen in sera with elevated titers to *Pseudomonas pseudomallei*. J Clin Microbiol 1980;11:27-9.
49. Kohler RB, Winn WC Jr, Wheat LJ. Onset and duration of urinary antigen excretion in Legionnaires disease. J Clin Microbiol 1984;20:605-7.
50. Kuchta JM, States SJ, McGlaughlin JE, et al. Enhanced chlorine resistance of tap water-adapted *Legionella pneumophila* as compared with agar medium-passaged strains. Appl Environ Microbiol 1985;50:21-6.
51. Kurtz JB, Bartlett CL, Newton UA, White RA, Jones NL. *Legionella pneumophila* in cooling water systems. Report of a survey of cooling towers in London and a pilot trial of selected biocides. J Hyg (Lond) 1982;88:369-81.
52. Lattimer GL, Rhodes LV III, Salventi JS, et al. The Philadelphia epidemic of Legionnaire's disease: clinical, pulmonary, and serologic findings two years later. Ann Intern Med 1979;90:522-6.
53. Mangione EJ, Remis RS, Tait KA, et al. An outbreak of Pontiac fever related to whirlpool use, Michigan 1982. JAMA 1985;253:535-9.
54. Marrie TJ, Haldane EV, Noble MA, Faulkner RS, Martin RS, Lee SH. Causes of atypical pneumonia: results of a 1-year prospective study. Can Med Assoc J 1981;125:1118-23.
55. Mayock R, Skale B, Kohler RB. *Legionella pneumophila* pericarditis proved by culture of pericardial fluid. Am J Med 1983;75:534-6.

56. McCabe RE, Baldwin JC, McGregor CA, Miller DC, Vosti KL. Prosthetic valve endocarditis caused by *Legionella pneumophila*. Ann Intern Med 1984;100:525-7.
57. McDade JE, Shepard CC, Fraser DW, Tsai TR, Redus MA, Dowdle WR. Legionnaires' disease: isolation of a bacterium and demonstration of its role in other respiratory disease. N Engl J Med 1977;297:1197-1203.
58. Muder RR, Yu VL, McClure JK, Kroboth FJ, Kominos SD, Lumish RM. Nosocomial Legionnaires' disease uncovered in a prospective pneumonia study. JAMA 1983;249:3184-8.
59. Nagington J, Wreghitt TG, Tobin JO, Macrae AD. The antibody response in Legionnaires' disease. J Hyg (Lond) 1979;83:377-81.
60. Neill MA, Gorman GW, Gibert C, et al. Nosocomial legionellosis, Paris, France. Evidence for transmission by potable water. Am J Med 1985;78:581-8.
61. Nolte FS, Conlin CA, Roisin AJ, Redmond SR. Plasmids as epidemiological markers in nosocomial Legionnaires' disease. J Infect Dis 1984;149:251-6.
62. Orrison LH, Cherry WB, Fliermans CB, Dees SB, McDougal LK, Dodd DJ. Characteristics of environmental isolates of *Legionella pneumophila*. Appl Environ Microbiol 1981;42:109-15.
63. Osterholm MT, Chin TD, Osborne DO, et al. A 1957 outbreak of Legionnaires' disease associated with a meat packing plant. Am J Epidemiol 1983;117:60-7.
64. Pasculle AW, Dowling JN, Frola FN, McDevitt DA, Levi MA. Antimicrobial therapy of experimental *Legionella micdadei* pneumonia in guinea pigs. Antimicrob Agents Chemother 1985;28:730-4.
65. Posner MR, Caudill MA, Brass R, Ellis E. Legionnaires' disease associated with rhabdomyolysis and myoglobinuria. Arch Intern Med 1980;140:848-50.
66. Reingold AL, Thomason BM, Brake BJ, Thacker L, Wilkinson HW, Kuritsky JN. *Legionella* pneumonia in the United States: the distribution of serogroups and species causing human illness. J Infect Dis 1984;149:819.
67. Rihs JD, Yu VL, Zuravleff JJ, Goetz A, Muder RR. Isolation of *Legionella pneumophila* from blood with the BACTEC system: a prospective study yielding positive results. J Clin Microbiol 1985;22:422-4.
68. Sathapatayavongs B, Kohler RB, Wheat LJ, White A, Winn WC Jr. Rapid diagnosis of Legionnaires' disease by latex agglutination. Am Rev Respir Dis 1983;127:559-62.
69. Selander RK, McKinney RM, Whittam TS, et al. Genetic structure of populations of *Legionella pneumophila*. J Bacteriol 1985;163:1021-37.
70. Shands KN, Ho JL, Meyer RD, et al. Potable water as a source of Legionnaires' disease. JAMA 1985;253:1412-16.
71. Storch G, Baine WB, Fraser DW, et al. Sporadic community- acquired Legionnaires' disease in the United States. A case-control study. Ann Intern Med 1979;90:596-600.
72. Terranova W, Cohen ML, Fraser DW. 1974 outbreak of Legionnaires' Disease diagnosed in 1977. Clinical and epidemiological features. Lancet 1978;2:122-4.
73. Thacker L, McKinney RM, Moss CW, Sommers HM, Spivack ML, O'Brien TF. Thermophilic sporeforming bacilli that mimic fastidious growth characteristics and colonial morphology of *Legionella*. J Clin Microbiol 1981;13:794-7.
74. Thacker WL, Plikaytis BB, Wilkinson HW. Identification of 22 *Legionella* species and 33 serogroups with the slide agglutination test. J Clin Microbiol 1985;21:779-82.
75. Vereerstraeten P, Stolear JC, Schoutens-Serruys E, et al. Erythromycin prophylaxis for Legionnaire's disease in immunosuppressed patients in a contaminated hospital environment. Transplantation 1986;41:52-4.
76. Vickers RM, Yu VL. Clinical laboratory differentiation of *Legionellaceae* family members with pigment production and fluorescence on media supplemented with aromatic substrates. J Clin Microbiol 1984;19:583-7.
77. Wadowsky RM, Wolford R, McNamara AM, Yee RB. Effect of temperature, pH, and oxygen level on the multiplication of naturally occurring *Legionella pneumophila* in potable water. Appl Environ Microbiol 1985;49:1197-1205.

78. Wadowsky RM, Yee RB, Mezmar L, Wing EJ, Dowling JN. Hot water systems as sources of *Legionella pneumophila* in hospital and nonhospital plumbing fixtures. Appl Environ Microbiol 1982;43:1104-10.
79. Westerman EL, McDonald J. Tularemia pneumonia mimicking Legionnaires' disease: isolation of organism on CYE agar and successful treatment with erythromycin. South Med J 1983;76:1169-70.
80. Wilkinson HW, Brake BJ. Formalin-killed versus heat-killed *Legionella pneumophila* serogroup 1 antigen in the indirect immunofluorescence assay for legionellosis. J Clin Microbiol 1982;16:979-81.
81. Wilkinson HW, Cruce DD, Broome CV. Validation of *Legionella pneumophila* indirect immunofluorescence assay with epidemic sera. J Clin Microbiol 1981;13:139-46.
82. Wilkinson HW, Farshy CE, Fikes BJ, Cruce DD, Yealy LP. Measure of immunoglobulin G-, M-, and A-specific titers against *Legionella pneumophila* and inhibition of titers against nonspecific, gram-negative bacterial antigens in the indirect immunofluorescence test for legionellosis. J Clin Microbiol 1979;10:685-9.
83. Wilkinson HW, Fikes BJ. Detection of cell-associated or soluble antigens of *Legionella pneumophila* serogroups 1 to 6, *Legionella bozmanii, Legionella dumoffii, Legionella gormanii* and *Legionella micdadei* by staphylococcal coagglutination tests. J Clin Microbiol 1981;14:322-5.
84. Wilkinson HW, Fikes BJ, Cruce DD. Indirect immunofluorescence test for serodiagnosis of Legionnaires' disease: evidence for serogroup diversity of Legionnaires' disease bacterial antigens and for multiple specificity of human antibodies. J Clin Microbiol 1979;9:379-83.
85. Wilkinson HW, Reingold AL, Brake BJ, McGiboney DL, Gorman GW, Broome CV. Reactivity of serum from patients with suspected legionellosis against 29 antigens of *Legionellaceae* and *Legionella*-like organisms by indirect immunofluorescence assay. J Infect Dis 1983;147:23-31.
86. Winn WC Jr, Myerowitz RL. The pathology of the *Legionella* pneumonias. A review of 74 cases and the literature. Hum Pathol 1981;12:401-22.
87. Winn WC Jr, Pasculle AW. Laboratory diagnosis of infections caused by *Legionella* species. Clin Lab Med 1982;2:343-69.
88. Yu VL, Zuravleff JJ, Gavlik L, Magnussen MH. Lack of evidence for person-to-person transmission of Legionnaires' disease. J Infect Dis 1983;147:362.
89. Zimmerman SE, French ML, Allen SD, Wilson E, Kohler RB. Immunoglobulin M antibody titers in the diagnosis of Legionnaires disease. J Clin Microbiol 1982;16:1007-11.
90. Zuravleff JJ, Yu VL, Shonnard JW, Davis BK, Rihs JD. Diagnosis of Legionnaires' disease. An update of laboratory methods with new emphasis on isolation by culture. JAMA 1983;250:1981-5.

CHAPTER 18

LEPTOSPIROSIS

Michael A. Saubolle, Ph.D.

INTRODUCTION

Leptospirosis, a protean clinical entity in humans, is a zoonosis with nearly worldwide distribution. Wild and domestic animals act as major reservoirs, with humans as accidental hosts. Although extensively studied since the beginning of this century, human leptospiral infections are infrequently diagnosed.

Leptospirosis was recognized a century ago as a severe, icteric disease in man. Thirty years later, the etiologic agent was isolated and named *Spirochaeta icterohemorrhagiae*. Morphologic similarity was noted between this clinical isolate and the environmental spirochete named *Spirochaeta biflexa* isolated at approximately the same time from water in the United States. Both groups of organisms differed morphologically from all other known genera of spirochetes and were placed in their own genus, *Leptospira*.[11,26]

The rodent population was almost immediately recognized as a major reservoir of *L. icterohemorrhagiae* in areas around the world, as well as in the United States.[26] Although the rat was initially believed to be the sole reservoir, a variety of other animal reservoirs were soon discovered, including dogs, cattle, swine, goats and hamsters. The rat, however, remains the primary source of human infection. It also became apparent that various animal species acted as natural reservoirs for leptospiral isolates having substantial serologic differences from *L. icterohemorrhagiae*. These serologically different organisms, now placed into separate serovars, were at first associated with specific animal reservoirs. It was later discovered that serovars were not limited to specific hosts, nor were individual animal hosts limited to parasitism by single serovars.[11,26]

Concomitant with the discovery of additional serovars of *Leptospira*, it became clear that the clinical manifestations of leptospirosis in man were extremely diverse. In the United States, leptospires were found to cause such clinical entities as Fort Bragg Fever, Wycon Fever and Bushy Creek Fever.[11] Approximately 25 different syndromes were directly linked to leptospires throughout the world.[11,26]

The leptospires were recently promoted to their own family, the *Leptospiraceae*, which together with the *Spirochaetaceae* family, are placed in the order *Spirochaetales*.[14] The *Spirochaetaceae* family contains four genera, while the *Leptospiraceae* family has only a single recognized genus, *Leptospira*. This genus is comprised of two well defined species, *L. interrogans* and *L. biflexa*, as well as a third poorly defined species, *L. illini*, included as a *species incertae sedis*. The new genus name *Leptonema* has been proposed but not yet accepted for this last leptospire.[14]

CAUSATIVE ORGANISMS

Leptospires are slender, helical, tightly-coiled rods normally 6-20 μm in length and 0.1-0.2 μm in width. The coils are so tightly wound that it is difficult to see them under darkfield microscopy or in stained films. The organisms are usually hooked at either one or both ends, although this characteristic is medium-dependent and may be absent. Because of their width and light-refractive properties, leptospires are not visible by ordinary light microscopy, but are easily visualized by darkfield and phase-contrast. These organisms stain poorly with aniline dyes, but may be stained with fluorescent antibody or with silver-impregnation techniques, although the latter often distorts cellular appearance.[2,8,26] Leptospires have both rotational and translational motility. In fluid media, organisms may show darting, back and forth movement. In more viscous environments or in semi-solid media, leptospiral motility is characterized as flexuous, serpentine and boring.[2,8,14,26]

Nutritional and growth requirements of leptospires are fairly simple. The organisms are strictly aerobic with a preference for microaerophilic conditions. They also require long-chain fatty acids, thiamine, vitamin B_{12} and ammonium, as well as inorganic salts. Optimal temperatures for growth range between 28-30°C, but a temperature of 37°C may be withstood for a few days. Leptospires prefer neutral or slightly alkaline environments with the optimal pH ranging between 7.2 and 7.4. They are extremely sensitive to dehydration and may not survive short exposure to dry conditions. Growth is usually slow, with generation times ranging between 6-16 hours. Overgrowth with other bacteria may occur easily.[2,8,14,26]

Species of *Leptospira* are morphologically identical and they are all capable of producing oxidase, catalase and/or peroxidase. Characteristic differences between *L. interrogans* and *L. biflexa* include the former's pathogenicity in animals, sensitivity to purine analogues and conversion to spherical forms by 1 M NaCl, and the latter's ability to grow at 13°C, as well as lipase activity. The species also differ in moles percent guanine plus cytosine content of DNA; DNA hybridization studies have described seven distinct groups within the genus.[14] Most recently, restriction endonuclease analysis of chromosomal DNA in leptospires has been proposed as the most accurate means for their characterization. [17,25]

The present standard for classification, however, rests primarily on antigenic analysis by a microscopic agglutination procedure. The basic taxon, the serovar, includes isolates which are shown by cross-absorption studies to share a majority of antigens. For convenience rather than for taxonomic purposes, serovars which crossreact partially, sharing common antigens, are combined into categories called serogroups.[2,8,14] At present, the pathogenic species *L. interrogans* contains 180 or more serovars assembled into 19 serogroups, while the free-living species *L. biflexa* contains more than 60 serovars assembled into 38 serogroups.[14]

Unfortunately, serologic criteria for classification are often complicated by the presence of heat-labile antigens in some leptospires, by the unavailability of standardized antisera and by the technical difficulty inherent in antigenic determination studies.[26] Improvements in isolation and characterization of leptospiral chromosomal DNA by restriction enzyme analysis may serve as a more standard means for classifying *Leptospira* in the future.[15,17,25]

CLINICAL MANIFESTATIONS

Clinical recognition of leptospirosis is difficult because of its protean manifestation in humans. Although totally asymptomatic disease may occur, the majority of cases present in the anicteric form.[6,11,13,24] Human infections usually result from exposure to leptospires in contaminated environments. The organisms gain entry via cutaneous abrasions or through contact with mucous membranes, including those around the nose, mouth or eyes.[11,27]

Normal incubation periods range from 7-13 days, although periods of 2-30 days have been reported.[13,21,24] Disease may vary from a mild, anicteric syndrome to severe manifestation of jaundice, impaired renal and hepatic function, vascular collapse, hemorrhage, azotemia, disturbance in consciousness and high mortality.[1,7,11,21] The severe form of the disease is much less common (5-10% of recognized cases) than the protean presentation (85% of recognized cases).[11] In either case, onset is abrupt in most patients. The most commonly reported symptom is fever (88% of cases), followed by headache (71%), myalgia (62%) and chills (55%).[1,10,18] According to some reports, a typical but often unrecognized symptom is conjunctival suffusion.[21] Less frequently recognized symptoms include nonproductive cough, nausea and/or vomiting, diarrhea, conjunctivitis, pharyngitis, lymphadenopathy and rash or cutaneous hypersensitivity.

The difficulty in recognition of leptospirosis is reflected in the reports made to the Centers for Disease Control (CDC) for the years 1974-1978.[18] Of the 160 confirmed cases, only 26.9% were initially diagnosed correctly. The presence and recognition of symptoms may depend on the severity of the disease, presently thought to be related more to the disposition and age of the patient than to the infecting leptospiral serovar. Icteric and anicteric forms of leptospirosis are typically biphasic in their course. The incubation period culminates abruptly in an initial febrile period of 4-9 days duration, followed first by an afebrile interval with symptomatic improvement for 1-3 days and then a secondary febrile period.[7,21] The first febrile phase is an acute manifestation of systemic disease, with leptospires present in blood and cerebrospinal fluid (CSF) but not yet recoverable in urine. The second phase occurs concomitantly with the disappearance of leptospires from blood and spinal fluid, with their appearance in urine and with appearance of IgM antibodies. The symptoms in the second phase may be extremely variable, ranging from few recognizable symptoms of short duration to extended periods of morbidity. It is in the second phase that aseptic meningitis becomes a principle manifestation. It is also in the second phase that the Weil's form of the disease becomes recognizable in severe cases.[7] In a few cases, myocarditis may develop. Renal failure may occur, and recently, a patient with leptospirosis was reported to develop hemolytic uremic syndrome.[12,21]

Prognosis is good in most cases, depending on patient age and the presence or absence of jaundice. The case fatality rate is higher for patients older than 60 years of age.[18] In the United States, the overall fatality rate for the period 1971-1979 ranged from 2.2% to 9.7%.[21]

THERAPY

The role of antimicrobial therapy in leptospirosis has been controversial. In vitro and animal studies suggest that leptospires are susceptible to most of the penicillins, cephalosporins, tetracyclines, erythromycin and streptomycin, while being resistant to chloramphenicol, the sulfa agents and neomycin. Generally, it is believed that therapy is beneficial only if initiated within 2-4 days of clinical presentation.[1,4,10]

The most popular therapy includes either high dose parenteral penicillin G or oral tetracycline.[10] Reports of a Jarisch-Herxheimer reaction in patients receiving penicillin suggests that agent's activity against leptospires.[21] However, penicillin does not seem to eliminate the organisms from the kidney whereas tetracycline does.[10] Oral amoxicillin and ampicillin have also been reported to be of benefit.[10] In severe cases, general supportive therapy is paramount and probably of greater benefit to the patient than antimicrobial therapy.

Although penicillin has been commonly used in therapy of leptospirosis, its role in prophylaxis is questionable.[4] Recent studies indicate the efficacy of doxycycline for prophylaxis and support its effectiveness in therapy of leptospirosis if administered within the first three days of illness.[19,24]

EPIDEMIOLOGY

The pathogenic leptospiral serovars are almost all members of the species *L. interrogans*. Serovars of *L. biflexa*[1] are normally saprophytic water leptospires and considered incapable of infecting animals and humans.[8] Although a few *L. biflexa* serovars have recently been isolated from animals, including rats and horses, their role in disease is uncertain.[8]

Leptospirosis due to serovars of *L. interrogans* is one of the most extensive zoonoses in the world. Over 181 species of animals are known to harbor leptospires and almost every known mammal may carry and disseminate these organisms.[26] The importance of certain animals in transmission of disease to humans depends on the degree of association between man and animal, as well as on the virulence of the leptospires.

Pathogenic leptospires are perpetuated in animals within the convoluted tubules of the kidney. Infected animals may remain asymptomatic, may not show any serologic conversion and may shed organisms in urine for extensive periods. Immunized pet dogs with documented high antibody titers have been shown to still excrete and transmit organisms to humans.[11]

Transmission to humans occurs most frequently by exposure to environments contaminated by infected urine, and less commonly by direct contact with infected materials from animals. Shed leptospires may remain viable and infectious from a few days to several weeks in appropriate natural environments, including water and soil. Neutral or alkaline pH, moderate temperatures and the presence of moisture are especially conducive to leptospiral viability and infectivity. Human to human transmission occurs rarely, if ever. However, infection during pregnancy may lead to fetal death and spontaneous abortion.[8,11]

The average number of leptospiral cases reported annually to the CDC has been less than 100 during the past three decades. [5] The greatest number of cases reported in that time period occurred in 1978 (110 cases); the lowest number in 1983 (61 cases). Peak incidence occurs between July and October.[5,18] Most cases occur in males between the ages of 20-30 years.[18]

Considered a vocational disease for many years, leptospirosis has become more commonly recognized in individuals with no vocational exposures. Although occupational exposures such as those experienced by farmers, ranchers, trappers and veterinarians, as well as by abattoir and sewer workers, still pose a significant risk, the majority of recently reported cases are sporadic and apparently unrelated to job exposure.[11,18] Disease usually occurs following contact with contaminated recreational water, pets and livestock.[11,18,27] Serogroups most commonly implicated in human disease in the United States include icterohaemorrhagiae, canicola, autumnalis, grippotyphosa, hebdomadis, australis, pomona and ballum (Table 18:1).[18]

PUBLIC HEALTH SIGNIFICANCE, PREVENTION AND CONTROL

Leptospirosis is a major public health problem in many developing or agricultural countries, although not presently an important public health problem in the United States.[8] It does, however, have an impact on veterinary medicine and poses a substantial animal health problem in this country.

The changing epidemiology of leptospirosis in the United States is due in part to measures to control hazards in the occupational environment. Decontamination programs have been successful in reducing the infection rate in such righ risk environments as rat-infested sewers and fishgutting sheds.[11] Worker awareness and use of safety precautions may also have contributed to the decline in common source outbreaks.[11] Rodent control is more difficult to achieve, but may help to decrease the prevalence of infection even further.[8,11]

Immunization of humans is not routinely recommended in the United States, but is used to control leptospirosis in domestic animal populations. Serovar-specific vaccines usually employ two or more serovars reflecting the predominant leptospires found in the area. Immunized animals may still shed leptospires and are susceptible to infection by serovars not included in vaccines. Use of doxycycline for human prophylaxis has been suggested,

Table 18:1. Important Serogroups of *Leptospira interrogans* in the United States with their Primary and Secondary Animal Hosts

Serogroup (Occurrence)*—Primary; (secondary animal hosts)†
Icterohaemorrhagiae (35%)—rats; (cattle, dogs, foxes, hedgehogs, horses, mice, muskrats, raccoons, skunks, woodchucks)
Canicola (14%)—dogs; (armadillos, cats, cattle, hamsters, hedgehogs, horses, pigs, raccoons, rats, skunks, voles)
Autumnalis (13%)—mice; (cattle, dogs, opossums, raccoons, rats)
Grippotyphosa (17%)—rodents; (cats, cattle, dogs, foxes, goats, hedgehogs, mice, muskrats, opossums, pigs, rabbits, raccoons, rats, other rodents, sheep, shrews, skunks, weasels)
Hebdomadis (7%)—rodents; (cattle, dogs, other rodents)
Australis (6%)—rats; (cattle, dogs, foxes, horses, opossums, other rodents, raccoons, skunks, weasels)
Pomona (5%)—pigs, cattle; (horses, rodents, skunks, wildcats)
Ballum (3%)—mice; (cattle, dogs, foxes, horses, rabbits, raccoons, other rodents)

* Based on % of total reported serogroups by Martone,[18] exclusive of cases in which serogroups were unknown.

† Compiled from Alexander[1] and Sonnewirth.[22]

and may be warranted in areas where attack rates are five percent or greater, but not in areas where rates are less than one percent.[21,24]

DIAGNOSTIC PROCEDURES

Diagnostic confirmation of leptospirosis can be made by direct microscopic visualization of the organism, by recovery of organisms in culture or by serology. The practicality and efficiency of different microscopic, cultural and serologic techniques depends on their availability and on the period of the disease under study. Laboratories having little experience with leptospirosis should seek the assistance of either reference or public health laboratories with appropriate expertise when processing specimens from patients suspected of having leptospirosis. All laboratories should, however, be capable of selecting, processing and properly submitting appropriate specimens to reference laboratories.

Selection and Processing of Specimens

Blood, CSF, urine and serum are most frequently tested. Selection depends on the course of the infectious process. Blood and CSF specimens may yield leptospires during the first febrile period and should be collected within the first seven to ten days of illness. Detection in urine is possible during the second week of illness and shedding continues intermittently for several months or longer. Tissue specimens collected by biopsy or at autopsy may also be productive; kidney and liver tissues are preferred. Antibody, which begins to appear during the second week of illness, reaches highest levels during the third or fourth week. Detectable antibody titers may persist for years. Muliple specimens are recommended for detecting leptospires and/or for demonstrating leptospiral antibody. Because of the frequent presence of leptospiral inhibitors in specimens, small amounts of blood and CSF are cultured and urine is serially diluted prior to culture.[2,8,11]

Blood should be defibrinated or collected with anticoagulants such as heparin, sodium oxalate, or sodium polyanetholesulfonate, but not citrate.[2,8,22] Clotted blood may also be used if the clot is first asceptically dispersed and a 10% suspension prepared in physiologic saline. Leptospires may remain viable for up to 10 days in such specimens held at room temperature.

Cerebrospinal fluid can be centrifuged to concentrate the leptospires prior to culturing. Biopsy or autopsy tissue should be ground and may be stored for short periods at 4°C and for longer periods by rapid freezing. Addition of glycerol may enhance survival of organisms in tissues. Clean-catch midstream urine should be collected carefully to avoid contamination by other bacteria. The pH of the urine should be checked and adjusted to neutrality if necessary.[8] Addition of bovine serum albumin to diluted urine may enhance leptospiral survival.[8] Filtration through 0.22 μm or 0.45 μm filters is not recommended, as the procedure may drastically lower the numbers of leptospires.[26]

Blood collected for serologic analysis should be allowed to clot, the serum harvested and processed as for other serologic procedures.

Rapid Methods

Rapid methods for detection of leptospires in human infections are not routinely available at present. Direct microscopic evaluations of specimens are the quickest to perform but have marked disadvantages. Enzyme-linked immunosorbent assays (ELISA) have been suggested as rapid methods for detection of both soluble leptospiral antigens in tissues as well as specific IgM class antibody in serum during the acute phase of illness.[9,20]

Microscopy

Darkfield microscopy has been used to detect leptospires in CSF, body fluids and tissue preparations, while direct fluorescent-antibody staining and silver impregnation techniques have been used to demonstrate organisms in tissue and urine.[1] The latter have been especially useful for autopsy specimens or specimens requiring extended periods of time for transport. However, these methods are often plagued by their low sensitivity and specificity; leptospires usually occur in low concentrations in human specimens, and artifacts caused by cellular extrusions may confuse the inexperienced microscopist. When performing darkfield microscopy, the worker must observe typical morphology as well as motility for accurate identification.[8] Differential centrifugation of unclotted blood for darkfield microscopy and addition of formalin to centrifuged urine for fluorescent microscopy may increase the chance of demonstrating leptospires in these specimens. However, negative findings should not be construed as precluding the presence of *Leptospira*. Both positive and negative microscopic findings should be confirmed by cultural and serologic means.[1,8]

Primary Isolation and Culture

Leptospira may be cultured fairly easily if appropriate fresh specimens and media are used.[23] Cultures are essential for epidemiologic characterization. Single specimens may not always yield the organism and multiple, serial specimens are recommended. Leptospires are slow-growing, requiring incubation periods of 1.5 to 4 weeks for detection by conventional culture methods. Radiometric methods for culture and detection may prove to substantially reduce time for recovery.[16]

Media for growth of pathogenic leptospires require supplementation with bovine serum albumin and polysorbate 80 (e.g., Ellinghausen & McCullough medium and its modification by Johnson and Harris) or with buffered salts and rabbit serum (e.g., Fletcher's, Stuart's, Korthof's media).[1,8,14] Semi-solid media are preferred and many are commercially available. [,8,10] Antimicrobials such as 5-fluorouracil may be added to media to prevent bacterial contamination, but such supplemented media should only be used in conjunction with, and not as a replacement for, regular media. Some authors recommend inoculating multiple tubes of media, preferably media from at least two different lots.[8] In all cases, careful quality control must be exercised to assure the growth capabilities of various media.

Normally sterile, uncontaminated specimens may be cultured directly in tubes containing 5-10 mL of media. Blood specimens may be cultured by transferring 1-4 drops to the surface of each of 3-5 tubes of media. Approximately 0.5 mL of appropriately processed CSF may likewise be cultured directly.[8,22]

Urine must be serially diluted with either liquid medium or buffered physiologic saline prior to tube inoculation. One drop of each urine dilution (ranging from undiluted to a $1{:}10^5$ dilution) should be inoculated in the same manner as for blood specimens. Sterile urine collected by suprapubic aspiration should be cultured undiluted and at 1:10 and 1:100 dilutions. Tissues should be ground, diluted 1:10 to 1:100[4] and cultured in the same manner as urines.[5,8,22]

All cultures should be incubated at 30°C in the dark.[10,22] Tubes should be examined at 5 to 7 day intervals both macroscopically for growth in the form of a ring approximately 1-3 cm below the surface of the medium, and by darkfield microscopy. Although growth usually appears within the first two weeks, cultures should be examined for a minimum of four weeks and preferably up to 5-6 weeks before being reported as negative.[1,8,22]

Positive cultures should be transferred to fresh medium. Stock cultures survive well in medium for 6-8 weeks at room temperature; freezing at low temperatures[1] is needed for longer storage.

Intraperitoneal inoculation of animals such as weanling hamsters, young guinea pigs, chinchillas and gerbils has been advocated to enhance leptospiral recovery, especially from contaminated specimens. Superiority of animal inoculation over culture is controversial.[8] Although animal inoculation may increase isolation rates, availability of this service is not common.

Methods for Identification

Isolation of morphologically typical organisms showing characteristic growth and motility patterns is usually adequate for confirmation of leptospirosis.[1] Leptospires within the species *L. interrogans* cannot be differentiated biochemically, nor is virulence for animals a reliable means of identification.[22] Further identification is accomplished by serologic techniques. Tentative characterization to serogroup level may be obtained by microscopic agglutination studies using live or formalin-fixed organisms. Formalin-killed organisms may also be studied by macroscopic slide agglutination, a method not as sensitive as the microscopic test but probably adequate and simpler to perform.[22]

Reciprocal agglutinin-absorption studies are needed for definitive identification to the serovar level. These should be performed by the leptospiral reference laboratory at the CDC. Isolates and patient sera can be submitted to the CDC through local and state health laboratories. Although definitive identification is not necessary for patient care, serovar identity is important for epidemiologic investigations and surveillance.

Serologic Procedures

Diagnosis of leptospirosis is most commonly made by serologic means, since cultures are infrequently attempted. Antibodies to leptospires usually appear by the end of the first week of illness and peak by the third to fourth week.[10] Response may be variable among individual patients and may be suppressed or delayed by antimicrobial therapy.[10,20] Evaluation of paired, acute and convalescent (collected 2-4 weeks or longer after onset of illness) sera is most helpful in diagnosis of recent infection.[8] The presence of antibody in single serum specimens is indicative of past infection and may remain variably elevated for years.[20] Although serologic studies provide clues to the identity of the infecting serovar, definitive establishment of the etiologic serovar can only be made by isolation and serologic typing of the leptospiral organism.[3]

Several serologic methods have been described, including microscopic agglutination, macroscopic (slide or plate) agglutination, hemolytic, indirect hemagglutination and complement fixation tests, as well as ELISA.[3,8,20,22]

The microscopic agglutination test, being the most sensitive and serovar specific, has become the standard reference procedure. Because of its high serovar specificity, multiple serovar antigens must be tested to assure detection of antibody against specific serovars. Although at least 15 serovar antigens have been recommended for testing, use of 8 specific serovar anigens would probably detect the majority of leptospiral cases in the United States.[3] Serum titers of 1:20 or more are often considered evidence of exposure or possible previous infection.[6] Titers of 1:100 or more are considered significant, while single serum titers greater than or equal to 1:1,600 are strong presumptive evidence of recent infection.[2,3] The test is time-consuming, technically difficult and may require maintenance of a large variety of live leptospiral serovars.[3]

Currently, the macroscopic slide agglutination test is the simplest alternative to microscopic agglutination. Its practicality is enhanced by the availability of commercial antigen preparations, while its sensitivity and specificity are adequate to diagnose acute or recent leptospirosis. However, it is not as sensitive as microscopic agglutination, and titers range to approximately 1:160.[3]

Other serologic techniques such as indirect hemagglutination, hemolytic, complement fixation and ELISA tests, suffer from the lack of commercially available entigens. These methods, however, show promise for detecting acute leptospirosis and are far simpler and less technically demanding than the standard reference method. Generally, these studies detect genus specific rather than species or serovar specific antibodies. There are several in-depth reviews dealing with specific serologic methods.[2,3,5,8,22]

REFERENCES

1. Alexander AD. Leptospirosis. In: Hoeprich PD, ed. Infectious diseases. 3rd ed. Philadelphia: Harper and Row, 1983;751-9.
2. Alexander AD. Leptospira. In: Lennette EH, Balows A, Hausler WJ Jr, Shadomy HJ, eds. Manual of clinical microbiology. 4th ed. Washington, DC: American Society for Microbiology, 1985:473-8.
3. Alexander AD. Serologic diagnosis of leptospirosis. In: Rose NR, Friedman H, Fahey JL, eds. Manual of clinical immunology. 3rd ed. Washington, DC: American Society for Microbiology, 1986:435-9.
4. Broom JC, Norris TStM. Failure of prophylactic oral penicillin to inhibit a human laboratory case of leptospirosis. Lancet 1957;1:721-2.
5. Centers for Disease Control. Annual summary 1983: reported morbidity and mortality in the United States. Morbid Mortal Weekly Rep 1984;32:3-6,30.
6. Demers RY, Frank R, Demers P, Clay M. Leptospiral exposure in Detroit rodent control workers. Am J Public Health 1985;75:1090-1.
7. Edwards GA, Domm BM. Human leptospirosis. Medicine 1960;39:117-21.
8. Ellinghausen HC Jr, Thiermann AB, Sulzer CR. Leptospirosis. In: Balows A, Hausler WJ Jr, eds. Diagnostic procedures for bacterial, mycotic and parasitic infections. 6th ed. Washington, DC: American Public Health Association, 1981:463-99.
9. Fairbrother JM. Effects of autolysis of tissue and urine on the viability, morphology, and antigenicity of *Leptospira interrogans* serovar *pomona*. J Clin Microbiol 1985;21:189-94.
10. Farrar WE. *Leptospira* species (leptospirosis). In: Mandell GL, Douglas RG Jr, Bennett JE, eds. Principles and practice of infectious diseases. 2nd ed. New York: John Wiley, 1985:1338-41.
11. Feigin RD, Anderson DC. Human leptospirosis. In: Heath CW, ed. Critical reviews in clinical laboratory sciences; vol 5. Washington, DC: U.S. Department of Health Education and Welfare, Public Health Service, 1975:413-67.
12. Hanvanich M, Moolaor P, Suwangool P, Sitprija V. Hemolytic uremic syndrome in leptospirosis bataviae. Nephron 1985;40:230-1.
13. Jacobs R. Leptospirosis-medical staff conference. University of California, San Francisco. West J Med 1980;132:440-50.
14. Johnson RC, Faine S. Family II. *Leptospiraceae* Hovind-Hougen 1979,245. In: Krieg NR, Holt JG, eds. Bergey's manual of systematic bacteriology; vol 1. Baltimore: Williams and Wilkins, 1984:62-7.

15. Le Febvre RB, Foley JW, Thiermann AB. Rapid and simplified protocol for isolation and characterization of leptospiral chromosomal DNA for taxonomy and diagnosis. J Clin Microbiol 1985;22:606-8.
16. Manca N, Verardi R, Colombrita D, Ravizzola G, Savoldi E, Turano A. Radiometric method for the rapid detection of *Leptospira* organisms. J Clin Microbiol 1986;23:401-3.
17. Marshall RB, Winter PJ, Yanagawa R. Restriction endonuclease DNA analysis of *Leptospira interrogans* serovars *icterohaemorrhagiae* and *hebdomadis*. J Clin Microbiol 1984;20:808-10.
18. Martone WJ, Kaufman AF. Leptospirosis in humans in the United States, 1974-1978. J Infect Dis 1979;140:1020-2.
19. McClaine JBL, Ballou WR, Harrison SM, Steinweg DL. Doxycycline therapy for leptospirosis. Ann Intern Med 1984;100:,696-8.
20. Milner AR, Jackson KB, Woodruff K, Smart IJ. Enzyme-linked immunosorbent assay for determining specific immunoglobulin M in infections caused by *Leptospira interrogans* serovar *hardjo*. J Clin Microbiol 1985;22:539-42.
21. Sanford JP. Leptospirosis-time for a booster. N Engl J Med 1984;310:524-5.
22. Sonnenwirth AC. The spirochetes. In: Sonnenwirth AC, Jarrett L, eds. Gradwohl's clinical laboratory methods and diagnosis; vol 2. 8th ed. St Louis: C.V. Mosby, 1980:1853-69.
23. Sulzer CZ, Jones WL. Leptospirosis: methods in laboratory diagnosis. Washington, DC: Public Health Service, U.S. Department of Health, Education and Welfare, Publ. No. (CDC),76-8275,1976.
24. Takafuji ET, Kirkpatrick JW, Miller RN, et al. An efficacy trial of doxycycline chemoprophylaxis against leptospirosis. N Engl J Med 1984;310:497-500.
25. Thiermann AB, Handsaker AL, Moseley SL, Kingscote B. New method for classification of leptospiral isolates belonging to serogroup pomona by restriction endonuclease analysis: serovar *kennewicki*. J Clin Microbiol 1985;21:585-7.
26. Torten M. Leptospirosis. In: Steele JH, ed. CRC handbook series in zoonoses; vol 1. Boca Raton, FL: CRC Press, 1979:363-421.
27. Waitkens SA. Update on leptospirosis. Br Med J 1985;290:1502-3.

CHAPTER 19

LISTERIOSIS

Mary J. R. Gilchrist, Ph.D.

INTRODUCTION

Since its first description in 1926 as a cause of monocytosis in laboratory animals,[14] this organism has come to be known as a cause of disease in humans and many animals and has been named *Bacterium monocytogenes, Listerella hepatolytica* and finally *Listeria monocytogenes*. This facultative intracellular parasite has long intrigued scientists because of its elicitation of unique host cellular and humoral immune responses. The epidemiology of disease in man and animals caused by this namesake of Lord Lister remains an enigma. Implicated but not proven to cause repeated abortions in humans, the organism has been hypothesized to have affected the course of history. Queen Anne conceived as many as 17 times but was unable to produce an heir to the throne, leaving 18th century England without a Protestant monarch and effecting the rise of Parliament to its present status.[20]

Within the genus *Listeria* are a number of species found in the environment or in animals, some of which are known to cause disease in animals. This chapter will deal almost exlusively with *Listeria monocytogenes*, since it is the only known human pathogen in this group with the rare exception of *L. ivanovii*.

CAUSATIVE ORGANISM

Although *L. monocytogenes* has a tendency to be pleomorphic and appear as cocci or coccobacilli in purulent exudates, the morphology of the organism is most characteristically that of a small, non-acidfast, nonsporeforming rod, 0.5 μm x 1-2 μm,[1,8] that has a tendency to occur in palisade formation, resembling "diphtheroids" (see color plate Fig. 19:1A). Gram-positive in young cultures, *Listeria* organisms are often gram-variable when detected in clinical material and in older cultures.

Listeria monocytogenes is a facultative anaerobe and grows best in the moderate (30-37°C) temperature range.[21] Colonies of *L. monocytogenes* on the surface of blood agar are small, entire, convex, bluish-grey and translucent. Most strains produce a narrow zone of hemolysis (Color plate Fig. 19:1B) that is more pronounced on rabbit than on sheep blood agar. In some cases, it may be necessary to scrape off the colony to visualize the hemolysis underneath. Hemolysis is not constant, particularly in laboratory strains.[21] The Henry effect[10] is observed with colonies grown on clear agar: they appear blue-green when examined with light transmitted through the agar at an oblique angle.

Listeria monocytogenes exhibits a characteristic tumbling motility when growing in broth at room temperature; organisms in wet mounts or hanging drop preparations exhibit end-over-end movement. When the organism is grown in semisolid agar at room temperature, motility is expressed in an "umbrella" shaped turbid area a few millimeters below the surface of the agar (Color plate Fig. 19:1C). When organisms are grown at 35-37°C, flagellar structure and function are compromised and the organisms are nonmotile or weakly motile.

CLINICAL MANIFESTATIONS

Protean in its manifestations, listeriosis is not a disease but a group of diseases.[8] The species of animal and its immune status may detemine clinical manifestations. Ruminants experience encephalitis (circling disease) whereas monogastric animals and young ruminants with a nonfunctional rumen experience septicemia and focal hepatic necrosis.[8] In adult humans, meningitis is the most common form of listeriosis;[16] bacteremia, empyema, endocarditis, encephalitis, endophthalmitis, peritonitis[15] and hepatitis[33] have also been reported. Immunocompromised adults are those most commonly affected, particularly those undergoing renal transplant or cancer chemotherapy.[4,7,16,24] In humans (and other mammals), *Listeria* infections are a common cause of abortion, stillbirth and perinatal disease. Whereas the mother is often asymptomatic or may report a mild, flu-like illness, disease in the infant is associated with considerable morbidity and mortality. Not unlike group B streptococcal infections in neonates, there is an early (<1 week) or delayed (>1 month) onset of septicemia and/or meningitis. Infants born with early, fulminant *Listeria* sepsis (granulomatosis infantiseptica) usually have evidence of transplacental infection (abscesses in placental tissue) and usually exhibit multisystem (liver, spleen, central nervous system, lung, intestine) infection.[1] Primary cutaneous listeric infections have been described in veterinarians and animal handlers. Monocytosis is an atypical feature of human infection with *L. monocytogenes*; human infections are characterized by a polymorphonuclear response in peripheral blood, cerebrospinal fluid (CSF) and tissue.[22]

THERAPY

The results of in vitro antimicrobial susceptibility tests of clinical isolates of *L. monocytogenes* are depicted in Table 19:1. Newer methods of antimicrobial susceptibility testing involving decreased incubation periods may be invalid for *L. monocytogenes*, since one such system has been shown to falsely predict resistance to penicillin.[17]

As with all microorganisms, in vitro antimicrobial susceptibility data do not necessarily predict therapeutic success. Since *Listeria* is an intracellular parasite with a propensity to invade sequestered sites (central nervous system, placenta), an antibiotic that penetrates host cells and crosses the blood-brain barrier or placenta may be required. In devising therapy for immunocompromised patients, it is often considered necessary to include a bactericidal antibiotic since host defenses do not adequately complement the action of a bacteriostatic agent. *L. monocytogenes* is not killed by penicillin and ampicillin; bactericidal concentrations at least four two-fold dilutions above the minimum inhibitory concentration have been observed with these antimicrobials.[31] Synergistic action of combinations of antimicrobials has been documented.[31,27] For renal transplant recipients, intravenous therapy with ampicillin and gentamicin has been recommended; prolonged duration of therapy (3 weeks) may be necessary to avoid relapses.[25] Tetracycline, erythromycin and chloramphenicol are bacteriostatic and should be avoided.[32] Trimethoprim-sulfamethoxazole is usually bactericidal to *L. monocytogenes* and may ultimately prove to provide adequate alternative therapy.[24]

Table 19:1. Antibiotic Susceptibility (MIC_{90}) of *Listeria monocytogenes**

Antibiotic	Wiggins, et al.[31] 178 strains, U.S.A.	Larsson, et al.[12] 175 strains, Sweden	Tuazon, et al.[27] 12 strains, U.S.A.
Erythromycin	0.25	0.25	0.312
Penicillin	0.5	0.5	0.625
Ampicillin	0.5	0.5	0.25
Tetracycline	2.0	0.25	—
Chloramphenicol	8.0	8.0	5.0
Gentamicin	4.0	1.0	5.0
Cotrimoxazole		0.5	1.25

* Concentration (μg/ml) required to inhibit growth of 90% of strains tested. Adapted from data in references cited.

EPIDEMIOLOGY

Widespread in nature, *L. monocytogenes* has been isolated from many different mammals, both feral and domesticated, and from fish, fowl, water, mud and sewage. Human fecal carriage has been demonstrated to occur in 1-12% of healthy adults and 44% of pregnant females to whom normal infants were delivered.[18] Several recent epidemics in which a common source was culturally documented and/or epidemiologically implicated have helped to elucidate the mechanisms of transmission. In 1981 in Nova Scotia, an outbreak occurred that was traced to cole-slaw made from cabbage grown on ground fertilized with manure from infected sheep and stored over winter in a cool storage area. In 1983 in Massachusetts, pasteurized milk was found to be the source of an outbreak. In 1985 in Los Angeles, an outbreak was traced to the consumption of Mexican-type soft cheese from a Los Angeles county processor. In these three outbreaks, even though exposure to the incriminated product was experienced by a diverse population of humans, affected individuals were primarily those in the perinatal period and immunocompromised adults.

PUBLIC HEALTH SIGNIFICANCE

Since listeriosis is not a reportable disease in the United States nor in most other countries, the extent and significance of infections may go unrecognized unless a large outbreak occurs. Manifest largely in the immunocompromised, listeriosis is of considerable public health significance. As intervention strategies such as cancer chemotherapy and organ transplantation increase the number of immunocompromised patients, control of transmission of this agent will be of increasing importance. Studies underway to determine how cheese and pasteurized milk became contaminated with *Listeria* may lead to improvements in surveillance and monitoring of procedures for food preparation, thus subsequently decreasing the incidence of human fecal carriage and of human disease.

DIAGNOSTIC PROCEDURES

Selection and Processing of Specimens

The clinical manifestations of meningitis and septicemia due to *Listeria* are not unique. Thus, in most cases the laboratory will not be alerted to culture specifically for the organism but rather will be sent CSF or blood for routine culture. Fortunately, the organism grows readily on media routinely employed for the evaluation of such specimens, appearing within 24 hours of aerobic incubation at 35°C. Therefore, no special processing of specimens is indicated for specimens from sterile body fluids. When *Listeria* occurs in sites contaminated with other microorganisms, such as feces, vagina, placenta and food, selective enrichment techniques may be necessary to ensure recovery. Specimens awaiting transport to a public health laboratory should be maintained at 4°C to minimize overgrowth by other organisms.

Rapid Methods

Present at low numbers in CSF, *Listeria* is often not detected by Gram stain. Pleomorphic and gram-variable when present, it may be misread as a coccus or gram-negative bacillus. The application of fluorescent antibody techniques to human clinical material has been used as a rapid method; problems include crossreactions with gram-positive cocci, subjectivity in interpretation of appropriate fluorescence intensity and the labor-intensive nature of the work. New technologies, e.g., flow cytometry and nucleic acid probes, may ultimately provide means for screening foods or clinical materials rapidly.

Primary Isolation and Culture

The organism grows readily on blood agar plates inoculated with sterile body fluids. It may be detected as a small colony with a narrow zone of hemolysis on sheep, rabbit or horse blood agar. Special selective media should accompany non-selective primary media for examination of contaminated specimens. Columbia colistin-nalidixic acid (CNA) agar[5] or tellurite blood agar [6] may be employed as a selective medium. In public health and research laboratories, enrichment broths and selective media appropriate to the microbiologic milieu have been devised[13,29] to detect the organism in food, feces and the environment. For tissues and environmental specimens, cold enrichment, i.e., incubation in broth at 4°C with plating onto selective and/or differential media at intervals, may be superior to direct plating on selective or differential media.[6,29]

Methods for Identification

Identification of *Listeria* is not difficult; the greatest problem lies in producing a protocol which assures that the organism is not overlooked. As it is often coccoid, is esculin-positive, bile and 6.5% NaCl tolerant, hippurate-positive and CAMP-positive, it is potentially misidentified as enterococcus[30] or as group B *Streptococcus*.[11] Subtle differences in colonial morphology and hemolysis, and drastic differences in CAMP reactions (Figure 19:1d) would often be clues to its identity. Nevertheless, it is prudent to include a test for catalase in every protocol for the identification of streptococci. *Listeria* is catalase-positive whereas streptococci are catalase-negative.

To ensure that *Listeria* is not discarded as a contaminating "diphtheroid," laboratory protocols should require that all gram-positive, asporogenous rods forming beta-hemolytic, catalase-positive colonies be tested for motility at room temperature, particularly those from cultures of sterile body fluids. If the isolate is motile at room temperature, a presumptive *Listeria* is present. To distinguish *L. monocytogenes* from other genera of asporogenous gram-positive bacilli, consult Table 19:2. Although *L. monocytogenes* is the most common species of *Listeria* recovered from human clinical material, other beta-hemolytic *Listeria* species have been reported. *Listeria monocytogenes* may be distinguished from these by fermentation tests. *Listeria monocytogenes* uniquely produces acid from rhamnose but not xylose.[21] Isolates of *Listeria* spp. other than *L. monocytogenes* should be submitted to a reference laboratory for characterization.

Markers of Epidemiologic Importance

Available in public health laboratories, serotyping involves detection of both O and H antigens.[21] Serotypes 1/2a, 1/2b and 4b are commonly found as causes of epidemics and account for the majority of the cases of listeriosis in humans; serotypes 3a, 3b, 4d and 4e are less common isolates from humans. Serotyping may not be used to identify the organism since other members of the genus *Listeria* are known to possess the O and H antigens of *L. monocytogenes*. Serotyping is useful to establish that *L. monocytogenes* isolates of different serotypes are not from a common source. Since there are so few serotypes, two isolates of the same serotype cannot be presumed a priori to have a common source. Phage typing schemes for *L. monocytogenes* permit typing of many serotype 4 and 1/2 strains.[26] These schemes

Table 19:2. Differentiation Among *Listeria* and Similar Genera of Asporogenous Gram-Positive Bacilli*

	Motile	Oxygen Require-ments	Catalase Activity	Hydrogen Sulfide Produced	Acid from Glucose
Listeria	+†	Facultative	+	−	+
Erysipelothrix	−	Facultative	−	+	+
Lactobacillus	−‡	Facultative	−‡	−	+
Kurthia	+	Aerobic	+	−‡	−

* Adapted from References 2, 21 and 28. *L. monocytogenes,* because of its motility, catalase positivity and beta hemolysis, is readily distinguished from *Corynebacterium* spp., *Bacterionema* spp. and *Oerskovia* spp., because none possess all three of these characteristics.
† Motile 20-25°C, reduced or no motility 35-37°C.
‡ Few strains positive.

may be applied to isolates of the same serotype from apparent outbreaks to document a common source; they have yielded results implying cross-infection among neonates in a hospital setting.[26] Isoenzyme analysis has been developed as an adjunct to phage typing to discriminate strains within a serotype.[3]

Serology

Serologic procedures have little value in the diagnosis of listeriosis. Individuals with no known history of listeric infection often have low titers of antibody to *Listeria*, at least partially due to the presence on *Listeria* of antigens that crossreact with other gram-positive organisms, such as *Staphylococcus aureus* and *Streptococcus faecalis*. Thus, it is necessary to demonstrate a four-fold rise in titer to document infection. Unique to *L. monocytogenes* infections, the humoral immune response of humans is of the IgM class. Since these antibodies persist, the presence of IgM cannot be used as a marker for acute disease. Finally, neonates and immunocompromised patients may not mount a humoral immune response.

REFERENCES

1. Ahlfors CE, Goetzman BW, Halstead CC, Sherman MP, Wennberg RP. Neonatal listeriosis. Am J Dis Child 1977;131:405-8.
2. Bortolussi R, Schlech WF III, Albritton WL. Listeria. In: Lennette EH, Balows A, Hausler WJ Jr, Shadomy HJ, eds. Manual of clinical microbiology. 4th ed. Washington, DC: American Society for Microbiology. 1985:205-8.
3. Bibb WF, Kuffner TA, Weaver RE. Typing of *Listeria monocytogenes* by isoenzyme analysis [Abstract]. Annual meeting of the American Society for Microbiology. Washington, DC: American Society for Microbiology, 1986.
4. Cherubin CE, Marr JS, Sierra MF, Becker S. *Listeria* and gram-negative bacillary meningitis in New York City, 1972-1979: frequent causes of meningitis in adults. Am J Med 1981;71:199-209.
5. Clarridge JE, Weissfeld AS. *Listeria monocytogenes*. Clin Microbiol Newsletter 1985;7:59-62.
6. Finegold SM, Baron EJ. Bailey and Scott's diagnostic microbiology. St. Louis: C.V. Mosby Company, 1986.
7. Gantz NM, Myerowitz RL, Medeiros AA, Carrera GF, Wilson RE, O'Brien TF. Am J Med 1975;58:637-43.
8. Gray JL, Killinger AH. *Listeria monocytogenes* and listeric infections. Bacteriol Rev 1966;30:309-82.
9. Issekutz TB, Lee SHS, Bortolussi R. Immune response to *Listeria monocytogenes*. In: Rose NR, Friedman H, Fahey JL, eds. Manual of clinical immunology. 3rd ed. Washington, DC: American Society for Microbiology. 1986:402-7.
10. Henry BS. Dissociation in the genus *Brucella*. J Infect Dis 1933;52:374-402.
11. Kontnick C, von Graevenitz A, Piscitelli V. Differential diagnosis between *Streptococcus agalactiae* and *Listeria monocytogenes* in the clinical laboratory. Ann Clin Lab Sci 1977;7:269-76.

12. Larsson S, Walder MH, Cronberg SN, Forsgren AB, Moestrup T. Antimicrobial susceptibilities of *Listeria monocytogenes* strains isolated from 1958 to 1982 in Sweden. Antimicrob Agents Chemother 1985;28:12-14.
13. Mavrothalassitis P. A method for the rapid isolation of *Listeria monocytogenes* from infected material. J Appl Bacteriol 1977;43:47-52.
14. Murray EGD, Webb RA, Swann MBR. A disease of rabbits characterized by large mononuclear leucocytosis, caused by a hitherto undescribed bacillus *Bacterium monocytogenes* . J Pathol Bacteriol 1926;29:407-39.
15. Myers JP, Peterson G, Rashid A. Peritonitis due to *Listeria monocytogenes* complicating chronic ambulatory peritoneal dialysis. J Infect Dis 1983;148:1130.
16. Nieman RE, Lorber B. Listeriosis in adults: a changing pattern. Report of eight cases and review of the literature, 1968-1978. Rev Infect Dis 1980;2:207-27.
17. Overman TL, Dillon PA. False resistance of *Listeria monocytogenes* to penicillin G with the Autobac AIS test [Abstract]. Annual meeting of the American Society for Microbiology. Washington, DC: American Society for Microbiology, 1986.
18. Relier JP. Listeriosis. J Antimicrob Chemother 1979;5(suppl A):51-7.
19. Recourt J, Grimont PAD. *Listeria welshimeri* sp. nov. and *Listeria seeligeri* sp. nov. Int J Syst Bacteriol. 1983;33:866-9.
20. Saxbe WB. *Listeria monocytogenes* and Queen Anne. Pediatrics 1972;49:97-101.
21. Seeliger HPR, Jones D. Listeria. In: Sneath PHA, Mair NS, Sharpe E, eds. Bergey's manual of systematic bacteriology; vol 2. Baltimore: Williams and Wilkins, 1986:1235-45.
22. Shackelford PG, Feigin RD. *Listeria* revisited. Am J Dis Child 1977;131:391-2.
23. Skalka B, Smola J, Elischerova K. Routine test for in vitro differentiation of pathogenic and apathogenic *Listeria monocytogenes* strains. J Clin Microbiol 1982;15:503-7.
24. Spitzer PG, Hammer SM, Karchmer AW. Treatment of *Listeria monocytogenes* infection with trimethoprim-sulfamethoxazole: case report and review of the literature. Rev Infect Dis 1986;8:427-30.
25. Stamm AM, Dismukes WE, Simmons BP, Cobbs CG, Elliott A, Budick P, Harmon J. Listeriosis in renal transplant recipients: report of an outbreak and review of 102 cases. Rev Infect Dis 1982;4:665-82.
26. Taylor AG, McLauchlin J, Green HT, Macaulay MB, Audurier A. Hospital cross-infection with *Listeria monocytogenes* confirmed by phage-typing. Lancet 1981;1:1106.
27. Tauzon CU, Shamsuddin D, Miller H. Antibiotic susceptibility and synergy of clinical isolates of *Listeria monocytogenes*. Antimicrob Agents Chemother 1982;21:525-7.
28. Weaver RE, Hollis DG. Gram-positive organisms: a guide to presumptive identification. Atlanta: Centers for Disease Control, 1983.
29. Welshimer HJ. The genus *Listeria* and related organisms. In: Starr MP, ed. The prokaryotes: A handbook on habitats, isolation and identification of bacteria; vol 2. New York: Springer-Verlag, 1981:1680-7.
30. Wetzler TF, Freeman NR, French ML, Renkowski LA, Eveland WC, Carver BJ. Biological characterization of *Listeria monocytogenes*. Health Lab Sci 1968;5:46-62.
31. Wiggins GL, Albritton WL, Feeley JC. Antibiotic susceptibility of clinical isolates of *Listeria monocytogenes*. Antimicrob Agents Chemother 1978;13:854-60.
32. Winslow DL, Damme J, Dieckman E. Delayed bactericidal activity of betalactam antibiotics against *Listeria monocytogenes*: antagonism of chloramphenicol and rifampin. Antimicrob Agents Chemother 1983;23:555-8.
33. Yu VL, Miller WP, Wing EJ, Romano JM, Ruiz CA, Bruns FJ. Disseminated listeriosis presenting as acute hepatitis. Case reports and review of hepatic involvement in listeriosis. Am J Med 1982;73:773-7.

CHAPTER 20

MISCELLANEOUS GRAM-NEGATIVE ROD INFECTIONS: FASTIDIOUS ORGANISMS

J. R. Greenwood, Ph.D. and Sydney Harvey, Ph.D.

INTRODUCTION

The bacteria covered in this chapter, although different in their metabolism, morphology and biochemical features, are unified by their gram-negative cell wall, fastidious nature and limited pathogenicity. The identification approach and tables used here are adapted from Clark et al.[5]

Actinobacillus

CAUSATIVE ORGANISMS

The genus *Actinobacillus* consists of nonmotile, facultatively anaerobic, fastidious gram-negative coccoid to rod-shaped organisms which have a fermentative type of metabolism. Published reports of the guanine plus cytosine ratio (G+C) of the DNA range from 40-48 mol%. At present, there are five recognized species in the genus: *A. actinomycetemcomitans, A. equuli, A. suis, A. lignieresii* and *A. capsulatus*. *A. capsulatus* is the only species not reported as isolated from man. It has been described as the etiological agent of arthritis in rabbits and it is not known to infect any other animal.

CLINICAL MANIFESTATIONS

A. actinomycetemcomitans is found primarily in man. It has been considered a member of the normal flora of the upper respiratory tract and oral cavity since a 1959 report by Heinrich and Pulverer.[7] Recent evidence, however, appears to implicate it as a major pathogen of destructive periodontal disease.[15] Prior to this linkage, *A. actinomycetemcomitans* was most frequently reported as an agent of bacterial endocarditis or as an isolate from actinomycotic or actinomycotic-like lesions. The pathogenic role of this organism in mixed infections remains unclear.

A. suis is mainly a pathogen of pigs, although it has been reported as a pathogen as well as a commensal of horses. Human isolations of *A. suis* are not frequent but have been obtained from a variety of sources such as animal bite wounds, blood and the upper respiratory tract.

A. equuli has been reported as a commensal at various sites in the horse but it is considered to be primarily a pathogen for both horses and pigs, causing a variety of conditions. It has been isolated only rarely from human sources.

A. lignieresii is the causative agent of a granulomatous disease in cattle and sheep. In cattle, the lesions are found most frequently in the tongue, from which the appellation "wooden tongue" was derived. Granulomatous lesions caused by *A. lignieresii* have also been described in dogs, horses, rats and ducks. The commensal role of *A. lignieresii* has been demonstrated by isolations from the mouth and rumen of normal cattle and sheep. The organism has been isolated from a variety of sources in man (sputum of individuals with infected cervical lymph nodes, from wounds, a brain abscess, blood and animal bites).

THERAPY

In vitro antimicrobial susceptibility data for *Actinobacillus* species are limited. The majority of the data is for *A. actinomycetemcomitans*. Strains of this species are reported as susceptible to chloramphenicol, streptomycin, erythromycin, tetracycline, kanamycin, gentamicin and polymyxin B. Susceptibility to ampicillin and penicillin G has been variable. Strains of *A. suis* are reported ɛ susceptible to ampicillin, chloramphenicol, streptomycin, tetracycline, penicillin G and gentamicin. *A. equuli* and *A. lignieresii* are susceptible to chloramphenicol but variable in their susceptibility to other antibiotics.

EPIDEMIOLOGY AND PUBLIC HEALTH SIGNIFICANCE

Because all species of *Actinobacillus* known to infect man can be found as commensals in humans or animals, disease in man has been ascribed primarily to animal contact or to endogenous origin. Experimental pathogenicity of the actinobacilli is low and no public health significance has yet been demonstrated for any of these organisms.

DIAGNOSTIC PROCEDURES

Microscopic Examination

With the exception of *A. actinomycetemcomitans*, most actinobacilli are usually rod-shaped, although considerable size variation may occur, depending on the medium. *A. actinomycetemcomitans* is similar in morphology to *Haemophilus aphrophilus* with a size comparable to that of *Brucella* species. Characteristically, *A. actinomycetemcomitans* is coccoid to coccobacillary, although rod forms may be present, particularly in agar cultures.

Primary Isolation and Culture

Specimens are inoculated onto blood agar or chocolate agar, or into blood culture broth, depending on the source. Incubation of plates at 35-37°C in an atmosphere containing additional CO_2 promotes growth. Agar colonies of all species tend to be sticky and to adhere to the medium. Growth in broth is usually viscous for all species except *A. actinomycetemcomitans*. Typically, this species forms granules at the bottom and sides of the tube, although occasionally uniform turbidity will prevail. Growth in blood culture bottles may be delayed for 6 days.

Identification Procedures

Biochemical reactions for the genus are listed in Table 20:1. Because of the variability in characteristics, there are no key reactions for placement of an isolate in the genus, *Actinobacillus*. Confirmation of an isolate as an *Actinobacillus* species necessitates a fairly comprehensive biochemical profile.

Strains of *A. suis* are usually β-hemolytic on sheep blood agar; strains of *A. equuli* may be hemolytic on this medium also. No hemolysis is produced by any other members of the genus.

Fermentation of carbohydrates usually occurs within 24 hours, but observation should be extended for at least 1 week, since strain and species variation does occur and acid production may be delayed. Although gas production from glucose is negative for most species, approximately 1/3 of strains of *A. actinomycetemcomitans* produce small quantities of gas.

Markers for Epidemiology

Because of the variability in carbohydrate fermentation exhibited by most species, a number of biotypes have been described. Within the species *A. actinomycetemcomitans*, eight biotypes have been identified on the basis of galactose, mannitol and xylose fermentation.

Table 20:1. Biochemical reactions of *Actinobacillus* species

Feature	*A. actino-mycetemcomitans*	*A. equuli*	*A. lignieresii*	*A. suis*
Catalase	+	+ (73% +)	+ (89% +)	+ (85% +)
Esculin hydrolysis	−	−	−	+
Growth on: SS agar	−	−	−	− (3% +)
MacConkey agar	−	V (89% +)	V (75% +)	+
Motility	−	−	−	−
Nitrate reduction	+	+	+	+
Oxidase	V (19% +)	+	+	+
Simmons Citrate	−	−	−	−
Urea, Christensen's	−	+	+	+
Acid from: Glucose	+	+	+	+
Xylose	+ (42% +)	+	+	+
Mannitol	+	+	+	+ (54% +)
Lactose	−	+	+ (78% +)	+
Sucrose	−	+	+	+
Maltose	+	+	+	+
TSI* slant, acid	+	+	+	+
TSI* butt, acid	+	+	+	+

* Triple sugar iron agar

Serologic Procedures

Antisera are not commercially available for identification, although antigenic types have been described for all species. Antigenic relationships exist among *A. lignieresii, A. equuli* and *A. suis*. Using immunodiffusion techniques,[10] it was shown that heat-stable antigenic complexes have at least one antigenic determinant shared by *A. ligniersii, A. equuli* and *A. suis*. A number of serotypes have been detected in *A. actinomycetemcomitans* but, thus far, no patterns of clinical relevance have emerged.

Moraxella

CAUSATIVE ORGANISMS

Genus *Moraxella* consists of 10 species of aerobic gram-negative rods and cocci. Species are assigned to subgenera on the basis of microscopic morphology; subgenus *Moraxella* containing rod-shaped organisms and subgenus *Branhamella* containing coccal organisms. (A separate genus has been proposed for *Branhamella catarrhalis*, see Chapter 10, "*Branhamella*," for discussion of this organism). The G+C of the DNA ranges from 40.0-47.5 mol%.

CLINICAL MANIFESTATIONS

Moraxella lacunata has been a significant cause of human conjunctivitis and keratitis. Other species such as *M. nonliquefaciens, M. osloensis* and *M. catarrhalis* are considered to be opportunistic pathogens of man. *M. bovis* can cause eye infections in cattle while *M. ovis* causes similar infections in sheep.

THERAPY

Traditionally, all strains assigned genus *Moraxella* are very sensitive to penicillin, but β-lactamase producing isolates have been reported recently.

EPIDEMIOLOGY AND PUBLIC HEALTH SIGNIFICANCE

Moraxella are found on the mucous membranes of man and other warm-blooded animals. Consequently, in the compromised host they have access to the respiratory tract and other sites in the head and neck region. From a disease control standpoint, *Moraxella* are presently of little public health significance. They can, however, present a diagnostic problem in sexually

Table 20:2. Biochemical reactions of selected *Moraxella* species

Feature	*M. phenylpyruvica*	*M. urethralis*	*M. atlantae*	*M. nonliquifaciens*	*M. osloensis*	*M. lacunata*	*M. catarrhalis*
Catalase	+	+	+	+	+	+	+
Esculin hydrolysis	–	–	–	–	–	–	–
Growth on: SS agar	–	– (9% +)	–	–	–	–	–
MacConkey agar	V (86% +)	+	+	–	V (70% +)	–	–
Motility	–	–	–	–	–	–	–
Nitrate reduction	–	+	V (20% +)	+	V (24% +)	+	+
Oxidase	+	+	+	+	+	+	+
Phenylalanine deaminase	+	+	–	–	– (14% +)	V (31% +)	V (68% +)
Simmons Citrate	–	V (46% +)	–	–	–	–	–
Urea, Christensens	+	–	–	–	–	–	–
TSI* acid, slant	–	–	–	–	–	–	–
TSI* acid, butt	–	–	–	–	–	–	–

* Triple sugar iron agar

transmitted diseases clinics if they are misidentified as *Neisseria gonorrhoeae*.

DIAGNOSTIC PROCEDURES

Microscopic Morphology

Members of subgenus *Moraxella* are gram-negative rods that can often be short and plump (1.0-1.5 by 1.5-2.5 μm). They can also occur in pairs or short chains. Members of subgenus *Branhamella* are relatively small gram-negative cocci (0.6-1.0 μm in diameter), occurring either as single cells or pairs. It is not uncommon for both subgenera to resist decolorization of the crystal violet in the Gram stain.

Isolation Methods

All clinically significant *Moraxella* grow on sheep blood agar incubated at 35°C. Isolation of some of the more fastidious strains of *M. lacunata*, however, are facilitated on chocolate agar incubated in a humid atmosphere containing CO_2. Growth on MacConkey agar is variable, with some *Moraxella* species unable to grow on this medium.

Methods for Identification and Markers for Epidemiology

Moraxella species are relatively inert biochemically and distinguishing between species can be difficult. Table 20:2 lists pertinent biochemical features. Sensitivity to a 10-unit penicillin disk can be a useful feature as it helps to separate *Moraxella* and *Moraxella*-like species from other fastidious, oxidase-positive, gram-negative rods and cocci. Genetic transformation techniques for *Moraxella* have been thoroughly described[1] and can be used to recognize strain differences for epidemiological purposes.

Cardiobacterium

CAUSATIVE ORGANISMS

The genus *Cardiobacterium* consists of one species, *Cardiobacterium hominis*, originally designated "group II D organisms" until described and named by Slotnick and Dougherty in 1964.[12] This organism is a fastidious, facultatively anaerobic, nonmotile, pleomorphic gram-negative rod with a fermentative type of metabolism. The G+C ratio of the DNA is 59-60 mol%.

CLINICAL MANIFESTATIONS AND THERAPY

C. hominis causes bacterial endocarditis in humans. No evidence has been found to link this organism with disease in any animal. Few antimicrobial susceptibility studies have been done. Data on nine strains showed susceptibility to penicillin, ampicillin, carbenicillin, cephalothin, chloramphenicol, streptomycin, tetracycline, erythromycin, kanamycin, gentamicin and colistin.[18]

EPIDEMIOLOGY AND PUBLIC HEALTH SIGNIFICANCE

In man, *C. hominis* appears to be part of the normal flora of the upper respiratory tract. In limited studies, this organism was isolated from human fecal specimens as well as from the female genital tract.[14] Endocarditis has occurred subsequent to periodontal disease, dental procedures or other trauma that would allow entry of the organism into the bloodstream. At this time, there is no known public health significance. Prophylactic measures similar to those taken to prevent endocarditis from other oral bacteria would presumably be effective with *C. hominis*.

DIAGNOSTIC PROCEDURES

Microscopic Methods

Cells of *C. hominis* are pleomorphic gram-negative rods which may show retention of crystal violet in the central portion or in the enlarged ends. Teardrop cells and filaments of varying lengths may occur. There is evidence that the degree of pleomorphism is related to the medium on which the organism is grown.

Primary Isolation and Culture

Since blood is the usual specimen for isolation of *C. hominis*, routine blood culture techniques are applicable to primary isolation. Subculture to 5% sheep blood agar is satisfactory and growth is enhanced by high humidity or 3-5% CO_2. Good growth occurs between 30-37°C. The upper and lower limits of growth are 42°C and 22°C. There is no growth on MacConkey or SS agar.

Identification Procedures

On blood agar, colonies are punctate after 24 h at 37°C and achieve a maximum size of 1-2 mm after 48 h. Colonies are unremarkable in appearance;

they are circular, smooth, moist, convex, opaque and nonhemolytic. Indole formation is an important distinguishing characteristic of *C. hominis*; however, indole production may be weak and not detected unless the indole is concentrated by xylene extraction. Additional biochemical features of *C. hominis* are listed in Table 20:3.

Serologic Procedures

There are no commercially available antisera. Slotnick et al[13] used antisera prepared in rabbits to detect *C. hominis* in mixed culture by fluorescent antibody techniques. Antibodies to *C. hominis* have not been detected in individuals from whom the organism was isolated as part of the normal flora. Sera of individuals with *C. hominis* endocarditis, however, have been shown to agglutinate the infecting strain.

EVALUATION OF LABORATORY FINDINGS

At present, only isolates of *C. hominis* from blood are considered significant; isolates from the upper respiratory, the intestinal or the genital tract are deemed insignificant.

Kingella

CAUSATIVE ORGANISM

Kingella is a relatively new genus of fastidious gram-negative organisms previously considered to be *Moraxella*.[8] The three species now in genus *Kingella, K. kingae, K. indologenes* and *K. denitrificans* (previously designated as CDC TM-1) differ from *Moraxella* in that *Kingella* species are catalase-negative and saccharolytic.

CLINICAL MANIFESTATIONS AND THERAPY

K. kingae is increasingly being recognized as an organism that can cause osteomyelitis, endocarditis, septic arthritis and bacteremia. *K. indologenes* and *K. denitrificans* are considered to have limited pathogenic potential. *K. kingae* is susceptible to benzyl- and phenoxymethyl penicillin, ampicillin, oxacillin, piperacillin, doxycycline, chloramphenicol, streptomycin, tobramycin, gentamicin and carbenicillin. Increased resistance to erythromycin has been reported in a treatment failure of a 56-year old patient with *K. kingae* endocarditis.[4]

Table 20:3. Biochemical reactions of *Cardiobacterium hominus*, genus *Capnocytophaga*, *Eikenella corrodens* and *Kingella* species

Feature	*C. hominis*	*K. denitrificans*	*K. indologenes*	*K. kingae*	*Capnocyto-phaga*	*Eikenella corrodens*
Catalase	–	– (10% +)	–	–	– (7% +)	– (8% +)
Esculin hydrolysis	NA†	NA	NA	NA	V (83% +)	–
Growth on: SS agar	–	–	–	–	–	–
McConkey agar	–	–	–	– (36% +)	–	–
Indole	+	–	+	–	NA	NA
Motility	–	–	–	–	V (gliding)	–
Nitrate reduction	–	+	–	– (6% +)	V (63% +)	+
Oxidase	+	+	+	+	– (7% +)	+
Simmons Citrate	–	–	–	–	–	–
Urea, Christensen's	–	–	–	–	–	–
Acid from: Glucose	+	+ (92% +)	+	+ (90% +)	+	–
Lactose	–	–	–	–	+ (88% +)	–
Maltose	+	–	+	+	+	–
Mannitol	+	–	–	–	–	–
Sucrose	+	–	+	–	+	–
Xylose	–	–	–	–	–	–
TSI*, slant acid	+	NA	NA	NA	V (73% +)	–
TSI*, butt acid	V (84% +)	NA	NA	NA	V (55% +)	–
Arginine dihydrolase	NA	NA	NA	NA	NA	–
Lysine decarboxylase	NA	NA	NA	NA	NA	V (82% +)
Ornithine decarboxylase	NA	NA	NA	NA	NA	+

* Triple sugar iron agar
† Not Applicable

EPIDEMIOLOGY AND PUBLIC HEALTH SIGNIFICANCE

K. kingae and *K. denitrificans* are normal flora of the oral and nasopharyngeal tracts. It appears that clinical infections by these organisms can be initiated through damage to the mucosa at these body sites. *Kingella* have little, if any, public health significance. *K. denitrificans* has caused diagnostic problems, however, when it has been misidentified as *N. gonorrhoeae*.

DIAGNOSTIC PROCEDURES

Microscopic Methods

Kingella are straight gram-negative rods, approximately 1 μm by 2-3 μm in size with rounded or square ends. They can appear in pairs or short chains. There is some tendency to resist Gram stain decolorization.

Primary Isolation, Culture and Methods for Identification

Kingella strains grow on sheep blood agar and colonies generally reach 0.1-0.5 mm in diameter after 24 hours of incubation at 35°C. Although CO_2 is not required, a humid atmosphere can improve growth. *K. kingae*, the most frequently encountered species of *Kingella*, is strongly beta-hemolytic on sheep blood agar. *K. denitrificans* (TM-1) can be selectively isolated on Thayer-Martin medium. Table 20:3 lists pertinent biochemical reactions that distinguish the three *Kingella* species.

EVALUATION OF LABORATORY FINDINGS

K. kingae can be considered as pathogenic when isolated in pure culture from normally sterile body sites. Other species should be evaluated on a case-by-case basis.

Capnocytophaga

CAUSATIVE ORGANISM

Genus *Capnocytophaga* was proposed in 1982 and, although it does not appear in Bergey's Manual, volume 1, 1984,[2] it is considered to be validly published. Three species have been described: *C. ochracea* (synonymous with *Bacteroides ochraceus*), *C. gingivalis* and *C. sputigena*. These organisms were originally designated the DF-1 (dysgonic fermenter) group. *Capnocytophaga* species are fastidious, gram-negative, fusiform bacteria which exhibit gliding motility, have a fermentative metabolism and require CO_2 for either aerobic or anaerobic growth. The G+C ratio of the DNA is 39-41 mol%.

CLINICAL MANIFESTATIONS AND THERAPY

Capnocytophaga species are associated with diseases of the oral cavity (particularly periodontal disease) as well as systemic diseases in compromised hosts. These species appear to have an antimicrobial profile similar to that of true anaerobes. Aminoglycosides are routinely inactive and cephalosporins, with the exception of cefoxitin, can be ineffective or only bacteriostatic. The organisms are susceptible to penicillin, carbenicillin, clindamycin, erythromycin, tetracycline, metronidazole, cefoxitin and chloramphenicol. Most strains are resistant to oxacillin and vancomycin.

EPIDEMIOLOGY AND PUBLIC HEALTH SIGNIFICANCE

Because *Capnocytophaga* species have been isolated from supragingival dental plaque of asymptomatic individuals, these organisms are considered to be part of the normal flora of the upper respiratory tract. In a recent study,[11] 500 clinical specimens from a variety of sources (throat, sputum, sinus, skin, urine, stool, wound, vagina and cervix) were screened for *Capnocytophaga* species. All 75 isolates were recovered from respiratory tract specimens only. The Centers for Disease Control, however, has received isolates from a variety of anatomical sites in addition to the respiratory tract. At this time there is no public health significance to isolations of *Capnocytophaga*.

DIAGNOSTIC PROCEDURES

Microscopic Examinations

Capnocytophaga species are gram-negative fusiform bacteria which may vary in length from 2-6 μm depending upon the medium of growth. Organisms do not demonstrate motility in wet mount preparations because the cells are usually nonflagellated, although an occasional cell may have a single polar or lateral flagellum-like structure. The gliding motility of log-phase cultures can be observed by darkfield microscopy.

Primary Isolation and Culture

Capnocytophaga species require primary culture on 5% sheep blood agar plates incubated anaerobically at 35-37°C. Although the organisms grow in atmospheres of increased CO_2, comparative studies have shown optimal recovery occurs under anaerobic conditions.[6] Plates should be held for 5 days before being discarded as negative.

Identification Procedures

The colonial morphology varies, depending to some extent on the medium and the atmospheric conditions. Some isolates form mucoid and nonadherent colonies whereas others form colonies that adhere so tightly to the medium that the growth is extremely difficult to remove. Some colonies appear to "pit" the agar. Depending on the medium, colonies may exhibit flat, spreading, finger-like projections indicative of the organism's gliding motility. Although colony color may be white-gray, pink or yellow, almost all strains are yellow-pigmented when scraped from the agar surface and viewed under direct light.

Motility medium is not used to detect the gliding motility of *Capnocytophaga* species, although some strains will grow out slightly from the stab line. Biochemical tests for distinguishing among the species of *Capnocytophaga* are listed in Tables 20:3 and 20:4.

Serological Procedures

Studies have demonstrated a common antigen in all *Capnocytophaga* species which does not crossreact with other gram-negative oral bacteria and a second antigen which distinguishes among strains.[17]

EVALUATION OF LABORATORY FINDINGS

At present, isolations of *Capnocytophaga* species from blood and oral lesions are considered to be significant, but the relevance of isolations from other sites has not yet been investigated.

Table 20:4. Differential features of *Capnocytophaga* species*

	C. ochracea		*C. sputigena*		*C. gingivalis*	
Feature	Reaction	%+	Reaction	%+	Reaction	%+
Acid from:						
Lactose	+	92	V	40	–	8
Galactose	V	83	–	0	–	0
Nitrate reduction	–	8	V	83	–	4

* Adapted from Reference 16.

Eikenella corrodens

CAUSATIVE ORGANISM

The genus *Eikenella* was established by Jackson and Goodman in 1972 to include organisms previously referred to as HB-1 or as *Bacteroides corrodens*.[9] As established, the genus contains a single, genetically uniform species, *E. corrodens*. The G+C ratio of the DNA is 56-58 mol%.

CLINICAL MANIFESTATIONS AND THERAPY

Although *E. corrodens* is apparently of low pathogenic potential, it does have the ability to infect virtually any body site. Reports in the literature demonstrate that *E. corrodens* has caused brain and liver abscesses, meningitis, fatal endocarditis, peritonitis and infections of the lips and face. Infections with *E. corrodens* after human bites have also been reported frequently.

Most *E. corrodens* isolates are sensitive to penicillin G, ampicillin and cefoxitin. Some strains are also sensitive to chloramphenicol, tetracycline and colistin. Variable resistance to cephalothin and aminoglycosides is reported, but all strains are resistant to clindamycin and metronidazole.

EPIDEMIOLOGY

E. corrodens is a normal inhabitant of the human mouth and intestine. It appears to be an opportunistic pathogen capable of producing disease in the compromised host or after trauma to the body sites where it commonly resides (e.g., dental procedures). A possible relationship to periodontal disease with bone destruction has also been reported.

DIAGNOSTIC PROCEDURES

Microscopic Morphology

E. corrodens is a straight, gram-negative rod approximately 0.3-0.4 by 1.5-4.0 μm in size. It has a uniform morphology with rounded ends.

Primary Isolation and Culture

Optimal conditions for isolation of *E. corrodens* from clinical specimens include the use of fresh sheep blood agar plates (preferably with Columbia agar base), 5-10% CO_2 and a temperature of 35°C. At 24 h, colonies are small (0.2-0.5 mm) but at 48 h can reach 0.5-1.0 mm. On continued incubation they can reach 3.0 mm. Two types of colonies may appear on blood agar. The first type, for which the species is named, appear to corrode the agar surface. The colonies are opaque, yellowish and appear as if they are in small pits in the surface of the agar. Stains that do not corrode are dome-shaped, translucent and 0.5-1.0 mm in diameter. A selective *E. corrodens* isolation medium has been described.[3]

Identification Methods

Table 20:3 lists the biochemical reactions of *E. corrodens*. The species is extremely uniform in its features with virtually all reactions being either 100% positive or negative. Positive ornithine and lysine decarboxylase reactions help to distinguish *Eikenella* from other fastidious gram-negative organisms.

REFERENCES

1. Bovre K. Transformation and DNA base composition in taxonomy with special reference to recent studies in *Moraxella* and *Neisseria*. Acta Pathol Microbiol Scand 1967;69:123-44.
2. Bovre K. Family VIII. *Neisseriaceae* Prevot 1933, 119[AL]. In: Krieg NR, Holt JC, eds. Bergey's manual of systematic bacteriology; vol 1. Baltimore: Williams and Wilkins, 1984;288-309.
3. Brooks GF, O'Donoghue JM, Rissing JP, Soapes K, Smith JW. *Eikenella corrodens*, a recently recognized pathogen: infections in medical-surgical patients and in association with methylphenidate abuse. Medicine 1974;53:325-42.
4. Claesson B, Falsen E, Bengt K. *Kingella kingae* infections: A review and a presentation of data from 10 Swedish cases. Scand J Infect Dis 1985;17:233-43.
5. Clark WA, Hollis DG, Weaver RE, Riley P. Identification of unusual pathogenic Gram-negative aerobic and facultatively anaerobic bacteria. Centers for Disease Control, USDHHS, 1984.
6. Forlenza S, Newman MG. *Capnocytophaga*. In: Bottone EJ, ed. Unusual microorganisms. New York: Marcel Dekker, 1983:45-66.
7. Heinrich S, Pulverer G. Zur atiologic and mikrobiologic der *Aktinomykose*. II. Difinition und praktische diagnostik des *Actinobacillus actinomycetemcomitans*. Zentral Bakteriol Parasit Infect Hyg Abt Orig 1959;174:123-36.
8. Henriksen SD, Bovre K. Transfer of *Moraxella kingae* Henriksen and Bovre to the genus *Kingella* gen. nov. in the family *Neisseriaceae*. Int J Syst Bacteriol 1976;26:447-50.
9. Jackson FL, Goodman YE. Transfer of the facultatively anaerobic organism *Bacteroides corrodens* Eiken to a new genus, *Eikenella*. Int J Syst Bacteriol 1972;22:73-7.
10. Kim BH. Studies on *Actinobacillus equuli* [Dissertation]. University of Edinburgh, 1976.
11. Marucha PT, Horikoshi AL, Newman MG, Martin W. Incidence of *Capnocytophaga* in oral and non-oral specimens [Abstract]. J Dental Res 1980;59:324.
12. Slotnick IJ, Dougherty M. Further characterization of an unclassified group of bacteria causing endocarditis in man: *Cardiobacterium hominis* gen. et sp. n. Antonie van Leeuwenhoek J Microbiol Serol 1964;30:261-72.
13. Slotnick IJ, Mertz JA, Dougherty M. Fluorescent antibody detection of human occurrence of an unclassified bacterial group causing endocarditis. J Infect Dis 1964;114:503-5.

14. Slotnick IJ. *Cardiobacterium hominis* in genitourinary specimens. J Bacteriol 1968;95:1175.
15. Slots J. The predominant cultivable organisms in juvenile periodontitis. Scand J Dental Res 1976;84:1-10.
16. Socransky SS, Holt SC, Leadbetter ER, Tanner ACR, Savott E, Hammond BF. *Capnocytophaga*: A new genus of Gram-negative gliding bacteria III. Physiological characterization. Arch Microbiol 1979;122:29-33.
17. Stevens RH, Hammond BF, Lai CH. Group and type antigens of *Capnocytophaga*. Infect Immun 1979;23:532-7.
18. Wormser GP, Bottone EJ. *Cardiobacterium hominis*. In: Bottone EJ, ed. Unusual organisms: Gram-negative fastidious species. New York: Marcel Dekker, 1983:67-86.

CHAPTER 21

MISCELLANEOUS GRAM-NEGATIVE ROD INFECTIONS: NONFASTIDIOUS ORGANISMS

Charles H. Zierdt, Ph.D.

INTRODUCTION

The genera and groups described in this chapter are *Acinetobacter, Achromobacterium, Alcaligenes, Chromobacterium, Flavobacterium, Agrobacterium, Sphingobacterium* and Centers for Disease Control (CDC) groups EO-2, IV-e and IVc-2. *Chromobacterium*, a glucose fermenter, is included with the genera of non-glucose fermenting gram-negative rods (NFB).

About 15% of all isolates in clinical microbiology laboratories are glucose nonfermenters and the majority of these are *Pseudomonas* spp. Though they are less frequently encountered, it is important that the remaining genera and species be accurately identified. Since some NFB grow better in 5-10% CO_2, blood plates should be incubated in that atmosphere or in a candle jar. It should be remembered that some NFB fail to grow well at 35-37°C, so that growth at 30°C or at room temperature may be required.

Acinetobacter

INTRODUCTION

Bouvet and Grimont[3] now assign to *Acinetobacter* 12 genospecies and 3 ungrouped strains, based first on DNA similarity groups and then on biochemical reactions. They have named only 6 of these genospecies: *A. calcoaceticus* (genospecies 1), *A. lwoffi (genospecies 8), A. haemolyticus* (genospecies 4), *A. baumannii* (genospecies 2), *A. johnsonii* (genospecies 7) and *A. junii* (genospecies 5). *A. alcaligenes* is absorbed into *A. haemo-*

lyticus. There is the probability of yet further named species. This scheme remains an option for those laboratories willing to utilize it. The other options are Gilardi's four biotypes,[11] or the currently widely used *A. calcoaceticus* var *anitratus, A. calcoaceticus* var *lwoffi*, or as many do, simply to report *A. calcoaceticus*. When the latter is done, it is understood that, stated or not, reference is to the classic *Bacterium anitratum*. Bouvet and Grimont[3] have combined *Acinetobacter calcoaceticus* biovars alcaligenes and haemolyticus as *A. haemolyticus*. By far the most common species isolated from infections is *A. calcoaceticus* var *anitratus*.

CAUSATIVE ORGANISM

Generally, *Acinetobacter* species are short or coccoid gram-negative rods that counterstain deep red, looking much like the *Neisseria*, with which they may be confused. Under decolorized strains may appear to be gram-positive cocci or coccobacilli. *A. calcoaceticus* may also be confused with *Haemophilus influenzae* or *Streptococcus pneumoniae*, causing delay in correct diagnosis and therapy. *Acinetobacter* are more typically rod-shaped during logarithmic growth. Capsules are present in mucoid strains. Flagella and spores are absent. They are strict aerobes, oxidase-negative, catalase-positive, grow readily on routinely used agars and grow at 20-30°C, with optimal growth at 33-35°C. *Acinetobacter* is ubiquitous in nature, except that it has not been found in sea water.

CLINICAL MANIFESTATIONS

A. calcoaceticus and its varieties are not strongly toxigenic. They are opportunistic pathogens, gaining entrance to the body via contaminated solutions, and indwelling bladder and intravenous catheters. *A. calcoaceticus* infects the increasing number of seriously ill, compromised patients in hospitals. It is now both a common commensal and an important pathogen of wounds. It causes pneumonia, urinary tract infections, meningitis and septicemia. Most of these infections are predisposed by various invasive procedures or by trauma. In a trauma center, it was observed[21] that severely injured patients frequently suffered *A. calcoaceticus* var *anitratus* septicemia but survived, compared to bacteremia caused by unrelated, more virulent organisms, leading to death.

Premature infants have shown *A. calcoaceticus* var *lwoffi* meningitis, evidently acquired during birth. *A. calcoaceticus* var *lwoffi* infections occur infrequently, predominently as meningitis that mimics meningococcal meningitis. Meningitis induced by head trauma and caused by *A. calcoaceticus* var *anitratus* was indolent and did not progress to fulminant disease, even when initial therapy was inappropriate and the organism persisted in the cerebrospinal fluid.[2]

THERAPY

Most strains are sensitive to carbenicillin, trimethoprim-sulfamethoxazole, aminoglycosides and polymyxins. The *Acinetobacter*, except the variable *A. lwoffi*, are resistant to penicillin. Aminoglycosides usually have a minimum inhibitory concentration (MIC) below the expected serum level. Rapid susceptibility testing is most important, as no single drug can be used with total confidence. Combinations of an aminoglycoside and ticarcillin or piperacillin should be used until susceptibility results are obtained. Synergism may occur.[10]

EPIDEMIOLOGY

Much like *Pseudomonas aeruginosa, A. calcoaceticus* is associated with water as wet environs—solutions, aerosols, baths, irrigation units, dialysis tanks and injectables. It also colonizes the mucosae and the skin of man. Up to 25% of healthy individuals may harbor it on the skin. It has been found in 7% of the respiratory tracts of healthy persons, but it is not usually found in the colon. *A. calcoaceticus* has been reported to cause urinary tract infection, but true infections are rare compared to frequent isolation from the urinary tract. Ear infections have been reported.[8]

A late summer peak of *A. calcoaceticus* var *anitratus*, both in clinical specimens generally and in infections, has been reported a number of times. Pneumonia is the most common nosocomial as well as community-acquired infection. Endemics and epidemics occur among seriously ill patients, requiring respiratory assistance. Bacteremia is common in these pneumonias, which affect men much more than women. Alcoholism often contributes to community-acquired pneumonia, where the fatality rate may approach 50%.

DIAGNOSTIC PROCEDURES

Acinetobacter grow well on ordinary media without enrichment. However, media selective for *Enterobacteriaceae* inhibit or eliminate some biovars and provide scant growth of others. There is no growth on cetrimide agar and most strains do not grow on *Salmonella-Shigella* (SS) agar. MacConkey agar is the best choice for isolation from heavily contaminated material, but 10% of *A. calcoaceticus* subsp. *lwoffi* are inhibited. In this case, reliance must be placed on selection of isolated colonies from blood agar. *A.*

Table 21:1. Characteristics for Identification of Six *Acinetobacter* Genospecies

Characters	8 strains *A. calcoaceticus*	121 strains *A. baumannii*	23 strains *A. haemolyticus*	23 strains *A. johnsonii*	34 strains *A. lwoffii*	17 strains *A. junii*
Growth at 44°	–	+	–	–	–	–
41°	–	+	+	–	–	90
37°	+	95*	+	–	+	+
Gelatin liquefaction	–	–	96	–	–	–
Hemolysis	–	–	+	–	–	–
-glutamyltransferase	+	99	4	–	–	–
Citrate (Simmons)	+	+	91	+	–	82
Acid from glucose	+	95	52	–	6	–
β-Xylosidase	–	95	52	–	–	–
Utilization of:						
D-L-lactate	+	+	–	+	+	+
Glutarate	+	+	–	–	–	–
L-phenylalanine	+	87	–	–	–	–
Phenylacetate	–	87	–	–	94	–
Malonate	+	98	–	13	–	–
β-histidine	+	98	96	–	–	+
Azelate	+	90	–	–	+	–
D-malate	–	98	96	22	76	+
L-aspartate	+	+	64	61	–	40
L-leucine	38	97	96	–	–	11
Histamine	–	–	–	–	–	–
L-tyrosine	+	+	5	70	3	60
β-alanine	+	95	–	–	–	–
Ethanol	+	+	96	+	97	+
2, 3-butanediol	+	+	–	35	–	–
Transiconitate	+	99	52	–	–	–
L-arginine	+	98	96	35	–	95
L-ornithine	+	93	–	4	2	–
DL-4-aminobutyrate	+	+	+	35	40	88
Catalase	+	+	+	+	+	+
Oxidase	–	–	–	–	–	–
Nitrate	–	–	–	–	–	–
Indole	–	–	–	–	–	–
TSI acid						
Slant	–	–	–	–	–	–
Butt	–	–	–	–	–	–
H_2S	–	–	–	–	–	–

calcoaceticus var *anitratus* forms colonies on blood agar that are high, convex, large, moist, whitish and possibly hemolytic.

All subspecies of *Acinetobacter* are nonmotile, nonsporing, gram-negative, oxidase-negative, aerobic coccobacilli. Table 21:1 shows that *A. calcoaceticus* subsp. *anitratus* oxidizes a number of sugars, while *A. calcoaceticus* subsp. *lwoffi* does not.

There is no established, readily available serotyping scheme. Over 30 capsular serotypes of *A. calcoaceticus* var *anitratus* and *A. calcoaceticus* var *lwoffi* have been described.[19]

Alcaligenes

HISTORY AND CLINICAL ASPECTS

This is an old genus name that has been stable in nomenclature and usage. The name *Alcaligenes* was chosen for the alkaline reaction produced in litmus milk. This organism is isolated infrequently now. The high rate of reporting in earlier years reflected the fact that most gram-negative rods growing on MacConkey agar with a "no change" reaction on Kligler's, Triple Sugar Iron (TSI) or Russell's Double Sugar slants were reported as *Alcaligenes faecalis*. For this reason, most early clinical reports of *Alcaligenes* in disease must be discounted. Only reports including unequivocal speciation can be assuredly used.

The three species are isolated from the same types of infection and specimens, such as septicemia, meningitis, ear discharge, urine, skin, sputum and feces, although *A. odorans* is recovered more often from urine and urinary tract infections than from other sources. Isolation from blood without symptoms of septicemia is frequent, as is recovery in mixed flora.

THERAPY

Susceptibility of *Alcaligenes* to such antimicrobial agents as ampicillin, carbenicillin, cephalothin, chloramphenicol and aminoglycosides is markedly variable. Most isolates are susceptible to trimethoprim-sulfamethoxazole and polymyxin B.

EPIDEMIOLOGY

Alcaligenes infections are usually acquired nosocomially. The primary species, *A. faecalis*, has been identified as an agent of disease, arising from the usual aqueous sources such as contaminated nebulizers, respirators, dialysis fluids, urological instruments, injectables and disinfectant solutions.

Surgery of various types has preceded infections. The hospital control of *Alcaligenes* infections is the same as that for *Acinetobacter, Pseudomonas, Achromobacter* and *Flavobacterium*. *A. faecalis* infections, often of the respiratory tract or meninges, far exceed those of *A. denitrificans* and *A. odorans*. Septicemia is common during *A. faecalis* infections. *A. odorans* is isolated frequently from urine and pus.

CAUSATIVE ORGANISMS

As a genus, *Alcaligenes* includes gram-negative, nonsporing, peritrichously flagellated, short rods. They are obligate aerobes, nonsaccharolytic and oxidase-positive. The three *Alcaligenes* species are very similar, and it has been proposed that the genus could be reduced to two, or even to one, species. *A. faecalis* is divided into biovar 1, with small, low, convex, glistening colonies having an entire edge, similar to *A. denitrificans*; and biovar 2, with larger, umbonate, granular colonies having a spreading periphery, similar to *A. odorans*, but lacking the dark green coloration of *A. odorans* on rabbit blood agar. All three species grow well on MacConkey agar and use citrate as a carbon source.

DIAGNOSTIC PROCEDURES

Since *A. faecalis, A. denitrificans* and *A. odorans* are inert in most biochemical tests, only a few tests separate the species (Table 21:2).

Bordetella bronchiseptica and unnamed groups IVc-2 and IVe may be confused with *Alcaligenes*, but these groups can easily be distinguished by their immediate urea hydrolysis on prewarmed Christensen's medium. *Alcaligenes* and *Achromobacter* are also similar. *Achromobacter* species produce acid from xylose and usually from glucose, but *Alcaligenes* is inert. *A. denitrificans* colonies are tiny, about 0.5 mm in diameter, low, convex and glistening. It is distinguished from *A. odorans* by reducing both nitrate and nitrite to gas. *A. odorans* colonies are large, from 1.0 to 1.5 mm in diameter, umbonate, with a flat spreading edge. It fails to reduce nitrate, reduces nitrite to gas and always grows in medium with added 6% NaCl.

A. odorans has a fruity odor resembling apples or strawberries. It imparts a dark green coloration to rabbit blood agar. No serological differentiation of *Alcaligenes* species or strains has been developed.

Achromobacter

INTRODUCTION

Achomobacter is not listed in "Bergey's Manual of Determinative Bacteriology, 8th edition;"[4] it is not on Skerman's "Approved Lists of Bacterial

Table 21:2. Identification of *Alcaligenes* Species

Character	*A. faecalis*	*A. denitrificans*	*A. odorans*
Indophenol oxidase	+	+	+
Motility	+	+	+
Peritrichous flagella	+	+	+
Glucose, xylose, acid (OFBM)*	−	−	−
Nitrate to gas	−	+	−
Nitrite to gas	−	+	−
Fruity odor	−	−	+
NaCl 6%	v†	v	+
Gelatin	−	−	−
Tween 80	v	v	−
Urea hydrolysis	−	−	−
Indole	−	−	−
ONPG‡	−	−	−
Lysine decarboxylase	−	−	−
Arginine dihydrolase	−	−	−
Ornithine decarboxylase	−	−	−

* OFBM = OF basal medium
† v = variable
‡ ONPG = O-nitrophenyl-β-D-galactosidase

Names;''[29] it is without status in ''Bergey's Manual of Systematic Bacteriology, volume 1.''[15] Other genera have slowly acquired its species. But yet it lingers on. Yabuuchi and Yano[35] provided impetus to its survival by proposing *Achromobacter* as a legitimate genus with the type species *A. xylosoxidans*. By this, it may survive indefinitely. Bergey's volume 1[15] places *Achomobacter xylosoxidans* as *Alcaligenes denitrificans* subspecies *xylosoxydans*. Note the difference in spelling. The Special Bacteriology Laboratory of the CDC lists *Achromobacter xylosoxidans* and the unnamed species *Achromobacter* Vd.[6]

CAUSATIVE ORGANISMS

Achromobacter species are peritrichously flagellated, oxidase-positive, use glucose and xylose aerobically and do not produce 3-ketolactose from lactose. Cellular morphology is typically rod-shaped and an appearance of barring may be seen in Gram stains of young cultures. The genus, at present, has the species *A. xylosoxidans*, of which biovar IIIa reduces nitrate to nitrite, while biovar IIIb reduces nitrate to gas. Strains of *Achromobacter* Vd-1 do not oxidize sucrose, maltose nor mannitol, while strains of *Achromobacter* Vd-2 do, but the two are identical in fatty acid composition and production of keto acids.[7]

CLINICAL MANIFESTATIONS

A. xylosoxidans may cause purulent outer or inner ear infection, urinary tract infection, tonsillitis, pulmonary infection, pulmonary infections associated with cystic fibrosis, pneumonia associated with IgM deficiency, purulent meningitis and septicemia with lymphadenopathy. Many are mixed infections, and most patients are at risk for one of a variety of possible reasons, including immune dyscrasia, cancer, previous infection or injury, anatomical abnormality, organ replacement, alcoholism, smoking, hereditary disease, plastic prosthetic devices and intravenous devices.

Before *Achromobacter* is accepted as the cause of infections described in the literature, the description of the organism should be examined for adequacy to determine the genus. Literature prior to 1965 may be generally disregarded as a source of information on *Achromobacter* infections and subsequent reports should be checked for adequate species identification. One *Achromobacter* Vd infection has been described.[1]

Achromobacter species are not aggressive pathogens causing fulminant infections with high fatality rates. Spontaneous recovery is common. Recovery occurs regularly in the face of inappropriate therapy.[13] Infections often persist during catheter use and disappear immediately when the catheter is removed. Nosocomial outbreaks occur in immunocompromised patients.[20,25]

THERAPY

Antibiogram data for this genus are limited. *Achromobacter* species are remarkably variable in susceptibility to antibiotics. Even those drugs that are usually effective in vitro are ineffective for a significant percentage of infections. *A. xylosoxidans* is susceptible to minocycline, doxycycline, carbenicillin, polymyxin B, trimethoprim-sulfamethoxazole, cefoperazone, ceftazidime and the ureidopenicillins. It is resistant to tetracycline. *Achromobacter* Vd-1 and Vd-2 are susceptible to tetracycline, aminoglycosides, carbenicillin, nalidixic acid and trimethoprim-sulfamethoxazole, but resistant to other antibiotics.

EPIDEMIOLOGY

In the older literature, many clinical reports of *Pseudomonas* species other than *P. aeruginosa* may have been misidentifications of *Achromobacter*, especially when flagellar staining was not done. Therefore, the role of *Achromobacter* as a significant pathogen may be underestimated. The habitat of *Achromobacter* in "wet" areas of hospitals is probably similar to that of *Pseudomonas, Acinetobacter, Alcaligenes* and *Flavobacterium*. Most *Achromobacter* infections are hospital-acquired, from the usual long list of "wet" sources, including saline and hemodialysis fluids. The rate of colonization of humans has not been established.

DIAGNOSTIC PROCEDURES

Colonies on blood agar are 1 mm in diameter, smooth, glistening and entire. Oxidation of glucose is weak. Xylose is oxidized strongly by *A. xylosoxidans*, which grows on MacConkey, SS and cetrimide agars, although *Achromobacter* Vd-1 and Vd-2 do not.

Formulations for differential media and reagents are provided by Greenwood.[12] Table 21:3 depicts differential characteristics for *Achromobacter* species. It also distinguishes the related bacterium, *Agrobacterium radiobacter*. Since this organism is isolated from clinical specimens such as sputum, blood and urine, and has been reported to have caused endocarditis in a patient with a prosthetic valve,[24] it must be differentiated from *Achromobacter* species. The production of 3-ketolactose by *Agrobacterium* separates it from *Achromobacter*. *A. radiobacter* is nonpigmented and is much more active biochemically than the achromobacters. Oxidation of glucose by *Achromobacter* in OF medium may be weak or delayed. Seven serotypes of *A. xylosoxidans* have been described.[28]

Flavobacterium

INTRODUCTION

Before flagellar stains[16,33] and careful motility testing were widely used in bacterial identification, the yellow pigmented pseudomonads from water faucets and wet areas were often falsely reported to be *Flavobacterium*. Since then, the genus has become better defined, but is in a continuing state of flux. Elizabeth King and her successors at CDC have used numbers and letters to designate unassigned bacteria. Some of these have been entered into the genus as *Flavobacterium indologenes* (CDC IIb), with the transfer of *F. multivorum* and *F. spiritivorum* to the genus *Sphingobacterium* as *S. multivorum* and *S. spiritivorum*. *Sphingobacterium* is characterized by its high concentration of sphingophospholipids. CDC numbers IIe, IIf, IIh, IIi and IIj are now assigned to *Flavobacterium*. *Flavobacterium* is discussed in detail by Holmes et al[13] and by Clark et al.[6] A new species, *F. thalpophilum*, has been proposed by Holmes et al.[13]

CAUSATIVE ORGANISMS

Flavobacteria and sphingobacteria are free-living, nonsporing, nonmotile, gram-negative rods occurring in soil and water. Except for *F. meningosepticum*, they seldom cause disease, but are occasionally found in clinical specimens. Yellow pigmentation is present on appropriate media, but the carotenoid pigment is very pale in some species. Pigmented, oxidase-positive

Table 21:3. Identification of *Achromobacter xylosoxidans* biovar IIIa, *Achromobacter xylosoxidans* biovar IIIb, *Achromobacter* Vd-1, *Achromobacter Vd-2*, and *Agrobacterium radiobacter*

Character	*A. xylosoxidans* Biovar IIIa	*A. xylosoxidans* Biovar IIIb	*Achromobacter* Sp. Vd - 1	*Achromobacter* Sp. Vd -2	*A. radiobacter*
Gram-negative, rod-shaped, asporogenous	+	+	+	+	+
Indophenol oxidase	+	+	+	+	+
Motility	+	+	+	+	+
Peritrichous flagella	+	+	+	+	+
Xylose, acid (OFBM)*	+	+	+	+	+
Glucose, acid	+	+	+	+	+
Lactose	−	−	−	−	+
Sucrose, maltose	−	−	−	+	+
Mannitol	−	−	−	+ or −	+
Nitrate to nitrite	+	−	−	−	−
Nitrate to gas	−	+	+	+	−
Urease	−	−	+(r)‡	+(r)	+(r)
3-Ketolactose	−	−	−	−	+
ONPG†	−	−	−	−	+
Indole	−	−	−	−	+
Arginine dihydrolase	−	−	v§	v	−
Lysine decarboxylase	−	−	−	−	−
Ornithine decarboxylase	−	−	−	−	−
Phenylalanine deaminase	−	−	+	+	+
Esculin	−	−	v	v	+
Gelatin	−	−	−	−	−
Motile	+	+	+	+	+
Flagellation	p‖	p	p	p	p

* OFMB = OF basal medium
† ONPG = O-nitrophenyl-β-D-galatosidase
‡ (r) = rapid
§ v = variable
‖ P = peritrichous

colonies on blood agar suggest flavobacteria. Gram stain reveals long, thin rods which may have slightly bulbous ends. Growth on MacConkey agar is variable and growth is absent on SS and cetrimide agars. A lavender-green discoloration is produced on blood agar within 18-24 h incubation. This is more marked with a few strains.

CLINICAL MANIFESTATIONS AND EPIDEMIOLOGY

The natural habitat of the flavobacteria is similar to that of the other genera described in this chapter. Humans are not usually colonized with *Flavobacterium* species but may be transiently colonized in hospital environments, from water systems generally, and specifically from nebulizers, water baths, distilled water, irrigation solutions, faucets, fountains, humidifiers and hemodialysis systems.

F. meningosepticum occurs far more often than other flavobacteria in nosocomial outbreaks, infecting mostly premature infants, but isolated infections in compromised adults have occurred as meningitis, pneumonia or endocarditis.[9,30] Infection in the newborn is usually fatal. Blood cultures are usually positive in meningitis.

Flavobacterium IIf, *F. indologenes, S. multivorum* and *F. odoratum* have not been reported in hospital epidemics, but have been isolated from blood and other clinical samples. *F. odoratum* is often isolated from human urine samples. Infections caused by *Flavobacterium* IIj have been traced to bites or scratches from dogs or cats. The remaining *Flavobacterium* species are rarely involved with human disease. *Flavobacterium* IIh is isolated primarily from the respiratory tracts of animals.

THERAPY

Strains of most *Flavobacterium* species are resistant to penicillin and polymyxin. The antibiogram is essential to successful treatment because human isolates are resistant to most antimicrobial agents. Isolates may be sensitive to trimethoprim-sulfamethoxazole, erythromycin, novobiocin, nalidixic acid and rifampin. Spontaneous recovery in adults is usual. Rapid recovery from infections may occur even when inappropriate therapy, such as penicillin and streptomycin, is used.

DIAGNOSTIC PROCEDURES

The genus may be divided into those species that produce acid oxidatively from maltose and other carbohydrates and those that do not. Most species liquefy gelatin. Differential reactions are seen in Table 21:4. Indole is formed

Table 21:4. Identification of *Flavobacterium* and *Sphingobacterium* Species*

Character	Acid-Producing *Flavobacterium*						Non-Acid-Producing *Flavobacterium*				*Sphingobacterium*		
	F. meningo-septicum	*F. thalpo-philum*	*F. breve*	*F. indolo-genes*	*F.* sp. IIh	*F.* sp. IIi	*F. odor-atum*	*F.* sp. IIe	*F.* sp. IIf	*F.* sp. IIj	*S. multi-vorum*	*S. spiriti-vorum*	*S. mizutae*
Gram-negative, rod-shaped, asporogenous	+	+	+	+	+	+	+	+	+	+	+	+	+
Indophenol oxidase	+	+	+	+	+	+	+	+	+	+	+	+	+
Motility	−	−	−	−	−	−	−	−	−	−	−	−	−
Glucose (OFBM)†	+	+	+	+	+	+	−	−	−	−	+	+	+
Maltose, acid (OFBM)	+	+	+	+	+	+	−	−	−	−	+	+	+
Mannitol	+	−	−	v§	−	−	−	−	−	−	−	+	−
Adonitol	−	+	−	−	−	−	−	−	−	−	−	−	−
Rhamnose	−	−	−	−	−	−	−	−	−	−	−	+	+
Xylose	−	+	−	v	−	+	−	−	−	−	+	+	+
Inulin											+	v	−
Glycogen											+	−	−
Ethanol (3%)											−	+	−
ONPG‡ reaction	+	+	−	v	v	+	−	−	−	−	+	+	+
Indole	+	−	+	+	+	+	−	+	+	+	−	−	−
Nitrate	−	+	−	−	−	−	−	−	−	−	−	−	−
Urease	−	+	v	v	−	−	+	−	−	+(r)‖	+	+	v
Esculin Hydrolysis	+	+	−	+	+	+	−	−	−	−	+	+	+
Tween 80 hydrolysis	−	−	−	+	−	v	v	+	−	−	v	v	v
Starch hydrolysis	v	−	−	+	+	v	−	+	−	−	v	v	v
Deoxyribonucleic acid hydrolysis	+	+	+	−	+	−	+	−	−	−	−	−	−
Gelatin hydrolysis	+	+	+	+	+	−	+	−	+	+	−	−	−
Growth at 42°C	v	+	−	v	v	−	−	+	+	+	−	−	−
Penicillin susceptible							−	+	+	+			
Polymyxin susceptible							−	+	+	−			

* Taken from Gilardi
† OFBM = OF basal medium
‡ ONPG = O-Nitrophenyl-β-D-galactosidase
§ v = variable
‖ (r) = rapid

by all but one species, although xylene extraction is required before testing with Ehrlich's reagent.

Acid-producing Flavobacteria

F. meningosepticum produces smooth, convex, butyrous, glistening colonies with entire edges, that may have a pale yellow pigment. *F. breve* colonies are glistening, with yellow centers and greenish edges. The culture has a fruity odor. *F. indologenes* colonies produce a bright yellow pigment. *F. thalpophilum* is distinct by its ability to reduce nitrate, grow at 42°C and produce acid from adonitol as well as from various other carbohydrates and alcohols. *Flavobacterium* IIh has no distinctive pigment. *Flavobacterium* IIi is not proteolytic and is separated from *Sphingobacterium multivorum* by being indole-positive and urea-negative.

Non-acid-producing Flavobacteria

Flavobacterium IIe does not grow on basal medium nor on nutrient agars without blood. A faint yellow pigment may be seen in growth on blood agar. *Flavobacterium* IIf isolates are usually from vaginal or urine specimens. Greening of blood agar occurs. Colonies are large, mucoid, sticky and difficult to scrape off the agar. Growth is heavy on blood agar, with pale yellow pigmentation. An amber to brown soluble pigment is produced. Good growth occurs on OF medium, with an alkaline reaction. There is usually no growth on MacConkey agar. This organism is sensitive to penicillin and polymyxin, a further differential from *F. meningosepticum*. (Table 21:4)

F. odoratum exhibits colonial pleomorphism. Large, rough, spreading colonies with a raised center and smaller, convex, smooth colonies (which may be the only form present) occur. A yellow pigment is produced. Growth occurs in OF medium. *Flavobacterium* IIj has been isolated from the respiratory tract of dogs and cats. It may have a greening reaction on blood agar. There is no growth on OF basal medium nor on MacConkey agar. Pigmentation is scant. The colonies are sticky and difficult to remove from the agar surface.

Sphingobacterium (Cytophagaceae) includes *S. multivorum* (mannitol-negative) and *S. spiritivorum* (mannitol-positive). Table 21:4 includes reactions for three species, including *S. mizutae*, proposed by Yabuuchi et al.[34] *S. multivorum* includes pale yellow species that are oxidase-positive but are nonproteolytic and indole-negative. All three species are isolated from clinical specimens and from the hospital environment. *S. mizutae* was isolated from the spinal fluid of a premature infant with meningitis. These species are notably resistant to most antibiotics but exceptions are noticed. Most strains are susceptible to trimethoprim-sulfamethoxazole as well as to sulfadiazine.

Serology

Antisera are available for six serotypes of *F. meningosepticum* (Difco Laboratories). Crossreactions have been seen among the six, as well as with *Flavobacterium* IIb.

Chromobacterium

CAUSATIVE ORGANISMS

Chromobacterium has two species, the fermentative mesophile, *C. violaceum*, and oxidative psychrophilic *C. lividum*, now *Janthinobacterium lividum*. Only *C. violaceum* causes disease in man and further discussion is confined to this species. Flagellation (in young agar colonies) is of unusual morphology, with one faintly-staining polar flagellum of long wavelength and 1-4 normal-staining subpolar or lateral flagella with shorter wavelengths. Cells of *C. violaceum* are short rods with rounded ends. They occur singly or in pairs and typically show bipolar staining. The pigment, violacein, is a water-soluble, violet, indole-pyrrole. It is markedly antibacterial to both gram-negative and gram-positive bacteria. Open lesions in patients may yield pure cultures of *C. violaceum* because of this antibiotic property. Violacein is too toxic for use in animals or man. The mouse lethal dose (LD^{50}) is just over the dose that protects mice from pneumococcus challenge. Nonpigmented *C. violaceum* has not been reported to cause disease, although about 8% of isolates from nature are nonpigmented. Whether this is due to misidentification of nonpigmented strains is not known.

CLINICAL MANIFESTATIONS

The rare *C. violaceum* infections inspire an unusual interest, particularly because of a high fatality rate and the beautiful violet pigment produced by the bacterium. The earliest symptoms are fever and lymphadenopathy, with a skin lesion or lesions. Terminal bronchopneumonia is usual, as the infection becomes systemic. Subcutaneous, pulmonary and liver abscesses and diarrhea are usual. In its late stages, the disease may present as respiratory disease syndrome, tuberculosis or urinary tract infection. Manifestations of the disease are so varied that early presumptive evidence of the etiologic agent may best be obtained from the patient's history—often indications of immunodeficiency in the young and contact with water and/or soil in an appropriate geographical location. Blood cultures are positive early in the disease. Previously healthy adults have acquired the disease, but case reports for the few survivors record no immunological surveys.

Lee and Wright[17] considered respiratory distress syndrome to be a standard malignant development in *C. violaceum* infections. They successfully used high positive end-expiratory pressure (PEEP) to bring arterial oxygenation to normal and save a comatose 3-year old who had required resuscitation following 3 cardiopulmonary arrests.

THERAPY

An antibiogram should be obtained as rapidly as possible on *C. violaceum* isolates. Combined chloramphenicol-gentamicin therapy has been successful. The organism is also sensitive to tetracycline, streptomycin, kanamycin, erythromycin and trimethoprim-sulfamethoxazole.[17] It is resistant to ampicillin, penicillin, clindamycin, cephalothin, carbenicillin (some strains) and the polymyxins. Aminoglycosides may or may not be effective.[23,32] There may be need for extended therapy even beyond 30 days because of multiple, hidden abscesses that resist treatment.

EPIDEMIOLOGY

C. violaceum is an abundant soil and water organism occurring between 35° S and 35° N latitude around the world. There have been 12 infections (8 fatal) reported in the United States, 10 in Florida and 2 in Louisiana.[5] One patient, a 49-year old male, acquired infection after a near drowning, having incurred a massive challenge with *C. violaceum*. Of those patients most recently examined, 3 were young (mean age 15 years) and had chronic granulomatosis disease.[18]

DIAGNOSTIC PROCEDURES

Strains produce pigmentation aerobically on MacConkey's and most diagnostic media. The TSI slant reaction is no-change/acid for *C. violaceum* and acid/no change for *C. lividum*. The pigment, violacein, develops over a period of days through beautiful shades of blue-violet to purple to black.

Table 21:5. Biochemical Reactions of *Chromobacterium violaceum*

Pigment violet	Gelatinase +	ONPG* −	
Oxidase +	Citrate (Simmons) v†	Acid from:	glucose +
Motility +,	Esculin hydrolysis −		trehalose +
Indole −	Lysine decarboxylase −		sucrose v
Catalase +	Arginine dihydrolase +		maltose −
Nitrate reduction +	Ornithine decarboxylase −		lactose −

* ONPG = O-nitrophenyl-β-D-galatosidase
† v = variable

Growth on blood agar may smell of cyanide (odor of bitter almonds). Growth is rapid on all the usual nonselective media. Identification of *C. violaceum* is simple and straightforward, especially since all clinical strains isolated to date have been pigmented and can be identified adequately by kit systems. No clearcut antigenic groups have been established.

UNCLASSIFIED CDC GROUPS IVc-2, IVe and EO-2

Group IVe is similar to oxidase-positive, strictly aerobic, motile and nonsaccharolytic *Alcaligenes*, but Group IVe immediately hydrolyzes warm Christensen's urea agar. Cellular morphology may be cocobacillary, rod-shaped or filamentous. These groups are similar to *Achromobacter* but do not produce acid from xylose and, except for EO-2, not from glucose.

Pseudomonas species that are nonsaccharolytic have polar flagella. Group IVc-2 strains are motile with peritrichous flagella. Group IVe strains may be nonmotile or weakly motile. Motile IVe strains have polar flagella as well as long lateral flagella with long wavelength and low amplitude. *Bordetella bronchiseptica* resembles IVe but has peritrichous flagella. Also Group IVe strains usually reduce nitrate to nitrite and gas, while fewer than half of *B. bronchiseptica* strains reduce nitrate and none produce gas. Group IVe strains have been recovered exclusively from human urine except for one septicemia strain from a patient with obstructive uropathy.[26]

In laboratory practice, these three groups are also recovered from sources such as catheters, body surfaces and as "contaminants" on blood plates and Isolator (Dupont Company) blood culture plates, which perhaps indicates shedding from human body surfaces.

Unnamed group EO-2 comprises oxidase-positive, nonmotile, glucose-oxidizing rods, with often mucoid colonies, similar to *Acinetobacter* but different in the oxidase reaction and acidity from fructose. Three of four strains break down urea and are nitrate-positive. Growth on MacConkey agar is variable. The organism is active on carbohydrates but otherwise rather inactive biochemically (Table 21:6). EO-2 is usually susceptible to aminoglycosides, tetracycline, chloramphenicol, polymyxin and trimethoprim-sulfamethoxazole. It is resistant to cephalothin.

Experience is limited but IVc-2 strains are usually sensitive to tetracycline, polymyxin, carbenicillin, cefoxitin, cefamandole and trimethoprim-sulfamethoxazole; usually resistant to aminoglycosides, penicillin, ampicillin, cephalothin and chloramphenicol. IVe isolates are sensitive to cephalosporins, aminoglycosides, colistin, gentamicin, kanamycin, tetracycline and trimethoprim-sulfamethoxazole; resistant to carbenicillin, ampicillin, chloramphenicol and often to tetracycline.

Table 21:6. Characteristics of *Bordetella bronchiseptica*, Group EO-2, Group IVe, and Group IVc-2

	EO-2	IVe	IVc-2	*Bordetella bronchiseptica*
Gram-negative asporogenous rods	+	+	+	+
Motility	–	+	+	+
Indophenol oxidase	+	+	+	+
Simmons citrate	v*	v	+	v
Urea, Christensen	v	+(r)†	+(r)	+(r)
Nitrate to nitrite	v	+	–	+
Nitrate to gas	–	+	–	–
Pigment	v (soluble yellow)	v (soluble yellow)	v (soluble yellow-tan)	–
Growth on:				
MacConkey agar	v	v	+	+
SS‡ agar	–	v	–	+
Growth at 42°C	v	–	v	v
Acid from:				
Glucose	+	–	–	–
Xylose	+	–	–	–
Mannitol	v	–	–	–
Lactose	+	–	–	–
Sucrose	–	–	–	–
Maltose	v	–	–	–
TSI§ (slant and butt)	–	–	–	–
Gelatin hydrolysis	–	–	–	–
Esculin hydrolysis	–	–	–	–
Arginine dihydrolase	–	–	–	–
Ornithine decarboxylase	–	–	–	–
Lysine decarboxylase	–	–	–	–
Flagella:				
Peritrichous	–	–	+	+
Polar and lateral	–	+	–	–
Phenylalanine deaminase	–	+	–	v

* v = variable
† (r) = Rapid
‡ SS = *Salmonella-Shigella*
§ TSI = Triple sugar iron

COMMERCIAL SYSTEMS—AUTOMATED IDENTIFICATION SYSTEMS

About a dozen automated or semi-automated instruments for bacterial speciation and antimicrobic susceptibility testing are on the market or are being developed. These include ALADIN and Uniscept (Analytab Products), Autoscan (Microscan), Autobac IDX-C (General Diagnostics), Auto Microbic System (Vitek Systems), MS-2 and Avantage (Abbott Laboratories), Micro-Coder I (Micro-Media Systems), Pasco (Difco Laboratories), Prescept (Austin Biological Laboratories), Sensititre (Gibco Laboratories) and Sceptor (BBL Microbiology Systems). The sophistication, cost and advancement in the marketplace of these systems varies greatly. A few are in process of being phased out.

COMMERCIAL SYSTEMS—KIT OR MINIATURIZED IDENTIFICATION SYSTEMS

One system is the Oxi-Ferm (Roche Diagnostics), a plastic tube with 8 compartments and 8 media, generating at least 9 test results, and finally a 4-digit code. Genus but not species identification is available for *Moraxella, Alcaligenes* and *Flavobacterium*, but the system does speciate the more common NFB.

The API 20 E (Analytab Products) system can also be used for NFB, but their new strip, the API Rapid NFT, is now recommended for nonfermenters. It combines 8 conventional tests with 12 carbon assimilation, or growth, tests. Von Graevenitz[31] reported that only 3% of 431 strains of NFB could not be identified by this system. It is identical to API 20 NE (API System N.A.). The Minitek System (BBL Microbiology Systems) is a plastic plate containing 20 wells to hold dried disks impregnated with biochemicals and substrates for NFB. This 48-hour system is flexible in that different substrate disks may be used, such as the esculin disk for *P. maltophilia* or *Flavobacterium*. As with all systems, identification of many uncommon NFB may require 15-60% supplemental tests.

The Flow N/F System (Flow Laboratories) includes 2 screening tubes (GNF and 42P) for oxidase-positive organisms and a circular plate divided into 12 sections containing conventional agar media. This system is used successfully by many laboratories.

Basic comparative and guideline information about rapid identification using commercial miniaturized kits may be found in publications by Oberhofer[22] and Sherris and Ryan.[27]

REFERENCES

1. Appelbaum PC, Campbell DB. Pancreatic abscess associated with *Achromobacter* group Vd biovar 1. J Clin Microbiol 1980;12:282-3.
2. Berk SL, McCabe WR. Meningitis caused by *Acinetobacter calcoaceticus* var *anitratus*. Arch Neurol 1981;38:95-8.
3. Bouvet PJM, Grimont PAD. Taxonomy of the genus *Acinetobacter* with the recognition of *Acinetobacter baumannii* sp. nov., *Acinetobacter johnsonii* sp. nov., and *Acinetobacter junii* sp. nov., and emended description of *Acinetobacter calcoaceticus* and *Acinetobacter lwoffi*. Int J Syst Bacteriol 1986;36:228-40.
4. Buchanan RE, Gibbons NE, eds. Bergey's manual of determinative bacteriology. 8th ed. Baltimore: Williams and Wilkins, 1974.
5. Centers for Disease Control. Chromobacteriosis - Florida. Morbid Mortal Weekly Rep 1981;29:613-15.

6. Clark WA, Hollis DG, Weaver RE, Riley P. Identification of unusual pathogenic gram-negative aerobic and facultatively anaerobic bacteria. Atlanta: Centers for Disease Control, 1984.
7. Dees SB, Moss CW. Identification of *Achromobacter* species by cellular fatty acids and by production of keto acids. J Clin Microbiol 1978;8:61-6.
8. Dadswell JV. *Acinetobacter* and similar organisms in ear infections. J Med Microbiol 1976;9:45-53.
9. Dooley JR, Nims LJ, Lipp VH, Beard A, Delaney LT. Meningitis of infants caused by *Flavobacterium meningosepticum*. J Trop Pediatr 1980;26:24-30.
10. Feigin RD, Shearer WT. Opportunistic infection in children. J Pediatr 1975;87:852-66.
11. Gilardi GL. Cultural and biochemical aspects for identification of glucose nonfermenting gram-negative rods. In: Gilardi GL, ed. Nonfermentative gram-negative rods. New York: Marcel Dekker, 1985:17-84
12. Greenwood JR. Methods of isolation and identification of glucose-nonfermenting gram-negative rods. In: Gilardi GL, ed. Nonfermentative gram-negative rods. New York: Marcel Dekker, 1985:1-16
13. Holmes B, Hollis DG, Steigerwalt AG, Pickett MJ, Brenner DJ. *Flavobacterium thalpophilum*, a new species recovered from human clinical material. Int J Syst Bacteriol 1983;33:677-82.
14. Igra-Siegman Y, Chmel H, Cobbs C. Clinical and laboratory characteristics of *Achromobacter xylosoxidans* infection. J Clin Microbiol 1980;11:141-5.
15. Krieg NR, Holt JG, eds. Bergey's manual of systematic bacteriology; vol 1. Baltimore: Williams and Wilkins, 1984.
16. Kodaka H, Armfield AY, Lombard GL, Dowell VR. Practical procedure for demonstrating bacterial flagella. J Clin Microbiol 1982;16:948-52.
17. Lee TS, Wright BD. Fulminating chromobacterial septicaemia presenting as respiratory distress syndrome. Thorax (England) 1981;36:557-9.
18. Macher AM, Casale TB, Fauci AS. Chronic granulomatous disease of childhood and *Chromobacterium violaceum* infections in the southeastern United States. Ann Intern Med 1982;97:51-5.
19. Marcus BB, Samuels SB, Pittman B, Cherry WB. A serologic study of *Herellea vaginicola* and its identification by immunoflorescent staining. Am J Clin Pathol 1969;52:309-19.
20. McGluckin MB, Thorpe RJ, Koch KM, Alavi A, Staum M, Abrutyn E. An outbreak of *Achromobacter xylosoxidans* related to diagnostic tracer procedures. Am J Epidemiol 1982;115:785-93.
21. Miller RM, Polakavetz SH, Hornick RB, et al. Analysis of infections acquired by the severely injured patient. Surg Gynecol Obstet 1973;137:7-10.
22. Oberhofer TR. Rapid identification of glucose-nonfermenting gram-negative rods with commercial miniaturized kits. In: Gilardi GL, ed. Nonfermentative gram-negative rods. New York: Marcel Dekker, 1985:85-116.
23. Ognibene AJ, Thomas E. Fatal infections due to *Chromobacterium violaceum* in Vietnam. Am J Clin Pathol 1970;54:607-10.
24. Plotkin GR. *Agrobacterium radiobacter* prosthetic valve endocarditis. Ann Intern Med 1980;93:839-40.
25. Reverdy ME, Freny J, Fleurette J, et al. Nosocomial colonization and infection by *Achromobacter xylosoxidans*. J Clin Microbiol 1984;19:140-3.
26. Rockhill RC, Lutwick LJ. Group IVe-like gram negative bacillemia in a patient with obstructive uropathy. J Clin Microbiol 1978;8:108-9.
27. Sherris JC, Ryan KJ. Evaluation of automated rapid methods. In: Tilton RC, ed. Methods and automation in microbiology. Washington, DC: American Society for Microbiology, 1981:1-5.
28. Shigeta S, Hyodo S, Chonan E, Yabuuchi E. Serological classification of *Achromobacter xylosoxidans*. J Clin Microbiol 1983;17:181-6.

29. Skerman VBD, McGowan V, Sneath PHA. Approved lists of bacterial names. Int J Syst Bacteriol 1980;30:225-420.
30. Thong ML, Puthucheary SD, Lee EL. *Flavobacterium meningosepticum* infection; an epidemiological study in a newborn nursery. J Clin Pathol 1981;34:429-33.
31. Von Graevenitz A, Zollingen-Iten J. Evaluation of pertinent parameters of a new identification system for non-enteric gram-negative rods. Eur J Clin Microbiol 1985;4:108-12.
32. Victorica B, Baer H, Ayoud EM. Successful treatment of systemic *Chromobacterium violaceum* infection. JAMA 1974;230:578-80.
33. West M, Burdash NM, Freimuth F. Simplified silverplating stain for flagella. J Clin Microbiol 1977;6:414-18.
34. Yabuuchi E, Kaneko T, Yano I, Moss CW, Myoshi N. *Sphingobacterium* gen. nov., *Sphingobacterium spiritivorum* comb. nov., *Sphingobacterium multivorum* comb. nov., *Sphingobacterium mizutae* sp. nov. and *Flavobacterium indologenes* sp. nov.: Glucose nonfermenting rods in CDC groups IIk-2 and IIb. Int J Syst Bacteriol 1983;33:580-98.
35. Yabuuchi E, Yano I. *Achromobacter* gen. nov. and *Achromobacter xylosoxidans* (ex Yabuuchi and Ohyami 1971) nom. rev. Int J Syst Bacteriol 1981;31:477-8.

CHAPTER 22

MYCOPLASMAL INFECTIONS

Wallace A. Clyde, Jr., M.D.

INTRODUCTION

Mycoplasma(s) is the trivial name given to the heterogeneous members of bacterial class *Mollicutes*. The prototype species, *Mycoplasma mycoides*, was established as the cause of bovine pleuropneumonia in 1898.[35] Subsequently, more than 90 species have been grouped taxonomically into 3 families and 6 genera.[29] These organisms produce a wide variety of diseases in man, animals, birds, insects and plants. Some species occur as normal microbial flora on mucous membranes, while others may be found in soil and sewage. Their small genome (5 x 10^8-10^9 daltons) and absence of cell wall material are the cardinal features distinguishing mycoplasmas from classical bacteria. The organisms are bound only by trilaminar unit membranes. These properties contribute to their small size, limited metabolic activities, requirement for precursor substances in media, absence of reactivity with organic dyes used in many staining procedures and absolute insensitivity to the penicillin antibiotics. On solid media, typical colonial growth is embedded into the agar, more deeply at the center, producing a "fried egg" morphology. Generally only faint turbidity is produced by growth in liquid or semi-solid media.

This chapter will focus on mycoplasma species that are human pathogens, but other indigenous species will be mentioned relative to laboratory identification requirements (Table 22:1). Certain non-human species have public health significance in terms of foodstuff production and diagnostic laboratory quality control.

CAUSATIVE ORGANISMS

Four mycoplasma species have been implicated in human diseases. Foremost among these is *M. pneumoniae*, originally isolated by Eaton from

Table 22:1. Mycoplasma Species Indigenous to Man*

Species	Habitat	Pathobiology	Distinctive features
M. pneumoniae	Respiratory tract	Tracheobronchitis, pneumonia	Slow-growing; ferments carbohydrates; β-hemolysis of sheep erythrocytes
M. orale	Pharynx	Normal flora	Hydrolyzes arginine; colony resembles *M. pneumoniae*
M. buccale	Oropharynx	Normal flora	Isolated rarely
M. faucium	Oropharynx	Normal flora	Isolated rarely
M. salivarium	Gingiva, oropharynx	Normal flora	Hydrolyzes arginine; large fried-egg colony
M. fermentans	Genital tract, rarely pharynx	Normal flora	Ferments carbohydrates, hydrolyzes arginine
M. genitalium	Genital tract	Urethritis	Similar to *M. pneumoniae;* primary isolation difficult
M. hominis	Genital tract, oropharynx occasionally	Normal flora, salpingitis, pyelonephritis, postpartum sepsis neonatal abcesses	Hydrolyzes arginine; large fried-egg colony; grows rapidly
U. urealyticum	Genital tract, oropharynx occasionally	Normal flora, urethritis, congenital pneumonia, amnionitis	Tiny colonies grow rapidly; acid pH optimum for growth; produces urease

* Other species which have been isolated include *M. lipophilum, M. primatum,* and *A. laidlawii*

patients with atypical pneumonia.[18] Several genitourinary tract syndromes have been ascribed to *M. hominis* and *Ureaplasma urealyticum*; the strength of etiologic associations is less clear than for *M. pneumoniae* and is summarized in proceedings of recent symposia devoted to them.[4,32] A newly described species, *M. genitalium*, also has been related to genitourinary diseases but has not been studied adequately to define its significance. Other species listed in Table 22:1 have been found occasionally in suppurative processes where they appear to be opportunists.

Mycoplasma pneumoniae

M. pneumoniae is a minute filament (0.1 X 2.0 μm) having the capacity for gliding motility. A differentiated terminal organelle attaches the organism to host cell membranes with a neuraminic acid receptor mechanism. Growth on solid medium requires the presence of serum and heat-stable components from aqueous extracts of baker's yeast. Spherical, slightly granular colonies measuring 10-100 μm in diameter can be seen after 7-10 days at 37°C.

Growth in broth medium produces no gross turbidity, but when viewed microscopically (100 X) refractile "spherules" are seen attached to the culture vessel surfaces. Many carbohydrates are fermented by these organisms, and the pH reduction accompanying acid metabolite production is a convenient reflection of growth in liquid medium containing a suitable substrate and indicator dye. Production of peroxide is another metabolic feature useful in identification of the species. Although various phenotypic strain variations have been described, only one serotype of *M. pneumoniae* is recognized.

Mycoplasma hominis

M. hominis is generally a spherical organism or short filament in the size range of 0.2 μm. Growth requirements are less stringent than for *M. pneumoniae*, although serum must be present as a source of sterol. Solid media incubated at 35-37°C yield colonies measuring 0.1-1.0 mm in diameter within 2-4 days. If well separated, the colonies show the classical "fried egg" morphology of mycoplasmas. In older colonies, the periphery takes on a vacuolated appearance due to production of large, probably degenerative forms. Growth in liquid media results in a faint homogeneous turbidity best visualized with oblique fluorescent illumination. Carbohydrates are not fermented, but arginine deaminase activity results in production of ammonia with a consequent pH rise accompanying growth. There is evidence that there are multiple serotypes of *M. hominis*.[30]

Ureaplasma urealyticum

U. urealyticum is a small spherical organism which, like *M. pneumoniae* has the ability to attach to host cells. Members of this genus were formally called "T" (for tiny) strains because of small colony size (5-25 μm) on solid media. This may represent medium deficiency rather than a fixed characteristic, since larger colonies can be achieved using special buffering systems. After anaerobic incubation for 24-48 h at 35-37°C colonies are seen as thin, rather granular fried-egg or round forms on solid media. Organisms grow with similar rapidity in liquid media but no turbidity is evident. As the species name implies, these organisms produce a urease, which is a unique metabolic feature among the mycoplasmas. Cleavage of urea with production of ammonia raises medium pH rapidly and constitutes a visible reflection of growth in the presence of appropriate indicators. At least 14 distinct serotypes of *U. urealyticum* have been described.[38]

Mycoplasma genitalium

M. genitalium is a flask-shaped organism sharing several biologic properties with *M. pneumoniae* although the two species are genetically distinct.[45,46] A broad differentiated portion of the cell membrane mediates attachment to cells. Carbohydrates are utilized and peroxide is produced by this species. The first isolations in liquid SP4 medium required 60-90 days incubation, although more rapid growth is achieved after laboratory subcultivation. The prolonged incubation required for primary isolation is a major technical problem that has impeded ecologic and epidemiologic study. Cultures may be overgrown readily with more rapidly proliferating forms, particularly *M. hominis*.

CLINICAL MANIFESTATIONS

The expression of *M. pneumoniae* infections ranges from entirely subclinical disease through tracheobronchitis to pneumonia. This mycoplasma was identified originally as the causative agent of "primary atypical pneumonia" and infection has been characterized most completely in this syndrome. After a 2-4 week incubation period, symptoms begin insidiously with dry throat, fever and malaise. This influenza-like illness continues with development of persistent dry, then productive, cough and headache. Physical examination may be unremarkable initially, but as cough becomes productive, fine rales sometimes associated with localized wheezing may be heard. Chest x-ray usually reveals a patchy bronchopneumonia involving one of the lower lobes, but a wide spectrum of changes including segmental atelectasis and lobar consolidation have been described. Unusual manifestations include frank hemoptysis, pleuritic pain, large pleural effusions, and a variety of nonrespiratory findings such as nondescript rashes, erythema multiforme, hemolytic anemia, arthritis and several neurologic syndromes. Disease is usually mild and self-limited, running its course in 2-4 weeks. Resolution of symptoms and signs is accelerated by appropriate antibiotic therapy.

The manifestations of *M. hominis* infection are less well defined, since the organism is found frequently as a component of the normal pharyngeal and genital tract flora. Instances of postpartum fever have been associated with *M. hominis* sepsis, presumably resulting from opportunistic invasion of the compromised female genital tract; this is a self-limited process without known complications or sequelae.[43] The frequency of this cause of postpartum fever is unknown, but it is important to establish this etiology from the standpoint of differential diagnosis and for therapeutic considerations. Isolated cases of "sterile" meningitis and scalp abcesses in newborn infants yielding only *M. hominis* on culture have been described. Reports of pyelonephritis, salpingitis, wound infections and arthritis suggest the potential pathogenicity of this species.[32] *Ureaplasma urealyticum* is another common inhabitant of the genital tracts of both sexes. Venereal transmission is suggested by the observation that frequency of colonization is directly proportional to degree of sexual activity.[43] A relationship has been noted between *U. urealyticum* and nongonococcal urethritis in males, and between amnionitis, fetal wastage and congenital or neonatal pneumonia: the etiologic association between organisms and these diseases is a matter of unresolved controversy.[4]

Specimens from men with urethritis yielded the original *M. genitalium* strains. Experimental infections in chimpanzees producing urethritis, and sepsis in a few instances, strongly suggest the pathogenicity of this species.[44,47]

THERAPY

Generally, mycoplasmas are susceptible to the tetracyclines and "resistant" to the penicillins, polymyxin, neomycin and bacitracin in vitro. Sensitivity to aminoglycosides and chloramphenicol is variable, and selected species are inhibited by the macrolide group. Antibiotic effects appear to be mycoplasmastatic and resistance develops readily due to incompletely understood mechanisms.

Clinical trials have established that the natural course of *M. pneumoniae* pneumonia is shortened significantly by treatment with either tetracycline or erythromycin; resistance to these antibiotics has been reported, but has not been a significant clinical problem. Infection and/or colonization with *U. urealyticum* usually responds to erythromycin or tetracycline, although recent surveys suggest increasing resistance of isolates. Tetracycline has been the treatment of choice for *M. hominis* infections; this species is insensitive to erythromycin, but clindamycin provides a possible alternative. No information is available on treatment of *M. genitalium* infections.

EPIDEMIOLOGY

Respiratory disease due to *M. pneumoniae* occurs both endemically and in irregular, protracted epidemics. Although the disease may occur in any season, it has been observed frequently in the fall months when other causes of tracheobronchitis and pneumonia are less common. Transmission is presumed to occur by a person-to-person droplet route. Studies in families suggest that communicability is of high order, although not all infected individuals manifest overt clinical disease.[24] Pneumonia due to *M. pneumoniae* has its peak incidence in late childhood and adolescence. Disease is uncommon below age 5.[23] In studies of college populations, this organism has accounted for up to 50% of all cases of pneumonia. Many outbreaks have been described in institutional settings and among the Armed Forces. In a metropolitan study, the yearly incidence of *M. pneumoniae* pneumonia was estimated to be as high as 3.2/1,000 population/yr; depending upon age grouping concerned, this represented the cause of 6-28% of all pneumonia cases observed.[1] Prospective studies have shown that infections, including those associated with pneumonia, can recur within 2-4 years.

The epidemiology of *M. hominis* and *U. urealyticum* infection is less clearly defined, since, unlike *M. pneumoniae*, they can be found as normal mucosal flora. Surveillance studies have shown a low incidence in children and among nuns and a high incidence among adults with multiple consorts, suggesting that genital colonization is by venereal transmission.[43] The fact that sexually transmitted diseases of all kinds follow this same pattern has complicated assessment of the relationship between *U. urealyticum* and disease in epidemiologic studies. Transmission of mycoplasmas from mother to newborn infant has been demonstrated, but generally there has been no associated morbidity except for a trend toward lower birth weight.[43] Technical problems have precluded definition of the epidemiology of *M. genitalium* infections and the importance of this organism as a cause of human disease cannot be ascertained from available data. Serologic study of women with pelvic inflammatory disease has implicated *M. genitalium* in that syndrome.[34] However, reports of antibody crossreactivity with *M. pneumoniae* complicate interpretation of seroepidemiologic information.[13,31]

PUBLIC HEALTH SIGNIFICANCE, PREVENTION AND CONTROL

M. pneumoniae is a major contributor to the lower respiratory tract disease of adolescents and young adults, thereby constituting a significant health problem among students, the work force and military personnel. Since the disease is rarely fatal, impact is measured more in terms of lost school and work days and in health care effort and cost. The impact of other mycoplasmas as agents of sexually transmitted and perinatal disease is difficult to estimate with available data.

Mycoplasmas have other implications for public health in addition to their role in human disease. It is now known that a variety of diseases affecting the quality and yield of grains and citrus fruits are caused by *Spiroplasma* species transmitted via insect vectors. The many mycoplasmal diseases of avian, bovine, ovine and porcine species can influence the production of these important protein sources. The prototype mycoplasmal disease -- bovine pleuropneumonia, caused by *M. mycoides* -- remains a problem among cattle in underdeveloped areas of the world, although it has been controlled by quarantine measures in more advanced countries. Less progress has been made in control of swine pneumonias (*M. hyorhinis, M. hyopneumoniae*) and in control of respiratory diseases of poultry (*M. gallisepticum* and others).

The importance of viral diagnosis to public health represents another point where mycoplasmas exert a more subtle but nevertheless significant influence. Mycoplasmas persist in tissue cultures in the presence of antimicrobials which inhibit bacteria and fungi, creating a problem for laboratories, especially in the maintenance of continuous cell lines. Depending upon species involved, these organisms can interfere with either cell or viral growth, or may themselves produce confusing cytopathic effects. Formerly, cell cultures were often contaminated with human oropharyngeal mycoplasma species. Recognition of this problem with consequent improvement in technique has altered the epidemiology of cell culture contamination so that currently the main sources of such contamination are other infected cell lines and biologic supplements such as sera. Guidelines for control of mycoplasmal contamination in cell culture are available.[33]

Prevention and control of mycoplasmal infections have been longterm goals for animal and poultry industries and are desirable among populations of humans at high risk for respiratory infections. Although some vaccines have proven effective experimentally or in selected field trials, application of this approach to prevention is limited at present. Use of antibiotics as a control measure has been more successful in reducing clinical disease than in eliminating infection or colonization. The current status of work in this area is the subject of a recent review.[2]

DIAGNOSTIC PROCEDURES

In general dimensions, mycoplasma are near the resolving power of light microscopes (0.2 μm), tend to be pleomorphic and react poorly or not at all with organic dyes. For these reasons, direct examination of specimens is nonproductive. Organisms may be visualized with phase-contrast or darkfield microscopy, but cannot be distinguished from debris in clinical samples. Only limited experience with immunofluorescence techniques has been reported. Although progress is being made in development of rapid diagnostic methods, isolation and serology remain important reference standards. These time-consuming techniques are not helpful for therapeutic decision-making in most instances, but are useful in retrospective diagnosis and for epidemiologic purposes. Many diagnostic techniques have been described but will not be reviewed in detail here. Choices among methods depend upon study purpose and laboratory resources. The following methods are popular ones for the organisms of principle interest.

Primary Isolation and Culture

Respiratory or genital mucosal secretions, sputa, body fluids and biopsy samples are suitable for culture. Transport media have not been evaluated systematically for all mycoplasma species. If possible, direct inoculation of agar or broth growth media is recommended. Tubed media are most practical for field studies but should be capped tightly to prevent leakage during transport and evaporation during extended incubation.

Media used for the original identification of *M. pneumoniae*,[5,26] (see Chapter 45, "Media, Reagents and Stains") patterned after those described by Edward,[19] have been used most widely for human isolation work. Recent experience suggests enhanced isolation of *M. pneumoniae* with the formula SP-4,[10] which was first used for identification of *Spiroplasma mirum* (formerly known as suckling mouse cataract agent) and also *M. genitalium*.[45,48] Use of "diphasic" media (broth over an agar layer) has been reported to increase isolation sensitivity.[15] Agar formula A8 and broth medium U10C of Shepard[40] are recommended for ureaplasma isolation. Careful quality control of all ingredients is essential to successful isolation; particular attention should be paid to the sera, yeast extract and medium base.

Media are made selective for mycoplasmas by incorporation of antibiotics that inhibit classical bacteria and fungi but allow mycoplasmal growth (penicillins, amphotericin B, polymyxin). Use of thallium acetate as an antibacterial agent is no longer recommended since it inhibits *U. urealyticum* and *M. genitalium* and is a dangerous poison.[11] Except for variations in nutritional requirements or incubation conditions that facilitate mycoplasmal growth, the media are not selective for particular species and further identification steps are required. Due to the softness of mycoplasma agar media, swab specimens should be rolled carefully back and forth over the surface to inoculate plates. Liquid inocula are spread conveniently with a sterile bent glass rod. Broth media in small tubes may be inoculated by dipping the swab several times into the broth and pressing the tip around the inside of the tube lip to express fluid. Swabs should not remain in the broth due to inhibitory effects of cotton and wooden sticks and the need to inspect tubes for clarity, color changes and microscopic evidence of growth. Synthetic fiber swabs on plastic handles are preferred.

Sputa can be homogenized by grinding or repeated drawing through a needle and syringe, but should not be treated with enzymes or detergents which are deleterious to mycoplasmas. Tissues may be finely minced in enough sterile saline, buffer or medium to produce a 10% w/v suspension. It is prudent to prepare one or two serial 10-fold dilutions of tissue suspensions to inoculate media, since mycoplasmal growth inhibitors often are present (hemoglobin, lysolecithin, antibodies, complement or antibiotics).

After inoculation, agar plates must be incubated in well humidified conditions to prevent drying. Aerobic incubation allows growth of *M. pneumoniae* and reduces recovery of the microaerophilic normal flora species. Anaerobic conditions are preferred for ureaplasma cultivation. Tightly capped broth tubes may be placed in standard incubators.

Identification Procedures

Mycoplasma colonies are nearly transparent and are most easily seen at 30-100 X magnification with the microscope illumination slightly off-center.

For more detailed examination at 100-1000 X, small blocks (1 cm square) bearing colonies can be cut from the agar and transferred surface up to microscope slides.

Coverslip fragments coated with Dienes' stain[17] and allowed to dry are then carefully inverted over the agar blocks. The supravital dyes diffuse rapidly through the moist agar and react with the colonies, producing a lavender or blue coloring. Nonviable artifacts do not stain with this procedure. For further propagation, similar agar blocks can be dropped into broth media or pushed (surface down) across fresh agar.

In broth media, growth of *M. pneumoniae* is suggested by gradual (1-3 weeks) acid pH shift during incubation, while the liquid remains clear and free of sediment. Microcolonies grow on the tube wall and may be seen microscopically (50-100 X) as refractile "spherules" or stellate forms. An alkaline pH shift occurs with growth of *M. hominis*, due to arginine hydrolysis and production of ammonia, and with *U. urealyticum* due to urea cleavage. Subculture to agar is required for proof of growth and use of one of the following methods is necessary for species identification.

Colonies of *M. pneumoniae* may be identified directly on agar by demonstration of hemadsorption or hemolytic reactions. Although *M. genitalium* also has these properties, it is unlikely to be confused with *M. pneumoniae* due to the protracted time required for its primary isolation in SP-4 broth. The few strains of *M. genitalium* available are from male urethritis cases, and there is no information about occurrence of this species at other sites, particularly the respiratory tract. The hemadsorption test[25] employs a 0.2% suspension of washed guinea pig or sheep erythrocytes which is overlaid on agar bearing suspect colonies. After 15-30 min at 37°C, the agar is rinsed with saline several times to remove excess cells. Microscopic examination reveals adsorption of erythrocytes to *M. pneumoniae* colony surfaces. Baby chick erythrocytes are adsorbed by *M. orale* and should not be used in this test. The hemolytic reaction of *M. pneumoniae*[7] is due to production of peroxide which diffuses into the agar. It can be demonstrated by adding a thin layer of melted sheep or guinea pig blood agar (5% cells made up in a 1% agar-0.85% saline mixture, melted and cooled to 56°C) to plate cultures. After reincubation for 24-48 h at 37°C, clear beta-hemolyzed zones with greenish edges are seen over *M. pneumoniae* colonies. Larger than the colonies, these lytic plaques may be seen grossly with transmitted illumination of the plate. Some strains of *M. salivarium* produce green alpha or green-gray alpha hemolysis, but usually are easily distinguished by the larger fried-egg colony morphology of this species.

Since *U. urealyticum* is the only human mycoplasma which possesses urease activity, demonstration of urea hydrolysis provides positive identification for this species. Characteristic colonies on agar can be tested by adding a drop of $MnCl_2$-urea solution which results in a dark brown reaction product on and around the colonies.[41] A differential agar containing $CaCl_2$ also can be used for growth of colonies, resulting in a reaction product which appears brown with transmitted light and white by reflected light. Since $MnCl_2$ inhibits one biogroup of *U. urealyticum* strains, it should not be used in primary isolation media.[37]

Definitive species identification of mycoplasmas requires the use of specific antisera. Convenient methods that have been described are applications of immunofluorescence and inhibition of growth by antiserum (which is a species-specific phenomenon). The immunofluorescence method can be used on agar plate cultures or blocks of agar with colonies, providing the most rapid identification as well as detection of mixed species.[16] After fixation and reaction of agar with fluorescein-labelled antisera, samples are examined with ultraviolet light by epi-illumination for specific fluorescence. Disadvantages of this method are requirements for large volumes of reagents that are not available commercially and for special microscopic equipment.

Mycoplasmal growth inhibition by antiserum has been used for many years for species identification.[8,9] In one method, agar plates are inoculated with a broth culture of the test organism and filter paper disks saturated with antisera are placed on the surfaces. After appropriate incubation for colony development, a zone of inhibited growth will be seen surrounding the homologous species serum disk, but not in the presence of heterologous antisera. Careful control of the inoculum density is important for meaningful results, since too few organisms may not yield distinct zones and too many may overpower the antiserum. Confusion can result if mixed species are present in the inoculum. Reagents can be conserved by selecting antisera to match the biologic properties of the isolate: for example, a fermenting strain could be tested with sera against *M. pneumoniae, M. fermentans* or *M. genitalium*; an arginine-cleaving strain against *M. orale, M. salivarium, M. hominis*, etc. For convenience, antiserum disks can be prepared, dessicated and stored in sterile containers at 4°C. Although highly specific, this method of growth inhibition is too insensitive to use as a measure of antibodies in sera.

Growth inhibition also can be measured in broth culture systems, where pH indicator color changes reflect growth and metabolic activity of the mycoplasma that can be suppressed by antibody.[42] This procedure has been used mainly as a serologic test, since it is more sensitive than the agar plate growth inhibition method. Each mycoplasma species has a characteristic protein profile demonstrable by high resolution gel electrophoresis which could be used as a species identification method, although this is unnecessarily complex for routine laboratory applications.

MARKERS FOR EPIDEMIOLOGIC INVESTIGATIONS

Features of mycoplasmas that could be used as markers for epidemiologic investigations are limited. Biologic properties such as growth rate and colony morphology are variable depending upon subculture history, medium quality and incubation conditions. Antibiotic sensitivity patterns also may change as strains are subcultured. Studies thus far of *M. pneumoniae* have not revealed any stable characteristics which differentiate strains. By serologic methods, at least 6 types of *M. hominis* and 14 types of *U. urealyticum* have been described. Coexistence of more than one type in a clinical sample, especially of *U. urealyticum*, complicates the use of typing schemes for studying transmission. Evidence to date does not relate particular serotypes of these mycoplasmas to pathogenicity.[4]

SEROLOGIC TESTS

A wide variety of techniques has been described to measure immune response to mycoplasmas, including complement fixation procedures, agglutination and hemagglutination (direct and indirect) methods, various types of inhibition of either mycoplasma growth or metabolism, radioimmunoprecipitation,complement-dependent mycoplasmacidal assays, indirect immunofluorescence antibody titrations, immunoblotting and enzyme-linked immunosorbent assays (ELISA). These tests represent extremes of sensitivity, specificity and complexity; choices for use will require consideration of study purpose and laboratory capability. Immune responses to *M. pneumoniae* have been studied most extensively, but indications for serologic tests against *M. hominis* and ureaplasmas are less clear and optimal methodology is the subject of ongoing research. Accordingly, only tests useful for diagnosis of *M. pneumoniae* infections will be discussed. These include the cold hemagglutination test, complement fixation method and others mentioned briefly.

Cold hemagglutination was described originally in relation to "primary atypical pneumonia," now known to be caused by *M. pneumoniae*.[36] Dilutions of patients' sera are mixed with a suspension of human erythrocytes (either from the patient, or Group O/Rh-negative cells) and incubated at 4°C overnight. Hemagglutination which disappears on warming the test to 37°C is a positive reaction. The phenomenon is based on development of antibodies in the IgM class which react with the I-antigen of the erythrocyte membrane.[21] Significant reactions are represented by a 4-fold rise (or fall) in titers between paired sera, or single values equal to or greater than a dilution endpoint of 1:128.

Cold hemagglutinins are useful diagnostically since they rise during the first and second weeks of illness and disappear around the sixth week. However, as they develop in only half of patients proven to be infected with *M. pneumoniae*, their absence by no means excludes the diagnosis. Cold hemagglutinins also have been reported to occur in nonmycoplasmal diseases, although frequently the titers are less than 1:128. Continued use of the procedure is justified by its simplicity, availability in most serology laboratories and the early appearance of cold hemagglutinins relative to more specific antibodies.

Complement fixation procedures for *M. pneumoniae* serology became practicable soon after organism propagation in artificial media was first described.[6] Standard methodology used with other test antigens is suitable, thus the procedure is readily added to existing laboratory routines. It has been popular to incubate serum dilutions with 2 units of complement and 4 units of antigen at 4°C overnight before addition of the hemolytic system. Antibodies of the IgM and IgG classes contribute to this reaction, developing in the second or third weeks of illness and persisting often for 6-12 months.[22] As in other serologic procedures, demonstration of a 4-fold or greater titer rise between paired sera is more meaningful than a single value. Relationship to acute illness is suggested by single titers exceeding 1:128, or by demonstration of IgM class antibodies, which may predominate early in the course of disease.[20]

Complement is fixed in the reaction between antibodies and a glycolipid moiety of *M. pneumoniae*. A workable antigen can be prepared by suspending washed organisms in saline and heating the product at 100°C for 10 min to reduce anticomplementary properties. A superior, more specific antigen is obtained by the chloroform-methanol extraction procedure described by Kenny and Grayston;[28] a simplified variation of this process is recommended.[14]

Other serologic tests may be appropriate in certain applications. A growth inhibition method involves adding a known quantity of organisms to serum dilutions in broth medium containing dextrose and phenol red indicator.[42] The endpoint is the serum level preventing organism growth, otherwise reflected by production of an acid pH. Careful control of the many variables influencing the reaction is required. A similar test is based on the ability of *M. pneumoniae* to reduce colorless triphenyl-tetrazolium chloride to red formazan, a reaction inhibited by the presence of antiserum.[39] These methods are more sensitive than the complement fixation test, and measure predominantly IgG developing late in convalescence.[22] For these reasons they are useful in assessing prior experience with *M. pneumoniae* and for seroepidemiologic investigations. More recently, ELISA technology has been used to detect *M. pneumoniae* antibodies.[3,27] These methods hold promise of greater sensitivity and specificity than the complement fixation test, allow measurement of immunoglobulin class-specific antibodies if desired and lend themselves to automation in laboratories doing large volume work.

CLINICAL SIGNIFICANCE OF LABORATORY TESTS

Despite the specialized techniques and time required for mycoplasma isolation and identification, culture remains the "gold standard" against which other diagnostic approaches are evaluated. Experience has shown the necessity for careful quality control of media to provide the greatest possible sensitivity.

Mycoplasmas are fastidious organisms requiring complex media that contain biological products which vary from lot to lot. It is advisable to store frozen aliquots of media to allow comparative testing when new stocks are prepared. These, in turn, should be subjected to quantitative growth testing using appropriate reference cultures. Ideally, media would be tested with known positive clinical material since primary isolation is more difficult than subsequent propagation. In the future, biotechnological developments based on antigen detection may obviate some of these problems.

The significance of mycoplasma isolation also depends upon differentiation of colonization and active infection. This is a special problem in genitourinary and perinatal disease, where colonization with *M. hominis* and *U. urealyticum* is frequently encountered in the absence of disease. Since *M. pneumoniae* is carried in the upper respiratory tract several weeks after overt disease, and asymptomatic infections are known to occur, recovery of this pathogen also must be correlated with clinical data for interpretation. This problem may not be solved with the development of antigen detection methodology.

The wide variety of serologic techniques described in the literature attests to the continuing quest for methods having greater sensitivity and specificity. The cold hemagglutination test has been shown to be about 50% sensitive and specific for detecting cases due to *M. pneumoniae*. The widely used complement fixation test for *M. pneumoniae* antibodies also is nonspecific in the sense that the antigen used is identical or similar to substances found in vegetables, other bacteria and several human tissues. As more is learned about the antigenic structure of the mycoplasmas, better serodiagnostic methods can be expected.

Another problem complicating seroepidemiologic studies is the tendency for certain common infections to produce perturbations of host immune responsiveness, particularly polyclonal B-cell activation and T-helper cell suppression. Examples of these diseases are measles, cytomegalovirus and Epstein-Barr virus infections. Several mycoplasmal diseases also show these features; *M. pneumoniae* infections may be accompanied by serologic responses to other microbial agents and host tissues, and by tuberculin anergy.[12] As with mycoplasma isolation methods, interpretation of immunologic response must include careful correlation with clinical and epidemiologic data.

REFERENCES

1. Alexander ER, Foy HM, Kenny GE, et al. Pneumonia due to *Mycoplasma pneumoniae*. Its incidence in the membership of a co-operative medical group. N Engl J Med 1966;275: 131-6.

2. Barile MF, Bové JM, Bradbury JM, et al. Current status on control of mycoplasmal diseases of man, animals, plants and insects. Bull Inst Pasteur 1985;83:339-73.
3. Busolo F, Meloni GA. Serodiagnosis of *M. pneumoniae* infections by enzyme-linked immunosorbent assay (ELISA). Yale J Biol Med 1983;56:517-21.
4. Cassell GH, Clyde WA Jr, Kenny GE, McCormack WM, Taylor-Robinson D, eds. International symposium on ureaplasmas of humans with emphasis upon maternal and neonatal infections. Pediatr Infect Dis 1986;5(Suppl):221-354.
5. Chanock RM, Hayflick L, Barile MF. Growth on artificial medium of an agent associated with atypical pneumonia and its identification as PPLO. Proc Nat Acad Sci 1962;48:41-8.
6. Chanock RM, James MD, Fox HH, Turner HC, Mufson MA, Hayflick L. Growth of Eaton PPLO in broth and preparation of complement fixing antigen. Proc Soc Exp Biol Med 1962;110:884-8.
7. Clyde WA Jr. Hemolysis in identifying Eaton's pleuropneumonia-like organism. Science 1963;139:55.
8. Clyde WA, Jr. Mycoplasma species identification based upon growth inhibition by specific antisera. J Immunol 1964;92:958-65.
9. Clyde WA Jr. Growth inhibition tests. In: Razin S, Tully JG, eds. Methods in mycoplasmology I: Mycoplasma characterization. New York: Academic Press, 1983:405-10.
10. Clyde WA Jr. Recovery of mycoplasmas from the respiratory tract. In: Tully JG, Razin S, eds. Methods in mycoplasmology II: Diagnostic mycoplasmology. New York: Academic Press, 1983:9-17.
11. Clyde WA Jr. Letter to the editors. Clin Microbiol Newsletter 1985;7:164-5.
12. Clyde WA Jr, Fernald GW. Mycoplasmas: the pathogens' pathogens. Cellular Immunol 1983;82:88-97.
13. Clyde WA Jr, Hu PC. Antigenic determinants of the attachment protein of *Mycoplasma pneumoniae* shared by other pathogenic *Mycoplasma* species. Infect Immun 1986;51:690-2.
14. Clyde WA Jr, Senterfit LB. The complement fixation test for diagnosis of *Mycoplasma pneumoniae* infection. In: Tully JG, Razin S, eds. Methods in mycoplasmology II: Diagnostic mycoplasmology. New York: Academic Press, 1983:47-56.
15. Craven RB, Wenzel RP, Calhoun AM, Hendley JO, Hamory BH, Gwaltney JM. Comparison of the sensitivity of two methods for isolation of *Mycoplasma pneumoniae*. J Clin Microbiol 1976;4:225-6.
16. DelGiudice RA, Robillard NF, Carski TR. Immunoflourescence identification of mycoplasma on agar by use of incident illumination. J Bacteriol 1967;93:1205-8.
17. Dienes L. Morphology and nature of the pleuropneumonia group of organisms. J Bacteriol 1945;50:441-58.
18. Eaton MD, Meiklejohn G, van Herick W. Studies on the etiology of primary atypical pneumonia. I. A filterable agent transmissible to cotton rats, hamsters and chick embryos. J Exp Med 1944;79:649-68.
19. Edward DG. A selective medium for pleuropneumonia-like organisms. J Gen Microbiol 1947;1:238-43
20. Emmons J, Schluederberg A, Cordero L. An aid to the rapid diagnosis of *Mycoplasma pneumoniae* infections. J Infect Dis 1969;119:650-3.
21. Feizi T, Taylor-Robinson D. Cold agglutinins, anti-I and *Mycoplasma pneumoniae*. Immunology 1967;13:405-8.
22. Fernald GW, Clyde WA Jr, Denny FW. Nature of the immune response to *Mycoplasma pneumoniae*. J Immunol 1967;98:1028-38.
23. Fernald GW, Collier AM, Clyde WA Jr. Respiratory infections due to *Mycoplasma pneumoniae* in infants and children. Pediatrics 1975;55:327-35.
24. Foy HM, Grayston JT, Kenny GE, Alexander ER, McMahan R. Epidemiology of *Mycoplasma pneumoniae* infection in families. JAMA 1966;197:859-66.
25. Gardella RS, DelGiudice RA. Hemagglutination, hemadsorption, and hemolysis. In: Razin S, Tully JG, eds. Methods in mycoplasmology I: Mycoplasma characterization. New York: Academic Press, 1983:379-84.

26. Hayflick L. Tissue cultures and mycoplasmas. Texas Rep Biol Med 1965;23:285-303.
27. Jacobs E, Bennewitz A, Bredt W. Reaction pattern of human anti-*Mycoplasma pneumoniae* antibodies in enzyme-linked immunosorbent assays and immunoblotting. J Clin Microbiol 1986;23:517-22.
28. Kenny GE, Grayston JT. Eaton PPLO (*Mycoplasma pneumoniae*) complement fixing antigen: extraction with organic solvents. J Immunol 1965;95:19-25.
29. Krieg NR, Holt JG, eds. Bergey's manual of systematic bacteriology; vol 1. Baltimore: Williams and Wilkins, 1984:740-93.
30. Lin J S-L, Alpert S, Radnay KM. Combined type-specific antisera in the identification of *Mycoplasma hominis*. J Infect Dis 1975;131:727-30.
31. Lind K, Lindhardt BO, Schutten HJ, Blom J, Christiansen C. Serological cross-reactions between *Mycoplasma genitalium* and *Mycoplasma pneumoniae*. J Clin Microbiol 1984;20: 1036-43.
32. Mardh P-A, Moller BR, McCormack WM, eds. International symposium on *Mycoplasma hominis* - a human pathogen. Sex Transm Dis 1983;112(Suppl):225-385.
33. McGarrity GJ, Murphy DG, Nichols WW, eds. Mycoplasma infection of cell cultures. New York: Plenum Press, 1978:1-342.
34. Moller BR, Taylor-Robinson D, Furr PM. Serological evidence implicating *Mycoplasma genitalium* in pelvic inflammatory disease. Lancet 1984;1:1102-3.
35. Nocard E, Roux ER. Le microbe de la peripneumonie. Ann Inst Pasteur 1898;12:240-62.
36. Peterson OL, Ham TH, Finland M. Cold agglutinins (autohemagglutinins) in primary atypical pneumonia. Science 1943;97:167.
37. Robertson JA, Chen MH. The effect of manganese on the growth and morphology of *Ureaplasma urealyticum*. J Clin Microbiol 1984;19:857-64.
38. Robertson JA, Stemke GW. An expanded serotyping scheme for strains of *Ureaplasma urealyticum* isolated from humans. J Clin Microbiol 1982;15:873-8.
39. Senterfit LB, Jensen KE. Antimetabolic antibodies to *Mycoplasma pneumoniae* measured by tetrazolium reduction inhibition. Proc Soc Exp Biol Med 1966;122:786-90.
40. Shepard MC. Culture media for ureaplasmas. In: Razin S, Tully JG, eds. Methods in mycoplasmology I: Mycoplasma characterization. New York: Academic Press, 1983: 137-46.
41. Shepard MC, Howard DR. Identification of "T" mycoplasmas in primary agar cultures by means of a direct test for urease. Ann NY Acad Sci 1970;174:809-19
42. Taylor-Robinson D, Purcell RH, Wong DC, Chanock RM. A colour test for the measurement of antibody to certain mycoplasma species based upon the inhibition of acid production. J Hyg(Camb) 1966;64:91-104.
43. Taylor-Robinson D, McCormack WM. Mycoplasmas in human genitourinary infections. In: Tully JG, Whitcomb RF, eds. The mycoplasmas II: Human and animal mycoplasmas. New York: Academic Press, 1979:307-366.
44. Taylor-Robinson D, Tully JG, Barile MF. Urethral infection in male chimpanzees produced experimentally by *Mycoplasma genitalium*. Br J Exp Pathol 1985;66:95-101.
45. Taylor-Robinson D, Tully JG, Furr PM, Cole RM, Rose DL, Hanna NF. Urogenital mycoplasma infections of man: a review with observations on a recently discovered mycoplasma. Israel J Med Sci 1981:524-30.
46. Tully JG, Taylor-Robinson D, Rose DL, Cole RM, Bové JM. *Mycoplasma genitalium*, a new species from the human urogenital tract. Int J Syst Bact 1983;33:387-96.
47. Tully JG, Taylor-Robinson D, Rose DL, Furr PM, Graham CE, Barile MF. Urogenital challenge of primate species with *Mycoplasma genitalium* and characteristics of infection induced in chimpanzees. J Infect Dis 1986;153:1046-54.
48. Tully JG, Whitcomb RF, Clark HF, Williamson DL. Pathogenic mycoplasmas: cultivation and vertebrate pathogenicity of a new spiroplasma. Science 1977;195:892-4.

CHAPTER 23

NEISSERIAL INFECTIONS

Stephen A. Morse, Ph.D. and Joan S. Knapp, Ph.D.

INTRODUCTION

The genus *Neisseria* is the type genus of the family *Neisseriaceae*, which currently contains four genera, *Neisseria, Moraxella, Kingella* and *Acinetobacter*.[6] The genus *Branhamella*, which was listed as a separate genus in the 8th edition of Bergey's Manual,[10] was included in the genus *Moraxella* in the 9th edition.[6] Although the *Neisseria* spp. are not closely related to *B. catarrhalis*,[6] the latter are isolated from the same sites and can be confused with *Neisseria* spp.; they are therefore considered here with *Neisseria* spp. for purposes of identification. However, *Branhamella* is discussed in detail in chapter 10, "Branhamella Infections." *Neisseria* spp. are gram-negative diplococci whose adjacent sides are flattened to give a characteristic "kidney bean" shape. Dividing diplococci occur in tetrads. Species are nonmotile, oxidase-positive, catalase-positive and are identified by their ability to produce acid from carbohydrates, reduce nitrate, produce deoxyribonuclease and produce polysaccharide from sucrose. *Neisseria* spp. and *B. catarrhalis* may be identified using the characteristics listed in Table 23:1.

Most *Neisseria* spp. are normal flora in the oro- and nasopharynx and are rarely isolated from other sites.[3,38,70,80] Two species of the genus *Neisseria* cause worldwide endemic and epidemic infections. *N. gonorrhoeae* causes genitourinary tract infections. *N. meningitidis* may colonize the pharynx as normal flora; however, certain serogroups and serotypes may cause epidemics or pandemics of meningitis.

GONORRHEA

CAUSATIVE ORGANISM

Neisseria gonorrhoeae, commonly called the gonococcus, is the etiologic agent of gonorrhea, a disease which occurs only in humans. The organism

Table 23:1 Characteristics Differentiating between *Neisseria* spp., *Branhamella catarrhalis* and *Kingella denitrificans*

Species	Pigment*	Catalase*	Acid from: Glucose	Maltose	Fructose	Sucrose	Lactose (ONPG)*
N. gonorrhoeae	–‡	–‡	+	–	–	–	–
N. meningitidis	–	+	+	+	–	–	–
N. lactamica	+	+	+	+	–	–	+
N. cinerea	–	+	–	–	–	–	–
N. sicca	+	+	+	+	+	+	–
N. subflava							
biovar *subflava*¶	+	+	+	+	–	–	–
biovar *flava*	+	+	+	+	+	–	–
biovar *perflava*	+	+	+	+	+	+	–
N. mucosa	+	+	+	+	+	+	–
N. flavescens	+	+	–	–	–	–	–
*N. polysaccharea***	–	+	+	+	–	–	–
B. catarrhalis	–	+	–	–	–	–	–
K. denitrificans	NG	–	+	–	–	–	–

Species	Polysaccharide from 5% sucrose†	Reduction: NO_3^-	Reduction: NO_2^-	DNase*	Extra CO_2	Growth: MTM, ML or NYC medium*	Growth: Chocolate, blood agar at 22°C	Growth: Nutrient agar at 35°C
N. gonorrhoeae	NG	–	–§	–	VI‖	+	–	–
N. meningitidis	NG	–	d‡	–	I	+	–	–
N. lactamica	–	–	d	–	d	+	–	–
N. cinerea	–	–	d	–	d	–	–	+
N. sicca	+	–	+	–	No	–	+	+
N. subflava								
biovar *subflava*¶	–	–	+	–	No	–	+	+
biovar *flava*	–	–	+	–	No	–	+	+
biovar *perflava*	+	–	+	–	No	–	+	+
N. mucosa	+	+	+	–	No	–	+	+
N. flavescens	+	–	+	–	No	–	+	+
*N. polysacchareae***	+	–	d	–	No	–	+	+
B. catarrhalis	–	+	+	+	No	d	+	+
K. denitrificans	NG	+	+	–	I	+	–	–

* On nutrient agar.
Catalase test using 3% H_2O_2; *N. gonorrhoeae* reactions stronger using 30% H_2O_2 (Superoxol).
ONPG = O-nitrophenyl-β-D-pyranoside
DNase = Deoxyribonuclease
MTM = Modified Thayer-Martin medium
ML = Martin-Lewis medium
NYC = New York City medium.
† Some strains may be inhibited by 5% sucrose (1% sucrose may be used).
‡ + = Most strains positive (>90%)
– = Most strains negative (>90%)
d = Some strains positive, some negative
NG = No growth
§ Results for tests in 0.1% nitrite; *N. gonorrhoeae* will reduce 0.01% nitrite.
‖ VI = Extra CO_2 very important for growth
I = Extra CO_2 important for growth
No = Extra CO_2 not important for growth
¶ Strains of *N. subflava* biovars have consistent acid reactions.[69]
** New species.[98]

was first described by Albert Neisser in 1889. Gonococci infect the columnar epithelial cells of exposed mucosal surfaces, causing uncomplicated gonorrhea. They may spread to adjacent organs or disseminate via the blood stream. Primary isolates are small (0.5-0.8 μm diameter) diplococci which form colonies 0.5-1.0 mm in diameter, named T_1 and T_2. The cells comprising T_1 and T_2 colonies are virulent, a property conferred, in part, by pili which aid in the attachment of gonococci to epithelial cells. Within one or two nonselected subcultures from a primary culture, larger colonies (1.0-2.0 mm diameter) termed T_3 or T_4 are observed.[59,60] Cells composing T_3 and T_4 colonies are avirulent and lack pili. Optimal growth requires aerobic incubation at 35-37°C in an atmosphere of increased CO_2 tension (ca. 5%) on moist enriched media in which toxic fatty acids are bound by starch. Gonococci will not normally grow on nutrient agar and do not survive well at refrigerator temperature or at -20°C.

N. gonorrhoeae does not grow on chocolate agar under anaerobic conditions,[16] although some strains of *N. gonorrhoeae* have been isolated under these conditions.[102] Subcultures will not grow anaerobically unless nitrite is provided as an exogenous terminal electron acceptor.[65]

CLINICAL MANIFESTATIONS

After an incubation period of 2 to 7 days, most infected men develop symptoms. The initial symptom may be mild dysuria or urethral discharge, but often both occur. The urethral discharge can range from a scanty clear fluid to a profoundly purulent, copious one. The discharge in gonococcal urethritis is usually more purulent and profuse than the discharge in nongonococcal urethritis, but this difference is not diagnostic. Approximately 3% of newly infected men develop asymptomatic urethral infection and thus serve as an important reservoir of gonorrhea.[23,44] The prevalence of infection among asymptomatic men who are consorts of women with salpingitis and disseminated infection or are identified by routine screening can range from 40% to 60%.[23,44]

In women, the endocervix is the primary site of genital gonococcal infection. The clinical picture in women with endocervical infection largely depends on the epidemiologic setting in which they are diagnosed.[74] Women who go to emergency rooms or to sexually transmitted disease (STD) clinics most often have symptoms. Women who are diagnosed because of positive screening cultures, or who are seen because of contact tracing, are usually asymptomatic. The vaginal wall of the postpubertal woman is relatively resistant to gonococcal infection, but Bartholin's glands and Skene's glands occasionally may become infected, causing inflammation with a purulent mucous exudate.

The clinical spectrum of rectal gonococcal infection ranges from asymptomatic infection to severe symptoms with a profuse, purulent anal discharge, marked stinging or burning rectal pain, tenesmus, pus and occasionally, blood in the stool. There are minimal differences in symptoms between men and women, although there are differences in the percentages who are asymptomatic. Anorectal gonococcal infection in homosexual men follows rectal intercourse.[63] Anorectal infections rarely, if ever, occur in men who are strictly heterosexual. Between 18% and 34% of men with rectal infection are asymptomatic.[36,71] Of the women with genital gonococcal infection, between 30% and 60% have positive rectal cultures;[12,100,101] about 5% of women with gonococcal infection have positive cultures only from the rectum.[84,101] Less than 5% of women with rectal gonococcal infection are symptomatic.

Pharyngeal infection with *N. gonorrhoeae* occurs predominantly in women and homosexual men who practice fellatio.[85,107,110] Less commonly, pharyngeal infection follows cunnilingus, mouth-to-mouth contact or presumed autoinoculation with infectious genital secretions.[85,107,110] Pharyngeal gonococcal infection is usually asymptomatic in approximately 80% of patients. Most of the patients with symptoms have very mild pharyngitis with minimal sore throat and pharyngeal erythema. Rarely, a patient may have acutely symptomatic exudative pharyngitis.[110] Pharyngeal infection may lead to disseminated infections.[76,110]

N. gonorrhoeae has been implicated as the cause of acute salpingitis in 20 to 80% of patients by data based on the recovery of organisms from endocervical cultures. When the data are based on cultures obtained during laparoscopy, gonococci have been implicated in 8% to 70%.[34] In many respects, gonococcal salpingitis cannot be differentiated from salpingitis caused by other agents. Acute salpingitis usually has a rapid onset of lower abdominal and pelvic pain. Onset is often associated with menstruation and vaginal discharge. About 50% of patients will have fever up to 38-39°C. Local scarring of the fallopian tubes may lead to ectopic pregnancy or infertility, even after a single episode of infection.

Salpingitis is one of the most common and potentially the most costly consequence of sexually transmitted diseases. Previous salpingitis predisposes a woman to recurrent infections. However, recurrent salpingitis is less likely to be caused by *N. gonorrhoeae* than are initial episodes. The terms salpingitis and pelvic inflammatory disease are often used interchangeably to describe pelvic infections in women. Pelvic inflammatory disease also includes infections that occur outside the fallopian tubes. Gonococcal perihepatitis (Fitz-Hugh/Curtis Syndrome) occurs in 1% to 10% of women with pelvic infections.[33] Perihepatitis can also occur in men,[61] presumably from hematogenous dissemination.

Disseminated gonococcal infection (DGI) is a complication of infection of the mucosa and usually represents hematogenous spread from an asymptomatic urogenital, rectal or pharyngeal infection. The organisms may be cultured from the blood of bacteremic patients with fever and chills. Erythematous macular skin lesions appear which may evolve into pustular lesions, some becoming hemorrhagic or developing small necrotic centers. Joint symptoms ranging from mild tenosynovitis to polyarthritis appear at the same time as the skin lesions. If untreated, a single joint will often develop purulent arthritis, and gonococci may be found on culture of the joint fluid. On rare occasions, DGI may be followed by the more severe manifestation of endocarditis or meningitis.[58,73] Patients with repeated DGI may have a congenital deficiency in one of the late-acting complement components.[87]

Gonococcal ophthalmia neonatorum is still responsible for an occasional infection of the eye in a newborn baby. Infection follows contamination of the infant's conjunctiva by direct contact with the infected cervix during birth. The incubation period is usually 2 to 4 days, although it may be longer in cases where ineffective prophylactic measures have been used.[89,105] Silver nitrate prophylaxis at the time of birth has almost eliminated this clinical form of gonorrhea. Adults seldom get gonococcal ophthalmia, but when it occurs it can be severe. The purulent conjunctivitis which occurs following the inoculation of the conjunctiva with infectious genital secretions may proceed to involve and damage the cornea.

EPIDEMIOLOGY

Gonorrhea is the most commonly reported infectious disease in the United States. During the 10-year period 1975-1984, reported gonorrhea in the United States declined from nearly 1 million to 878,600 cases a year; this produced a corresponding decrease in rates from 468/100,000 to 375/100,000 - a drop of nearly 20%.[18] However, in 1985 reported cases increased 4% nationwide over the previous year. Gonococcal infection has been reported more frequently in younger persons than in older adults, with most of the cases in those less than 35 years of age.

Disseminated infection is more common in women than in men.[48,73] Approximately 75% of the cases occur in women in association with menstruation or in pregnancy. In men, DGI can follow either homosexual or heterosexual activity. There are no known specific racial factors predisposing individuals to DGI. DGI tends to occur in much higher incidence in certain geographical areas, apparently associated with certain *N. gonorrhoeae* strains.[66]

Gonococci that produce beta-lactamase (PPNG) have been isolated around the world. In the United States, PPNG accounted for 1% of national gonococcal morbidity in 1985.[111] Current data indicate that this proportion will increase.

PUBLIC HEALTH SIGNIFICANCE

From the 1960s through 1975, incidence of gonococcal infections in the United States increased annually.[2] These increases were attributed to both qualitative and quantitative factors. Qualitatively, the "sexual revolution" resulted in substantial liberalization of sexual practices, and quantitatively, the postwar baby boom produced a large cohort of teenagers reaching sexual maturity in those years.[14]

The recognition of gonorrhea as an increasing public health problem, particularly for women, was the impetus for instituting a gonorrhea control program during the 1970s. This consisted of public education, clinical screening and disease intervention (contact tracing) activities. These broad-based programs are felt to have contributed substantially to the decline in disease which occurred in the late 1970s and early 1980s. Reported rates of gonorrhea increased in 1985, reversing a decade-long trend. The reasons for this resurgence are probably a combination of variables including the diversion of control resources into other priority STD efforts, primarily AIDS and *Chlamydia*, and by the increasing number and variety of antibiotic-resistant strains. Research towards the development of an effective vaccine for gonorrhea continues in a number of laboratories around the world. The likelihood of a successful vaccine is enhanced as knowledge of the pathobiology of the gonococcus increases.

DIAGNOSTIC PROCEDURES

Microscopic Examination of Stained Smears

A presumptive diagnosis of gonorrhea may be made if intracellular and extracellular gram-negative diplococci are observed in leukocytes from exudates. Gonococci are generally present in large numbers in urethral specimens from symptomatic men. In contrast, gonococci generally occur in low numbers in cervical specimens and in early and late infections in symptomatic and asymptomatic men. Presumptive diagnosis of gonorrhea cannot be made on the basis of gram-negative diplococci in pharyngeal smears because other *Neisseria* spp. are normal flora of this site.

Procedure:

Immediately after the specimen is collected, prepare a thin smear on a clean microscope slide clearly marked with a patient identification number. Take care not to disrupt pus cells. Air-dry and heat-fix the smear. A heat-fixed slide may be shipped to a laboratory in a container that will protect the smear from damage. Gram stain the smear, using Hucker's violet,[45] and examine the stained smear under an oil immersion (100 X) objective. Record the presence and quantity of polymorphonuclear leukocytes and epithelial cells, and the morphology, Gram reaction, and intra- or extracellular location of diplococci. The report should include all findings and whether the bacteria "resemble *Neisseria* spp." Gram stains of synovial fluid sediments, urine sediments and conjunctival pus may also be done. Interpretation of Gram-stained conjunctival smears should be made with care, because *N. meningitidis, N. cinerea* and *B. catarrhalis* have been isolated from this site.

Fluorescent antibody (FA) staining procedures may be used to confirm the presence of gonococci in direct smears. Some polyvalent antisera previously thought to be specific for the gonococcus may contain antibodies which crossreact with antigenically related species, including *N. cinerea*. Fluorescent antibody reagents prepared with gonococcal Protein I-specific monoclonal antibodies appear to be highly specific for the gonococcus, and provide a means for direct confirmed identification of *N. gonorrhoeae*.

Culture and Confirmed Identification of *N. gonorrhoeae*

Type of Specimen:

The choice of specimens for culture is made on the basis of the sex and sexual preference of the patient and the site(s) of exposure. Normally, only urethral specimens are obtained from heterosexual men. Cervical, rectal and pharyngeal specimens are obtained from heterosexual women; urethral, rectal and pharyngeal specimens from homosexual men. All specimens should be obtained before administration of antigonococcal therapy. Specimens may also be obtained from the urethra, and Skene's and Bartholin's glands of infected women. Exudate may be obtained by applying pressure to these sites with a swab. Synovial aspirates should be obtained from patients with arthritis or tenosynovitis. Occasionally, *N. gonorrhoeae* may be isolated from centrifuged or even uncentrifuged first-voided urine from infected men and women.[35]

Blood cultures for *N. gonorrhoeae* should be attempted for any patient with suspected disseminated infection. The blood may be inoculated directly onto selective and nonselective media. Alternatively, the blood may be sent to the laboratory in a vacutainer containing sodium polyanetholsulfonate and gelatin.[31,32] It should be noted, however, that sodium polyanetholsulfonate is toxic for some strains of *N. gonorrhoeae* and the specimen should be plated within one hour of collection.

N. gonorrhoeae may often be cultured from specimens which are negative by Gram stain. Gonococci are most successfully cultured when the specimen is processed rapidly. Specimens from mucosal sites may be obtained with cotton, polyester or calcium alginate swabs. Ideally, the specimen should be cultured on an appropriate medium and incubated immediately at 35-37°C in a humid, CO_2-enriched atmosphere.

Culture Media:

Urethral, cervical and pharyngeal specimens are plated on selective medium, i.e., Thayer-Martin medium, modified Thayer-Martin medium and Martin-Lewis medium. These media consist of supplemented GC basal medium plus heated hemoglobin and various antibiotics. A clear medium, New York City medium, is also used for the primary isolation of *N. gonorrhoeae*.

Rectal specimens are plated on modified Thayer-Martin medium or equivalent media containing trimethoprim lactate which suppresses swarming organisms such as *Proteus* spp.

Specimens from sites that are normally sterile may be plated on chocolate agar in addition to selective media to enhance recovery of the organism. Growth of gram-negative diplococci on nonselective medium but not on selective medium may indicate that the organism is either a vancomycin-sensitive gonococcus or is a commensal species.

Media should be quality-controlled for their ability to support growth of fastidious gonococci such as the vancomycin-sensitive strains which are associated with asymptomatic gonorrhea and DGI. Quality control of inhibitors using strains with known susceptibilities, should also be performed on each batch of medium.

Inoculation:

Specimens are inoculated over the entire surface of the plate. The initial inoculum may be applied in a "Z" pattern, and then crossstreaked with a sterile loop. Inoculation methods which will yield isolated colonies are desirable, especially when processing pharyngeal specimens that may also contain colistin-resistant species, e.g., *N. meningitidis* and *N. lactamica*, or the coccobacillus *K. denitrificans*.

Incubation:

Immediately after inoculation, plates should be incubated at 35-37°C in a chamber with ca. 70% relative humidity and ca. 5% CO_2. A CO_2-enriched atmosphere may be provided by either a CO_2 incubator, candle-extinction jar or a sealed container with a CO_2-generating tablet. Only unscented, white candles should be used in a candle jar. Scented candles may contain volatile substances that are toxic for gonococci.

Transport:

If specimens must be shipped to a laboratory, they should be inoculated onto a growth medium (Jembec plate or bottled Transgrow) and incubated for 24 h before transport. The plate system allows the growth of isolated colonies, which in turn permits the separation of gonococci from contaminants. Liquid in the bottle or plate which facilitates overgrowth by contaminants may prevent isolation of the gonococci. Transport of specimens in traditional transport media such as Amies[1] or Stuart[104] is discouraged unless no other means is available. Specimens should be transported to microbiology laboratories by courier or by overnight mail because gonococci generally will not survive in the transport medium for longer than 48 h.

Examination of Cultures:

Plates should be inspected after 24 h of incubation. A culture is not reported as negative unless no suspicious growth is observed after incubation for 48 h.

Suspicious colonies are Gram stained and tested for oxidase production using a 1% aqueous solution of tetramethyl-paraphenylenediamine-dihydrochloride.[45] The oxidase reagent may be placed directly on colonies on the plate, or alternatively, growth harvested on a loop may be placed on reagent-impregnated filter paper and examined for color change. If the organism is oxidase-positive, the growth will turn purple within 10 s. The oxidase reagent is toxic for the gonococci, and should not be placed on all colonies, or the cells should be removed immediately and inoculated onto chocolate agar. A presumptive identification of *N. gonorrhoeae* may be made on the basis of gram-negative, oxidase-positive diplococci in urethral cultures from heterosexual men. Since *N. meningitidis* may also be isolated in urethral cultures from homosexual men,[56] cells from a selective medium shoud be stained with a gonococcal-specific FA reagent, and additional tests performed for confirming identification of *N. gonorrhoeae*.

Identification of Isolates:

Isolation of *N. gonorrhoeae* can be reported only after the isolate has been confirmed by biochemical or specific serologic tests. Pure cultures of isolated colonies must be obtained on chocolate agar for identification. The purity of subcultures must be confirmed by both Gram stain and oxidase reaction. Two types of biochemical tests are currently available for identifying *N. gonorrhoeae*. These are 1) tests that detect acid production from carbohydrates and 2) tests that determine the presence of various enzymes.

The traditional method for detecting acid production from carbohydrates is inoculation of cystine trypticase agar (CTA) containing 1% reagent grade, filter-sterilized glucose, maltose, sucrose, lactose, or fructose. Growth from an 18-24 h culture on chocolate agar medium is inoculated into CTA tubes by pipetting an aliquot of a dense suspension of cells in saline onto the medium, followed by stabbing the upper third of the tube with a needle or loop. Alternatively, the growth is heavily inoculated into the medium using cotton-tipped applicators. The tubes are incubated 16-20 h at 35-37°C in a non-CO_2 incubator. If tubes must be incubated in a CO_2 incubator, the caps should be sealed to prevent exposure of the media to the CO_2, which will produce an acid reaction in the media.

Several rapid tests have been developed which give results within 2-4 h.[8] Differentiation of *N. gonorrhoeae* from most *Neisseria* spp. is made on the basis of acid production from glucose, but not from the other carbohydrates.[104] Negative reactions with glucose must be interpreted with caution because some strains of *N. gonorrhoeae* produce only small amounts of acid and may appear to be glucose-negative. *N. cinerea, N. flavescens* and *B. catarrhalis* do not produce detectable acid from carbohydrates and may be misidentified as "glucose-negative" *N. gonorrhoeae*.[26,70] A radiometric test which detects $^{14}CO_2$ from ^{14}C-labeled carbohydrates has also been used. However, strains of *N. cinerea* produce $^{14}CO_2$ from glucose.[9,91,103]

Rapid enzyme tests are only recommended for confirmation of strains isolated on selective media. *N. gonorrhoeae* produces only prolyl aminopeptidase, *N. meningitidis* produces both prolyl aminopeptidase and gamma glutamyl aminopeptidase and *N. lactamica* produces β-galactosidase in addition to the other two enzymes. In contrast, *B. catarrhalis*, which may occasionally be isolated on a selective medium, produces none of these enzymes.[21] It must be remembered, however, that other *Neisseria* spp. and *K. denitrificans* may occasionally be isolated on selective media as well, especially from pharyngeal specimens.[6,7,47] *N. cinerea* produces prolyl aminopeptidase and has been misidentified as *N. gonorrhoeae*.[8] Careful examination of Gram-stained smears and penicillin-elongation[15] will distinguish the coccobacilli of *K. denitrificans*, and the use of adjunct tests including catalase production, colistin susceptibility and growth on simple culture media such as tryptic soy agar will aid in differentiating *N. gonorrhoeae* from other *Neisseriaceae*.

Serologic Procedures:

Currently, there are no reliable commercially available tests that can indicate current infection by detecting the presence of antigonococcal antibodies in patient sera.[82] Three techniques have been used to identify gonococci serologically in direct specimens or in cultures. A fluorescent antibody (FA) staining technique using an absorbed polyvalent antibody has been used for many years.[82] Recently, it has been found that some FA reagents thought to be specific for the gonococcus also react with the recently described species *N. cinerea*. Thus, these reagents should only be used in conjunction with tests that will differentiate between these species. A new FA reagent using monoclonal antibodies appears to be both sensitive and specific for *N. gonorrhoeae*. An ELISA test using absorbed polyvalent antibodies has been used to detect gonococcal antigens in direct specimens.[99] The sensitivity and specificity of this test approaches that of the Gram stain for men. The test is not as sensitive for detecting gonococcal antigens in women.[99] A coagglutination test using absorbed polyvalent antibodies has been available for several years.[82] However, this reagent also crossreacts with *N. lactamica* and *N. cinerea*. Recently, a coagglutination test using monoclonal antibodies directed against protein I has been introduced. These tests can be used as confirmatory tests, using growth from the initial isolation plate or from a pure culture. The sensitivity of these tests may vary, depending upon the strains studied.[77]

Because of the limitations of these techniques, the need to use other confirmatory tests must be emphasized. Biochemical tests, colistin susceptibility and growth on simple media are useful in differentiating *N. gonorrhoeae* from other *Neisseriaceae*, especially for strains obtained from the pharynx, from sites that are normally sterile and from children at low risk for gonorrhea.

Antimicrobial Susceptibility

Gonococcal resistance to antimicrobial agents has been evolving since the introduction of sulfonamides in the 1930s and penicillin in the 1940s. Early reports[72,92] documented steady increases in chromosomal penicillin resistance from 1944 through 1969, accompanied by the requisite increasing doses of penicillin necessary to treat infections. In 1976, beta-lactamase-producing *N. gonorrhoeae* strains were reported.[3,88] Penicillinase-producing *N. gonorrhoeae* (PPNG) are gonococcal strains that have acquired either a 2.9, 3.2 or 4.4 Mdal plasmid which encodes for the synthesis of beta-lactamase.[28] The plasmids resemble R plasmids found in *Enterobacteriaceae* and *Haemophilus influenzae*.[30,97] Gonococcal strains which also possess a 24.5 Mdal conjugative plasmid can transfer the beta-lactamase plasmid via conjugation.[62] Chromosomally-mediated resistance to penicillin, tetracycline and cefoxitin has also been reported.[93] The basis for this resistance may involve alterations in the cell envelope permeability and penicillin-binding proteins. Resistance to spectinomycin, a drug used to treat PPNG, has been reported.[19] Recently, high-level tetracycline-resistant strains of *N. gonorrhoeae* (MIC 16-64 μg/mL) (TRNG) have been isolated.[20] These strains are also resistant to doxycycline and minocycline. Tetracycline resistance is plasmid-mediated and is due to the presence of a 25.2 Mdal plasmid containing the streptococcal *tetM* determinant.[81]

As a general rule, test-of-cure isolates should be tested for antimicrobial resistance and during an epidemic it may be desirable to test all isolates. Beta-lactamase production can be detected using commercially available methodology, including acidometric tests, chromogenic cephalosporin or an iodometric test.[106] Clinical resistance to penicillin can be determined by placing a 10-unit penicillin disk on a plate containing GC agar plus supplements or chocolate agar, inoculated according to the National Committee for Clinical Laboratory Standards (NCCLS) proceedings for disk diffusion susceptibility testing. Zones of inhibition of less than 25 mm (20 mm on chocolate agar) indicate clinical penicillin resistance. Clinical resistance to tetracycline can be determined in a similar manner, using a 30-μg tetracycline disk. Zones of inhibition of less than 30 mm (25 mm on chocolate agar) suggest clinical tetracycline resistance. Spectinomycin resistance can be determined by placing a 100-μg spectinomycin differential disk (Difco Laboratories) on the surface of a GC agar or chocolate agar plate inoculated as described. Strains exhibiting zones of inhibition of less than 18 mm indicate resistance and should be examined by a standardized test. It is recommended that all PPNG, TRNG and spectinomycin-resistant strains be forwarded to a reference health department laboratory for confirmation and epidemiologic follow-up. The agar-dilution test is the reference method of choice for determining MICs.[5] The use of selective media for susceptibility testing is not recommended.

EVALUATION OF LABORATORY FINDINGS

There is a high degree of correlation (up to 90%) between observation of gram-negative diplococci in urethral smears from men with classical signs of gonorrhea and the presence of *N. gonorrhoeae*.[54] However, a presumptive diagnosis of gonorrhea cannot be made by examining smears from sites which have a normal flora, and particularly from the pharynx which is the normal habitat of commensal *Neisseria* spp. Also, a presumptive diagnosis of gonorrhea cannot be made by Gram stain from patients who have been taking antibiotics.

Cultures may be falsely negative if antibacterial agents such as detergents or disinfectants contaminate the specimen or the instruments used to take them. Toxic materials, such as certain cotton-tipped applicators or scented candles, may also influence culture results. Technical problems including inappropriate transport media, outdated media, insufficient inoculum for biochemical or serologic tests and the use of impure carbohydrates in biochemical tests may result in misidentification. The inhibitor content of selective media must also be monitored. Inhibitory concentrations of vancomycin are believed to have played a role in the selection of certain auxotypes in some geographic areas.[78] Successful isolation and identification are dependent on properly trained personnel, adequate procedures and appropriate interpretation of results.

EPIDEMIOLOGIC MARKERS

Phenotypic markers used to characterize strains aid in studying epidemiologic correlates of gonococcal infection, including the association of specific strains with various syndromes, monitoring antimicrobial susceptibility patterns and ascertaining the effectiveness of control measures. These classification techniques are not practical for routine laboratories, but can be used by reference laboratories.

Before 1973, antimicrobial susceptibility patterns were used to study test-of-cure isolates from patients with apparent treatment failures and specific strains associated with DGI.[109] The validity of such analyses was questionable, because it was not known whether changes resulted from the selection of resistant mutants or to the introduction of more resistant strains. Thus, there was a need for stable epidemiologic markers.

Auxotyping was introduced in 1973 as a method for classifying strains of *N. gonorrhoeae*.[17] Strains were grouped into auxotypes based on their requirements for amino acids, vitamins and pyrimidines. Of the auxotypes described, the arginine, hypoxanthine, uracil-requiring (AHU^-) strains were shown to be associated with DGI and asymptomatic infections.[64] However, the majority of isolates were prototrophic or required proline (Pro^-).[29] Although some prototrophic and Pro^- strains were isolated from DGI in certain geographic areas, it was not possible to subdivide these strains using other markers.[66,68]

Gonococcal isolates have been divided into 46 different serovars using a panel of 6 protein IA- and 6 protein IB-specific monoclonal antibody coagglutination reagents.[69] Use of a dual classification system, auxotype and serovar (A/S) which uses two unrelated phenotypic characteristics, provides a refined method for typing gonococcal strains. A/S classification has been used to study geographic and temporal distribution of gonococcal strains,[68] the association of individual strains with different syndromes and the distribution of antimicrobial resistance in nonPPNG strain populations.[50] A/S classification has been used in conjunction with plasmid analysis to study the frequency and distribution of PPNG strains[90] and of TRNG strains.[81]

MENINGOCOCCAL AND OTHER NEISSERIAL INFECTIONS

CAUSATIVE ORGANISMS

N. meningitidis is the causative agent of meningococcal meningitis (formerly called epidemic cerebrospinal meningitis). The disease can occur in epidemic form. It was first recognized as a contagious disease early in the 19th century. The causative organism was first described by Marchiafava and Celli (1884) in meningeal exudate. In 1887, Weichselbaum isolated the organism from purulent meningeal exudate. Like the gonococcus, *N. meningitidis* (meningococcus), is a small, gram-negative diplococcus which exhibits different colony types and piliation when grown on agar medium.

In contrast to *N. gonorrhoeae*, there is no consistent relationship between pili and colony morphology.[75] Freshly isolated strains may be encapsulated.

Meningococci are not as nutritionally fastidious as gonococci, but specimens from patients with suspected meningococcal disease must be cultured on enriched medium. The optimum growth temperature for *N. meningitidis* is 35-37°C; a moist environment of 50% or higher humidity is required. CO_2 concentrations of 3% to 10% will stimulate growth and are necessary for some strains. Although laboratory strains may grow on simple synthetic media, freshly isolated strains will not form colonies on nutrient agar. Meningococci autolyze easily and are sensitive to desiccation and sunlight.

The primary habitat of *Neisseria* species that colonize humans is the nasopharynx. *N. lactamica* has been infrequently implicated in meningitis, bacteremia or respiratory infections, but has been isolated from the urogenital tract.[57] Its primary habitat is the nasopharynx of infants and young children, 3 months to 6 years of age. The other species which colonize humans include *N. sicca, N. subflava, N. flavescens, N. cinerea, N. mucosa* and *N. elongata*. Although they are considered normal flora, they have been implicated rarely as the etiologic agent of meningitis, bacteremia, endocarditis, empyema, pericarditis and pneumonia.[46] When they are isolated from blood, cerebrospinal fluid (CSF) or other normally sterile body fluids and secretions, they must be identified and distinguished from *N. meningitidis* and *N. gonorrhoeae* (see Table 23:1).

Clinical Manifestations

Meningococcal infection typically presents as meningitis and/or bacteremia. Meningococcemia without meningitis begins with sudden high fever, prostration, myalgias and a petechial or purpuric skin rash. In fulminant infection (Waterhouse-Friderichsen Syndrome), there is widespread intravascular coagulation with resulting shock and usually death. In those who recover from fulminant meningococcemia, loss of gangrenous skin or digits is common. The pathogenic mechanism of fulminant meningococcemia is not entirely clear, but presumably it is initiated by meningococcal endotoxin.

Meningococcal meningitis may occur alone or with meningococcemia. Symptoms of an upper respiratory tract infection frequently precede the onset of meningitis. The sudden appearance of high fever, headache, vomiting and confusion occurs in over 50% of cases, along with the petechial or purpuric rash of meningococcemia.

Meningococci have also been implicated as agents of arthritis, a relatively common complication of meningococcemia. Chronic meningococcemia with fever, rash, and arthritis may last for weeks or months. Meningococci have rarely been implicated as the causative agent of purulent conjunctivitis, sinusitis, pericarditis, endocarditis, primary pneumonia or urethritis.[11,52,55]

EPIDEMIOLOGY

Humans are the only known reservoir for *N. meningitidis*. Meningococci are isolated most commonly from the throat or nasopharynx of asymptomatic persons who carry the organism for variable time periods, usually only a few weeks. The carrier state is important because it provides a reservoir for meningococcal infection and enhances the immunity of the host. From 3% to 30% of normal individuals are carriers at any given time, yet few develop meningococcal disease. Even during epidemics of meningococcal meningitis in military recruits where the carrier rate may reach 95%, the incidence of systemic disease is less than 1%.[39,40] Person-to-person transmission occurs by direct contact with respiratory secretions or with airborne droplets contaminated with the organism.

Meningococci are subdivided into serogroups depending on the presence of capsular antigens. Thirteen serogroups are currently recognized and include A, B, C, D, H, I, K, L, X, Y, Z, W-135 and 29E.[112] Classically, serogroup A strains are responsible for epidemic meningococcal disease; serogroups B and C strains are responsible for infections during interepidemic periods. However, serogroups B and C have also been implicated in epidemics. The other serogroups are isolated sporadically from both carriers and patients with disease. During epidemics, carriers tend to be colonized with the prevailing serogroup.

Meningococcal infections reach peak incidence in late winter and early spring; the lowest incidence is in the summer. Infants between 6 months and 1 year of age have the highest attack rate. Persons under 20 years of age account for 75% of cases.

PUBLIC HEALTH SIGNIFICANCE

At present, mono- or polyvalent group A, C, Y and/or W-135 polysaccharide vaccines are commercially available.[112] The group A and C vaccines are highly immunogenic[41] and effective[4] in adults, but the seroresponse in young children is less marked and of shorter duration.[41,79] Protection is provided through complement-mediated bactericidal antibodies that persist for at least 5 years after a single parenteral injection of vaccine. The capsular polysaccharide from serogroup B organisms is not immunogenic. The vaccines should be used to control outbreaks of serogroup A or C infection, and they may be used as an adjunctive measure in preventing the spread of infection among household contacts of case-patients.

Chemoprophylaxis was an easily implemented and reportedly effective tool in meningococcal epidemics until resistance to the sulfonamides became widespread.[49,83] The most effective alternatives are now minocycline and/or rifampin.[22,83] However, because of objections to the large-scale use of such broad-spectrum antibiotics, these drugs should be administered only rarely, and then to restricted and well-controlled populations.

DIAGNOSTIC PROCEDURES

Specimen Selection and Transport

Specimens for the diagnosis of meningococcal infections include cerebrospinal fluid, blood, aspirate from petechial lesions, nasopharyngeal swabs, sputum, aspirates from effusions, etc.

Transporting Specimens

Ideally, all specimens obtained by aspiration and swabs should be inoculated onto culture media at the patient's bedside. If necessary, specimens from patients with suspected meningitis should be maintained at a neutral pH and transported to the laboratory as quickly as possible under conditions that avoid desiccation and cold. Blood cultures should also be inoculated immediately. If cultures are to be sent to a central laboratory for identification, methods similar to those for gonococci should be used.

Laboratory Processing

Because these infections are life-threatening, processing of specimens from patients with suspected meningitis or meningococcemia is an emergency procedure in the microbiology laboratory. Meningococci are extremely susceptible to chilling and desiccation, so their viability will decline rapidly. Immediate processing of the specimen will avoid loss of viability and reduce the reporting time. If the fluid specimen is not turbid, it should be centrifuged at 1000 X g for up to 60 min, and the sediment used to prepare a smear and to inoculate media.[53] CIE can be used to detect soluble capsular material from group A and group C strains in CSF (and sometimes other fluids).[42,80] CIE results for other meningococcal groups are much less satisfactory, and meningococcal disease should not be ruled out on the basis of a negative test. Both latex agglutination and coagglutination tests for detecting meningococcal antigens in body fluids are commercially available. Both tests are considerably more sensitive for detecting antigen than is CIE.[27,51] Antigen detection tests should always be used in conjunction with Gram stain and culture. Positive results of antigen detection tests provide a rapid, presumptive diagnosis and permit early administration of appropriate therapy. Negative results do not exclude a meningococcal etiology.

Microscopic Examination

Presumptive diagnosis of *Neisseria* spp. can be made by direct microscopic examination of specimens such as CSF, buffy coat preparations and petechial aspirations, as well as liquid cultures and colonies growing on a solid medium.

Preparation and Staining:

Make thin smears of specimens on a clean microscope slide, air-dry, and heat-kill or fix in absolute methanol for 10 min to preserve the leucocyte morphology.[16] Stain smears by the Gram method. A methylene blue-stained smear may be prepared; such stains are rapid and permit recognition of the characteristic "kidney bean" shaped diplococci.

If many gram-negative diplococci are present in the specimen, presumptive identification of serogroup A or C meningococci can be made using a capsular swelling (Quellung) test. Diplococci in body fluids or in culture can be tested with homologous group-specific antisera.

The observation of gram-negative diplococci in specimens from sites such as the oro- or nasopharynx, or in sputum, is not specific for *N. meningitidis* because other *Neisseria* spp. are part of the normal flora of these sites.[70,80] Fluorescent antibody staining techniques are not recommended for examination of direct smears from these sites because the polyvalent antisera crossreact with other *Neisseria* spp.

Examination and Report:

Exhaustive, field-by-field examination of stained smears of CSF under oil immersion (1000 X magnification) must be done before the specimen is reported as negative. The presence, type and number of leukocytes are noted. Gram-negative, intracellular diplococci (0.6 μm x 0.8 μm) may be present as single diplococci or in tetrads. In fulminating infections, few leukocytes may be seen and the diplococci may be mainly extracellular. If patients have been treated with antimicrobial agents that inhibit peptidoglycan synthesis, the cells may be highly pleomorphic. Occasionally, the smear will be negative but the specimen will be culture-positive. Lightly stained, extracellular diplococci may represent a secondary contaminant in the specimen. Meningococci present in direct smears from petechiae appear as intracellular diplococci. Exact observations on direct smears should be reported to the physician immediately. Although the report may indicate that organisms resembling meningococci have been seen, it should be noted that other *Neisseria* spp. including the gonococci have been isolated from CSF[94] and skin lesions.

In early cultures, the diplococci may be pleomorphic. Many tetrads, and sometimes short chains of cells, may be observed. Diplococci may vary greatly in size from very small cells to giant cells, and may stain with varying intensity. A positive reaction of cells with group-specific antiserum may be reported presumptively as *N. meningitidis*.

Culture Procedures

Media:

An enriched solid medium such as chocolate agar or blood agar, and a tube of enriched broth medium such as nutrient broth or brain heart infusion broth supplemented with 10% to 20% serum or ascitic fluid should be used for isolating *N. meningitidis* from body fluids. For isolation from sites with normal flora or contaminated by other bacteria, a selective medium such as Thayer-Martin medium is recommended. All agar plates should be fresh and moist (but not wet), and be prewarmed to 25°C before inoculation. All media selected should be quality controlled to show they can support growth of *N. meningitidis*.

Thioglycolate may inhibit the growth of *N. meningitidis* and should not be used in media. Some strains of *N. meningitidis* are inhibited by the sodium polyanetholsulfonate contained in blood culture media.[32] Toxicity may be overcome by the addition of gelatin.[31] Sodium amylosulfate is not toxic for the meningococcus.[95]

Inoculation:

CSF or other body fluids, including blood, are inoculated onto agar plates. Any remaining fluid should be added to broth medium in a ratio of 1:5 to 1:10.

Blood specimens are inoculated in 10-15 mL aliquots into each of 3 blood bottles to give a final concentration of 10% (v/v). Evacuated bottles must be vented. Blood cultures are subcultured blindly onto chocolate or blood agar for confirmation even when the BACTEC radiometric method is used. A buffy coat prepared for smears may also be inoculated into blood culture medium or onto chocolate agar.

Swab specimens are inoculated onto a selective medium such as Thayer-Martin medium. The specimen is inoculated over the entire surface of the agar while rotating the swab. If nonselective media are used, one-third of the plate is inoculated with the swab and a loop is then used to streak the plate for isolated colonies.

Incubation:

Plate and broth media are incubated at 35-37°C in an atmosphere enriched with ca. 5% CO_2. A CO_2-enriched atmosphere is required for growth of some strains of *N. meningitidis*.

Examination of Cultures:

N. meningitidis normally forms colonies ca. 1 mm diameter in 18-20 h. Plates which show no suspicious growth should be reincubated for 48 h before discarding. Colonies of *N. meningitidis* are circular, smooth, glistening, translucent and nonpigmented. Some strains may begin to lyse within 18-24 h and the growth will be sticky. Nonlysed colonies can be easily emulsified in saline.

Strains of the species *N. mucosa, N. sicca, N. subflava* biovars *subflava, flava* and *perflava* and *N. flavescens* will normally develop pigmented or nonpigmented, opaque colonies upon extended incubation. Strains of *B. catarrhalis* are whitish in appearance, and growth will be dry and slightly friable, unlike the smooth growth of the pathogenic species. Strains of *N. cinerea* will appear identical to *N. gonorrhoeae*.

Identification of Isolates

Strains of *N. meningitidis* may be differentiated from most other *Neisseria* spp. and from *B. catarrhalis* on the basis of their ability to produce acid from glucose and maltose, but not from lactose or sucrose. Strains of *N. meningitidis* may still be confused with colistin-resistant, poorly pigmented strains of both *N. subflava* biovars *subflava* and *flava*,[67] or with *N. polysacchareae*,[7] when acid production from fructose is not used as a differential test. There have also been some reports of maltose-negative meningococci.[98] However, like maltose-positive meningococci, maltose-negative isolates produce gamma-glutamyl aminopeptidase. According to Diena et al,[24] meningococci form colonies on Dubos oleic-acid agar whereas gonococci will not. Phosphate-buffered saline should not be used to make suspensions of *N. meningitidis* because phosphate may be toxic to meningococci.[80]

Presumptive tests must be reported on all isolates from life-threatening infections, including meningitis and septicemia. Although information about the clinical, cytologic and chemical results may aid the microbiologist in presumptively identifying meningococci, it must be remembered that strains of other species can also cause meningitis and bacteremia. Meningococci may also be found in unusual sites such as the urethra, vagina or rectum.[43,56]

Serologic Procedures and Epidemiologic Markers

Isolates of *N. meningitidis* can be grouped according to their capsular polysaccharide. The most commonly encountered serogroups in the United States are groups B, C and Y. Group A strains have been responsible for major epidemics.[86] The additional serogroups (X, Z, W-135, 29E, D, H, E, K and L) are rarely associated with disease.

Some grouping sera are commercially available. A number of serologic methods have been used to group meningococci; however, agglutination is the most reliable and routinely used technique.[108] For epidemiologic studies, group B and group C meningococci can be subdivided into serotypes[37,112] based on specific outer membrane proteins.

The detection of antibodies against meningococci is mainly of epidemiologic interest. The passive hemagglutination test can be used for the detection of group-specific antibody response to infection or to polysaccharide immunization. However, negative results should be interpreted with caution.[112] A bactericidal assay has been used to measure the immune status of an individual, whereas a solid-phase immunoassay has been used for the determination of the immune response to noncapsular antigens such as lipopolysaccharide and serotype proteins of the outer membrane.[112]

Antimicrobial Susceptibility

Routine animicrobial susceptibility testing of meningococci is not yet required since these organisms remain susceptible to penicillin. This may not be the situation for long, however, as a strain of *N. meningitidis* harboring a gonococcal beta-lactamase plasmid has been reported from Canada,[25] and strains of *N. meningitidis* harboring the gonococcal 25.2 Mdal plasmid which encodes for high-level tetracycline resistance have been isolated in the United States. These reports suggest that antibiotic-resistance plasmids can be transferred in vivo from *N. gonorrhoeae* to *N. meningitidis*. Isolates from patients who are not responding well to antimicrobial therapy should be examined by an agar dilution susceptibility or beta-lactamase test to detect possible resistance.

Sulfadiazine susceptibility can be determined by the agar dilution method on Mueller-Hinton agar plates containing 1, 5 or 10 μg of sulfadiazine per mL. Isolates growing at the highest concentration of sulfadiazine are considered resistant.[80] Growth of *N. meningitidis* on Mueller-Hinton agar plates containing 0.25 μg of rifampicin per mL is considered evidence of rifampicin resistance.[80]

EVALUATION OF LABORATORY FINDINGS

N. meningitidis may be suspected on the basis of clinical symptoms, but a meningococcal infection must be confirmed by isolation and identification of the meningococcus. It should be remembered that in the early stages of bacterial meningitis, the symptoms are vague and flu-like, and many classical symptoms may not be present in very young, old or debilitated patients. In these cases, the clinician will rely on the laboratory results for a diagnosis. Four rapid laboratory tests will guide the clinician in treating the patient: a

Gram stain, cytologic examination, glucose and protein content of spinal fluid and a serologic test for meningococcal antigens in blood or spinal fluid.

The Gram stain can reveal the presence of gram-negative diplococci located either intracellularly or extracellularly. If the patient has been treated with antimicrobial agents, the bacteria may be pleomorphic and might be easily mistaken for artifacts. Secondary contamination of the specimen, of containers or of microscope slides may result in the presence of bacterial "ghosts" in the smear and erroneous interpretation of the results. Bacteria in spinal fluid may not be observed if the specimen is contaminated with blood. A presumptive diagnosis of meningitis may be made when gram-negative diplococci are present in the smear, there is an increased white cell count predominated by polymorphonuclear leucocytes and a decreased glucose level with concomitant increase in protein in the spinal fluid.

The results of the microbiologic cultures will depend on proper handling procedures in the laboratory. Specimens must be cultured promptly before desiccation, cooling, phagocytosis, and post-phagocytic killing result in a negative culture. However, it is more common that negative cultures result when specimens are obtained from a patient who has already received antimicrobial therapy. In such cases, the detection of meningococcal antigens by serologic tests can confirm meningococcal meningitis. All isolates must be identified to confirm that the organism is *N. meningitidis* and not another *Neisseria* spp., and for public health and infection control purposes.

REFERENCES

1. Amies CR, Douglas JL. Some defects in bacteriological transport media. Can J Public Health 1965;56:27.
2. Aral SO, Holmes KK. Epidemiology of sexually transmitted diseases. Holmes KK, Mardh PA, Sparling PF, Wiesner PJ, eds. In: Sexually Transmitted Diseases. New York: McGraw Hill, 1984:85-9.
3. Ashford WA, Golash RD, Hemming VG. Penicillinase-producing *Neisseria gonorrhoeae*. Lancet 1965;2:657-8.
4. Ayme G, Etienne J, Gotschlich EC, et al. Cerebrospinal meningitis control. WHO Tech Rep Ser 588, 1976:29.
5. Biddle JW, Swenson JM, Thornsberrry C. Disc agar diffusion antimicrobiol susceptibility tests with β-lactamase producing *Neisseria gonorrhoeae*. J Antibiot 1978;3:352-8.
6. Bovre K. Family VII. *Neisseriaceae* Prevot 1933. In: Krieg NR, Holt JG, eds. Bergey's manual of systematic bacteriology; vol 1. 9th ed. Baltimore: Williams & Wilkins, 1984:288-309.
7. Boquete MT, Marcos C, Saez-Nieto JA. Characterization of *Neisseria polysacchareae* sp. nov. (Riou, 1983) in previously identified noncapsular strains of *Neisseria meningitidis*. J Clin Microbiol 1986;23:973-5.
8. Boyce JM, Mitchell EB Jr. Difficulties in differentiating *Neisseria cinerea* from *Neisseria gonorrhoeae* in rapid systems used for identifying pathogenic *Neisseria* species. J Clin Microbiol 1985;22:731-4.
9. Boyce JM, Mitchell EB Jr, Knapp JS, Buttke TM. Production of ^{14}C-labeled gas in BACTEC *Neisseria* differentiation kits by *Neisseria cinerea*. J Clin Microbiol 1985;22:416-18.

10. Buchanan RE, Gibbons NE, eds. Bergey's manual of determinative bacteriology. 8th ed. Baltimore: Williams and Wilkins, 1974:427-33.
11. Byeff PD, Suskiewica L. Meningococcal arthritis. JAMA 1976;235:2572.
12. Caldwell JG, Price EV, Pazin GJ, Cornelius CE. Sensitivity and reproducibility of Thayer-Martin culture medium in diagnosing gonorrhea in women. Am J Obstet Gynecol 1971;109:463-8.
13. Carrington GO. Unusual isolates of *Neisseria* from blood. In: Von Graevenitz A, Sal T, eds. Pathogenic microorganisms from atypical clinical sources. New York: M. Dekker, 1975:41-8.
14. Cates W Jr, Rauh JL. Adolescents and sexually transmitted diseases - an expanding problem. J Adolesc Health Care 1985;6:257-61.
15. Catlin BW. Cellular elongation under the influence of antibacterial agents: way to differentiate coccobacilli from cocci. J Clin Microbiol 1975;1:102-5.
16. Catlin BW. *Neisseria meningitidis* (meningococcus). In: Lennette EH, Spaulding EH, Truant JP, eds. Manual of clinical microbiology. 2nd ed. Washington, DC: American Society for Microbiology, 1974:116-23.
17. Catlin BW. Nutritional profiles of *Neisseria gonorrhoeae, Neisseria meningitidis* and *Neisseria lactamica* in chemically defined media and the use of growth requirements for gonococcal typing. J Infect Dis 1975;128:178-94.
18. Centers for Disease Control. Sexually Transmitted Diseases Statistics. Atlanta: DHHS(CDC)No. 134, 1984.
19. Centers for Disease Control. Spectinomycin-resistant penicillinase-producing *Neisseria gonorrhoeae*. Morbid Mortal Weekly Rep 1983;32:51-2.
20. Centers for Disease Control. Tetracycline-resistant *Neisseria gonorrhoeae*. Morbid Mortal Weekly Rep 1985;34:563-70.
21. D'Amato RF, Eriquez LA, Thomforde KM, Singerman E. Rapid identification of *Neisseria gonorrhoeae* and *Neisseria meningitidis* by using enzymatic profiles. J Clin Microbiol 1978;7:77-81.
22. Devine LF, Pollard RB, Krumpe PE, et al. Field trial of the efficacy of a previously proposed regimen using minocycline and rifampin sequentially for the elimination of meningococci from healthy carriers. Am J Epidemiol 1973;97:394-401.
23. Dexter DD, Cave VG, Faur YC, Weisburd MH, Wilson ME. Asymptomatic urethral gonorrhea among men in public New York City social hygiene clinics. Sex Trans Dis 1976;12:7-11.
24. Diena BB, Wallace R, Kenny CP, Greenberg L. Dubos oleic acid agar medium in the differentiation of meningococci and gonococci. Appl Microbiol 1970;19:1025.
25. Dillon JR, Pauzé M, Yeung K-H. Spread of penicillinase-producing and transfer plasmids from the gonococcus to *Neisseria meningitidis*. Lancet 1983;1:779-81.
26. Dossett JH, Appelbaum PC, Knapp JS, Totten PA. Proctitis in a child associated with *Neisseria cinerea* misidentified as *Neisseria gonorrhoeae*. J Clin Microbiol 1985;21:575-7.
27. Drow DL, Welch DF, Hensel D, Eisenach K, Long E, Slifkin M. Evaluation of the Phadebact CSF test for the detection of the four most common causes of meningitidis. J Clin Microbiol 1983;18:1358-61.
28. Easmon CSF. Gonococcal resistance to antibiotics. J Antimicrob Chemother 1985;16:409-12.
29. Eisenstein BL, Lee TJ, Sparling PF. Penicillin sensitivity and serum resistance are independent attributes of strains of *Neisseria gonorrhoeae* causing disseminated gonococcal infections. Infect Immun 1977;15:834-41.
30. Elwell LP, Roberts M, Mayer LW, Falkow S. Plasmid-mediated beta-lactamase production in *Neisseria gonorrhoeae*. Antimicrob Agents Chemother 1977;11:528-33.
31. Eng J, Holten E. Gelatin neutralization of the inhibitory effect of sodium polyanethol sulfonate on *Neisseria meningitidis* in blood culture media. J Clin Microbiol 1977;6:1-3.
32. Eng J, Iveland H. Inhibitory effect in vitro of sodium polyanethol sulfonate on the growth of *Neisseria meningitidis*. J Clin Microbiol 1975;1:444-7.

33. Eschenbach DA, Holmes KK. Acute pelvic inflammatory disease: current concepts of pathogenesis, etiology and management. Clin Obstet Gynecol 1975;18:35-56.
34. Eschenbach DA, Holmes KK. The etiology of acute pelvic inflammatory disease. Sex Transm Dis 1979;6:244-7.
35. Feng WC, Madeiros AA, Murray ES. Diagnosis of gonorrhea in male patients by culture of uncentrifuged first-voided urine. JAMA 1977;237:896-7.
36. Fluker JL, Deherogoda P, Platt DJ, Gerlen A. Rectal gonorrhea in male homosexuals: presentation and therapy. Br J Vener Dis 1980;56:397-9.
37. Frasch CE. Noncapsular surface antigens of *Neisseria meningitidis*. In: Weinstein L, Fields BN, eds. Seminar on infectious disease; vol 2. New York: Stratton Intercontinental Medical Book Corp, 1979:304-37
38. Gay RM, Sevier RE. *Neisseria sicca* endocarditis: report of a case and review of the literature. J Clin Microbiol 1978;8:729-32.
39. Goldschneider I, Gotschlich EC, Artenstein MS. Human immunity to the meningococcus. I. The role of humoral antibodies. J Exp Med 1969;129:1307-26.
40. Goldschneider I, Gotschlich EC, Artenstein MS. Human immunity to the meningococcus. II. Development of natural immunity. J Exp Med 1969;129:1327-40.
41. Gotschlich EC, Rey M, Triau R. Sparks KJ. Quantitative determination of the human immune response to immunization with meningococcal vaccines. J Clin Invest 1972;51:89-96.
42. Greenwood BM, Whittle HC, Dominic-Rajkovic O. Countercurrent immunoelectrophoresis in the diagnosis of meningococcal infections. Lancet 1971;3:519-21.
43. Gregory JE, Abramson E. Meningococci in vaginitis. Am J Dis Child 1971;121:423.
44. Handsfield HH, Lipman TO, Harnisch JP, Tronca E, Holmes KK. Asymptomatic gonorrhea in men. N Engl J Med 1974;290:117-23.
45. Hendrickson DA. Reagents and stains. In: Lennette EH, Balows A, Hausler WJ Jr, Shadomy HJ, eds. Manual of clinical microbiology. 4th ed. Washington, DC: American Society for Microbiology, 1985:1093-1107.
46. Herbert DA, Ruskin J. Are the "nonpathogenic" neisseriae pathogenic? Am J Clin Pathol 1981;75:739-42.
47. Hollis GD, Wiggens GL, Weaver RE. An unclassified Gram-negative rod isolated from the pharynx on Thayer-Martin medium (selective agar). Appl Microbiol 1972;17:71-7.
48. Holmes KK, Counts GW, Beaty HN. Disseminated gonococcal infection. Ann Intern Med 1971;74:979-93.
49. Holten E, Vaage L, Neess C, Midtvedt T, Jyssum K. Sulphonamide-resistant meningococci after sulphonamide prophylaxis among naval recruits in Norway. Scand J Infect Dis 1969;1:185-98.
50. Hook EW III, Knapp JS, Hale JA, Bonin P, Handsfield HH. Prevalence of chromosomal penicillin and tetracycline resistance in Seattle, WA. In: Schoolnik GK, Brooks GF, Falkow S, et al, eds. The pathogenic neisseriae. Washington, DC: American Society for Microbiology, 1985:96-100.
51. Ingram DL, Pearson AW, Occhiuti AR. Detection of bacterial antigens in body fluids with the Wellcogen *Haemophilus influenzae* b, *Streptococcus pneumoniae*, and *Neisseria meningitidis* (ACYW135) latex agglutination tests. J Clin Microbiol 1983;18:1119-21.
52. Irwin RS, Woelk WK, Coudon WL. Primary meningococcal pneumonia. Ann Intern Med 1975;82:493-8.
53. Isenberg HD, Washington JA II, Balows A, Sonnenwirth AC. Collection, handling and processing of specimens. In: Lennette EH, Balows A, Hausler WJ Jr, Shadomy HJ, eds. Manual of clinical microbiology. 4th ed. Washington, DC: American Society for Microbiology, 1985:73-98.
54. Jacobs NF, Kraus S. Gonococcal and nongonococcal urethritis in man. Clinical and laboratory differentiation. Ann Intern Med 1975;82:7-12.
55. Jacobs SA, Norden CW. Pneumonia caused by *Neisseria meningitidis*. JAMA 1974;227:67-78.

56. Janda WM, Bohnhoff M, Morello JA, Lerner SA. Prevalence and site-pathogen studies of *Neisseria meningitidis* and *N. gonorrhoeae* in homosexual men. JAMA 1980;244:2060-4.
57. Jephcott AE, Morton RS. Isolation of *Neisseria lactamica* from a genital site. Lancet 1972;2:739-40.
58. John JF, Nichols JT, Eisenhower EA, Farrar WE. Gonococcal endocarditis. Sex Transm Dis 1977;4:84-8.
59. Kellogg DS, Cohen IR, Norins LC, Schroeter AL, Reising G. *Neisseria gonorrhoeae*. II. Colonial variation and pathogenicity during 36 months in vitro. J Bacteriol 1968;95:596-605.
60. Kellogg DS, Peacock WL, Deacon WE, Brown L, Pirkle CI. *Neisseria gonorrhoeae*. I. Virulence genetically linked to clonal variation. J. Bacteriol 1963;85:1274-9.
61. Kimball MW, Knee S. Gonococcal perihepatitis in a male: the Fitz-Hugh/Curtis Syndrome. New Engl J Med 1970;282:1082-4.
62. Kirven LA, Thornsberry C. Transfer of beta-lactamase genes of *Neisseria gonorrhoeae* by conjugation. Antimicrob Agents Chemother 1977;11:1004-6.
63. Klein EJ, Fisher LS, Chow AW, Guze LB. Anorectal gonococcal infection. Ann Int Med 1977;18:340-6.
64. Knapp JS. Typing of gonococci. In: Brooks GF, Donegan EA, eds. Gonococcal infection. London: Edward Arnold 1985:159-67.
65. Knapp JS, Clark VL. Anaerobic growth of *Neisseria gonorrhoeae* coupled to nitrite reduction. Infect Immun 1984;45:176-81.
66. Knapp JS, Holmes KK. Disseminated gonococcal infections caused by *Neisseria gonorrhoeae* with unique nutritional requirements. J Infect Dis 1975;132:204-8.
67. Knapp JS, Holmes KK. Modified oxidation-fermentation medium for detection of acid production by *Neisseria* spp. and *Branhamella catarrhalis*. J Clin Microbiol 1983;18:56-62.
68. Knapp JS, Sandstrom EG, Holmes KK. Overview of epidemiologic and clinical applications of the auxotype/serovar classification of *Neisseria gonorrhoeae*. In: Schoolnik GK, Brooks GF, Falkow S, et al, eds. The pathogenic neisseriae. Washington, DC: American Society for Microbiology, 1985:6-12.
69. Knapp JS, Tam MR, Nowinski RC, Holmes KK, Sandstrom EG. Serological classification of *Neisseria gonorrhoeae* using monoclonal antibodies directed against gonococcal outer membrane protein I. J Infect Dis 1984;150:44-8.
70. Knapp JS, Totten PA, Mulks MH, Minshew BH. Characterization of *Neisseria cinerea* a nonpathogenic *Neisseria* spp. isolated on Martin-Lewis medium selective for pathogenic *Neisseria* spp. J Clin Microbiol 1984;19:63-7.
71. Lebedeff DA, Hochman EB. Rectal gonorrhea in men: diagnosis and treatment. Ann Int Med 1980;92:463-6.
72. Martin JE, Lester A, Price EV, Schmale JD. Comparative study of gonococcal susceptibility to penicillin in the US 1955-1968. J Infect Dis 1970;122:459-61.
73. Masi AT, Eisenstein RI. Disseminated gonococcal infection (DGI) and gonococcal arthritis (GCA). II. Clinical manifestations, diagnosis, complication, treatment and prevention. Seminars Arthritis Rheum 1981;10:173-97.
74. McCormack WM. Clinical spectrum of infection with *Neisseria gonorrhoeae*. Sex Transm Dis 1981;8:305-7.
75. McGee ZA, Dourmashkin RR, Gross JG, Clark JB, Taylor-Robinson D. Relationship of pili to colonial morphology among pathogenic and nonpathogenic species of *Neisseria*. Infect Immun 1977;15:594-600.
76. Metzger AL. Gonococcal arthritis complicating gonorrheal pharyngitis. Ann Int Med 1970;73:267-9.
77. Minshew BH, Beardsley JL, Knapp JS. Evaluation of GonoGen coagglutination test for serodiagnosis of *Neisseria gonorrhoeae*: Identification of problem isolates by auxotyping, serotyping and with a fluorescent antibody reagent. Diagn Microbiol Infect Dis 1985;3:41-6.

78. Mirrett S, Reller LB, Knapp JS. *Neisseria gonorrhoeae* inhibited by vancomycin in selective media. J Clin Microbiol 1981;14:94-9.
79. Monto AS, Brandt BL, Artenstein MS. Response of children to *Neisseria meningitidis* polysaccharide vaccines. J Infect Dis 1973;127:394-400.
80. Morello JA, Janda WM, Bohnhoff M. *Neisseria* and *Branhamella*. In: Lennette EH, Balows A, Hausler WJ Jr, Shadomy HJ, eds. Manual of clinical microbiology. 4th ed. Washington, DC: American Society for Microbiology, 1985:176-92.
81. Morse SA, Johnson SR, Biddle JW, Robert MC. High-level tetracycline resistance in *Neisseria gonorrhoeae* is due to the acquisition of the streptococcal *tetM* determinant. Antimicrob Agents Chemother. 1986;30:664-70.
82. Morse SA, Kellogg DS Jr. *Neisseria gonorrhoeae*: Role of antibodies in diagnosis and identification. In: Rose NR, Friedman H, Fahey JL, eds. Manual of clinical laboratory immunology. 3rd ed. Washington, DC: American Society for Microbiology, 1986:353-8.
83. Munford RS, de Vasconcelos ZJS, Phillips CJ, et al. Eradication of carriage of *Neisseria meningitidis* in families. A study in Brazil. J Infect Dis 1974;129:644-9.
84. Nicol CS. Some aspects of gonorrhea in the female, with special reference to infection of the rectum. Br J Vener Dis 1948;24:26-37.
85. Osborne NG, Grubin L. Colonization of the pharynx with *Neisseria gonorrhoeae*: experience in a clinic for sexually transmitted diseases. Sex Transm Dis 1979;6:253-6.
86. Peltola H. Meningococcal disease still with us. Rev Infect Dis 1983;5:71-91.
87. Petersen BH, Lee TJ, Synderman R, Brooks GF. *Neisseria meningitidis* and *Neisseria gonorrhoeae* bacteremia associated with C6, C7 or C8 deficiency. Ann Int Med 1979;90:917-20.
88. Phillips I. Beta-lactamase-producing penicillin-resistant gonococcus. Lancet 1976;2:656-7.
89. Pierig S, Nigam S, Marasigan DC, Dube SK. Gonococcal ophthalmia neonatorum: relationship of maternal factors and delivery room practices to effective control measures. Am J Obstet Gynecol 1975;122:589-92.
90. Plummer FA, Lourcies J, D'Costa J, et al. Development of endemic penicillinase-producing *Neisseria gonorrhoeae* in Kenya. In: Schoolnik GK, Brooks GF, Falkow S, et al, eds. The pathogenic neisseriae. Washington, DC: American Society for Microbiology, 1985:101-6.
91. Rapacz S, Kasper J. Comparison of a radiometric method with a carbohydrate fermentation method in the speciation of *Neisseria* [Abstract]. Annual Meeting American Society for Microbiology. Washington, DC: American Society for Microbiology, 1976;38:76.
92. Reyn A, Komer B, Bentzon MW. Effects of penicillin, streptomycin and tetracycline on *N. gonorrhoeae* isolated in 1944 and in 1957. Br J Vener Dis 1958;34:227-39.
93. Rice RJ, Biddle JW, JeanLouis YA, DeWitt WE, Blount JH, Morse SA. Chromosomally mediated resistance in *Neisseria gonorrhoeae* in the United States: results of surveillance and reporting, 1983-1984. J Infect Dis 1986;153:340-5.
94. Rice RJ, Schalla WO, Whittington WL, et al. Phenotypic characterization of *Neisseria gonorrhoeae* isolated from three cases of meningitis. J Infect Dis 1986;158:362-5.
95. Rintala L, Pollock HM. Effects of two blood culture anticoagulants on growth of *Neisseria meningitidis*. J Clin Microbiol 1978;7:332-6.
96. Riou JY, Guibourdenche M, Popoff MY. A new taxon in the genus *Neisseria*. Ann Microbiol (Paris) 1983;134:257-67.
97. Roberts M, Falkow S. Conjugal transfer of R plasmids in *Neisseria gonorrhoeae*. Nature 1977;226:630-1.
98. Saez-Nieto JA, Fenoll A, Vazquez J, Casal J. Prevalence of maltose-negative *Neisseria meningitidis* variants during an epidemic period in Spain. J Clin Microbiol 1982;15:78-81.
99. Schachter J, McCormack WM, Smith RF, Parks RM, Bailey R, Ohlin AC. Enzyme immunoassay for diagnosis of gonorrhea. J Clin Microbiol 1984;19:57-9.
100. Schmale JD, Martin JE, Domescik G. Observations on the culture diagnosis of gonorrhea in women. JAMA 1969;210:312-4.

101. Schroeter AL, Reynolds G. The rectal culture as a test of cure of gonorrhea in the female. J Infect Dis 1972;125:499-503.
102. Short HB, Clark VL, Kellogg DS Jr, Young FE. Anaerobic survival of clinical isolates and laboratory strains of *Neisseria gonorrhoeae*: use in transfer and storage. J Clin Microbiol 1982;15:915-19.
103. Strauss RR, Holderbach J, Friedman H. Comparison of a radiometric procedure with conventional methods for identification of *Neisseria*. J Clin Microbiol 1978;7:419-22.
104. Stuart RD, Toshach SR, Patsula TM. The problem of transport specimens for culture of gonococci. Can J Public Health 1954;45:73-83.
105. Thompson TR, Swanson RE, Wiesner PJ. Gonococcal ophthalmia neonatorum: relationship of time of infection to relevant control measures. JAMA 1974;228:186-8.
106. Thornsberry C, Gavan TL, Gerlach EH. New developments in antimicrobial agent susceptibility testing. In: Sherris JC, ed. Cumitech 6. Washington, DC: American Society for Microbiology, 1977:1-13.
107. Tice AW, Rodriguez VL. Pharyngeal gonorrhea. JAMA 1981;246:2717-19.
108. Vedros NA. Serology of the meningococcus. In: Bergen T, Norris JR, eds. Methods in microbiology; vol 10. New York: Academic Press, 1978:293-314.
109. Wiesner PJ, Handsfield HH, Holmes KK. Low antibiotic resistance of gonococci causing disseminated infection. N Engl J Med 1973;288:1221-2.
110. Wiesner PJ, Tronca E, Bonin P, Pederson AHB, Holmes KK. Clinical spectrum of pharyngeal gonococcal infection. New Engl J Med 1973;228:181-5.
111. Zenilman JM, Cates W Jr, Morse SA. *Neisseria gonorrhoeae*: an old enemy rearms. Obstet Gynecol 1986;8(suppl):2-11.
112. Zollinger COD, Brandt BL, Tramont EC. Immune response to *Neisseria meningitidis*. In: Rose NR, Friedman H, Fahey JL, eds. Manual of clinical laboratory immunology. 3rd ed. Washington, DC: American Society for Microbiology, 1986:346-58.

CHAPTER 24

PASTEURELLOSIS AND OTHER BITE WOUND INFECTIONS

Alfred E. Bacon, M.D. and Stephen C. Ross, M.D.

INTRODUCTION

Injuries from animal bites affect an estimated one to three million individuals annually, although fewer than one-fourth are seen by physicians or reported.[30,36] Dogs are clearly the most significant culprit, responsible for well over 80% of injuries.[12] Cats account for an estimated 5-19% of bites.[19] Bites from almost every conceivable animal have been described, including farm animals, wild rodents and carnivores, laboratory animals and pets.

The pediatric population is involved in over half of animal bites.[30,36] Occupations with high risk exposure include animal control officers, who have an estimated 175-500 times greater risk of sustaining a dog bite than the general population,[35] and research laboratory employees in daily contact with a multitude of animals, including monkeys, rabbits, rats and other small rodents.

Variable data exist with respect to the incidence of infection following a bite. Earlier literature suggests an infection rate of 29% following dog bites, with an increased rate of infection to 47% if suturing of the wound is attempted.[34] Recently, however, a number of investigators have prospectively evaluated the incidence and risk factors of infection following bites by animals. These studies suggest overall infection rates of 3.6% to 41%.[7,13,25] Although suturing of wounds continues to be controversial, most authors reported decreased risk of infection if aggressive debridement and wound irrigation are undertaken.[12,13,24,34] Bites from cats are at a significantly higher risk of infection, with up to 50% becoming infected.[20]

CAUSATIVE ORGANISMS

The organisms causing infection after animal bites reflect the skin flora of the victim as well as the oral and gingival flora of the animal. Dog and cat bites have been the most studied and form the basis of the discussion here. Traditionally, *Pasteurella multocida* has been the organism of concern, but other *Pasteurella* spp., particularly *P. pneumotropica*, have been implicated in bite-transmitted disease as well.[30]

The genus *Pasteurella* has undergone taxonomic reclassification leading to three new species which may be associated with animal bites. These include *P. canis* (formerly *P.* "gas" and some *P. pneumotropica*) and *P. stomatis* (formerly considered *P. multocida*) from the oral flora of dogs and cats.[46] As yet, no clinical correlation exists for these organisms since they have not previously been distinguished as separate entities. Recent studies of gingival flora of canines and clinical experience with dog bites identify gram-negative pathogens not previously recognized nor classified. These include the Centers for Disease Control (CDC) alphanumeric groups IIj, M-5, DF-2, EF 4a and 4b.[2,11,49]

Pasteurella multocida

P. multocida is a nonmotile, gram-negative coccobacillus which is facultatively anaerobic and nonsporeforming. It has a worldwide distribution and causes disease in many animals, including hemorrhagic sepsis and pneumonia in farm animals and fowl cholera.[9] It has been found in many domestic animals, including cattle, horses and swine, as well as rabbits, hamsters and opossums.[1] *P. multocida* has been isolated from the oral secretions of over 70% of cats[1] and 22-66% of dogs.[2,49] Infections of bite wounds have been reported to occur at rates from 7% to 50%.[20,22,34] The fact that cats more often carry *P. multocida* and that cat bites more frequently become infected agrees with the observation that the majority of clinical isolates of *P. multocida* (72%) come from cat bites.[1] Other animals implicated in bite infections with *P. multocida* include lions, opossums, rats, panthers and rabbits.[22]

Bite wounds infected with *P. multocida* typically present within 24 hours with local swelling, erythema and purulence: 36% have regional lymphadenopathy but not always fever.[22] In one large series, 30% of patients exhibited significant underlying disease which may have predisposed them to infection.[54] Other manifestations of bite infections with *P. multocida* include sepsis,[3] septic arthritis,[40,54] osteomyelitis[56] and meningitis.[17] Nonbite infections of humans are predominantly respiratory diseases. *P. multocida* is often a secondary invader of the respiratory tract with underlying disease such as bronchiectasis.[40,56] Lung abscess has also been described.[53] Meningitis, without wound infection, has been seen in adults[17] and neonates.[54]

Isolation of *P. multocida* from bite wounds does not require specialized techniques. Swabs of purulent material or aspirates of absesses, if promptly transported to the laboratory and streaked on media containing 5% blood (sheep or horse) will yield recovery of the organism. Recently, a selective medium has been described that can facilitate the isolation of *P. multocida* from clinical specimens. It includes clindamycin, gentamicin and amphotericin B.[33] Gram stain of infected tissue often more clearly demonstrates the coccobacillary nature of the gram-negative organism (Figure 24:1) than do Gram stains of laboratory isolates.

P. multocida forms smooth, gray colonies 0.5 to 1.0 mm in diameter on 5% sheep and other blood agars (See color plate, Fig. 24:1). No hemolysis occurs. More mucoid colonies are often noted in cultures of respiratory tract isolates. A prominent characteristic is lack of growth on media containing bile salts. Biochemical markers are shown in Table 24:1.[55] Consistent reactions include nitrate reduction and catalase positivity. All strains ferment sucrose and glucose. Poor growth results in inconsistency of indole production in peptone broth, whereas the results of the spot indole tests are more consistent.[45]

The oxidase reaction can be inconsistent as well, particularly if commercial test kits are utilized. An 18- to 24-hour colony should be used with a 5% tetramethyl-D-phenylenediamine dihydrochloride solution to reliably demonstrate this attribute.[55] Differentiation from other species of *Pasteurella* depends on lack of acid production from maltose, on the absence of urease activity and the presence of ornithine decarboxylase.

Eleven different biotypes of *P. multocida* have been proposed, based on fermentative characteristics with maltose, mannitol, xylose, sorbitol and trehalose.[45] Others have limited the number of biotypes to five and utilized xylose, mannitol, lactose, sucrose and maltose.[54] Serotyping of *P. multocida* strains can also be performed.[14]

P. canis (formerly *P. multocida* biotype 6) is similar in biochemical reactivity to *P. multocida*, with the presence of ornithine decarboxylase, lack of urease activity and the inability to produce acid from lactose, maltose and variably from xylose. *P. multocida* produces acid from mannitol whereas *P. canis* does not. *P. canis* contains biotypes 1 (indole positive) and 2 (indole negative). Its separation from *P. multocida* is based on DNA homology studies.[42] *P. stomatis* may be distinguished from *P. multocida* by the lack of ornithine decarboxylase and inability to produce acid from xylose, mannitol and sorbitol.

Virulence factors for *P. multocida* are probably related to lipopolysaccharide in the cell wall, as would be expected in a gram-negative bacillus. In addition, a dermatonecrotic toxin has been identified in isolates from pigs and from the swine disease, atrophic rhinitis.[44] Toxin-mediated disease in humans has not been described.

Antibiotic susceptibility testing indicates uniform susceptibility to penicillin G, ampicillin, tetracycline, chloramphenicol and cephalothin.[45,52] More recently, improved activity has been noted with second and third generation cephalosporins. Poor minimum inhibitory concentration (MIC) values with cephalothin and oxacillin should be noted.[52] Pending laboratory in vitro studies, oral therapy with ampicillin or penicillin VK appears adequate for

Table 24:1. Differential Characteristics of *Pasteurella* Species

	*P. multocida**	*P. canis*†	*P. dagmatis*†	*P. stomatis*†	*P. (Actino-bacillus)* pneumotropica*	*P. (Actino-bacillus)* ureae*	*P. (Actino-bacillus)* hemolytica*	*P. aerogenes**
Hemolysis	−	−	−	−	−	−	+/−	−
Motility	−	−	−	−	−	−	−	−
Gas from Glucose	−	−	−	−	−	−	−	+
Acid production								
glucose	+	+	+	+	+	+	+	+
xylose	+/−	+/−	−	−	+	−	+/−	+/−
mannitol	+	−	−	−	−	+	+/−	−
maltose	−	−	+	−	+	+	+	+
Catalase	+	+	+	+	+	+/−	+/−	+
Oxidase	+	+	+	+	+	+	+	+
Urease	−	−	+	−	+	+	−	+
Indole	+	+/−	+	+	+	−	−	−
Ornithine decarboxylase	+	+	−	−	+	−	−	+/−

* Adapted from reference 55.
† Adapted from reference 47

P. multocida infections. Trimethoprim-sulfamethoxazole may be an alternative for patients with significant penicillin allergy. Intravenous therapy with penicillin or cephalothin is appropriate for more serious infections.

Pasteurella pneumotropica (Actinobacillus pneumotropica)

This species was first introduced by Jawetz as an organism causing pneumonia in laboratory mice.[31] Subsequently, the organism has clearly been associated with human disease. Recent studies of DNA homology have led to the proposed reclassification of *P. pneumotropica* in the genus *Actinobacillus*. It is isolated as normal flora from cats, dogs, mice and rats:[23] 4% of dogs harbor the organism[2] and it has been found as a pathogen in bite wounds from dogs as well as in cases of sepsis associated with animal bites.[39,47] As with *P. multocida*, bone and joint infections following bite wounds can occur.[24] The organism can cause disease not associated with bites, predominantly upper respiratory in nature, including pharyngitis.

P. pneumotropica can be differentiated biochemically from *P. multocida* by the presence of urease and the formation of acid from maltose but not from mannitol (Table 24:1). In addition, 36% of strains will grow on MacConkey agar. A species classified by some along with *P. pneumotropica* is termed "*Pasteurella* sp new species." It is clearly associated with animal bites and has many reactions similar to *P. pneumotropica* including urease and maltose reactions.[55] Unlike *P. multocida* and *P. pneumotropica*, it does not possess ornithine decarboxylase activity. This organism, in addition to some isolates of *P. pneumotropica* identified by Hendrickson, has been reclassified on the basis of DNA homology with the species *P. dagmatis*.[42] *P. dagmatis* has biochemical activity similar to *P. pneumotropica* but is unable to produce acid from xylose or mannitol and does not contain ornithine decarboxylase.

Antibiotic susceptibility studies of *P. pneumotropica* are limited but suggest in vitro sensitivity to penicillin, ampicillin, tetracycline, aminoglycosides, erythromycin and cephalosporins.[47] Limited clinical experience has included successful therapy with penicillin, amoxicillin, chloramphenicol and cefuroxime.[23,47]

Pasteurella ureae (Actinobacillus ureae)

First described in 1960, *P. ureae*, unlike the majority of *Pasteurella* species, has been found only in humans.[29] *P. ureae* has been taxonomically related to *Actinobacillus* species and transfer to the genus *Actinobacillus* has been proposed.[43] It is very rarely isolated as a primary pathogen, but the respiratory tract appears to be its usual site of colonization. It is not surprising, therefore, that *P. ureae* has occasionally been implicated in pneumonia and in episodes of bronchitis and bronchiectasis.[48] A few cases of meningitis, bacteremia and neonatal conjunctivitis have been described.[8,10,28,35,37] A number of patients have had possible predisposing diseases.

P. ureae is distinguished biochemically from *P. multocida* by the presence of urease activity and from *P. pneumotropica* by the absence of ornithine decarboxylase. Unlike *P. pneumotropica, P. ureae* will not grow on MacConkey agar.[23,51]

Antibiotic susceptibility testing has been limited but by most accounts the organism is susceptible to penicillin, ampicillin, cephalothin, aminoglycosides and chloramphenicol.[10,28,51] Clinical experience has shown response to penicillin G, ampicillin, cephalothin, chloramphenicol and cefoxitin.

Pasteurella haemolytica (Actinobacillus haemolyticus)

DNA homology studies suggest that *P. haemolytica* should be a member of the genus *Actinobacillus*.[42] It is included here and in Table 24:1 because it will undoubtedly continue to be referred to as *P. haemolytica*. It causes infection predominantly in cattle and sheep. The CDC had received only 11 isolates from humans as of 1985.[55] This organism has been isolated from deer, cattle and sheep, with animal to human transmission poorly documented except in a report of a wound infection following cleaning of a deer.[41]

Distinguishing features of *P. haemolytica* include beta hemolysis on blood agar (72% of isolates),[55] the lack of indole production and growth on MacConkey agar.

P. haemolytica is divided into two biotypes, A and T, based on colonial morphology, carbohydrate fermentation, growth and penicillin susceptibility.[4] These biotypes correlate with colonization of cattle and sheep, respectively.[5] Serological typing based on rabbit antisera to surface antigens has identified twelve different serotypes. Some controversy exists concerning the reliability of various typing methods.[16]

Limited antibiotic susceptibility testing suggests typical susceptibility to penicillin, streptomycin, chloramphenicol and erythromycin.

Pasteurella aerogenes

The taxonomic classification of *P. aerogenes* is unclear; however, it appears to lack adequate DNA homology with the genus *Pasteurella* as reason for continuing to so classify it.[42] It is included here for reference.

A pathogen predominantly in swine, this organism has caused infection following bites from these animals.[55] First described in 1974,[38] it appears biochemically to be similar to *P. ureae* except that it will grow on MacConkey agar and often contains ornithine decarboxylase. It has urease activity and, unlike the other *Pasteurella* spp., it readily produces gas from glucose and sucrose.[61] This organism is an unusual primary pathogen in man but should be considered in swine bite wounds.

DF-2

DF-2 was first reported in 1975 by Bobo and Newton as a cause of meningitis and sepsis in a veterinary worker following a dog bite.[6] Subsequently, 17 cases of DF-2 sepsis following dog bites were described by Butler et al.[11] Despite the presence of DF-2 in only 8% of the oral flora of canines,[2] the association with human infection and dog bites has been well documented through retrospective, epidemiological data.[6,11,21,32]

The clinical manifestations of infection with DF-2 relate to its apparent propensity for bacteremia, particularly in individuals with a history of alcohol abuse or splenectomy.[11,21,32] Meningitis, the Waterhouse-Friderichsen syndrome and disseminated intravascular coagulopathies have been described.[11,15]

DF-2 is a filamentous, gram-negative rod, which can appear curved. The ability of different blood culture media to support its growth is not well defined[53] and the best growth has been reported for heart infusion agar with 5% blood in the presence of 10% CO_2.[11] The organism does not grow on MacConkey agar. DF-2 is a designation of the Special Bacterial Pathogens Laboratory of CDC and represents the term dysgonic fermenter, indicating that the fermentation properties of the organism are difficult to ascertain in routine media. Lack of growth in triple-sugar iron and oxidation fermentation media make determining glucose fermentation difficult.[11,55] Broth with 1% peptone and 3% beef extract with a petrolatum seal enables acid production from glucose.[11]

DF-2 is characterized biochemically by oxidase and catalase positivity. It does not reduce nitrate nor produce urease. Cellular fatty acid analysis by gas liquid chromotography will differentiate it from other dog bite pathogens, including IIj, EF-4, M-5 and *P. multocida*.[18]

Antibiotic susceptibility studies have demonstrated that clindamycin, penicillin and erythromycin are effective agents. Trimethoprim-sulfamethoxazole does not appear consistently effective and the MIC for cephalothin at 4-8 μg/mL argues that it may not be optimal for therapy. Resistance to gentamicin is usually found.[11]

EF-4a and EF-4b

These organisms are short, gram-negative, rod-shaped bacteria, termed EF because their growth is eugonic and because carbohydrate metabolism is fermentative. They have been isolated from both cat and dog oral flora.[55] In the CDC collection of 97 strains of EF-4a, 77 were recovered from human wounds, 32 of which were dog bites and 7 were cat bites.[55]

Separation of the original EF-4 group into EF-4a and -4b is based on the ability of EF-4a to ferment glucose whereas EF-4b does not.[46] Arginine hydrolysis (absent in EF-4b) also distinguishes the subgroups. They are catalase- and oxidase-positive[55] and 42% grow on MacConkey agar. Unlike DF-2, EF-4a utilizes glucose in oxidation fermentation media.[2] Nitrate reduction and lack of utilization of lactose and maltose also distinguish it from DF-2. EF-4b is able to produce acid from glucose in the open oxidation fermentation tube but is incapable of fermenting it.[46]

Antibiotic susceptibilities of a limited number of strains indicate variable sensitivity to cephalothin, but usual resistance to penicillin and susceptibility to ampicillin.[2]

IIj

IIj is classified by the alphanumeric system of CDC. It is an aerobic, gram-negative rod of medium length,[49] with two colony types, one viscous and one butyrous in nature.[2] It has been found in 38-90% of oral secretions of dogs.[2,49] This organism is distinct from DF-2 and EF-4 in its inability to ferment carbohydrates including glucose, and it has been reclassified as a *Flavobacterium* species.[46] It does not grow on MacConkey agar but does grow well on Christensen-urea agar, which helps to differentiate it from other *Flavobacterium* spp. It is catalase- and oxidase-positive and grows best at 35°C. Antibiotic studies have demonstrated sensitivity to ampicillin, cephalothin, erythromycin, tetracycline and gentamicin.[2]

M-5

Group M-5 is also a nonfermenting, aerobic, nonmotile, gram-negative rod. It is an uncommon isolate from dog bite wounds and is not considered a major pathogen.[25] It is similar to *Moraxella* species and grows well on MacConkey agar.[46] It is nonhemolytic on blood agar, producing tan colonies. Its growth on MacConkey agar differentiates it from IIj and the lack of nitrate reduction separates it from EF-4.[49] It is oxidase- and catalase-positive and is susceptible to penicillin.[46]

MANAGEMENT

The management of bite wounds should include debridement of devitalized tissue, copious irrigation of the wound and tetanus prophylaxis. Primary closure of wounds should be attempted only for facial wounds.

Infection as a sequela of bite wounds is common. Since similar organisms are identified in bite wounds, whether clinically infected or noninfected, all wounds should be treated as contaminated and patients should receive antibiotic therapy.[24,26] No empiric choice of antibiotic will cover all potential pathogens in bite wounds. Traditionally, penicillin has been considered the drug of choice for all bite wounds. However, *Staphylococcus aureus* is present in up to 20% of such wounds,[25] suggesting that antistaphylococcal coverage may be necessary. The relatively weak activity of oxacillin against *P. multocida* in vitro and its low oral absorption make it a poor choice for empiric therapy in both cat and dog bites.[27,50] The combination antimicrobial agent, amoxicillin-clavulanic acid deserves consideration, since it has in vitro activity against *S. aureus*, streptococci and *P. multocida*. If sepsis appears likely, blood cultures are indicated and DF-2 should be considered following dog bites, *P. multocida* in cat and dog bites and *Streptobacillus moniliformis* and *Spirillum minor* following rat bites. All are sensitive to penicillin G and this antibiotic would be an appropriate choice for therapy pending laboratory results. Examination of buffy coat smears may be helpful in these situations. As soon as possible, therapy should be guided by identification of specific pathogens and the results of in vitro susceptibility testing.

REFERENCES

1. Arons MS, Fernando L, Polayes IM. *Pasteurella multocida*: The major cause of hand infections following domestic animal bites. J Hand Surg 1982;7:47-52.
2. Bailie WE, Stowe EL, Schmitt AM. Aerobic bacterial flora of oral and nasal fluids of canines with reference to bacteria associated with bites. J Clin Microbiol 1978;7:223-31.
3. Bearn AG, Jacobs K, McCarty M. *Pasteurella multocida* septicemia in man. Am J Med 1955;18:167-8.
4. Biberstein EL, Gills MG. The relation of antigenic types of the A and T types of *Pasteurella haemolytica*. J Comp Pathol 1962;72:316-20.
5. Biberstein EL, Francis CK. Nucleic acid homologies between the A and T types of *Pasteurella haemolytica*. Am J Med Microbiol 1968;1:105-8.
6. Bobo RA, Newton EJ. A previously undescribed gram-negative bacillus causing septicemia and meningitis. Am J Clin Pathol 1975;65:564-9.
7. Boenning DA, Fleisher GR, Campos JM. Dog bites in children: Epidemiology, microbiology and penicillin prophylactic therapy. Am J Emerg Med 1983;1:17-21.
8. Bogaerts J, Lepage P, Kestelyn P, Vandepitte J. Neonatal conjunctivitis caused by *Pasteurella ureae*. Eur J Clin Microbiol 1985;4:427-8.
9. Boyce J. *Pasteurella* species. In: Mandell GL, Douglas RG Jr, Bennett JE, eds. Principles and practice of infectious diseases. 2nd ed. New York: John Wiley, 1985:1294-6.
10. Brass EP, Wray LM, McDuff T. *Pasteurella ureae* meningitis associated with endocarditis. Eur Neurol 1983;22:138-41.
11. Butler T, Weaver RE, Ramani V, et al. Unidentified gram-negative rod infection. Ann Int Med 1977;86:1-8.
12. Callahan M. Dog bite wounds. JAMA 1980;244:2327-8.
13. Callahan M. Prophylactic antibiotics in common dog bite wounds; a controlled study. Ann Emerg Med 1980;9:410-14.
14. Cary CJ, Peter GK, Chrisp CE, Keren D. Serological analysis of five serotypes of *Pasteurella multocida* of rabbit origin by use of an enzyme linked immunosorbent assay with LPS as antigen. J Clin Microbiol 1984;20:191-4.
15. Chaudhuri AK, Hartley RB, Maddock AL. Waterhouse-Friderichsen syndrome caused by a DF-2 bacterium in a splenectomized patient. J Clin Pathol 1981;34:172-3.
16. Chengappa MM, Carter GR, Bailie WE. Comparison of indirect hemagglutination and

rapid plate agglutination tests with counter immunoelectrophoresis for typing *Pasteurella haemolytica*. J Clin Microbiol 1984;20:660-3.
17. Controni G, Jones RS. *Pasteurella* meningitis: a review of the literature. Am J Med Technol 1967;33:379-86.
18. Dees SB, Powell J, Moss CW, Hollis DG, Weaver RE. Cellular fatty acid composition of organisms frequently associated with human infections resulting from dog bites: *Pasteurella multocida* and groups *EF-4, IIj, M5* and *DF-2*. J Clin Microbiol 1981;14:612-16.
19. Elenbaas RM, McNabney WK, Robinson WA. Evaluation of prophylactic oxacillin in cat bite wounds. Ann Emerg Med 1984;13:155-7.
20. Elliott DL, Tolle SW, Goldberg L, Miller JB. Pet-associated illness. N Engl J Med 1985;313:985-95.
21. Findling JW, Pohlmann GP, Rose HD. Fulminant gram-negative bacillemia (DF-2) following a dog bite in an asplenic women. Am J Med 1980;68:154-6.
22. Francis DP, Holmes MA, Brandon G. *Pasteurella multocida* infections after domestic animal bites and scratches. JAMA 1975;233:42-5.
23. Gadburry JL, Zipper R, Taylor JA, Wink C. *Pasteurella pneumotropica* isolated from bone and joint infections. J Clin Microbiol 1984;19:926-7.
24. Goldstein EJ. Animal bites. In: Mandell GL, Douglas RG Jr, Bennett JE, eds. Principles and practice of infectious diseases. 2nd ed. New York: John Wiley, 1985:632-5.
25. Goldstein EJ, Citron DM, Wield B, et al. Bacteriology of human and animal bite wounds. J Clin Microbiol 1978;8:667-72.
26. Goldstein EJ, Citron DM, Finegold SM. Dog bite wounds and infection: A prospective clinical study. Ann Emerg Med 1980;9:508-12.
27. Goldstein EJ, Citron DM, Vagvolgyi AE, Finegold SM. Susceptibility of bite wound bacteria to seven oral antimicrobial agents, including RU-985, a new erythromycin: considerations in choosing empiric therapy. Antimicrob Agents Chemother 1986;29:556-9.
28. Grewal P, Fonseca K, Andrews HJ. *Pasteurella ureae* meningitis and septicemia. J Infection 1983;7:74-6.
29. Hook EW, Hooten TM, Horten CA, Coyle MB, Ramsey PG, Turck M. Microbiologic evaluation of cutaneous cellulitis in adults. Arch Int Med 1986;146:295-7.
30. Jaffe AL. Animal bites. Pediatr Clin N Am 1983;30:405-13.
31. Jawetz E. A pneumotropic *Pasteurella* of laboratory animals I. Bacteriological and serological characteristics of the organism. J Infect Dis 1950;86:172-83.
32. Kalb R, Kaplan NH, Tenenbaum MJ, Joachim GR, Samuels S. Cutaneous infection at dog bite wounds associated with fulminant DF-2 septicemia. Am J Med 1985;78:687-90.
33. Knight DP, Paine JE, Speller DLE. A selective medium for *Pasteurella multocida* and its use with animal and human specimens. J Clin Pathol 1983;36:591-4.
34. Lee MLH, Buhr AJ. Dog bites and local infection with *Pasteurella septica*. Br Med J 1960;2:169-71.
35. Mann NM, Rollag OJ, Hull HF, Montes JM. Animal bites as an occupational hazard among animal control officers. Am J Public Health 1984;74:255-6.
36. Marcy MS. Infections due to dog and cat bites. Pediatr Infect Dis 1982;1:351-6.
37. Marriott DJ, Brady LM. *Pasteurella ureae* meningitis. Med J Aust 1983;2:455-6.
38. McAllister HA, Carter GR. An aerogenic *Pasteurella*-like organism recovered from swine. Am J Vet Res 1974;35:917-22.
39. Medley S. A dog bite wound infected with *Pasteurella pneumotropica*. Med J Aust 1977;2:224-5.
40. Mitchell H, Travers R, Barraclough D. Septic arthritis caused by *Pasteurella multocida*. Med J Aust 1982;1:137.
41. Muraschi TF, Smith CK, Miller JK. Primary cutaneous (ulceroglandular) infection due to *Pasteurella haemolytica*. NY State J Med 1962;62:3137-9.
42. Mutters R, Ihm P, Pohl S, Frederikson W, Mannheim W. Reclassification of the genus *Pasteurella* Trevisan 1887 on the basis of deoxyribonucleic acid homology with proposals

for the new species *Pasteurella dagmatis, Pasteurella canis, Pasteurella stomatis, Pasteurella anatis* and *Pasteurella langaa.* Int J Syst Bacteriol 1986;35:309-22.

43. Mutters R, Pohl S, Mannheim W. Transfer of *Pasteurella ureae* Jones 1962 to the genus *Actinobacillus ureae* Comb. nov. Int J Syst Bacteriol 1986;36:343-4.
44. Nakai T, Sawata A, Kume K. Intracellular locations of dermonecrotic toxins in *Pasteurella multocida* and *Bordetella bronchiseptica.* Am J Vet Res 1985;46:870-4.
45. Oberhofer TR. Characteristics and biotypes of *Pasteurella multocida* isolated from humans. J Clin Microbiol 1981;13:566-71.
46. Raffin BJ, Freemark M. Streptobacillary rat bite fever: A pediatric problem. Pediatrics 1979;64:214-17.
47. Rogers BT, Anderson JC, Palmer CA, Henderson WG. Septicemia due to *Pasteurella pneumotropica.* J Clin Pathol 1973;26:396-8.
48. Rubin SJ, Granato PA, Wasilaukas BL. Glucose-nonfermenting gram-negative bacteria. In: Lennette EH, Balows A, Hausler WJ Jr, Shadomy HJ, eds. Manual of clinical microbiology. 4th ed. Washington, DC: American Society for Microbiology, 1985:330-49.
49. Saphir DA, Carter GR. Gingival flora of the dog with special reference to bacteria associated with bites. J Clin Microbiol 1976;3:344-9.
50. Shanson DL, Gazzard BG, Midgley J, et al. *Streptobacillus moniliformis* isolated from blood in four cases of Haverhill fever. Lancet 1983;2:92-4.
51. Starkebaum GA, Plorde JJ. *Pasteurella* pneumonia: Report of a case and review of the literature. J Clin Microbiol 1977;5:332-5.
52. Stevens DL, Higbee JW, Oberhofer TR, Everett ED. Antibiotic susceptibilities of human isolates of *Pasteurella multocida.* Antimicrob Agents Chemother 1979;16:322-4.
53. Steyer BJ, Sobonya RE. *Pasteurella multocida* lung abscess. A case report and review of the literature. Arch Int Med 1986;144:1081-3.
54. Thompson CM, Pappu L, Levkoff AH, Herbert KH. Neonatal septicemia and meningitis due to *Pasteurella multocida.* Pediatr Infect Dis 1984;3:559-61.
55. Weaver RE, Hollis DG, Bottone EJ. Gram-negative fermentative bacteria and *Francisella tularensis.* In: Lennette EH, Balows A, Hausler WJ Jr, Shadomy HJ, eds. Manual of clinical microbiology. 4th ed. Washington, DC: American Society for Microbiology, 1985:309-29.
56. Weber DJ, Wolfson JS, Swartz MN, Hooper DC. *Pasteurella multocida* infections, report of 34 cases and review of the literature. Medicine 1984;63:133-54.

CHAPTER 25

PLAGUE

Thomas J. Quan, Ph.D.

INTRODUCTION

Perhaps the first written record of human plague was the "plague of the Philistines," recorded in 1 Samuel, Chapters 5 and 6, of the Bible. This episode occurred about 1320 BC. China is considered the ancestral home of plague, with the first record of a plague-like illness in humans in 224 BC.[17,30] Other noteworthy epidemics or pandemics include: one recorded by the poet Thucydides in 430 BC; the outbreak described by the physician Rufus of Ephesus in 100 AD; those during the reigns of the Roman emperors Marcus Aurelius and Justinian in 164-180 AD and 542-594 AD, respectively; the "Black Death" of the 14th century; and the pandemics of the 15th, 16th and 17th centuries. The current pandemic started in the mid-nineteenth century in central China and slowly spread across the world. The first recognized and reported cases in the United States occurred in 1899 in Hawaii and in 1900 in San Francisco. Other introductions occurred in port cities during the next 20 years. After its introduction into western states, the organism spread to native wild rodents, became established and is now enzootic in the western third of the United States. Only local, short-term outbreaks of the disease followed its introduction into eastern ports; the organism failed to become established in these areas, presumably because of the absence of one or more essential factors (suitable vectors, maintenance hosts, climatic conditions, etc.).[17,22]

Plague is now endemic in many other parts of the world with temperate climates, including Asia, Africa and South America. In the United States, plague poses a recurrent public health threat in states west of the 100th meridian—especially in New Mexico, Arizona and California. Since 1970, human infections have also occurred in Oregon, Colorado, Nevada, Texas, Utah, Wyoming and Washington. Plague epizootics have occurred in roughly

5-year cycles among rodent populations throughout these and other western states, with serologic evidence of expansion eastward to the 96th meridian in Texas.[14] Goldenberg et al[15] suggested that more human infections would occur in the United States as a result of increased exposure to plague-infected animals concomitant with increased use of the West for recreational purposes and for housing an expanding population. Indeed, in 1970-1985, there were 243 confirmed plague infections in humans (or a yearly average of 15.2) in contrast to 66 confirmed plague cases from 1925 to 1969 (or a yearly average of only 1.5).

CAUSATIVE ORGANISM

The etiologic agent of plague is a gram-negative, facultatively anaerobic bacterium, *Yersinia pestis*, of the family *Enterobacteriaceae*.[4] Although the organism is considered taxonomically a subspecies of *Yersinia pseudotuberculosis*, it is generally recommended that for clinical microbiologic purposes the specific epithet *Y. pestis* be retained and used.[3,5,23,25]

CLINICAL MANIFESTATIONS

Plague occurs in three principal clinical forms: bubonic, septicemic and pneumonic. Bubonic plague is the common form, resulting from the percutaneous inoculation of *Y. pestis* by the bite of an infective flea or from inoculation into skin lesions (such as cuts or abrasions exposed to infected animal exudates or tissues). The incubation period is 2-7 days, rarely longer. The disease is characterized by sudden onset of fever, shaking chills, headache, myalgia, prostration and pain in the area of involved lymph nodes. Untreated, bubonic plague can result in death. Gastrointestinal symptoms of nausea, vomiting, diarrhea and abdominal pain are frequent. Possible complications arising from hematogenous dissemination of *Y. pestis* include meningitis, pneumonitis and focal metastatic infections of the eye (endophthalmitis), skin (pustules), liver or spleen. Gram-negative endotoxemia may result in cardiovascular collapse, consumptive coagulopathy (i.e., disseminated intravascular coagulopathy) or cardiac failure. This latter event, although rare, may occur without warning when the patient seems almost well enough to be discharged from the hospital.[21]

Classic bubonic plague entails an inflammatory response in the regional lymph nodes. These enlarged nodes are referred to as buboes (singular: bubo). Primary buboes occur most commonly in the inguinal, axillary or cervical areas, but may occur in other regions such as epitrochlear, mediastinal, popliteal, supraclavicular or intra-abdominal areas. Multiple areas of lymphadenopathy may occur rarely as a result of hematogenous spread during intermittent bacteremia or septicemia. Untreated bubonic plague may become septicemic plague.

In all untreated septicemic plague patients, virtually all organs, including the lungs, are invaded. However, functionally transmissible pneumonic infection is estimated to occur in only 5% of such infections, because the patients die before alveolar pneumonitis develops or before respiratory spread is possible.[21] A chain of human-to-human infections may result, however, when plague pneumonia with productive cough ensues, since the agent is no longer dependent on the animal-flea-animal/human complex. The incubation period of primary pneumonic plague infection is 2-3 days. This clinical form is characterized by sudden onset of fever, cough, production of bloody sputum, headache, shaking chills and prostration. The infection is fulminant and the patient soon dies if not treated. Chances of recovery are markedly reduced if specific therapy is not initiated within 18 hours after onset of symptoms.

THERAPY

After appropriate specimens for bacteriologic tests have been obtained, patients diagnosed as having or suspected of having plague infection should be treated with tetracycline, streptomycin or chloramphenicol.[21] Certain sulfonamides, e.g., sulfadiazine, trimethoprim-sulfamethoxazole,[1,6] are also effective.

EPIDEMIOLOGY

Since 1925, all but one of the plague infections in humans have come from nonurban sources and no person-to-person pneumonic spread has been documented. Humans are usually infected by the bite of infective rodent fleas or by direct contact with the carcasses of infected animals. Rodents or their fleas are the most common direct source of infection, but human plague has been acquired from wild or domestic carnivores, specifically, bobcats,[8,13,20] coyotes,[24] domestic dogs[8] and house cats.[10-13,16]

Persons of both sexes, all ages and all races seem to be equally susceptible to plague infection. Recorded differences in age, sex or race distribution have represented differences in exposure to infection rather than differences in susceptibility. In the United States, the annual case-fatality rate has varied between 12% and 33.3% during the past two decades (1966-1985) and the average annual case-fatality rate for this period is 17%.

PUBLIC HEALTH SIGNIFICANCE, PREVENTION AND CONTROL

Plague is an internationally reportable disease. When plague is suspected, federal, state and local public health authorities must be notified. Confirmed

infections are reported to the World Health Organization.[28] Epidemiologic and epizootiologic investigations should be undertaken to ascertain the following:
(1) the source of infection for humans,
(2) the extent of the plague involvement in reservoir animal species,
(3) the potential for occurrence of additional infections in humans,
(4) the hazard to international travel and transport, and
(5) need for suitable animal and ectoparasite control measures.
Risk to humans can be reduced or eliminated by careful application of environmental health principles, animal population management practices and selective insecticidal measures.

Vaccination is generally recommended for laboratory and field personnel who are exposed to the plague organism, to infected mammals or to ectoparasites. The inactivated plague vaccine produced by Cutter Laboratories, Berkeley, California is the only vaccine available in the United States; other vaccines have been produced by various institutes in other countries.[18] However, vaccination of clinical laboratory personnel is not necessary if laboratory safety procedures are carefully followed and specimens and cultures are handled aseptically.

DIAGNOSTIC PROCEDURES

When plague is suspected, specimens should be obtained for laboratory analysis before the patient is given antibiotic therapy.[2] Examination of bubo aspirate by using stained slides or by a fluorescent antibody technique must be done immediately to differentiate gram-positive coccal from gram-negative rod etiologies of lymphadenitis. Proper therapy can be initiated when this examination is done immediately; however, therapy should not await laboratory confirmation or even early culture results when *Y. pestis* is seriously suspected.

In addition to the symptoms listed above, clinical laboratory findings for plague infections may include a polymorphonuclear leucocytosis (20,000 to 60,000/mm^3), lowered platelet counts and occurrence of fibrin split products. Although intermittent bacteremia is commonly recognized even during the first 2 or 3 days of illness, progressive bacteremia is usually present only in patients with septicemic plague or in terminal stages of fatal infections. In bubonic plague, large numbers of organisms are localized in the inflamed, enlarged lymph nodes. Numerous organisms are usually present in sputa from pneumonic plague patients. In either circumstance, dye-stained smears can provide supportive, but not presumptive, evidence of *Y. pestis*, and fluorescent antibody test results can provide specific, presumptive evidence of *Y. pestis*.

Rapid Methodology

Detection of plague antibody in sera by an enzyme-linked immunosorbent assay (ELISA) is sensitive and specific for human diagnostic use,[7] but because species-specific antibodies are required for the best ELISA results, specimens of nonhuman origin are easier and more economically tested by passive hemagglutination.[29] Detection of plague antigen in early clinical specimens (sera or bubo aspirates) by ELISA is based on the use of monoclonal antibodies to *Y. pestis* Fraction 1 antigen.[26] Reagents for either ELISA application are not commercially available and, at present, are available only in limited quantities from plague reference laboratories.

Fluorescent antibody tests for demonstrating plague organisms in specimens or for confirming culture identity are rapid (about 1 h after receipt of suitable specimen or culture grown at 37°C) and specific when performed with fluorescence inhibition tests.[19,27] False positive tests are rare; false negative tests are more common and may occur when specimens have been refrigerated for more than 24-30 h or when cultures have been grown at temperatures lower than 35°C. Fluorescent antibody reagents and protocols for their use are available to state health laboratories from plague reference laboratories.

Microscopic Methods

The plague organism is nonflagellated and nonsporulating. Organisms grown at 37°C on blood agar or seen in tissue smear preparations usually have definite envelopes but are not truly encapsulated. Envelopes of organisms grown in culture can be seen on standard India ink preparations.

On Gram staining, *Y. pestis* appears as a gram-negative rod or coccobacillus. Characteristic bipolar staining is best demonstrated with Wayson stain or another suitable polychromatic stain such as Giemsa. With Wayson stain, *Y. pestis* cells are characteristically light blue to reddish with dark blue polar bodies; cells appear swollen, barrel-shaped, or like ''closed safety pins.'' Microscopic pleomorphism is not uncommon and is determined in part by physiologic and/or environmental factors such as oxygen tension, drugs, chemicals, age and pH.

Primary Isolation and Culture

Identification of *Y. pestis* depends upon isolation in pure culture from human, animal or flea specimens and biochemical and biological characterization of the isolate.

Cultivation:

Inoculate 0.5-1.0 mL of a fluid specimen (blood, bubo aspirate, spinal fluid) into each of several tubes of sterile broth (infusion, brain heart infusion, tryptic soy or similar broths). An aliquot of the specimen (0.25-0.5 mL) is inoculated onto 3-4 blood agar plates or slants. Inoculated media are incubated at 28°C or 37°C (28°C for optimal growth; 37°C for cultures to be examined by fluorescent antibody tests) and examined for growth daily for 7-10 days. If no growth appears by 10 days, the specimen is reported as negative and discarded. Broths are subcultured at 18-24 h to blood agar or similar media. Colonies are picked from agar cultures for identification.

Tissue specimens of human or animal origin are triturated with a small volume of sterile saline or broth and the resulting suspension is processed in the same manner as fluid specimens.

Y. pestis can often be isolated from highly contaminated specimens (e.g., sputa, fleas, tissues from hosts in stages of post-mortem decomposition) by animal inoculation. From 0.1 to 0.5 mL of a saline suspension of the suspect material is inoculated subcutaneously into the inguinal region of a laboratory animal (e.g., mouse, rat or guinea pig). Suspensions of severely contaminated specimens may be inoculated percutaneously by rubbing a small amount of the material onto the scarified skin of the laboratory animal. Inoculated animals are observed daily for morbidity and mortality for at least 14 days. Tissues excised from animals which die or are killed when moribund are processed in the same manner as other specimens.

Methods for Identification

Y. pestis is aerobic and facultatively anaerobic with an optimal growth temperature of −25°-30°C (range = −2°-45°C). Best growth occurs within a pH range of 7.2 to 7.6, with tolerance limits of pH 5.0 to 9.6. The organism is nonfastidious and grows well but slowly on a wide variety of routinely used, commercially available media (e.g., brain heart infusion, tryptic soy broth, nutrient broth and their respective agar formulations). In stationary fluid cultures, *Y. pestis* exhibits a flocculent growth after 24 h of incubation at 28°C or 37°C. Turbid growth is never produced in broth; rather a "stalactite-type" pattern of growth is seen, with floccules that adhere to one side of the tube and settle to the bottom when the tube is jarred.

On agar plates, even after heavy inoculation, growth at 24 h incubation consists of pinpoint, thin, transparent colonies, detectable only with magnification. After an additional 24 h incubation, the colonies reach 1-1.5 mm in diameter and are grayish-white to gray. Under stereoscopic magnification, the colonies have a hammered metal appearance with undulated edges. Colonies grown at 37°C, especially those of fully virulent strains, are slightly mucoid.

Colonies suspected of being *Y. pestis* may be tested for lysis by specific bacteriophage. *Y. pestis* is lysed by the bacteriophage at 22°C and 37°C; other enteric organisms (e.g., *Y. pseudotuberculosis* serotype 1A, often used as a negative control strain) are lysed at only the higher temperature.

Bacteriophage preparations and protocols for their use are available from plague reference laboratories. Results of commonly used biochemical characterization tests are given in Table 25:1. Commercial, miniaturized biochemical test systems can be used for tentatively, but not conclusively, identifying *Y. pestis*. However, not all of these systems include *Y. pestis* in their numerical taxonomic keys. More than one colony may be required to prepare the inoculum and more than 24 h of incubation may be required by a miniaturized system to achieve correct results because *Y. pestis* grows slowly.

Serologic Tests

Diagnosis or confirmation of infection may be based on finding a 4-fold change in titer to specific plague antigens in 2 sera drawn 3 to 5 weeks apart, or in finding a significant titer (>1:10 or 1:16) in a single specimen from a patient with no history of prior vaccination against plague. Procedures for agglutination, complement fixation, passive hemagglutination and ELISA tests[2,7,26] can be obtained from plague reference laboratories. All required reagents are not commercially available and, unless large numbers of serologic tests are planned, reagent production is not cost-effective in terms

Table 25:1. Characteristics of *Yersinia pestis**

Gram Stain: Gram-negative rods or coccobacilli 0.5-1.0 by 1-2 μm
Growth temperature tolerances: −2°C to 45°C
Motility: Negative @ 37°C and @ 22°C

		Acid From:	*No Acid From:*
β-galactosidase	+		
Oxidase	−	Amygdalin (+)	Adonitol
Catalase	+	Arabinose	Cellobiose
Methyl red	+	Fructose	Dulcitol
Citrate utilization	−	Galactose	Erythritol
Nitrate reduction	V	Glucose	Fucose
Arginine dihydrol.	−	Maltose	Glycerol (v)
Arginine decarbox.	−	Mannitol	Glycogen
Lysine decarbox.	−	Mannose	Inositol
Ornithine decarbox.	−	Sorbitol (v)	Lactose
Phenylalanine deam.	−	Starch (w)	Melezitose
Gelatin hydrolysis	−	Trehalose	Melibiose (v)
Voges-Proskauer	−	Xylose (v)	Raffinose
Indol	−		Rhamnose (v)
Esculin hydrolysis	+		Sucrose
Urease	−		
Growth in KCN	−		
Malonate	−		
d-Tartrate	+		

* − = Negative; + = Positive; w = weak positive; (+) = delayed positive (v) = strains differ

Adapted from Bercovier and Mollaret[4]

of time and labor. Serum specimens can be sent to plague reference laboratories.

CLINICAL SIGNIFICANCE OF LABORATORY TESTS

Plague has a >60% fatality rate if untreated and it can be pneumonically spread; consequently, specific therapy should be initiated as soon as plague is suspected on the basis of medical history and clinical examination. However, specimens for laboratory diagnosis should be taken before antimicrobial agents are administered and examined immediately.

Because clinical diseases caused by *Y. pestis* and by *Francisella tularensis* (the tularemia agent) are similar, specimens should be cultured on media that will support growth and recovery of the latter agent as well, and serum specimens should be tested for tularemia antibodies as well as plague antibodies (see Chapter 31, "Tularemia").

REFERENCES

1. Ai NV, Hanh ND, Diem PV, Le NV. Co-trimoxazole in bubonic plague. Br Med J 1973;4:108-9.
2. Bahmanyar M, Cavanaugh DC. Plague manual. Geneva: World Health Organization, 1976.
3. Bercovier H, Mollaret HH, Alonso JM, Fanning GR, Brenner DJ. Intra- and interspecies relatedness of *Yersinia pestis* by DNA hybridization and its relationship to *Yersinia pseudotuberculosis*. Curr Microbiol 1980;4:225-9.
4. Bercovier H, Mollaret HH. Genus XIV *Yersinia*. In: Krieg NR, Holt JG, eds. Bergey's manual of systematic bacteriology; vol 1. Baltimore: Williams and Wilkins, 1984:498-506.
5. Brenner DJ, Feeley JC, Feldman R. Confusion in bacterial nomenclature. ASM News 1982;48:511-12.
6. Butler T, Bell WR, Linh NN, Tiep ND, Arnold K. *Yersinia pestis* infection in Viet Nam. I. Clinical and hematologic aspects. J Infect Dis 1974;129(Suppl):78-84.
7. Cavanaugh DC, Fortier MK, Robinson DM, Williams JE, Rust JH Jr. Application of the ELISA technique to problems in the serologic diagnosis of plague. Bull Pan Am Health Org 1979;13:399-402.
8. Centers for Disease Control. Plague surveillance, reference and research. Report for 1975. Division of Vector-Borne Viral Diseases, Center for Infectious Diseases, Fort Collins, CO.
9. Centers for Disease Control. Plague surveillance, reference and research. Report for 1980. Division of Vector-Borne Viral Diseases, Center for Infectious Diseases, Fort Collins, CO.
10. Centers for Disease Control. Plague surveillance, reference and research. Report for 1981. Division of Vector-Borne Viral Diseases, Center for Infectious Diseases, Fort Collins, CO.
11. Centers for Disease Control. Plague surveillance, reference and research. Report for 1981. Division of Vector-Borne Viral Diseases, Center for Infectious Diseases, Fort Collins, CO.
12. Centers for Disease Control. Plague surveillance, reference and research. Report for 1982. Division of Vector-Borne Viral Diseases, Center for Infectious Diseases, Fort Collins, CO.

13. Centers for Disease Control. Plague surveillance, reference and research. Report for 1983-1984. Division of Vector-Borne Viral Diseases, Center for Infectious Diseases, Fort Collins, CO.
14. Centers for Disease Control. Plague—United States 1976. Morbid Mortal Weekly Rep 1977;26:159.
15. Goldenberg MI, Hudson BW, Kartman L. *Pasteurella* infections. I. *Pasteurella pestis*. In: Bodily HL, Updyke EL, Mason JO, eds. Diagnostic procedures for bacterial, mycotic and parasitic infections. 5th ed. New York: American Public Health Association, 1970:422-39.
16. Isaacson M, Levy D, Pienaar B, Bubb HD, Louw JA, Genis DK. Unusual cases of human plague in Southern Africa. South Africa Med J 1973;4:2109-13.
17. Link VB. A history of plague in the United States. Washington, DC: Public Health Service Monograph No.26, Public Health Service Publication No 592. US Government Printing Office, 1955.
18. Meyer KF, Cavanaugh DC, Bartonelli PJ, Marshall JD Jr. Plague immunization. I. Past and present trends. J Infect Dis 1974;129(Suppl):13-8.
19. Moody MD, Winter CC. Rapid identification of *Pasteurella pestis* with fluorescent antibody. III. Staining *Pasteurella pestis* in tissue impression smears. J Infect Dis 1959;104:288-94.
20. Poland JD, Barnes AM, Herman JJ. Human bubonic plague from exposure to a naturally infected wild carnivore. Am J Epidemiol 1973;92:332-7.
21. Poland JD. Plague. In: Hoeprich PD, ed. Infectious diseases. 2nd ed. Hagerstown, MD: Harper and Row, 1977:1050-60.
22. Quan TJ. Plague. In: Starr MP, Stolp H, Truper HH, et al, eds. The prokaryotes. New York: Springer Verlag, 1981:1240-47.
23. Quan TJ, Poland JD, Barnes AM. Where has *pestis* gone? Dangerously egregious taxonomic recommendations. ASM News 1984;50:193-4.
24. Von Reyn CF, Barnes AM, Weber NS, Quan TJ, Dean WJ. Bubonic plague from direct exposure to a naturally infected wild coyote. Am J Trop Med Hyg 1976;25:626-9.
25. Williams JE. Warning on a new potential for laboratory acquired infection as a result of the new nomenclature for the plague bacillus. Bull WHO 1983;61:545-6.
26. Williams JE, Gentry MK, Braden CA, Leister F, Yolken RH. Use of an enzyme-linked immunosorbent assay to measure antigenemia during acute plague. Bull WHO 1984;62:463-6.
27. Winter CC, Moody MD. A rapid identification of *Pasteurella pestis* with fluorescent antibody. II. Specific identification of *Pasteurella pestis* in dried smears. J Infect Dis 1959;104:281-7.
28. World Health Organization. International health regulations. Geneva: World Health Organization, 1968.
29. World Health Organization Committee on Plague. Passive hemagglutination test. WHO Tech Rep Series 1970;447:23-5.
30. Wu LT. In: Scott HH, ed. A history of tropical medicine; vol II. Baltimore: Williams and Wilkins, 1939:712.

CHAPTER 26

PSEUDOMONAS INFECTIONS

David L. Sewell, Ph.D.

INTRODUCTION

Of the many members of the genus *Pseudomonas*, only a small number have been associated with disease in humans (Table 26:1). Although *Pseudomonas aeruginosa* was first isolated from a clinical infection in 1882 by Gessard, only in the last 30 years has it emerged as a significant pathogen. With the exception of *P. pseudomallei* and *P. mallei*, most other species are opportunistic pathogens or are encountered in clinical specimens as superficial colonizers or contaminants. The importance of *Pseudomonas* species in nosocomial infections is related to the increasing population of patients who are immunocompromised, are receiving broad-spectrum antimicrobial agents or are subject to invasive procedures.

The pseudomonads are a heterogeneous group of bacilli that are aerobic, asporogenous, oxidase-positive, gram-negative and usually motile by means of polar flagella. The *Pseudomonas* species metabolize carbohydrates via oxidative pathways. Some species can grow anaerobically using nitrate as an alternate electron acceptor for oxygen. The recent development and clarification of criteria for the practical identification of *Pseudomonas* species has led to greater clinical interest in their role as pathogens.

The extent to which a laboratory identifies *Pseudomonas* species depends on a number of factors including (1) the underlying condition of the patient (high risk for opportunistic infections); (2) the source of the specimen (sterile or colonized); (3) the sole or predominant isolate from the specimen; (4) the need for epidemiologic surveillance (same isolate from similar specimens suggests a common-source outbreak); and (5) available laboratory resources. The final determination of the clinical significance of a *Pseudomonas* species should involve both the clinician and the microbiologist.

Table 26:1. ***Pseudomonas*** **Species Isolated from Clinical Specimens**

Name	Disease	Frequency of Isolation
P. aeruginosa	Opportunistic	Frequent
P. fluorescens	Opportunistic	Infrequent
P. putida	Opportunistic	Infrequent
P. stutzeri	Opportunistic	Infrequent
P. cepacia	Opportunistic	Infrequent
P. maltophilia	Opportunistic	Infrequent
P. mallei	Glanders	Rare
P. pseudomallei	Melioidosis	Rare
P. alcaligenes	Opportunistic	Rare
P. pseudoalcaligenes	Opportunistic	Rare
P. pickettii	Opportunistic	Rare
P. acidovorans	Opportunistic	Rare
P. testosteroni	Opportunistic	Rare
P. species Group 1	Opportunistic	Rare
P. diminuta	Opportunistic	Rare
P. mesophilica	Opportunistic	Rare
P. paucimobilis	Opportunistic	Rare
P. putrefaciens	Opportunistic	Rare
P. sp Group Ve-1	Opportunistic	Rare
P. gladioli	None	Rare
P. mendocina	None	Rare
P. vesicularis	None	Rare
P. sp. Group Ve-2	None	Rare
P. sp. Group 2	None	Rare
P. delafieldii	None	Rare

CLINICAL MANIFESTATIONS

Members of the genus *Pseudomonas* produce a variety of opportunistic infections, usually in the immunocompromised, hospitalized patient or where there is environmental contamination of a wound.[21,22,23,28,67] Although many *Pseudomonas* species are frequently isolated from the hospital environment, *P. aeruginosa* is the most common isolate and it alone causes more infections than all the other species combined.

Major infections caused by *P. aeruginosa* and their predisposing factors are shown in Table 26:2. Common hospital-acquired infections include septicemia, lower respiratory, wound and urinary tract infections. Community acquired infections include folliculitis associated with use of whirlpools; otitis externa in divers, swimmers and diabetics; osteomyelitis associated with deep-puncture wounds; and endocarditis and vertebral osteomyelitis in drug addicts.

Despite the availability of effective antipseudomonal therapy, *P. aeruginosa* sepsis has an overall fatality rate of 38%; 33% in individuals receiving appropriate and 86% in patients receiving inappropriate therapy.[5] The poor response to therapy is associated with the severity of the underlying disease,

Table 26:2. *Pseudomonas aeruginosa* Associated Infections*

Predisposing Factor	Associated Infection
Immunocompromised	Bacteremia, penumonia, wound infections
Broad-spectrum antimicrobial therapy	Bacteremia, pneumonia, urinary tract infection
Intravenous infusion	Bacteremia, suppurative thrombophlebitis
Urinary catheter	Urinary tract infection, bacteremia
Burns	Bacteremia, pneumonia, wound infections
Tracheostomy	Pneumonia, tracheal and bronchial infection
CNS surgery	Meningitis
Corneal ulcer	Panophthalmitis
Cystic fibrosis	Bronchial and peribronchial infection
Puncture wounds	Osteomyelitis
Drug Addiction	Endocarditis, osteomyelitis
Diabetes	Malignant otitis externa
Swimmers and divers	Otitis externa
Whirlpool users	Folliculitis

*Adapted from[28]

a decreasing neutrophil count and a delay in the start of appropriate therapy. Patients at particular risk include those with malignant neoplastic disease, extensive burns, immune deficiency syndromes or other conditions treated with immunosuppression.[5,28,43,68]

Community-acquired pneumonia is seldom caused by *P. aeruginosa*, but hospitalized patients at risk for pneumonia include individuals with tracheostomies, neutropenia, neoplastic disease, chronic lung disease or heart disease.[28] Patients with cystic fibrosis are particularly susceptible to colonization of the respiratory tract by *P. aeruginosa* and subsequent deterioration of pulmonary function.[37,67] Colonization rates increase with the age of the patient, number of hospital admissions and use of antimicrobial agents. Isolates from patients with cystic fibrosis are most often mucoid, possibly reflecting organism response to a unique environment.[8] Recently, *P. cepacia* has been isolated with increasing frequency from patients with cystic fibrosis, an infection particularly refractory to therapy.[60,62]

Burn patients are especially susceptible to infection of the burn wound by *P. aeruginosa* and subsequent development of pneumonia or sepsis. Although topical treatment of the burn wound with antipseudomonal agents has improved the prognosis, burn patients are still at high risk.[39]

Osteomyelitis and septic arthritis caused by *P. aeruginosa* are usually secondary to trauma but are being seen with increasing frequency among abusers of intravenous drugs[40] where infection often involves the sternoclavicular joint or vertebra.[28] Endocarditis due to *P. aeruginosa* is rare, but may occur in drug addicts.[12,40] Infections of the eyelids and conjunctivitis caused by *P. aeruginosa* are often mild, but corneal infections can be catastrophic, requiring immediate diagnosis and treatment.[1,28]

A relatively new disease syndrome caused by *P. aeruginosa* is a self-limiting folliculitis related to the use of hot-tubs and whirlpools that have been inadequately disinfected.[32,53] Otitis externa in swimmers and deep-sea divers is often caused by *P. aeruginosa*. A severe form of the disease, malignant otitis externa, is seen most often in the diabetic patient.[9] *P. aeruginosa* rarely causes meningitis, but may occur in individuals following invasive diagnostic or therapeutic measures, e.g., those who have ventricular shunts, drains or reservoirs.[19]

Melioidosis, caused by *P. pseudomallei*, is a rare disease in North America occurring principally in military personnel returning from foreign travel in an endemic area. Serological studies indicate that most infections are asymptomatic. The disease usually presents as an acute pneumonia but may occur as a localized cutaneous lesion. Septicemia and dissemination are associated with high mortality.[18,30] Inapparent infections may reactivate following some type of stress years after the initial exposure.[56]

Glanders, caused by *P. mallei*, is a disease of horses and other mammals that has been eradicated from North America. Transmission to humans is extremely rare and, depending on the mode of transmission, the infection manfests as a local suppurative lesion or an acute pulmonary infection.[23]

P. cepacia is an important nosocomial pathogen.[11,42] In many respects the organism resembles *P. aeruginosa* in its ability to colonize various niches in the hospital environment. As a result, the types of infections and patients who are susceptible are similar to those seen with *P. aeruginosa*. *P. cepacia* has also been associated with infections in patients with chronic granulomatous disease.[10]

P. maltophilia has been isolated with increasing frequency from clinical specimens.[45] Although the organism is associated with a variety of disease states, it appears to have limited pathogenicity.

There are a large number of *Pseudomonas* species that are primarily colonizers and contaminants but have also been isolated from documented infections (Table 26:3).[28] The significance of the isolation of any of these species must be decided by the specific circumstances of each case.

THERAPY

Members of the genus *Pseudomonas* are a persistent therapeutic challenge to the medical community. Most species are resistant to the commonly used antimicrobics. Antimicrobial agents with antipseudomonal activity include aminoglycosides, extended spectrum penicillins, the third-generation cephalosporins, monobactams, thienamycins and quinolones. A troublesome aspect of the use of the newer broad-spectrum antimicrobics, including the quinolones, is the development of resistance during therapy.[24,55,58] In addition, the emergence of resistance to one antipseudomonal beta-lactam agent generally confers resistance to all such compounds.[55] The initial susceptibility

Table 26:3. Infections Associa*ted with *Pseudomonas* Species

Orgamism	Type of Infection	Selected references
P. cepacia	Bacteremia, wounds, urinary tract, respiratory tract, endocarditis, meningitis, peritonitis, conjunctivitis, septic arthritis	11, 17, 22, 48
P. maltophilia	Bacteremia, wounds, urinary tract, respiratory tract, endocarditis, conjunctivitis, acute mastoiditis, meningitis, cholangitis	21, 22, 23, 45, 70
P. fluorescens/putida	Wounds, urinary tract, bacteremia, septic arthritis	22, 23, 61
P. putrefaciens	Bacteremia, wounds, otitis media	22, 23, 64
P. stutzeri	Bacteremia, endocarditis, septic arthritis, wounds, urinary tract, conjunctivitis, otitis media	22, 23, 27
P. paucimobilis	Bacteremia, meningitis, wounds, peritonitis, urinary tract	23, 26
P. mesophilica	Bacteremia	25, 59
P. alcaligenes/ pseudoalcaligenes	Bacteremia, endocarditis, wounds, meningitis, pneumonitis	22, 23
Pseudomonas (other species)	Bacteremia, meningitis, urinary tract, respiratory tract, conjunctivitis	23, 52

test may fail to predict the emergence of resistant subpopulations during therapy.[54]

The variation in the divalent cation content (principally magnesium and calcium) of the susceptibility test medium affects results with tetracycline, polymyxin and aminoglycosides, particularly when testing *P. aeruginosa*. Mueller-Hinton medium containing a standardized concentration of these cations should be used for both dilution and disk diffusion susceptibility testing.[46,47] A useful characteristic for species identification is the inherent resistance of certain *Pseudomonas* species to the polymyxins.[23] In practice, the in vitro susceptibility of each isolate should be tested because of the unpredictable resistance to antimicrobial agents.

EPIDEMIOLOGY

The members of the genus *Pseudomonas* are ubiquitous in the environment and are commonly isolated from soil, water, vegetation or any moist location. The metabolic diversity and antimicrobial resistance of the *Pseudomonas* species, particularly of *P. aeruginosa*, has allowed them to colonize a variety of ecological niches, and has led to their emergence as important nosocomial pathogens. Hospital-associated outbreaks of *Pseudomonas* infections have been traced to a variety of reservoirs (Table 26:4), most often related to the contamination of sterile or clean solutions, disinfectants and equipment used for invasive procedures. *P. aeruginosa* was the second

Table 26:4. Reservoirs of *Pseudomonas* in Hospitals*

Group	Item
Sterile solutions or products	Dialysis fluid, nasopharyngeal irrigant, saline, transfusion products, infusion products, heparin solutions, eye drops, opthalmic ointments and fluorescein, anesthetics, coagulation solutions, blood drawing tubes, urinary catheterization kits
Disinfectants	Chlorhexidine, benzalkonium chloride, hexachlorophene soaps, dilute phenolic solutions, povidone iodine
Clean solutions	Contact lens solutions, hydrotherapy tanks, whirlpool baths
Equipment	Endoscopes, cardiopulmonary bypass equipment, pressure transducers, urological instruments, resuscitation apparatus, respiratory therapy equipment (humidifiers, nebulizers, oxygen analyzers), oral thermometers
Miscellaneous sources	Sinks, faucets, mops, plants, vegetables, baby formula, cosmetics, shaving brushes, soaps, hand creme, body lotions

* Adapted from[23,44]

most frequently reported organism causing a nosocomial infection in 1984. In decreasing order of frequency, *P. aeruginosa* was implicated in lower respiratory tract, urinary tract and wound infections. Approximately 8% of all nosocomial bacteremias were due to *P. aeruginosa*.[7] *P. aeruginosa* colonizes the skin, pharynx and gastrointestinal tract in 2-10% of healthy adults but generally does not cause disease in this population.[44] The rate of colonization is higher for hospitalized patients.[13,28,44] Transmission of *P. aeruginosa* in the hospital setting is believed to occur primarily from colonization of the patient, particularly the oropharynx and gastrointestinal tract, and subsequent infection with the same strain. Patient to patient exchange of *P. aeruginosa* strains is not a major route of transmission.[44,,50]

P. pseudomallei is found in the soil and water but is restricted geographically to southeast Asia and other tropical or subtropical parts of the world such as India, the Philippines, New Guinea, Australia and South and Central America. Transmission from the environment occurs primarily via breaks in the skin but may occur by inhalation or ingestion. Person-to-person transmission is extremely rare.

PUBLIC HEALTH SIGNIFICANCE, PREVENTION AND CONTROL

In general, the *Pseudomonas* species, as opportunistic pathogens, pose no threat to the general public health. The exception to this is the increasing problem of outbreaks of folliculitis due to the contamination of whirlpools and hot tubs by *P. aeruginosa*. The prevention of this infection rests with appropriate testing of the water for germicide concentration, pH and temperature as well as the proper maintenance of the units.[32]

The prevention of nosocomial infections caused by *Pseudomonas* species presently relies on minimizing exposure to environmental souces, especially contaminated equipment and products, limiting antimicrobial usage in hospitals and use of surveillance techniques to identify outbreaks.[69] Considering the ubiquitous presence of *Pseudomonas* species and the increase in the numbers of patients at risk, a significant decrease in the numbers of nosocomial *Pseudomonas* infections will occur only with the prevention of colonization of the patient and the development of effective immunizing technique.[44]

In recent years a polyvalent vaccine consisting of components from 16 serotypes of *P. aeruginosa* has been used to immunize patients with severe burns, cystic fibrosis or neutropenia. The vaccine proved useful in India for the prevention of bacteremia in burn patients where antibacterial chemoprophylaxis was not readily available, but did not appear to offer any significant advantage over existing methods used for patients in English hospitals.[34,35] The presently available vaccine did not significantly alter the course of cystic fibrosis in children[38] and produced variable results in patients with malignant disease.[2,31] Administration of hyperimmune globulin from immunized individuals proved useful in burn patients.[36]

DIAGNOSTIC PROCEDURES

Rapid Methodology

There is no commercially available, rapid (<1 h) system for the identification of *Pseudomonas* species. A relatively rapid (24 h) and cost-effective method for the identification of *P. aeruginosa* relies on the demonstration of pigment (pyocyanin) on differential primary plating medium.[14]

Microscopic Examination

Pseudomonas species are straight or slightly curved, gram-negative rods approximately 0.5-1.0 μm x 2-3 μm and have no morphologic features to consistently differentiate them from other common gram-negative rods on direct Gram stained smears. However, Bartlett et al[3] found that experienced observers can presumptively differentiate *P. aeruginosa* from members of the *Enterobacteriaceae* on direct Gram stained smears approximately 80% of the time.

Primary Isolation and Culture

Pseudomonas species grow well on all the usual media used for the routine isolation of nonfastidious bacteria. A noninhibitory medium, (e.g., sheep blood agar) and one of the less inhibitory selective-differential media (e.g., MacConkey or eosin methylene blue agar) should be used for primary isolation. Selective media, such as *Pseudomonas* isolation agar, cetrimide agar (Difco Laboratories, Detroit, MI), or Pseudosel agar (BBL Microbiology Systems, Cockeysville, MD), is useful for the isolation of *P. aeruginosa* from sources containing large numbers of other bacteria.

Most *Pseudomonas* species grow over a wide temperature range, but some fail to grow or grow slowly at 35°C. Therefore, media for the isolation of *Pseudomonas* from environmental sources or potentially contaminated hospital products should be incubated at 30°C or alternatively at 35°C for 1-2 days and reincubated at 30°C or room temperature (18-22°C) for an additional 1-2 days.[23]

Generally, *Pseudomonas* species produce well-formed colonies in 18-24 h. Colony morphology varies between species as well as within species. Wrinkled, rough colonies are usually produced by *P. pseudomallei, P. mallei* and *P. stutzeri*, but can be seen with *P. aeruginosa* and other species as well. Most strains of *P. aeruginosa* produce large, slightly convex grey colonies, smell grapelike and may be hemolytic on blood agar. Mucoid variants are frequently isolated from sputum of cystic fibrosis patients.

Most isolates of *P. aeruginosa* produce pyocyanin, a water and chloroform soluble, blue, phenazine pigment. Since *P. aeruginosa* is the only gram-negative rod that produces this pigment, the presence of pyocyanin is sufficient for the identification of this organism.[23] Apyocyanogenic strains may have altered biochemical characteristics, making their laboratory identification more difficult. *P. aeruginosa* strains can produce other pigments such as pyoverdin (fluorescein), pyorubin (red) and pyomelanin (brown to black) either alone or in combination with pyocyanin. Other *Pseudomonas* species may produce orange, pink, yellow, green or brown pigments. Flo agar (BBL Microbiological Systems, Cockeysville, MD) and *Pseudomonas* agar F (Difco Laboratories, Detroit, MI) enhance the production of pyoverdin. Pyocyanin production is improved with *Pseudomonas,* agar P (Difco Laboratories, Detroit, MI) and Tech agar (BBL Microbiological Systems, Cockeysville, MD).

Methods for Identification

Any system for the identification of *Pseudomonas* species should accurately identify the frequently isolated species and allow for progressive identification of the infrequently seen species. Most species can be identified by routine biochemical and morphologic characteristics from schemata developed by Gilardi,[23] Pickett[51] and King as modified by Weaver.[65,66] The minimal characteristics for identification of strains as *Pseudomonas* species are: gram-negative rod, asporogenous, polar monotrichous or tuft of flagella, motile, glucose oxidizer or nonoxidizer, oxidase-positive or -negative and catalase-positive.[23] *P. mallei* is nonmotile and void of flagella.

The initial tests used in the identification of nonfermentative bacteria separate similar genera and distinguish species within the genus *Pseudomonas*. Important information to collect includes: colony morphology, growth on MacConkey agar, pigmentation, odor; Gram reaction, somatic shape; motility and flagellar morphology; mode of glucose utilization, production of hydrogen sulfide, arginine dehydrolase, indophenol oxidase; growth at 42°C; oxidation of glucose, xylose, lactose, maltose; and an antibiogram. *Pseudomonas* species are straight or slightly curved gram-negative rods as opposed to the coccobacillary morphology seen with *Acinetobacter* and *Moraxella*. The majority of isolates grow on MacConkey agar and produce an alkaline slant and no change in the butt of triple sugar iron agar (TSIA) or Kligler iron agar (KIA). All strains with the exception of *P. mallei* are motile. Most strains are indophenol oxidase positive, the notable exception being *P. maltophilia*. Table 26:5 lists the characteristics of some *Pseudomonas* species. The performance of these tests is described by Gilardi.[23] For a complete listing of the characteristics of all *Pseudomonas* species, refer to Gilardi[23] and Weaver et al.[66] (See Chapters 20-21 for identification of nonfermentative organisms other than *Pseudomonas*.)

Table 26:5. Differential Characteristics of *Pseudomonas**

Characteristics†	*P. aeruginosa*	*P. fluorescens*	*P. putida*	*P. pseudomallei*	*P. cepacia*	*P. stutzeri*	*P. maltophilia*	*P. putrefaciens*
O-F Glucose	+	+	+	+	+	+	+	+
O-F Maltose	−/+	−/+	−/+	+	+	+	+	+/−
O-F Xylose	+/−	+/−	+/−	+/−	+	+	+/−	−
O-F Lactose	−	−/+	−/+	+	+	−	+/−	−
Oxidase	+	+	+	+/w	+/w	+	−	+
Motility	+	+	+	+	+	+	+	+
Polar flagella	1	>1	>1	>1	>1	1	>1	1
Gas from nitrate	+/−	−	−	+	−	+	−	−
Pyocyanin	+/−	−	−	−	−	−	−	−
Pyoverdin	+/−	+	+/−	−	−	−	−	−
Growth at 42°C	+	−	−	+	+/−	+/−	−/+	+/−
H_2S	−	−	−	−	−	−	−	+
Arginine dihydrolase	+	+	+	+	−	−	−	−
Lysine decarboxylase	−	−	−	−	+	−	+	−
Extracellular DNase	−/+	−	−	−	−	−	+	+
Polymyxin susceptibility	+	+	+	−	−	+	+	+
Gelatin hydrolysis	+/−	+	−	+	+/−	−	+	+/−

* Adapted from Gilardi[23]
† Signs: + = 90% or more positive; − = 90% or more negative; +/− = most strains positive; −/+ = most strains negative; w = weakly reactive

Some strains yield atypical reactions and their identification is beyond the scope of many clinical laboratories. Other laboratories may find it expedient to use one of the commercial systems designed for identification of nonfermenters. The accuracy of the identification of *Pseudomonas* species varies with the particular test system and the species.[49] More complicated techniques, such as determination of cellular fatty acid content, are more suitable for reference laboratories.[16]

The presumptive identification of the six most frequently isolated species can be accomplished with some routine diagnostic tests (Table 26:6). *P. aeruginosa, P. fluorescens, P. putida, P. maltophilia, P. cepacia* and *P. stutzeri* grow on MacConkey agar, oxidize glucose and are motile. *P. aeruginosa* produces a flat, dull-grey colony with an irregular edge on blood agar, has a grapelike odor, is often beta-hemolytic and is indophenol oxidase positive. Pyocyanogenic strains produce distinctive blue-green colonies and account for 70% of all glucose nonfermenting gram-negative rods isolated from clinical specimens.[23] The presence of pyocyanin pigment is sufficient for the identification of *P. aeruginosa*.

Most strains of *P. fluorescens* and *P. putida* produce a fluorescent pigment, are arginine dehydrolase positive and fail to grow at 42°C. The sole use of gelatin liquefaction to differentiate between these two strains has been questioned[23] and some laboratories report them as the *P. fluorescens/putida* group.

On blood agar, strains of *P. maltophilia* may produce an ammonia odor, a lavender-green colony and green discoloration around areas of confluent

Table 26:6. Key to the Presumptive Identification of Frequently Isolated *Pseudomonas* Species

Glucose oxidizer
MacConkey positive
Motile
- Oxidase positive
  - Pyocyanin positive: *P. aeruginosa*
  - Pyocyanin negative
    - 6.5% NaCl positive
      - Maltose positive: *P. stutzeri*
    - 6.5% NaCl negative
      - Arginine dehydrolase positive
        - 42°C growth positive: *P. aeruginosa*
        - 42°C growth negative
          - Pyoverdin positive
            - Gelatin positive: *P. fluorescens*
            - Gelatin negative: *P. putida*
      - Arginine dehydrolase negative
        - Lactose positive, lysine positive: *P. cepacia*
- Oxidase negative
  - DNase positive, maltose positive, lysine positive: *P. maltophilia*

growth. *P. maltophilia* is usually indcphenol oxidase negative and DNase, maltose and lactose positive.

Isolates of *P. cepacia* can produce a yellow, nonfluorescent, diffusible pigment and opaque colonies on blood agar. *P. cepacia* is lysine decarboxylase and lactose oxidation positive, and indophenol oxidase variable.

P. stutzeri produces a characteristic dry, wrinkled, leathery colony that may be confused with *P. pseudomallei*. Growth in 6.5% NaCl differentiates it from most other *Pseudomonas* species. Maltose oxidation separates *P. stutzeri* from *P. mendocina*.

Markers of Epidemiology

P. aeruginosa accounts for approximately 75% of all nonfermentative, gram-negative rods isolated from clinical specimens. Its importance as a nosocomial pathogen led to a variety of systems for subtyping or "fingerprinting" strains, including: serological typing, pyocin (aeruginocin) typing, bacteriophage typing, plasmid typing, enzyme profiling and antibiogram typing. Nonpigmented strains generally are not typable by antisera and demonstrate little pyocin activity.[23] The cost and complexity of serological, pyocin and bacteriophage typing generally restrict their use to reference and research laboratories.

Serological Typing

Seventeen commercial antisera (Difco Laboratories) against somatic 0 antigens are used to type *P. aeruginosa* strains by slide agglutination procedure.[6,41] The procedure types over 90% of the strains, but is usually unsatisfactory for typing mucoid strains.

Pyocin (Aeruginocin) Typing

Pyocin typing refers to specific bacteriocins produced by *P. aeruginosa* that inhibit or kill other strains of *P. aeruginosa* or closely related bacteria. The test strains are typed by determining their inhibitory or susceptibility pattern against known indicator strains.[20] Recently a similar method was reported for pyocin (cepaciacin) typing of *P. cepacia* strains.[29]

Bacteriophage Typing

Bacteriophage typing of *P. aeruginosa* strains is an epidemiological tool that can be used for subtyping strains encountered in hospital epidemics.[4]

Plasmid Typing

The value of plasmid typing is based on the observation that similar strains contain plasmids of identical number and size and will have a similar plasmid profile. This method is as sensitive as routine typing methods[57,63] and is used by larger clinical laboratories. A major drawback to the use of plasmids as the only typing method is the occurrance of some strains that lack plasmids.[40]

Enzyme Profiling

Enzyme profiling has been reported as an epidemiological aid for the differentiation of *P. aeruginosa* strains and warrants further study.[33,40]

Antibiogram Typing

Although most *P. aeruginosa* strains have similar susceptibility patterns, the unusual antibiogram is a useful tool for the early recognition of a potential nosocomial problem.[15]

Serological Tests

Serological testing for melioidosis by complement fixation or indirect hemagglutination is limited to reference laboratories due to the low incidence of disease in the United States. A hemagglutination titer greater than 1:40 is suggestive of active infection, but the definitive diagnosis of the disease rests with the isolation of *P. pseudomallei*. Serological tests for the diagnosis of infections caused by other *Pseudomonas* species are used in some research protocols, but are not available for the routine clinical microbiology laboratory.

REFERENCES

1. Allen HF. Current status of prevention, diagnosis and management of bacterial corneal ulcers. Ann Ophthalmol 1971;3:235-46.
2. Banister P, Mellor J. Serological failure of *Pseudomonas* vaccination in patients receiving multiple chemotherapy. J Biol Stand 1985;13:321-6.
3. Bartlett RC, Mazens MF, Testa MA. Differentiation of *Pseudomonas aeruginosa* and *Enterobacteriaceae* in direct smears based on measurements by scanning electron microscopy. Diagn Microbiol Infect Dis 1985;3:143-7.
4. Bergan T. Phage typing of *Pseudomonas aeruginosa*. In: Bergan T, Norris JR, eds. Methods in microbiology; vol 10. New York: Academic Press, 1978:169-99.
5. Bodey GP, Jadeja L, Elting L. *Pseudomonas* bacteremia. Arch Intern Med 1985;145:1621-9.
6. Brokopp CD, Gomez-Lus R, Farmer JJ III. Serological typing of *Pseudomonas aeruginosa*: use of commercial antisera and live antigens. J Clin Microbiol 1977;5:640-9.
7. Centers for Disease Control. Nosocomial infection surveillance, 1984. In: Surveillance Summaries. 1986;35(No 1SS):17-29.
8. Chan R, Lam JS, Lam K, Costerton JW. Influence of culture conditions on expression of the mucoid mode of growth of *Pseudomonas aeruginosa*. J Clin Microbiol 1984;19:8-16.
9. Chandler JR. Malignant external otitis and facial paralysis. Otolaryngol Clin North Am 1974;7:375-83.

10. Clegg HW, Newburger PE. *Pseudomonas cepacia* pneumonia in chronic granulomatous disease. Pediatr Infect Dis 1986;5:111.
11. Conly JM, Klass L, Larson L, Kennedy J, Low DE, Harding GM. *Pseudomonas cepacia*: colonization and infection in intensive care units. Can Med Assoc J 1986;134:363-6.
12. Crane LR, Levine DP, Zervous MJ, Cummings G. Bacteremia in narcotic addicts at the Detroit medical center. I. Microbiology, epidemiology, risk factors and empiric therapy. Rev Infect Dis 1986;8:364-73.
13. Cross AS. Evolving epidemiology of *Pseudomonas aeruginosa* infections. Eur J Clin Microbiol 1985;4:156-9.
14. Daly JA, Boshard R, Matsen JM. Differential primary plating medium for enhancement of pigment production by *Pseudomonas aeruginosa*. J Clin Microbiol 1984;19:742-3.
15. Dayton SL, Blasi D, Chipps DD, Smith RF. Epidemiological tracing of *Pseudomonas aeruginosa*: antibiogram and serotyping. Appl Microbiol 1974;27:1167-9.
16. Dees SB, Hollis DG, Weaver RE, Moss CW. Cellular fatty acid composition of *Pseudomonas marginata* and closely associated bacteria. J Clin Microbiol 1983;18:1073-8.
17. Ederer GM, Matsen JM. Colonization and infection with *Pseudomonas cepacia*. J Infect Dis 1972;125:613-18.
18. Everett ED, Nelson RA. Pulmonary melioidosis. Am Rev Respir Dis 1975;112:331-40.
19. Fong IW, Tomkins KB. Review of *Pseudomonas aeruginosa* meningitis with special emphasis on treatment with ceftazidime. Rev Infect Dis 1985;7:604-12.
20. Fyfe JA, Harris G, Goven JRW. Revised pyocin typing method for *Pseudomonas aeruginosa*. J Clin Microbiol 1984;20:47-50.
21. Gardner P, Griffin WB, Swartz MN, Kunz LJ. Nonfermentative gram-negative bacilli of nosocomial interest. Am J Med 1970;48:735-49.
22. Gilardi GL. Infrequently encountered *Pseudomonas* species causing infection in humans. Ann Intern Med 1972;77:211-15.
23. Gilardi GL. *Pseudomonas*. In: Lennette EH, Balows A, Hausler WJ Jr, Shadomy HJ, eds. Manual of clinical microbiology. Washington, DC: American Society for Microbiology, 1985;350-72.
24. Gilbert DN. An evaluation of antipseudomonal antimicrobic agents. Antibiot Chemother 1985;36:111-33.
25. Gilchrist MJR, Kraft JA, Hammond JG, Connelly BL, Myers MG. Detection of *Pseudomonas mesophilica* as a source of nosocomial infections in a bone marrow transplant unit. J Clin Microbiol 1986;23:1052-5.
26. Glupczynski Y, Hansen W, Dratwa M, et al. *Pseudomonas paucimobilis* peritonitis in patients treated by peritoneal dialysis. J Clin Microbiol 1984;20:1225-6.
27. Goetz A, Yu VL, Hanchett JE, Rihs JD. *Pseudomonas stutzeri* bacteremia associated with hemodialysis. Arch Intern Med 1983;143:1909-12.
28. Gould IM, Wise R. *Pseudomonas aeruginosa*: Clinical manifestations and management. Lancet 1985;2:1224-7.
29. Govan JRW, Harris G. Typing of *Pseudomonas cepacia* by bacteriocin susceptibility and production. J Clin Microbiol 1985;22:490-4.
30. Guard RW, Khafagi FA, Brigden MC, Ashdown LR. Melioidosis in far North Queensland. A clinical and epidemiological review of twenty cases. Am J Trop Med Hyg 1984;33:467-73.
31. Haghbin M, Armstrong D, Murphy M. Controlled trial of *Pseudomonas aeruginosa* vaccine in children with acute leukemia. Cancer 1973;32:761-6.
32. Highsmith AK, Favero MS. Microbiologic aspects of public whirlpools. Clin Microbiol Newsletter 1985;7:9-11.
33. Janda JM, Bottone EJ. *Pseudomonas aeruginosa* enzyme profiling: predictor of potential invasiveness and use as an epidemiological tool. J Clin Microbiol 1981;14:55-60.
34. Jones RJ, Roe EA, Gupta JL. Low mortality in burned patients in a *Pseudomonas* vaccine trial. Lancet 1978;2:401-3.
35. Jones RJ, Roe EA, Gupta JL. Controlled trials of a polyvalent *Pseudomonas* vaccine in burns. Lancet 1979;2:977-83.

36. Jones RJ, Roe EA. Controlled trial of *Pseudomonas* immunoglobulin and vaccine in burn patients. Lancet 1980;2:1263-5.
37. Kulczycki LL, Murphy TM, Bellanti JA. *Pseudomonas* colonization in cystic fibrosis. JAMA 1978;240:30-4.
38. Langford DT, Hiller J. Prospective, controlled study of polyvalent *Pseudomonas* vaccine in cystic fibrosis-three year result. Arch Dis Child 1984;59:1131-4.
39. Lawrence JC. The bacteriology of burns. J Hosp Infect 1985;6(Suppl B):3-17.
40. Levin MH, Weinstein RA, Nathan C, Selander RK, Ochman H, Kabins SA. Association of infection caused by *Pseudomonas aeruginosa* serotype 011 with intravenous abuse of pentazocine mixed with tripelennamine. J Clin Microbiol 1984;20:758-62.
41. Liu PV, Matsumoto H, Kusama H, Bergen T. Survey of heat-stable, major somatic antigens of *Pseudomonas aeruginosa*. Int J Syst Bacteriol 1983;33:256-64.
42. Martone WJ, Osterman CA, Fisher KA, Wenzel RP. *Pseudomonas cepacia*: implications and control of epidemic nosocomial colonization. Rev Infect Dis 1981;3:708-15.
43. McManus AT, Mason AD Jr, McManus WF, Pruitt BA Jr. Twenty-five year review of *Pseudomonas aeruginosa* bacteremia in a burn center. Eur J Clin Microbiol 1985:219-33.
44. Morrison AJ Jr, Wenzel RP. Epidemiology of infection due to *Pseudomonas aeruginosa*. Rev Infect Dis 1984;6(suppl 3):627-42.
45. Morrison AJ Jr, Hoffman KK, Wenzel RP. Associated mortality and clinical characteristics of nosocomial *Pseudomonas maltophilia* in a university hospital. J Clin Microbiol 1986;24:52-5.
46. National Committee for Clinical Laboratory Standards. Performance standards for antimicrobial disk susceptibility tests. 3rd ed. Approved standard M2-A3. Villanova, PA: National Committee for Clinical Laboratory Standards, 1984.
47. National Committee for Clinical Laboratory Standards. Methods for dilution antimicrobial susceptibility tests for bacteria that grow aerobically. Approved standard M7-4. Villanova, PA: National Committee for Clinical Laboratory Standards, 1985.
48. Noriega ER, Rubenstein E, Simberkoff MS, Rahal JJ. Subacute and acute endocarditis due to *Pseudomonas cepacia* in heroin addicts. Am J Med 1975;59:29-35.
49. Oberhofer TR. Use of the API 20E, Oxi/Ferm, and Minitek systems to identify nonfermentative and oxidase-positive fermentative bacteria: seven years of experience. Diagn Microbiol Infect Dis 1983;1:241-56.
50. Olson B, Weinstein RA, Nathan C, Chamberlin W, Kabins SA. Occult aminoglycoside resistance in *Pseudomonas aeruginosa*: epidemiology and implications for therapy and control. J Infect Dis 1985;152:769-74.
51. Pickett MJ, Pedersen MM. Nonfermentative bacilli associated with man. II. Detection and identification. Am J Clin Pathol 1970;54:164-77.
52. Pien FD, Chung EYS. Group Ve infection: case report of group Ve-2 septicemia and literature review. Diagn Microbiol Infect Dis 1986;5:177-80.
53. Ratnam S, Hogan K, March SB, Butler RW. Whirlpool-associated folliculitis caused by *Pseudomonas aeruginosa*: report of an outbreak and review. J Clin Microbiol 1986;23:655-9.
54. Sanders CC, Sanders WE Jr. Emergence of resistance during therapy with the newer beta-lactam antibiotics: role of inducible beta-lactamases and implications for the future. Rev Infect Dis 1983;5:639-48.
55. Sanders CC, Sanders WE Jr. Microbial resistance to newer generation beta-lactam antibiotics: clinical and laboratory implications. J Infect Dis 1985;151:399-406.
56. Sanford J, Moore W. Recrudescent melioidosis: a Southeast Asian legacy. Am Rev Respir Dis 1971;104:452-3.
57. Schaberg DR, Tompkins LS, Falkow S. Use of agarose gel electrophoresis of plasmid deoxyribonucleic acid to fingerprint gram-negative bacilli. J Clin Microbiol 1981;13:,1105-8.
58. Scully BE, Parry MF, Neu HC, Mandell W. Oral ciprofloxacin therapy of infections due to *Pseudomonas aeruginosa*. Lancet 1986;1:819-22.
59. Smith SM, Eng RHK, Forrester C. *Pseudomonas mesophilica* infections in humans. J Clin Microbiol 1985;21:314-17.

60. Tablan OC, Chorba TL, Schidlow DV, et al. *Pseudomonas cepacia* colonization in patients with cystic fibrosis: risk factors and clinical outcome. J Pediatr 1985;107:382-7.
61. Tabor E, Gerety RJ. Five cases of *Pseudomonas* sepsis transmitted by blood transfusions. Lancet 1984;1:1403.
62. Thomassen MJ, Demko CA, Klinger JD, Stern RC. *Pseudomonas cepacia* colonization among patients with cystic fibrosis. Am Rev Respir Dis 1985;131:791-6.
63. Tompkins L. DNA methods in clinical microbiology. In: Lennette EH, Balows A, Hausler WJ Jr, Shadomy HJ, eds. Manual of clinical microbiology. Washington, DC: American Society for Microbiology, 1985:1023-8.
64. Vandepitte J, Debois J. *Pseudomonas putrefaciens* as a cause of bacteremia in humans. J Clin Microbiol 1978;7:70-2.
65. Weaver RE, Hollis DG. Gram-negative organisms: an approach to identification. Atlanta: Centers for Disease Control, 1983.
66. Weaver RE, Hollis DG, Clark WA, Riley P. The identification of unusual pathogenic gram-negative bacteria. Atlanta: Centers for Disease Control, 1983.
67. Young LS, Armstrong D. *Pseudomonas aeruginosa* infections. In: King JW, Faulkner WR, eds. Critical reviews in clinical laboratory sciences. Cleveland: CRC Press, 1972:291-347.
68. Young LS. The clinical challenge of infections due to *Pseudomonas aeruginosa*. Rev Infect Dis 1984;6(suppl 3):603-36.
69. Young LS, Wenzel RP, Sabath LD, Pollack M, Pennington JE, Platt R. The outlook for prevention and treatment of infections due to *Pseudomonas aeruginosa*. Rev Infect Dis 1984;6(suppl 3):769-74.
70. Zuravleff JJ, Yu VL. Infections caused by *Pseudomonas maltophilia* with emphasis on bacteremia: case reports and a review of the literature. Rev Infect Dis 1982;4:1236-46.

CHAPTER 27

STAPHYLOCOCCAL INFECTIONS

James H. Jorgensen, Ph.D. and Wesley E. Kloos, Ph.D.

INTRODUCTION

"As a natural result of Lister's discovery of the antiseptic methods of treating wounds, the attention of nearly all operating surgeons and others was directed to the question: What is the cause of acute suppuration, of acute inflammation, and of blood poisoning after wounds and operations? . . .Often I meditated on the subject and became the more convinced that there was a single cause, and that cause was some special germ. But it was some time before it was possible for me to verify this conviction. At length I came upon a case of disease which promised to solve the problem. I had to attend . . . a young man suffering an extensive suppurating phlegmon of the leg. . . . Procuring a clean vial, I evacuated into it the matter from the phlegmon through the unbroken skin, proceeded home with it, and placed a little of the pus under an ordinary student's microscope. . . . My delight may be conceived when there were revealed to me beautiful tangles, tufts and chains of round organisms in great numbers, which stood out clear and distinct among the pus cells and debris . . . The pus on the microscope slide, which appeared to indicate the solution of a great puzzle, filled me with hope." Sir Alexander Ogston (1844-1929).[39] Several other independent workers had observed cocci in abscesses and pus; however, it was Ogston[38] who showed, in an impressive series of experiments, that cocci were the etiologic agents of most acute suppurative processes in man and that these could give rise to septicemia and pyemia. His lithographic illustrations showed that he could differentiate between the chain-micrococci or streptococci, a term coined by Billroth, and the group-micrococci or staphylococci, a term he coined himself. Ogston did not provide a formal description of the genus *Staphylococcus*, and so Rosenbach[44] is officially credited with proposing the genus and species *Staphylococcus aureus*.

Ogston suggested that different species of cocci with different pathogenic capabilities might exist and admitted the possibility that nonvirulent staphylococci might occur on skin surfaces. Investigations for several decades following his discoveries were mainly concerned with defining criteria of pathogenicity, virulence factors and differentiating potentially pathogenic *S. aureus* (also referred to as *S. pyogenes* or *S. pyogenes aureus*) from other less virulent or commensal staphylococci (named *S. albus, S. epidermidis* or *S. epidermidis albus*). The distinction was of considerable importance and practicality, since the host and clinical specimens often carried both types of organisms. The distinguishing characters used to identify *S. aureus* at the turn of the century were not completely reliable, though the most satisfactory criterion, i.e., their ability to clot blood plasma, was available but not recognized. Von Daranyi[14] demonstrated the practical value of the coagulating principle (coagulase) in identifying *S. aureus*, but the coagulase test did not gain general acceptance until the 1930s. Since that time, staphylococci have been divided into two major groups on the basis of coagulase activity. The coagulase-positive species, *S. aureus*, still remains one of our most common bacterial pathogens, although at the dawn of the antibiotic era it was thought that this species would no longer cause serious problems. Unfortunately, *S. aureus* has proved to be a most versatile species, counteracting many of the attempts to control it. It is remarkably equipped to colonize and invade breaks in the natural barriers (e.g., skin and mucous membranes) of the host, to protect itself from many of the host's defenses, thus gaining access to the blood stream and other sites and to develop resistance to a wide variety of antibacterial agents.

Until the 1960s, the coagulase-negative staphylococci, collectively called *S. epidermidis*, were regarded as part of the normal skin flora and thought to be harmless commensals. Smith et al,[50] Pulverer and Halswick[42] and Holt[22] were among the first investigators to draw attention to the pathogenicity of these organisms by demonstrating their occurrence in septicemia and bacterial endocarditis and their colonization of implanted ventriculoatrial or peritoneal shunts. It has become quite clear during the last two decades that certain coagulase-negative staphylococci, especially *S. epidermidis* (sensu stricto),[46] have emerged as pathogens in patients with artificial devices and in those with compromised host defenses.[6] Alteration of the integrity of skin by manipulation or trauma allows these normally commensal organisms to gain entrance to the body. Infection with these organisms is obviously related to the development of modern medical practices and appears to be steadily increasing.

CAUSATIVE ORGANISMS

Staphylococci are gram-positive cocci (0.5-1.5 μm in diameter), occur singly, in pairs, tetrads and short chains of three to four cells, and characteristically divide in more than one plane to form irregular "grape-like" clusters. They are nonmotile, nonsporeforming, usually catalase-positive and unencapsulated. Some encapsulated strains of *S. aureus* have been isolated from human sources.[37] Most species are facultative anaerobes. With the exception of the anaerobic species *S. saccharolyticus* and *S. aureus* subsp. *anaerobius*, growth is more rapid and abundant under aerobic conditions. Some uncommon strains of staphylococci may require the presence of CO_2, hemin or menadione for good growth.[49] Most strains grow well on noninhibitory media. Rare cell wall-deficient forms may require a hypertonic environment. Most strains grow in the presence of 10% NaCl and between 18 and 40°C.

The cell wall contains peptidoglycan and teichoic acid. The diamino acid present in the peptidoglycan is L-lysine. Staphylococci are susceptible to lysis by the endopeptidase lysostaphin, which cleaves glycine-glycine linkages in the interpeptide bridges of the peptidoglycan, while staphylococci are generally resistant to lysis or poorly lysed by the muramidase lysozyme.

Metabolism is respiratory and fermentative. Due to the presence of cytochromes, staphylococci are benzidine-positive by the standard test,[15] whereas streptococci are benzidine-negative. Carbohydrates and/or amino acids are utilized as carbon and energy sources. A variety of carbohydrates may be utilized aerobically with the production of acid.

Staphylococci are currently included with micrococci and planococci in the family *Micrococcaceae*, as a matter of historical and practical convenience. All three genera are catalase-positive, gram-positive cocci with a cell wall peptidoglycan containing L-lysine as the diamino acid. The guanine-cytosine content of DNA, nucleic acid hybridization and 16S rRNA cataloguing, however, indicate that the three genera are not closely related phylogenetically. In the clinical laboratory, it is sometimes necessary to distinguish staphylococci from micrococci as both are common inhabitants of the human cutaneous ecosystem and may be present in clinical specimens. They may be differentiated on the basis of (1) lysostaphin (staphylococci susceptible) and lysozyme (staphylococci resistant) susceptibilities,[47] (2) anaerobic acid production from glucose (positive for most staphylococci and negative for most micrococci),[52] (3) production of acid aerobically from glycerol in the presence of 0.4 μm/mL erythromycin (positive for most staphylococci and negative for most micrococci),[47] (4) growth on selective media (e.g., the SK medium of Schleifer and Kramer[48] supporting growth of staphylococci, or the FTO medium of Curry and Borovian[13] supporting growth of micrococci), (5) susceptibility to Taxo A bacitracin disks (staphylococci resistant),[16] and (6) modified oxidase and benzidine tests designed to identify the presence of cytochrome *c* (negative in most staphylococci and positive in micrococci).[17] Lysostaphin susceptibility may be tested by the commercial Lysostaphin Reagent Set (Remel Regional Medical Laboratories), and the commercially prepared Microdase Disk (Remel) can be used to detect oxidase in the modified oxidase test.

The genus *Staphylococcus* is presently composed of 23 species. Those found on humans include *S. aureus, S. epidermidis, S. hominis, S. haemolyticus, S. warneri, S. capitis, S. saccharolyticus, S. auricularis, S. simulans, S. saprophyticus, S. cohnii* and *S. xylosus*.[27,28,31,33,46] Other primates carry *S. aureus, S. simulans, S. saprophyticus, S. xylosus* and different subspecies of *S. auricularis, S. warneri, S. haemolyticus* and *S. cohnii* than are usually found on humans. *S. intermedius*, a coagulase-positive species and opportunistic pathogen of animals, is found frequently on carnivora and has also been isolated from certain other mammals and birds but not from man. *S. hyicus* subsp. *hyicus* is a coagulase-variable subspecies and opportunistic pathogen of pigs, while *S. hyicus* subsp. *chromogenes* is a coagulase-negative subspecies found predominantly on cattle. *S. sciuri, S. lentus, S. caprae, S. gallinarum, S. arlettae, S. equorum* and *S. kloosii* may be isolated from various animal species, while *S. caseolyticus* and *S. carnosus* are found in certain dairy and fermented meat products.

Most *Staphylococcus* species are common inhabitants of the human skin and mucous membranes. Some exhibit habitat or niche preferences.[28] *S. aureus* prefers the anterior nares as a principal area of colonization, especially in human adults. Ten to more than 40% of the general population carry this species in their nares and up to 70% of hospitalized patients and hospital personnel carry this organism. *S. epidermidis* is ecologically the most versatile human species, producing large populations in the anterior nares, axillae, inguinal and perineal areas, toe webs and on areas of the face. As a species, it is widely distributed over most of the skin area. *S. capitis* is found primarily on the human head, especially in regions of the scalp, forehead and external auditory meatus, where sebaceous glands are numerous and well developed. This species reaches a large population size following puberty and is usually the predominant species of the adult human scalp.[31] *S. auricularis* has a strong preference for the external auditory meatus.[33] *S. hominis* and *S. haemolyticus* prefer the moist axillae, inguinal and perineal areas and toe webs, which are richly supplied with apocrine glands, but also colonize the drier regions of the skin (e.g., arms and legs) more successfully than most species.[31,46] *S. hominis* is usually second to *S. epidermidis* in distribution over the skin surface and in population size. *S. saprophyticus* is rarely isolated from human skin, but appears to have a higher capacity to adhere to uroepithelial cells than to buccal or skin cells and does so better than other staphylococcal species.[4]

Certain *Staphylococcus* species are found frequently as etiological agents of a variety of human and animal infections. In this chapter we will be concerned primarily with the major human pathogens *S. aureus, S. epidermidis* and *S. saprophyticus*, and to a lesser extent with the opportunists *S. warneri, S. haemolyticus, S. hominis* and *S. simulans*, species exhibiting some though limited pathogenic potential.

CLINICAL FORMS OF STAPHYLOCOCCAL DISEASE

Staphylococci are responsible for a variety of human infections ranging from skin or integumentary infections to bacteremia and meningitis. The most common infections due to *S. aureus* are skin pustules, impetigo, cellulitis and postsurgical wound infections. More serious conditions attributable to *S. aureus* include bacteremia, osteomyelitis, renal abscess, pneumonia, endocarditis and meningitis.

S. aureus continues to be a prominent agent of hospital-acquired infections. Following the advent of penicillinase-resistant penicillins in the early 1960s, serious infections due to penicillin-resistant *S. aureus* could be treated with an effective group of antimicrobials. However, methicillin- and oxacillin-resistant strains (MRSA) were soon discovered in England and Europe and have emerged as a major epidemiologic problem in United States hospitals.[21,53] MRSA are frequently seen as opportunistic pathogens of debilitated patients undergoing prolonged hospitalization in large tertiary care facilities.[21] However, in recent years, MRSA have been seen with increasing frequency in smaller community hospitals, nursing homes, rehabilitation facilities and occasionally in outpatients. MRSA appear especially adept as colonizers of the nares, hands and gastrointestinal tract of patients and hospital staffs. The majority of MRSA strains exhibit multiple antimicrobial resistance, including resistance to macrolides, lincosamides, aminoglycosides, chloramphenicol, tetracycline and in some cases rifampin and trimethoprim-sulfamethoxazole. Despite occasional conflicting in vitro data, MRSA are effectively resistant to all current beta-lactam antibiotics, including the latest generation cephalosporins.[10,43] Serious MRSA infections have most often required treatment with vancomycin,[57] to which staphylococcal resistance has not yet been documented. Certain newer drugs, including teicoplanin and some of the newer quinolone antibiotics, offer the potential of additional choices for treatment.[1]

S. aureus has the capability of producing a number of extracellular toxins that cause significant human morbidity and mortality. One of the most common causes of food poisoning is the consumption of foods containing the thermostable enterotoxins produced by *S. aureus*. Classically, this results from contamination of foods with enterotoxin-producing *S. aureus* from the unwashed hands of kitchen workers. When contaminated foodstuffs are not stored under proper refrigeration, the staphylococci grow to large numbers and elaborate enterotoxin. Usually within a few hours of consumption of toxin-containing food, the individual suffers the sudden onset of nausea, vomiting and often diarrhea. Although usually self-limited, the symptoms of staphylococcal food poisoning can be temporarily incapacitating.

Another toxin-mediated condition of potentially serious consequence due to *S. aureus* is toxic shock syndrome (TSS). In situ production of a specific toxin (toxic shock syndrome toxin-1, TSST-1) has been demonstrated to produce a constellation of symptoms, including fever, skin rash, hypotension and possibly shock.[45] Most TSS patients have been young, menstruating women who have used certain highly absorbent tampons during menses. Vaginal colonization and production of TSST-1 appears to be the common sequence of the disease.[45] However, TSST-1 elaboration by *S. aureus* at other sites has resulted in TSS cases in nonmenstruating women and in men. In addition, there have been recent reports of staphylococcal enterotoxins (particularly enterotoxin B) resulting in nonmenstrual cases of TSS,[12] as well as TSST-1 production by coagulase-negative staphylococci.[11] It is clear that much is yet to be learned about this important syndrome.

The increasing clinical significance of the coagulase-negative species of *Staphylococcus* has been repeatedly documented in recent years. Although these species form a portion of the endogenous microbial flora of man and animals, a number of infectious processes may result from their introduction beyond the normal integumentary barriers. Our understanding of the importance of the individual species has in part been hampered by the common practice of designating all coagulase-negative isolates as *S. epidermidis*, or merely as coagulase-negative *Staphylococcus*, without species identification. Many times such isolates have been regarded as contaminants lacking clinical significance. However, more recent information has provided evidence of documented infections due to these species, including bacteremia, endocarditis, infection of intravascular catheters or patches, infection of internal prosthetic devices, cerebrospinal fluid shunts, peritonitis associated with dialysis, osteomyelitis and pyoarthritis, surgical wound and genitourinary infections.[6] Most of these infections arise as complications of invasive procedures such as surgery, catheterization or placement of a prosthesis.

S. epidermidis (sensu stricto) is the most prominent disease producer among the coagulase-negative species, probably causing slightly more than 50% of all infections due to this group. However, *S. saprophyticus* is unique among these species as one of the most common agents of lower urinary tract infections in young women, being second only to *Escherichia coli* in that setting. Because of this, useful diagnostic information results from species level identification of *S. saprophyticus* isolated from urine of reproductive age females.

Infections with methicillin-resistant, coagulase-negative staphylococci (especially *S. epidermidis* MRSE) have emerged as a therapeutic problem. Deep-seated infections, such as prosthetic valve endocarditis, often require multiple antibiotic therapy, usually with vancomycin, rifampin and often an aminoglycoside.[26] The clinical implications of apparent in vitro susceptibility of some MRSE to cephalosporin or carbapenem antibiotics is controversial and is compounded by technical difficulties involved in accurate beta-lactam susceptibility testing of coagulase-negative staphylococci.[8,26] Methicillin resistance and the ability to produce opportunistic infections also exists in the less commonly isolated species *S. haemolyticus, S. hominis, S. warneri* and *S. simulans*.

EPIDEMIOLOGY

Staphylococci are frequent causes of both community and hospital-acquired infections. Because colonization of the skin and mucous membranes and of the gastrointestinal tracts of humans with both coagulase-negative species and *S. aureus* is common, there are numerous opportunities for introduction of the organisms into wounds, interrupted body cavities or foodstuffs. Despite a high rate of nasal colonization in health care workers, most intrahospital spread of staphylococci undoubtedly results from patient to patient spread via the inadequately washed hands of hospital personnel. Thus, colonized or infected patients serve as the largest reservoir of staphylococci (particularly MRSA and MRSE).

Staphylococcal food poisoning results from unsanitary preparation of food by colonized or infected food handlers, compounded by inadequate refrigeration following introduction of *S. aureus* into food. The most commonly involved foods include potato salad, custards or custard-filled pastries, salads, dairy products and meats.

Although toxic shock syndrome results most often from inadvertent establishment of conditions suitable for TSST-1 production in otherwise healthy but colonized individuals, e.g., use of highly absorbent tampons during menses, the exact epidemiology of TSS is not always demonstrable. Approximately 20% of cases lack any obvious site of *S. aureus* infection or colonization. Perhaps such cases are due to *S. aureus* enterotoxin or TSST-1 production by coagulase-negative species.[11]

PUBLIC HEALTH SIGNIFICANCE

Because species of *Staphylococcus* are responsible for a wide variety of both community and institutionally acquired maladies, there is abundant opportunity for large clusters or outbreaks of staphylococcal disease. Particularly common are staphylococcal food poisonings in gatherings which range from small family functions to large business or social affairs involving hundreds of individuals. Outbreaks of nosocomial staphylococcal disease are generally confined to a single hospital. However, since patients may be transferred between different hospitals, from hospitals to extended care or rehabilitation facilities, or merely back into the community, it may at times be important to establish epidemiologic relatedness of staphylococcal isolates from different patient-care settings or to verify the antimicrobial resistance of certain strains (e.g., MRSA), to document the spread of infection. Intrahospital spread of MRSA has become a problem of growing concern, and might be lessened if an institution notified a second one when a patient with MRSA was transferred.

DIAGNOSTIC PROCEDURES

Selection and Processing of Specimens

The wide spectrum of human disease caused by species of *Staphylococcus* results in a diversity of specimen types being submitted for laboratory analysis. Common specimen types include wound exudates or aspirations, sputa or other lower respiratory secretions, tissues or bones, urine, blood and cerebrospinal fluid (CSF). As with all specimens for bacteriological analysis, samples should be taken from the offending site prior to antimicrobial therapy and so as to exclude normal microflora as much as possible. Transportation of specimens to and processing of specimens within the laboratory should be performed expediently. Specimens obtained with swabs should be transported in general purpose transport media.

To investigate an outbreak of staphylococcal foodborne disease, samples of suspect foods, as well as vomitus and feces from afflicted individuals, should be collected and submitted for culture and/or toxin testing. Any skin lesions and the anterior nares of food handlers should be cultured.

Microscopic Examination of Specimens

The examination of Gram-stained smears of body fluids may provide rapid, useful, presumptive evidence of staphylococcal infection. Of particular value are smears of CSF, other normally sterile fluids, tissues, sputa and wound exudates. Staphylococci usually appear as pairs or small clusters of gram-positive cocci, often associated with host inflammatory cells. *S. aureus* cannot be differentiated from coagulase-negative staphylococci, nor other species of gram-positive cocci (*Micrococcus, Streptococcus, Peptostreptococcus*) on the basis of Gram stain morphology. Thus, isolation remains the only definitive means for diagnosis of staphylococcal infection.

Primary Isolation and Culture

Clinical specimens should be inoculated onto at least nonselective blood agar (preferably sheep blood agar) and into a fluid medium such as thioglycolate broth. On blood agar, abundant growth of most species occurs within 18-24 h at 35-37°C. Colonies will be 1-3 mm in diameter and usually circular, smooth and raised, with a butyrous consistency. On sheep blood agar, colonies of *S. aureus* are usually surrounded by zones of hemolysis within 24 h. Most staphylococci of major medical or public health significance produce good growth in the lower anaerobic portions as well as in the upper more aerobic portions of thioglycolate broth or semisolid agar.[29]

Specimens from potentially contaminated sources such as wounds, feces or certain foods, where staphylococci are expected to be mixed with large populations of competing species, should be inoculated also onto a selective medium such as SK agar,[48] mannitol-salt agar, Columbia colistin-nalidixic acid agar (CNA), phenylethyl alcohol agar, lipase-salt-mannitol (LSM) agar or tellurite glycine agar. These media inhibit gram-negative organisms but allow growth of staphylococci and certain other gram-positive cocci. Incubation of selective media should be extended to at least 48 h for good colony development. Certain of these media may also offer differential capabilities. On mannitol-salt agar, species capable of producing acid from mannitol (*S. aureus, S. simulans, S. saprophyticus*) may be distinguished from the non-acid producing species, *S. epidermidis* and most strains of *S. hominis*. On LSM agar, most strains of *S. aureus* will produce a yellow (acid) zone due to acidification of mannitol and, in addition, will produce an opaque zone around the colony due to lipovitellin lipase activity. On tellurite glycine agar, *S. aureus* colonies become black after incubation for 24 h as a result of tellurite reduction.

Baird-Parker agar and Vogel and Johnson agar have gained wide acceptance[51] for the isolation of *S. aureus* from foods, especially for processed foods which may contain a small number of metabolically damaged cocci. On Baird-Parker agar, *S. aureus* colonies are typically dark gray to black with a light-colored margin and surrounded by an opaque zone (precipitate) with an outer clear edge, within 24-48 h of incubation. The blackening of colonies is due to tellurite reduction and the opaque zone to the presence of lipovitellin lipase activity. Most other species grow poorly on this medium or produce lighter gray colonies with no or only weak lipase activity. On Vogel and Johnson agar, *S. aureus* colonies are black and surrounded by a yellow zone within 24-48 h incubation. The blackening of colonies is due to tellurite reduction and the yellow zone to the acid produced from mannitol. Typical colonies should be tested for coagulase activity. Detailed procedures for preparing food samples and for isolating and enumerating *S. aureus* in foods can be found in the "Compendium of Methods for the Microbiological Examination of Foods"[51] and "FDA Bacteriological Analytical Manual for Foods."[18] It should be noted that isolation of *S. aureus* from foods is not, in itself, proof that it is responsible for the food poisoning. However, the presence of a large population of *S. aureus* does provide presumptive evidence. Etiology is confirmed by demonstrating the presence of staphylococcal entertoxin or by showing that the organisms cultured in high numbers are capable of producing enterotoxin.

Methods for Identification

Staphylococcus species can be identified on the basis of colony morphology, coagulase activity, oxygen requirements, hemolysis, novobiocin susceptibility, acetylmethylcarbinol (acetoin) production, aerobic acid production from certain carbohydrates and certain enzyme activities. Listings of the characteristics of the various species and methods for their determination may be found in the ''Manual of Clinical Microbiology, 4th edition''[29] and ''Bergey's Manual of Systematic Bacteriology, Volume 2.''[34] The more clinically significant species can be identified on the basis of several key characteristics (Table 27:1). There is current wide interest in using commercial biochemical test kits or instrument systems for the rapid identification of species,[5,35] in addition to, or in place of, the conventional methods described for the identification of staphylococcal species.[32] Several manufacturers have marketed products that can identify a number of staphylococcal species with an accuracy of 70-95% with relative speed and simplicity. For some of these systems, additional testing is recommended to increase accuracy (e.g., testing conventional coagulase production or resistance to novobiocin.[29,35]

Currently available identification systems include API STAPH-IDENT (Analytab Products), dms STAPH Trac (Analytab; DMS Laboratories), Pos Combo panel (American Micro Scan), Minitek Gram-Positive System (BBL Microbiology Systems) and the Vitek Gram-Positive Identification Card (Vitek).

In most clinical or public health laboratories, identification of *S. aureus* as an etiological agent or indicator of potential health risk is of primary importance. On nonselective blood agar, nutrient agar, tryptic soy agar, brain heart infusion agar or P agar,[31,46] colonies of *S. aureus* are relatively large, usually pigmented yellow or yellow-gray to orange and become translucent to nearly transparent with continued incubation. Some strains of *S. aureus* may not be pigmented. Some uncommon strains of this species may be cell wall-deficient or require media supplemented with specific metabolites (e.g., hemin, menadione, CO_2, etc.). They will produce dwarf colonies on routine media.[49] Rare encapsulated strains produce colonies smaller and more convex in profile than those of unencapsulated strains, and have a glistening-wet appearance.[37]

The ability to clot plasma continues to be the most widely used and generally accepted criterion for the initial identification of S. *aureus* from human sources. However, it should be noted that some strains of gram-negative enteric bacteria and *Enterococcus faecalis* also clot plasma; the enteric bacilli can be readily distinguished from staphylococci by Gram stain and *E. faecalis* is benzidine-and catalase-negative.

Two different coagulase tests can be performed: a tube test for free staphylocoagulase and a slide test for bound coagulase (clumping factor). Although the tube test is more definitive, the slide test may be used as a rapid screening technique. The standard tube coagulase test is performed by mixing 0.1 mL of an overnight brain heart infusion broth culture with 0.5 mL of reconstituted rabbit plasma anticoagulated with ethylenediami-

Table 27:1. Differentiation of Clinically-Relevant *Staphylococcus* Species

Character	*S. aureus*	*S. epidermidis*	*S. hominis*	*S. haemolyticus*	*S. warneri*	*S. saprophyticus*	*S. simulans*
Colony size (large)*	+†	−	−	+	d	+	+
Colony pigment‡	+	−	d	d	d	d	−
Anaerobic growth§	+	+	−	(+)	+	(+)	+
Coagulase	+	−	−	−	−	−	−
Deoxyribonuclease	+	−	−	−	−	−	±
Hemolysis	+	−	−	(+)	(d)	−	(d)
Phosphatase (alkaline)	+	+‖	−	−	−	−	(d)
Urease¶	+	+	+	−	+	+	+
β-Galactosidase¶	−	−	−	−	−	d	+
β-Glucuronidase¶	−	−	−	d	d	−	d
Novobiocin resistance**	−	−	−	−	−	+	−
Acid (aerobically) from:							
Maltose	+	+	+	+	(+)	+	−††
D-Trehalose	+	−	d	+	+	+	d
D-Mannitol	+	−	−	d	d	d	
D-Xylose	−	−	−	−	−	−	−
Xylitol	−	−	−	−	−	d	−
Sucrose	+	+	(+)	+	+	+	+
D-Turanose	+	d	d‡‡	d	d	+	−
D-Mannose	+	(+)	−	−	−	−	d

* Positive is defined as a colony diameter of ≥ 6 mm after incubation on P agar at 34 to 35°C for 3 days and at room temperature (ca. 25°C) for an additional 2 days (25, 27).

† +, 90% or more strains positive; −, 90% or more strains negative; d, 11–89% of strains positive; ±, 90% or more strains weak positive; ( ), delayed reaction requiring 48 to 72 hr. Data obtained from references 25 and 30.

‡ Positive is defined as the visual detection of carotenoid pigments during colony development at normal incubation or room temperatures. Usually less than 10% of strains of *S. aureus* are unpigmented; however, a significantly higher percentage of TSST-1 producing strains may be unpigmented or only weakly pigmented. Some uncommon strains of *S. epidermidis* may produce a violet pigment.

§ Anaerobic growth in a semisolid thioglycolate medium. Symbols +, moderate to heavy growth down tube within 16 to 24 hr; −, no visible anaerobic growth within 48 hr; (+), delayed growth appearing within 24 to 72 hr, sometimes as large discrete colonies in the anaerobic portion of tube.

‖ 10 to 20% of *S. epidermidis* strains isolated from clinical specimens may be alkaline phosphatase-negative.

¶ Shown to be useful characters in distinguishing species by the API STAPH-IDENT staphylococcal system.

** Positive as defined as a MIC of ≥ 1.6 μg/ml or growth inhibition zone diameter of ≤ 16 mm with a 5-μg novobiocin disk.

†† *S. simulans* strains range from having undetectable acid production to weak acid production from maltose.

‡‡ Most strains of *S. hominis* produce acid from turanose within 24 hr and demonstrate a stronger reaction than that found with positive strains of *S. epidermidis*, *S. warneri*, or *S. haemolyticus*.

netetraacetate (EDTA), incubating the mixture at 37°C in a water bath or heat block for 4 h, and observing the tube for clot formation (a positive test) by slowly tilting the tube 90°. Any degree of clotting constitutes a positive test. Reactions in which a flocculent precipitate forms or in which there are "strings" of cells should be considered negative. It is sometimes advisable to continue incubation for up to 24 h to identify those uncommon strains of *S. aureus* which show relatively weak coagulase activity. However, for those strains requiring a longer clotting period, other characters should be tested to support identification.

The slide test for bound coagulase is performed by making a heavy suspension of growth in distilled water, adding 1 drop of EDTA plasma, stirring the mixture and observing for clumping within 10 s (a positive test). The slide test is rapid and more economical than the tube test. However, 10-15% of *S. aureus* strains may yield a negative test, thus requiring reexamination by the tube test. Slide tests must be read quickly because false-positive results may appear with reaction times longer than 10 s. The test cannot be performed with cells taken directly from media containing a high concentration of salt (e.g., mannitol-salt agar), because autoagglutination and false-positive reactions may occur.

S. aureus can also be distinguished from other species on the basis of the following biochemical profile: positive coagulase, alkaline phosphatase, deoxyribonuclease (including a heat-stable nuclease); hemolysin activities, acetoin production, presence of protein A; and acid produced aerobically from sucrose, trehalose, maltose, mannose, and usually mannitol and lactose.

Newer alternative, commercially available methods for identification of *S. aureus* include a rapid hemagglutination slide test for clumping factor (Baltimore Biological Laboratories), latex agglutination tests that detect both clumping factor and protein A content of the cell wall of *S. aureus* (Scott Laboratories; American Micro Scan; Carr-Scarborough Microbiologicals; Wellcome Diagnostics) and some biochemical test systems for species identification of staphylococci from the same manufacturers. Certain of the methods may be chosen by individual laboratories for either primary or alternative identification of presumed *S. aureus* isolates.

On nonselective agars, colonies of *S. epidermidis* are usually slightly raised, gray or gray-white (nonpigmented) and become sticky with age. Some strains of this species produce a considerable amount of slime, especially when a metabolizable carbohydrate (e.g., glucose) is present.[11]

S. epidermidis can be identified on the basis of the following character profile: negative coagulase, usually positive alkaline phosphatase and urease, novobiocin-susceptible, rapid and strong anaerobic growth in thioglycolate semisolid medium (within 16-24 h), and acid produced aerobically from maltose, fructose and sucrose, but not from mannitol, trehalose, xylose nor xylitol. Acid from turanose is variable and acid is usually produced slowly (within 48-72 h) from mannose. Approximately 10-20% of strains from clinical specimens are negative for alkaline phosphatase activity. These can be distinguished from *S. hominis* on the basis of their strong overnight anaerobic growth in thioglycolate semi-solid agar medium.

Colonies of *S. saprophyticus* are entire, usually glistening, opaque, butyrous, sometimes pigmented and more convex than colonies of *S. aureus* or members of the *S. epidermidis* species group. *S. saprophyticus* is resistant to novobiocin, shows relatively slow anaerobic growth and poor anaerobic acid production from glucose (hence it was previously misclassified as a *Micrococcus*), usually is alkaline phosphatase-negative, and produces acid aerobically from turanose, sucrose and usually xylitol, but not from mannose nor xylose. Many strains of this species also produce acid from trehalose and mannitol and most strains demonstrate β-galactosidase activity. This species can be identified accurately using the rapid biochemical identification systems mentioned, if a novobiocin susceptibility test is included with the system. *S. saprophyticus*, as well as the other novobiocin-resistant human species (*S. cohnii* and *S. xylosus*) are generally resistant to novobiocin concentrations of 1.6 μg/mL or higher. A simple disk diffusion procedure for estimating novobiocin susceptibility can be performed using a 5μg novobiocin disk and either P,[29] Mueller-Hinton[2] or tryptic soy sheep blood agar.[20] With an inoculation suspension equivalent in turbidity to a 0.5 McFarland standard, a 5μg novobiocin disk, and incubation at 35-37°C for 16-20 h, novobiocin resistance is indicated by a zone diameter equal to or less than 16 mm on any of these media. A rapid disk-elution procedure using automated instrument interpretation has also been reported to reliably predict novobiocin resistance after only 4-5 h incubation.[3] Because novobiocin resistance is uncommon in the other clinically important species, it serves as a very useful test for the presumptive identification of *S. saprophyticus*.

EPIDEMIOLOGICAL MARKERS

Several epidemiological marker systems are currently used to recognize the strain distribution of staphylococci associated with infections. These include biotyping, antibiograms, bacteriophage typing and plasmid profiles. Typing is most often used to detect the source of an outbreak of staphylococcal food poisoning or to document the source of nosocomial infections.

Biotyping is the process of typing or grouping cultures of a species on the basis of similarities in their metabolic activities. It is used primarily with coagulase-negative *Staphylococcus* species, due to their marked heterogeneity. Accurate identification of biotypes (or biovars) requires the use of multiple character analyses, often more biochemical tests than may be required for species identification. Tests include those which determine various enzyme activities and aerobic acid production from various carbohydrates.[28] For *S. epidermidis*, alkaline phosphatase, β-glucosidase and arginine dihydrolase activities, as well as acid production from lactose, mannose, turanose, melezitose and ribose have been useful characters for the identification of biotypes. *S. saprophyticus* biotypes can be distinguished on the basis of β-glucosidase and β-galactosidase activities and acid production from lactose, mannitol and trehalose. Some of the uncommon human *S. aureus* biotypes can be resolved on the basis of differences in urease and arginine dihydrolase activities and acid production from lactose and mannitol, although most human *S. aureus* strains share rather similar characters, especially with regard to those used in taxonomic studies. One of the potential problems with biotyping is that of character instability or variation. Thus, biotyping by itself is often not sufficient for individual strain identity.

Antibiograms can be useful epidemiological markers, especially if restricted to isolates from a relatively confined area. They offer the practical advantages of being commonly determined in the laboratory and the wide availability of well standardized test procedures. An unusual susceptibility pattern may be useful to suggest similarity or dissimilarity of isolates. However, susceptibility patterns can be strongly influenced by the scope of antibiotic use within a given locale, with loss or acquisition of plasmids or other resistance factors, so that results may vary considerably from one setting to another. Susceptibility profiles may change within an institution over time or be different at different locations within the institution, making strain origin more difficult to identify. Thus, as with biotyping, antibiograms by themselves have somewhat limited value in strain identification, but taken together with other factors can assist in strain recognition.

The most established system for epidemiological studies of *S. aureus* is bacteriophage typing.[40] Since 1952, this technique has found widespread use with an established international system to control both the typing phages and the procedure. It is not a static system, since it must respond to the emergence of new nontypable strains. Thus the phages used in the standard typing set will vary over a period of years. Currently, the basic set includes: Group I - 29,52,52A,79,80; Group II - 3A,3C,55,71; Group III - 6,42E,47,53,54,75,77,83A,84,85; Misc. - 81,94,95,96. Most microbiology laboratories should not attempt to establish their own phage typing service because the procedures for maintenance, standardization and propagation of phages and propagating strains are expensive and require considerable experience. A few large hospitals and some state health department laboratories offer this service, as do the Centers for Disease Control (CDC), where a reference center is maintained. Several sets of bacteriophages for typing strains of *S. epidermidis* exist, but only a few laboratories maintain the phages and propagating strains. Unfortunately, the phage patterns of *S. epidermidis* are still not well defined. Since phages have only recently been isolated from *S. saprophyticus*, a typing set for this species has not yet been established.

The plasmid DNA profile of a staphylococcal isolate may provide a valuable epidemiological marker. Many of the *Staphylococcus* species demonstrate complex plasmid profiles, thus allowing for demonstrating differences between strains.[30] Some staphylococci may carry as many as 5 to 10 plasmids; however, most strains of the clinically important species carry from 1 to 4. On occasion, clonal variation in plasmid profile may be observed within a strain.[41] This is most often noted by the addition or deletion of a specific plasmid or by modifications resulting in a change of plasmid size. Some of the common antibiotic resistance plasmids are highly conserved in structure and therefore have a limited value in strain recognition. Although analysis of plasmid profiles is a useful epidemiological typing method, it should be used in conjunction with one or more other methods.[41]

TOXIGENICITY TESTS

At least five main classes of toxins are produced by *S. aureus*, including the hemolysins (α,β,γ,δ), leucocidin, enterotoxins (A,B,C,D,E), toxic shock sydrome toxin (TSST-1) and exfoliatin. Of these, the enterotoxins and TSST-1 are of major public health importance.

Most *S. aureus* strains produce enterotoxin A, though those producing enterotoxin E are also commonly associated with food poisoning outbreaks in the United States. At present, the diagnosis of staphylococcal food poisoning is done mostly on the basis of clinical, epidemiological and bacteriological evidence. However, it is also possible to detect the enterotoxins in contaminated foods directly. Because some purification or concentration procedure is often needed to detect low levels of toxin in foods by the conventional microslide test,[7] more sensitive, simplified tests have been developed, e.g., radioimmunoassay (RIA),[36] enzyme-linked immunosorbent assay (ELISA)[19] and reverse passive latex agglutination (RPLA).[24] An RPLA diagnostic kit is now commercially available (SET-RPLA, Oxoid USA) for detecting enterotoxins A,B,C and D, and an ELISA kit (Toxin Technology) is likewise available for the detection of low levels of entertoxins in cultures or foods.

The marker toxin TSST-1 is produced by more than 90% of *S. aureus* strains from toxic shock syndrome cases, although approximately 60% of these isolates also produce one or more staphylococcal enterotoxins.[12] Because TSST-1, when given intragastrically does not produce emesis in certain groups of monkeys, it does not strictly fit the criteria of a staphylococcal enterotoxin, though it was originally named enterotoxin F or pyrogenic exotoxin C. Presumably, the toxin is absorbed through mucous membranes or from subcutaneous tissue sites of colonization or infection, whereby the systemic symptoms of TSS are manifest. Most *S. aureus* strains producing TSST-1 are lysed by Group I phages (with phage types such as 29/52/80) and have several phenotypic properties in common.[55] The production of TSST-1 may be detected by an immunodiffusion assay[11] which utilizes TSST-1 hyperimmune rabbit sera, the test culture and purified TSST-1. A positive detection is indicated by identical precipitin lines between the test culture and purified TSST-1. As with the enterotoxins, newer tests for TSST-1 include RIA, ELISA and RPLA. Recently, an RPLA diagnostic kit (TST-RPLA, Oxoid USA)for detection of TSST-1 has been made commercially available.

SEROLOGICAL PROCEDURES

The serological typing of staphylococci has not been shown to have particular value in distinguishing species or strains, perhaps due to difficulties in producing specific antisera and the lack of standardization of methods. However, some progress has been made in the detection of antibodies to teichoic acids in the sera of patients with *S. aureus* endocarditis or bacteremia complicated by metastatic abscesses.[56] Teichoic acids are major cell wall components of staphylococci and in *S. aureus* are polymers of ribitol with α- or β-glycosidically-linked N-acetylglucosamine residues. Several methods have been utilized for the detection of elevated concentrations of antibodies against *S. aureus* teichoic acids, including gel diffusion counter-immunoelectrophoresis (CIE), RIA and ELISA.[58] All of these are relatively rapid (several hours to one day) and may allow a tentative diagnosis of infection before the results of cultures are available, or when cultures are inconclusive. A major disadvantage is the lack of a single standardized antigen. Most laboratories prepare extracts of the Lafferty strain of *S. aureus*. Sonicated or lysostaphin-treated cell preparations may be used as a source of teichoic acid antigen. Some progress has been made with *S. aureus* whole cell ELISA, as a more economical alternative to using purified antigen.[25] It was shown that 84% of patients with *S. aureus* endocarditis have positive test values. At present, two commercial diagnostic kits are available for the detection of *S. aureus* teichoic acid antibodies (Meridian Diagnostics).

ANTIMICROBIAL SUSCEPTIBILITY TESTS

The general procedures for performing antimicrobial susceptibility tests are described in Chapter 34, "Conventional Procedures for Antimicrobial Susceptibility Tests." It is important for a clinical laboratory to determine accurately the susceptibility of all clinically significant staphylococcal isolates, since resistance to the most commonly used antibiotics may occur. Particular care must be exercised in determining susceptibility to methicillin and other beta-lactam antibiotics since both false susceptibility and false resistance may occur under inadequate test conditions. Careful performance of disk diffusion tests or use of salt-containing media for dilution tests [54] appear to offer the most reliable results.

REFERENCES

1. Aldridge KE, Janney A, Sanders CV. Comparison of the activities of coumermycin, ciprofloxacin, teicoplanin and other non-β-lactam antibiotics against clinical isolates of methicillin-resistant *Staphylococcus aureus* from various geographical locations. Antimicrob Agents Chemother 1985;28:634-8.
2. Almeida RJ, Jorgensen JH. Use of Mueller-Hinton agar to determine novobiocin susceptibility of coagulase-negative staphylococci. J Clin Microbiol 1982;16:1155-6.
3. Almeida RJ, Jorgensen JH. Rapid determination of novobiocin resistance of coagulase-negative staphylococci with the MS-2 system. J Clin Microbiol 1983;17:558-60.
4. Almeida RJ, Jorgensen JH. Comparison of adherence and urine growth rate properties of *Staphylococcus saprophyticus* and *Staphylococcus epidermidis*. Eur J Clin Microbiol 1984;3:542-5.
5. Almeida RJ, Jorgensen JH, Johnson JE. Evaluation of the Automicrobic system Gram-positive Identification Card for species identification of coagulase-negative staphylococci. J Clin Microbiol 1983;18:438-9.
6. Archer GL. *Staphylococcus epidermidis*: the organism, its diseases and treatment. In: Remington JS, Swartz MN, eds. Current clinical topics in infectious diseases; vol. 5. New York: McGraw Hill, 1984:25-48.
7. Bergdoll MS. The enterotoxins. In: Cohen JO, ed. The staphylococci. New York: Wiley-Interscience, 1972:301-31.
8. Berry AJ, Johnston JL, Archer GL. Imipenem therapy of experimental *Staphylococcal epidermidis* endocarditis. Antimicrob Agents Chemother 1986;29:748-52.
9. Christensen GD, Simpson WA, Bisno AL, Beachey EH. Adherence of slime-producing strains of *Staphylococcus epidermidis* to smooth surfaces. Infect Immun 1982;37:318-26.
10. Collins JK, Mader JT, Kelly MT. Resistance of methicillin-resistant *Staphylococcus aureus* to third-generation cephalosporins. J Infect Dis 1983;147:159.
11. Crass BA, Bergdoll MS. Involvement of coagulase-negative staphylococci in toxic shock syndrome. J Clin Microbiol 1986;23:43-5.
12. Crass BA, Bergdoll MS. Involvement of staphylococcal enterotoxins in nonmenstrual toxic shock syndrome. J Clin Microbiol 1986;23:1138-9.
13. Curry JC, Borovian GE. Selective media for distinguishing micrococci from staphylococci in the clinical laboratory. J Clin Microbiol 1976;4:455-7.
14. Daranyi J von. Qualitative Untersuchung der Luftbakterien. Arch Hyg 1925;96:182-4.
15. Deibel RH, Evans JB. Modified benzidine test for the detection of cytochrome-containing respiratory systems in microorganisms. J Bacteriol 1960;79:356-60.
16. Falk D, Guering SJ. Differentiation of *Staphylococcus* and *Micrococcus* spp. with the Taxo A bacitracin disk. J Clin Microbiol 1983;18:719-21.
17. Faller A, Schleifer KH. Modified oxidase and benzidine tests for separation of staphylococci from micrococci. J Clin Microbiol 1981;13:1031-5.
18. Food and Drug Administration. FDA bacteriological analytical manual for foods. Washington, DC: Association of Official Analytical Chemists, 1976.
19. Freed RC, Evenson ML, Reiser RF, Bergdoll MS. Enzyme-linked immunosorbent assay for detection of staphylococcal enterotoxins in foods. Appl Envir Microbiol 1982;44:1349-55.

20. Goldstein J, Shulman R, Kelly E, McKinley G, Fung J. Effect of different media on determination of novobiocin resistance for differentiation of coagulase-negative staphylococci. J Clin Microbiol 1983;18:592-5.
21. Haley RW, Hightower AW, Khabbaz RF, et al. The emergence of methicillin-resistant *Staphylococcus aureus* infections in United States hospitals. Ann Intern Med 1982;97:297-308.
22. Holt R. The classification of staphylococci from colonized ventriculo-atrial shunts. J Clin Pathol 1969;22:475-82.
23. Hovelius B. Epidemiological and clinical aspects of urinary tract infections caused by *Staphylococcus saprophyticus*. In: Mardh PA, Schleifer KH, eds. Coagulase-negative staphylococci. Stockholm: Almqvist and Wiksell International, 1986:195-202.
24. Igarashi H, Shingaki M, Fujikawa H, Ushioda H, Terayama T. Detection of staphylococcal enterotoxins in food poisoning outbreaks by reversed passive latex agglutination. In: Jeljaszewicz J, ed. The staphylococci. New York: Gustav Fischer Verlag, 1985:255-7.
25. Jarv JO, Christensson B, Espersen F, Hertz JB, Hedstrom SA. Antibody response agsinst whole *Staphylococcus aureus* in patients with staphylococcal infections investigated by ELISA. In: Jeljaszewicz J, ed. The staphylococci. New York: Gustav Fischer Verlag, 1985:453-4.
26. Karchmer AW, Archer GL, Dismukes WE. *Staphylococcus epidermidis*: microbiologic and clinical observations as guides to therapy. Ann Intern Med 1983;98:447-55.
27. Kilpper-Balz R, Schleifer KH. Transfer of *Peptococcus saccharolyticus* Foubert and Douglas to the genus *Staphylococcus: Staphylococcus saccharolyticus* (Foubert and Douglas) comb. nov. Zentral Bakteriol Parasit Infek Hyg Abt 1 Orig 1981;2:324-31.
28. Kloos WE. Ecology of human skin. In: Mardh PA, Schleifer KH, eds. Coagulase-negative staphylococci. Stockholm: Almqvist and Wiksell International, 1986:37-50.
29. Kloos WE, Jorgensen JH. Staphylococci. In: Lennette EH, Balows A, Hausler WJ Jr, Shadomy HJ, eds. Manual of clinical microbiology. 4th ed. Washington, DC: American Society for Microbiology, 1985:143-53.
30. Kloos WE, Orban BS, Walker DD. Plasmid composition of *Staphylococcus* species. Can J Microbiol 1981;27:271-8.
31. Kloos WE, Schleifer KH. Isolation and characterization of staphylococci from human skin. II. Descriptions of four new species: *Staphylococcus warneri, Staphylococcus capitis, Staphylococcus hominis* and *Staphylococcus simulans*. Int J Syst Bacteriol 1975;25:62-79.
32. Kloos WE, Schleifer KH. Simplified scheme for routine identification of human *Staphylococcus* species. J Clin Microbiol 1975;1:82-8
33. Kloos WE, Schleifer KH. *Staphylococcus auricularis* sp. nov.: an inhabitant of the human external ear. Int J Syst Bacteriol 1983;33:9-14.
34. Kloos WE, Schleifer KH. Genus IV. *Staphylococcus* Rosenbach 1884. In: Sneath PHA, Mair NS, Sharpe ME, eds. Bergey's manual of systematic bacteriology; vol. 2. Baltimore: Williams and Wilkins, 1986:1031-5.
35. Kloos WE, Wolfshohl JF. Identification of *Staphylococcus* species with the API STAPH-IDENT system. J Clin Microbiol 1982;16:509-16.
36. Miller BA, Reiser RF, Bergdoll MS. Detection of staphylococcal enterotoxin A,B,C,D, and E in foods by radioimmunoassay, using staphylococcal cells containing protein A as immunoadsorbent. Appl Environ Microbiol 1978;36:421-6.
37. Notarinicola SM, Zamarchi GR, Onderdonk AB. Misidentification of mucoid variants of *Staphylococcus aureus* by standard laboratory techniques. J Clin Microbiol 1985;22:459-61.
38. Ogston A. Report upon micro-organisms in surgical diseases. Br Med J 1881;1:369-75.
39. Ogston WH, Cowan HH, Smith HE. Alexander Ogston, K.C.V.O. Aberdeen: Aberdeen University Press, 1943.
40. Parker MT. The significance of phage-typing patterns in *Staphylococcus aureus*. In: Easmon CSF, Adlam C, eds. Staphylococci and staphylococcal infections. London: Academic Press, 1983:33-62.

41. Parisi JT, Lampson BC, Hoover DL, Khan JA. Comparison of epidemiologic markers for *Staphylococcus epidermidis*. J Clin Microbiol 1986;24:56-60.
42. Pulverer G, Halswick R. Coagulase-negative staphylokokken (*Staphylococcus albus*) als Krankheitserreger. Dutsch Med Wschr 1967;92:1141-5.
43. Richmond AS, Simberkoff MS, Schaeffler S, Rahal JJ Jr. Resistance of *Staphyloccus aureus* semisynthetic penicillins and cephalothin. J Infect Dis 1977;135:108-12.
44. Rosenbach FJ. Micro-organisms bei den Wundinfectionskrankheiten des Menschen. Wiesbaden: J.F. Bergmann, 1884.
45. Shands KN, Schmid GP, Dan BB, et al. Toxic-shock syndrome in menstruating women. Association with tampon use and *Staphylococcus aureus* and clinical features in 52 cases. New Engl J Med 1980;303:1436-42.
46. Schleifer KH, Kloos WE. Isolation and characterization of staphylococci from human skin. I. Amended descriptions of *Staphylococcus epidermidis* and *Staphylococcus saprophyticus* and descriptions of three new species: *Staphylococcus cohnii, Staphylococcus haemolyticus* and *Staphylococcus xylosus*. Int J Syst Bacteriol 1975;25:50-61.
47. Schleifer KH, Kloos WE. A simple test system for the separation of staphylococci from micrococci. J Clin Microbiol 1975;1:337-8.
48. Schleifer KH, Kramer E. Selective medium for isolating staphylococci. Zentral Bakteriol Parasit Infekt Hyg Abt 1 Orig 1980;1:270-80.
49. Slifkin M, Merkow LP, Krevzberger SA, Engwall C, Pardo M. Characterization of CO_2 dependent microcolony variants of *Staphylococcus aureus*. Am J Clin Pathol 1971;56:584-92.
50. Smith IM, Beals PD, Kingsbury KR, Hasenclever NF. Observations on *Staphylococcus albus* septicemia in mice and men. Arch Intern Med 1985;102:375-88.
51. Speck ML, ed. Compendium of methods for the microbiological examination of foods. 2nd ed. Washington, DC: American Public Health Association, 1984.
52. Subcommittee on Taxonomy of Staphylococci and Micrococci. Recommendations. Int Bull Bacteriol Nomencl Taxon 1965;15:107-10.
53. Thompson RL, Cabezudo I, Wenzel RP. Epidemiology of nosocomial infections caused by methicillin-resistant *Staphylococcus aureus*. Ann Intern Med 1982;97:309-17.
54. Thornsberry C, McDougal LK. Successful use of broth microdilution in susceptibility tests for methicillin-resistant (heteroresistant) staphylococci. J Clin Microbiol 1983;18:1084-1.
55. Todd JK, Franko-Buff A, Lawellin DW, Vasil ML. Phenotypic distinctiveness of *Staphylococcus aureus* strains associated with toxic shock syndrome. Infect Immun 1984;45: 339-44.
56. Tuazon CU, Sheagren JN. Teichoic acid antibodies in the diagnosis of serious infections with *Staphylococcus aureus*. Ann Intern Med 1976;84:543-6.
57. Watanakunakorn C. Treatment of infections due to methicillin-resistant *Staphylococcus aureus*. Ann Intern Med 1982;97:376-8.
58. Wheat LJ, Kohler RB, White A. Diagnosis and management of deep seated infection. In: Easmon CSF, Adlam C, eds. Staphylococci and staphylococcal infections. London: Academic Press, 1983:121-48.

CHAPTER 28

STREPTOCOCCAL INFECTIONS

Kathryn L. Ruoff, Ph.D. and Carol V. Garner, M.D.

INTRODUCTION

The wide range of infections caused by streptococci is matched by the diversity of these microorganisms. Although the early fascination with the group A streptococcus and the pneumococcus persists, other streptococci, like those of group B and the enterococci, have more recently been recognized as significant pathogens. Streptococci of clinical importance are generally regarded as a group of related organisms which can conveniently be subdivided according to the hemolytic traits described by Brown in 1919 and the serological characteristics investigated by Lancefield, beginning in the 1930's. Although these criteria for identification and classification are still useful, they are not entirely satisfactory for accurate recognition of commonly encountered streptococci. Increased knowledge of the bacteriology and pathogenic mechanisms of these organisms is necessary; such knowledge is certain to reveal the streptococci as an even more remarkable group of pathogens than previously imagined.

CAUSATIVE ORGANISMS

The genus *Streptococcus* encompasses a heterogeneous collection of gram-positive coccoid organisms. Cells are typically arranged in pairs and chains. Glucose is degraded homofermentatively with lactic acid as the major endproduct.

Although oxygen is not used metabolically, most streptococci will grow in its presence. Thus these organisms have been referred to as "aerotolerant anaerobes." While streptococci are unable to synthesize heme and thus a true catalase, occasional strains can give false-positive catalase reactions due to production of peroxidase. Certain streptococci appear to be obligate anaerobes, but these organisms will often adapt to growth in the presence of oxygen when subcultured. Some of these apparently anaerobic streptococci are actually capnophiles (also referred to incorrectly as "microaerophiles") which grow in the presence of oxygen only if elevated (5-10%) amounts of carbon dioxide are present. The heterogeneous nature of the organisms is matched by their ability to reside in numerous sites in the human body (skin, alimentary, respiratory and genitourinary tracts) and by the types of infections as well as nonsuppurative sequelae they can cause.

Current Trends in Streptococcal Classification

Traditional streptococcal classification relies heavily on a minimal number of characteristics: hemolytic behavior, serological reaction, and in more recent times, one or a few simply performed physiological tests. It was recognized early that this system of classification was inadequate for certain groups of streptococci. For example, viridans streptococci cannot be subdivided into discreet groups on the basis of serology. As physiological characteristics were studied more intensively, it became apparent that unrelated streptococci may possess identical hemolytic and serologic characteristics and that physiologically similar strains may be heterogeneous with respect to serology and hemolytic behavior. Although reliance on hemolytic behavior and Lancefield serology is still feasible for classifying and identifying some groups of clinically important streptococci, laboratorians should be aware of the pitfalls of relying solely on these methods. The major divisions of streptococci reflect current taxonomic knowledge of these organisms, but it must be emphasized that classification still needs to be pursued and refined.

Major Divisions of Clinically Important Streptococci

Group A (Streptococcus pyogenes):

These streptococci, important in pharyngitis, respiratory and other infections, are also responsible for rheumatic fever and acute glomerulonephritis. Serologically, they are characterized by possession of the rhamnose and N-acetylglucosamine-containing group A polysaccharide and protein antigens. Host antibodies against the *S. pyogenes* M protein antigen offer protection against infection and recent research has suggested that adherence of group A streptococci to host cells is mediated by complexes of M protein and lipoteichoic acid.[13] These organisms produce extracellular enzymes (streptolysin O, deoxyribonuclease B, hyaluronidase, streptokinase, nicotinamide adenine dinucleotidase) and detection of antibodies to these proteins has been used as a method of diagnosis. Group A streptococci are characterized by their susceptibility to low concentrations of bacitracin and their ability to produce the enzyme, L-pyroglutamyl-peptidase hydrolase.[50]

Group B (Streptococcus agalactiae):

The majority of streptococci with Lancefield's group B polysaccharide antigen are beta-hemolytic, although nonhemolytic strains are not uncommon. Group B streptococci are important pathogens in neonates, but can also cause serious infection in adults. Serotyping of group B strains has been employed in epidemiological studies and a recent proposal for revising the nomenclature of the numerous antigens has been made.[61] In the clinical laboratory, these organisms are identified serologically, or by virtue of their ability to hydrolyze hippurate or produce a positive reaction in the CAMP test.

Group C and G "large colony" Streptococci:

Streptococci with Lancefield's group C or G antigen which form large colonies are differentiated here from "minute colony-forming" beta-hemolytic streptococci with group C or G antigen. Group C large colony strains have been traditionally subdivided into species (*S. equisimilis, S. zooepidemicus, S. equi, S. dysgalactiae*) on the basis of differing physiological reactions. *S. equisimilis* displays physiological properties similar to those of large colony group G streptococci[49] and recent taxonomic studies suggest that large colony group C and G streptococci are related at the species level.[51] Although these streptococci are important animal pathogens, they are often isolated from human throats[54] and have been implicated in infections in numerous body sites.[92] Evidence has also been presented that these streptococci can cause pharyngitis and sequelae in a manner similar to that of group A streptococci.[12,33,117] Although group C and G streptococci are usually beta-hemolytic, alpha and nonhemolytic strains have been described. In the clinical laboratory, organisms can be identified serologically as group C or G and further differentiation from "minute colony-forming" C and G streptococci by their inability to form acetoin.[23,79,110]

Group D Streptococci and Enterococci:

The group D Lancefield antigen, a lipoteichoic acid, is produced by diverse organisms. The enterococci, formerly considered group D streptococci, have been shown to comprise a separate genus.[111] Although *Streptococcus faecalis* and *Streptococcus faecium* are correctly called *Enterococcus faecalis* and *Enterococcus faecium*, they are still referred to as streptococci in common usage. In like manner, all organisms previously known as enterococcal streptococci are now considered to belong to the genus *Enterococcus*.[28] It is important clinically to be able to distinguish enterococci from streptococci because of enterococcal resistance to antimicrobial agents. This distinction is made easily in the laboratory with bile esculin and 6.5% salt-containing media or with a test for the enzyme, L-pyroglutamyl-peptidase hydrolase, possessed by enterococci but not by group D streptococci.[50] *Streptococcus bovis* and *Streptococcus equinus* remain as group D streptococci. Of these two species, *S. bovis* has been shown to be clinically important as a bacteremic indicator of gastrointestinal cancer.[76,95] A biotype of *S. bovis*, called *S. bovis* variant[40] or *S. bovis* II[98] has also been described, but its clinical significance as an indicator of bowel cancer is as yet unknown. *S. bovis* is identified presumptively as a bile esculin-positive, salt-intolerant, group D streptococcus which is unable to hydrolyze arginine, but extended characterization may be necessary for accurate identification.[108]

Pneumococci:

Streptococcus pneumoniae, a common agent of respiratory disease, is usually observed in the laboratory as an alpha-reacting, encapsulated diplococcus. This streptococcus can be easily identified by its susceptibility to optochin (ethylhydrocupreine) or its lysis in the presence of bile or deoxycholate. The antigens of pneumococci also provide a means for identifying these pathogens. Capsular polysaccharide antigens (of which over 80 types exist) can be detected with the use of polyvalent omniserum in the quellung reaction, counterimmunoelectrophoresis, immunofluorescence or with latex and coagglutination techniques. Crossreactions with nonpneumococcal, alpha-reacting streptococci may decrease the specificity of these methods.[64] Serological techniques have also been applied to direct detection of pneumococci and their antigens in sputum and body fluids. Serological tests for the pneumococcal C polysaccharide, thought to be a cell wall component of all pneumococcal capsular types have also been employed for direct detection.[65]

Viridans Streptococci:

The name "viridans streptococci" has been used to describe a heterogeneous collection of streptococci which cannot be categorized by traditional methods of identification (i.e., Lancefield's serology). These organisms are usually alpha-reacting or nonhemolytic, but beta-hemolytic strains also occur. They are serologically heterogeneous (Lancefield's groups A,C,E,F,G,H,K and O antigens have been found) but there is no correlation between possession of a given Lancefield's antigen and a characteristic biochemical profile.[42] Based on physiological characters, these streptococci can be divided into discreet groups which are currently given species status: *S. mutans, S. salivarius, S. sanguis* I, *S. sanguis* II, *S. mitis, S. morbillorum, S. acidominimus* and a group of organisms called *S. milleri* by British and

European authors.[10,29] *S. milleri* is divided on the basis of physiological and hemolytic reactions into 3 species, *S. intermedius, S. constellatus* and *S. anginosus* in the taxonomic scheme of Facklam.[43] Regardless of differences in nomenclature, the viridans streptococci are important causes of endocarditis and the organisms known as *S. milleri* are involved in pyogenic infections.[94,98,112] Nowhere is the confused state of streptococcal taxonomy more evident than in the *S. milleri* group, since they are serologically diverse and may be nonhemolytic, alpha-reacting or beta-hemolytic, but may constitute a genetically related group of streptococci.[74,124]

"Minute" Beta-Hemolytic Streptococci (S. anginosus, S. milleri):

These streptococci form tiny beta-hemolytic colonies on blood agar and may produce Lancefield's group A,C,F,G or no detectable antigen. First characterized by Long and Bliss,[84] these streptococci were later shown to be similar to nonhemolytic and alpha-reacting strains of *S. milleri*.[29,101] Thus these organisms are referred to as beta-hemolytic *S. milleri* or as *S. anginosus* in current nomenclatural terms.[43] Isolates with group A, C or G antigen are distinctly different from their "large colony" counterparts with identical antigens.[29,79,110]

Although these streptococci are considered normal inhabitants of the upper respiratory tract,[23] they can function as pathogens in various body sites.[101]

Nutritionally Variant Streptococci:

These organisms have been previously thought of as pyridoxal-requiring mutants of various viridans species.[30,106] However, recent studies of physiological traits and penicillin-binding proteins suggest that these streptococci may constitute a distinct species.[20] These organisms cause endocarditis and are usually recognized in the laboratory by their satelliting growth around other bacterial species.

CLINICAL MANIFESTATIONS AND THERAPY

Streptococci are extremely important pathogens in clinical medicine, capable of causing a wide variety of infections, including pharyngitis, otitis, tonsillitis, sinusitis, scarlet fever, erysipelas, pyoderma, pneumonia, endocarditis, meningitis, puerperal sepsis, urinary tract infection, arthritis and osteomyelitis. Beta-hemolytic streptococci tend to cause acute, suppurative infections, but also may reside in man as nonpathogens. Alpha- and gamma-hemolytic streptococci, normal inhabitants of the oropharynx and gastrointestinal tract, tend to be less virulent.

Group A streptococci, (*S. pyogenes*) are the most important human streptococcal pathogens, being a major cause of oropharyngeal skin and soft tissue infections. Streptococcal pharyngitis is characterized by a red, swollen, painful throat, tender anterior cervical nodes and constitutional symptoms of malaise, headache and fever. The clinical syndrome may range from a mild nonexudative pharyngitis, easily confused with a viral infection, to severe pharyngitis with fulminant septicemia. Cough and coryza, so common in viral upper respiratory tract infections, are not prominent signs in streptococcal pharyngitis. Culturing group A streptococci from a sore throat is helpful but not definitive, as asymptomatic carriage of these organisms occurs in 3-20% of persons, varying with age and geographical location.[71] A negative culture is helpful in avoiding unnecessary antibiotic therapy.

The major streptococcal skin infections are pyoderma and erysipelas. Pyoderma is a general term embracing all streptococcal skin infections except erysipelas, which is an acute infection of the skin and subcutaneous tissues, most commonly of the face, in which *S. pyogenes* may derive from an upper respiratory source.

Group A infections may be complicated by suppurative and nonsuppurative sequelae. Suppurative complications caused by spread of oropharyngeal infection to contiguous tissues include parapharyngeal space abscesses, otitis, sinusitis, mastoiditis, purulent lymphadenitis, meningitis, brain abscess and cavernous sinus thrombophlebitis. Bacteremic seeding of bones, joints or other metastatic foci may occur. *S. pyogenes* pneumonia is rare but often associated with antecedent viral infections and complicated by empyema.[57] The nonsuppurative sequelae of streptococcal disease are acute rheumatic fever and acute glomerulonephritis. Throat infections may give rise to either; skin infections may lead to glomerulonephritis but not rheumatic fever. *S. pyogenes* infections are diagnosed by clinical findings, culture and serology. The clinical presentation alone, particularly in a setting of epidemic disease, may direct antibiotic therapy while awaiting confirmatory studies. Serum antibodies to streptolysin O, deoxyribonuclease B, hyaluronidase or other streptococcal antigens provide retrospective evidence of infection and are particularly useful in cases of glomerulonephritis or rheumatic fever lacking a history of streptococcal disease.

Recognized for many years as important bovine pathogens, group B streptococci (*S. agalactiae*) have claimed a significant role in human disease since the 1970's. Human strains colonize the adult urogenital and gastrointestinal tracts, the pharynx and the rectum. *S. agalactiae* is a major cause of perinatal infections, including congenital pneumonia, chorioamnionitis, puerperal septicemia, neonatal sepsis and meningitis.[99] Two forms of neonatal disease are recognized. Early onset disease develops rapidly within the first few days of life, often within the first 24 hours, presents as sepsis or pneumonia and has a very high mortality. Late onset disease develops insidiously after 10 days of age, resembles other bacterial infections and frequently presents as meningitis. Although nosocomial spread of *S. agalactiae* may occur, neonates usually acquire the organism via maternal transmission on passage through a colonized or infected birth canal.[53] In older children, group B streptococci may cause otitis, adenitis, arthritis, osteomyelitis and cellulitis. The most common *S. agalactiae* infections in adults involve the urinary tract; but a variety of other infections have been described. Risk factors for adult group B infections include diabetes mellitus, alcoholic liver disease, vascular insufficiency, renal failure, malignancy and age over 60 years.[80]

The group C streptococci are important veterinary pathogens, but rarely cause disease in man. Human disease most often presents as pharyngitis or tonsillitis similar to the syndromes caused by group A streptococci, but a wide spectrum of serious infections have been described.[92] Group C pneumonia resembles group A disease in its frequent association with antecedent viral respiratory tract infection, high incidence of empyema and high morbidity. Infections may be acquired through animal exposure, but endogenous infection also occurs as the organism is a normal inhabitant of the nasopharynx, skin and genital tract. Alcohol or intravenous drug abuse, diabetes mellitus, cancer, immunosuppressive therapy and extremes of age (neonate, elderly) are conditions predisposing to severe group C infections.[92] Rarely, glomerulonephritis but not rheumatic fever may follow infections with these organisms.[33]

Group G streptococci are part of the normal flora of the pharynx, vagina, skin and gastrointestinal tract of humans. Group G organisms first were recognized as pathogens of domestic animals. The spectrum of group G infections includes puerperal and neonatal septicemia, otitis media, pharyngitis, pneumonia and empyema, meningitis, peritonitis, endocarditis, arthritis and cellulitis.[77] Although bacteremia is rare (0.3% of all bacteremia in one series[6]), it usually represents severe disease. The most frequent portal of entry is the skin,[121] often through cellulitic lesions or decubitus ulcers, so that conditions associated with skin breakdown may predispose to group G bacteremia. As with groups A and C, infections with group G streptococci elicit a rise in antistreptolysin O titers. There have been only two reports of nonsuppurative sequelae to group G infections.[34,105]

Group D streptococci have been traditionally divided into two major categories: enterococci (*S. faecalis, S. faecium*) and nonenterococci (*S. bovis, S. equinis*). This differentiation is important clinically. The enterococci are often resistant to many antibiotics, including penicillin, necessitating combination antimicrobial therapy for these infections. In contrast, the nonenterococcal group D streptococci have remained penicillin-susceptible. Recent classification elevates the enterococci to a separate genus, creating *Enterococcus faecalis* and *E. faecium*.

Enterococci are part of the normal oral and intestinal flora. They are frequent isolates in community-acquired and nosocomial sepsis, in endocarditis and in urinary tract infections associated with structural abnormalities. These organisms, particularly *E. faecalis*, are also commonly found in soft tissue infections and intra-abdominal abscesses, from which they may enter the blood as participants in a polymicrobial bacteremia.[62,73] Enterococci rarely cause meningitis, pneumonia or metastatic suppurative complications.

Although outnumbered by the enterococci, the nonenterococcal group D streptococci are also normal inhabitants of the gastrointestinal tract and may cause the same range of infections.[91] Taken together,the group D streptococci/enterococci account for 10-20% of bacterial endocarditis. *S. bovis* bacteremia is often associated with colonic lesions or gastrointestinal tract manipulation.[95] Although enterococcal urinary tract infections usually respond to penicillin or ampicillin therapy, more serious infections such as endocarditis require two-drug regimens such as pencillin (or vancomycin) and an aminoglycoside. Penicillin alone is adequate therapy for most *S. bovis* infections.

Group F streptococci normally reside in the gastrointestinal and genitourinary tracts, the mouth and the oropharynx.[11] Interpreting their clinical significance is difficult, as *S. milleri* cultures have often been included in studies seeking to characterize group F streptococcal infections.[112] Although some *S. milleri* carry the group F antigen, most are nongroupable in the Lancefield system and are placed with the viridans streptococci. One recent study eliminated most *S. milleri* by focusing on beta-hemolytic group F streptococci. These organisms were found to have a proclivity for suppurative infections, forming abscesses of the skin, oral cavity, cervicofacial area and abdomen. Serious illness related to these abscesses did not occur in otherwise healthy persons without concomitant trauma.[81] Most group F infections respond readily to penicillin therapy and abscess drainage.

The viridans group encompasses streptococci defying Lancefield's serological classification but sharing some physiological properties. The human mouth normally contains most viridans species, which comprise a high proportion of the oral bacterial flora.[21] Viridans streptococci have been implicated in infections of all organ systems, but are best known as the most frequent isolates in endocarditis.[106] The viridans species, *S. mutans*, is the major pathogen in dental caries.[83] Another viridans species, *S. milleri*, is known for its propensity to cause localized, purulent infections, such as intra-abdominal, cutaneous and central nervous system abscesses, and it is the most prominent streptococcus recovered from brain abscesses.[89] *S. milleri* endocarditis, unlike endocarditis caused by other viridans streptococci, is often associated with suppurative metastatic infections.[21] The nutritionally variant streptococci may also cause endocarditis and other serious infections. Failure to recover these organisms on standard media may account for many reported cases of "culture-negative" endocarditis.[106] Most viridans streptococci are susceptible to penicillin, but synergistic therapy with penicillin and an aminoglycoside has been found useful in endocarditis and other serious infections.

Streptococci of groups L-T are rarely isolated from clinical specimens. Even when cultured from blood or spinal fluid, these organisms seldom correlate with clinical disease and are usually contaminants.[22]

S. pneumoniae is one of the most important bacterial species pathogenic for man and the most frequent cause of bacterial pneumonia. Lobar pneumonia with consolidation is a common presentation of *S. pneumoniae* disease and is often accompanied by bacteremia. Complications of pneumococcal pulmonary infection include pleural effusion, empyema, pericarditis and lung abscess. *S. pneumoniae* may cause otitis, mastoiditis, sinusitis, meningitis, endocarditis, arthritis and peritonitis. Penicillin-resistant strains have been reported but fortunately are rare; and penicillin remains the drug of choice for therapy.

EPIDEMIOLOGY

The epidemiology of streptococcal infections reflects the microbiological diversity of the streptococci. Many streptococci are normal inhabitants of man, but can cause disease when the usual anatomical or immunological barriers are compromised. Even those groups not indigenous to man, such as group A, may be carried asymptomatically.[71] Pharyngitis due to group A streptococci is an extremely common infection, usually transmitted through direct personal contact via nasal or salivary secretory droplets. Extrahuman animal vectors or fomites are generally not involved in disease transmission, although outbreaks due to contaminated foods are well documented.[86,117] Conditions favoring crowding such as cold weather, poor housing and poverty enhance the spread of streptococcal pharyngitis.

Crowding also aids the spread of streptococcal pyoderma, but the most critical determinants are climate and level of hygiene. Although pharyngitis prevails in cold climates and seasons, pyoderma favors warm or tropical environments where increased skin exposure is associated with abrasions, insect bites and other minor trauma. The role of insects as possible vectors of disease remains to be clarified.[14] Skin colonization with group A streptococci has been documented in endemic and epidemic pyoderma, associated with eventual upper respiratory tract colonization with the same "skin" strains. In contrast, "throat" strains isolated in epidemic pharyngitis do not appear to colonize the skin.[16]

The epidemiology of acute rheumatic fever (ARF) parallels that of severe, exudative pharyngitis, which has been decreasing in frequency in the United States and western Europe over the last four decades. The attack rate for ARF has declined also, to as low as 0.3% or less. In developing countries, however, ARF remains a major post-pharyngitis complication.[15] Early studies of epidemic severe pharyngitis[102] identified two features associated with a high attack rate of ARF: (1) a prominent immune response as reflected in high antistreptolysin O titers and (2) a prolonged convalescent carriage of strains following untreated infection. Later studies identified M-types with a predilection for causing ARF, distinct from serotypes causing acute glomerulonephritis (AGN). Although additional M-types were identified with a high incidence of AGN, the association was not constant. The nature of the factor(s) endowing a streptococcus with "nephritogenic" or "rheumatogenic" potential is clearly more complex than serotype alone and remains to be elucidated.

Group B streptococcus has emerged in the last two decades as a major perinatal pathogen, causing severe disseminated infection in infants less than three months of age. The organism is carried in the genital and gastrointestinal tracts of pregnant women at rates of 2-40%, varying with such factors as socioeconomic status and geographic location.[2] Transmission to newborns occurs most frequently on passage through the birth canal, although nosocomial and community transmission are also documented.[56,97] The fulminant early onset form of group B streptococcal disease is much more common than the insidious late onset form. Exposure to group B streptococcus is the critical factor for disease development, but others include prematurity, premature rupture of maternal membranes, overt maternal peripartum infection and lack of type-specific antibody.[53] The importance of group B streptococci in neonatal disease has led to epidemiological studies using type antigens as markers. These investigations suggest that certain serotypes may have differing pathogenic potentials. Information of this kind will undoubtedly be important in control and prevention.[128]

Fecal carriage of *S. bovis* occurs in only 5-15% of normal adults, but an increased carriage rate has been noted in adults with colonic carcinoma. A study of patients for whom *S. bovis* bacteremia was the sole stimulus for evaluation of the gastrointestinal tract found a high proportion of patients harboring malignant or premalignant colonic lesions.[76] Recognition of this association warrants thorough gastrointestinal tract investigation in patients with otherwise unexplained *S. bovis* bacteremia.

S. pneumoniae is a common inhabitant of the upper respiratory tract, carried asymptomatically by 5-70% of normal adults.[60] Rates are higher in children, in closed populations such as those in schools and military barracks, and in persons with upper respiratory tract infections. Conditions interfering with normal pulmonary clearance mechanisms predispose to infection. An estimated 150,000 to 300,000 cases of pneumococcal pneumonia occur each year in the United States, making this the most common bacterial pneumonia. More cases occur in winter and spring than at other times in temperate climates and the disease has a male predominance (M:F = 3:2) in all age groups. Underlying conditions, such as chronic pulmonary, renal or hepatic disease, unstable diabetes mellitus, certain malignancies, immunodeficiency states and splenic dysfunction are associated with more invasive pneumococcal disease. Only a few of the more than 80 serotypes (types 1,3,4,6,7,8,12,14,18,19 and 23) cause the majority of severe pneumococcal infections, an epidemiologic finding with important implications for vaccine development.[7] The mortality of untreated pneumococcal pneumonia with bacteremia approaches 80%. The widespread use of penicillin has reduced this to 30%, where it has remained for the last 30 years despite technological improvements in intensive care.[24]

PUBLIC HEALTH SIGNIFICANCE, PREVENTION AND CONTROL

The streptococcus is a pathogen of worldwide distribution and unique clinical diversity, but data applicable to public health issues are often imprecise due to a lack of organized reporting systems for streptococcal illness. Group A streptococcal pharyngitis and pyoderma are the most common streptococcal infections and may occur in epidemics. Early therapy of pharyngitis may shorten the duration of symptoms, limit spread of the disease by eradicating the organism from the pharynx and prevent sequelae.[31] The decreased incidence of rheumatic fever and rheumatic heart disease in the United States and western Europe is used both as an argument for more selective treatment of patients with "sore throat" and as evidence of the efficacy of widespread, early penicillin therapy. Although controversy still exists, most authorities favor early treatment of any suspected streptococcal pharyngitis. The primary prevention of acute rheumatic fever requires diagnosis and therapy of streptococcal pharyngitis, although delay of treatment for a few days will not interfere with rheumatic fever prevention except in persons with a history of rheumatic fever. These patients are at increased risk of recurrent disease and have been shown to benefit from monthly prophylactic therapy with intramuscular penicillin. However, this prophylactic regimen is under reevaluation due to the decreased incidence of rheumatic fever and rheumatic heart disease.

Penicillin therapy does not alter the incidence nor severity of post-streptococcal glomerulonephritis, necessitating prevention of antecedent pharyngitis or pyoderma. Early recognition of epidemics with eradication of causative organisms, improvement of crowded living conditions and better personal hygiene have been helpful in limiting these diseases and the public health costs of their sequelae.

According to one national survey, the estimated number of pneumonia cases annually in the United States was 2,606,573. About one half of these were bacterial and *S. pneumoniae* was the most common bacterial cause.[63] Polyvalent polysaccharide pneumococcal vaccines capable of inducing protective immunity in immunocompetent and in some immunocompromised persons are now available. A recent study suggests use of these vaccines in several well-defined risk groups, including children with recurrent otitis media, patients with sickle cell anemia, Hodgkin's disease splenectomies or other immunodeficiencies, patients with chronic disorders such as chronic obstructive pulmonary disease, hepatic or renal disease and the elderly. Evidence for vaccine efficacy in the elder remains equivocal.[24]

The emergence of antibiotic-resistant *S. pneumoniae* makes pneumococcal disease potentially a major public health threat. These organisms have been recovered in many parts of the world, with the greatest number of penicillin-resistant and multiply-resistant pneumococci found in South Africa. Resistant organisms characteristically appear sporadically, often in immunocompromised patients, but may cause small epidemics within hospitals. Control measures include restricting use of antimicrobials, isolating infected patients, vaccinating susceptible patients if the strain is of a vaccine serotype and attempting to eliminate pharyngeal colonization with appropriate antimicrobial agents. The efficacy of these measures varies with the epidemiologic circumstances.[7,8]

Group B streptococcus has been recognized in recent years as a major perinatal pathogen. Efforts to limit neonatal group B disease have focused on identification of risk groups with early recognition and therapy of illness. Prophylactic penicillin therapy has been shown to reduce colonization and infection without altering neonatal flora to favor penicillin-resistant organisms in the first few days of life.[58] Studies using purified group B streptococcal capsular polysaccharides as immunogens in healthy adult volunteers have yielded promising results for development of an effective vaccine.

The public health impact of the remaining streptococci is impossible to assess accurately. Streptococcal endocarditis adds to public health costs through the two to six weeks of hospitalization required for adequate therapy and the occasional severe valvular damage necessitating surgical replacement. Antibiotic prophylaxis around procedures associated with significant bacteremia seems indicated for persons with known valvular disease, who are at particular risk for bacterial endocarditis.[1]

DIAGNOSTIC PROCEDURES

Selection and Processing of Specimens

Due to the variety of infections caused by streptococci and enterococci, these organisms may under appropriate conditions be considered as clinically significant when found in virtually any specimen type. Table 28:1 shows the types of streptococci that are often found as pathogens in a number of

Table 28:1. Types of Streptococci and Enterococci Commonly Isolated as Pathogens in Various Specimens*

Specimen type	Beta-hemolytic streptococci	Pneumococci	Enterococci	Viridans streptococci	Nutritionally variant streptococci
Respiratory	X	X			
Blood	X	X	X	X	X
Urine and genitourinary	X		X		
Body fluids other than blood	X	X	X		
Wounds	X		X	X*	
Eye	X	X			

* *Streptococcus milleri* (*Streptococcus intermedius*, *Streptococcus constellatus* or *Streptococcus anginosus*) is isolated from abscesses and other pyogenic infections.

major specimen categories. General principles of specimen collection (see Chapter 1, "Specimen Collection and Quality") should be observed.

Although streptococci are nutritionally fastidious, commonly used laboratory media usually support their growth and they are easily isolated in most cases. One notable exception is the failure of some commonly used blood culture media to support the growth of nutritionally variant streptococci. Reimer and Reller[104] noted that only a small percentage of the strains they examined grew in brain heart infusion or tryptic soy broth, though all strains grew in supplemented peptone, thioglycolate and thiol broths.

Microscopy and Other Rapid Methodology

Although most of these methods can be used for identification of pure cultures of streptococci, they are mainly methods for direct detection of organisms in body fluids or other specimens. Techniques of direct detection are covered in detail in Chapter 39, "Antigen Detection," so these methods and their application for streptococcal identification are only briefly summarized in tabular form in Table 28:2. Latex or coagglutination methods are probably the most widely used. It should be noted that, although the newer commercially available methods for direct extraction of group A polysaccharide (by nitrous acid or enzyme solutions) from throat swabs are specific, their sensitivity may be fairly low.[25] Thus specimens scored as negative in these tests should be cultured.

Primary Isolation and Culture

Media:

Rich nonselective broths and agars are excellent growth media. Trypticase soy, Columbia and Brucella agars supplemented with animal blood are

Table 28:2. Summary of Rapid Methods for Detection of Streptococci in Body Fluids and Other Specimens

Technique	Streptococci detected and specimen type	References
Immunofluorescence	Group A; throat swabs	93
	Group B; vaginal swabs	107
	Pneumococci; sputum	126
Quellung test	Pneumococci; sputum and CSF	90
Counterimmunoelectrophoresis	Pneumococci; CSF, blood, urine, sputum	72
	Group B; CSF	123
Agglutination (Latex or coaggultination	Pneumococci; sputum, CSF, blood	32,36,38
	Group B; CSF, blood, urine, urogenital swabs	69,70,114,123
	Group A,B,C,D,F,G,; blood	126
	Group A; throat swabs	25,87,115,118

examples of plated media for streptococcal culture. Although a number of animal bloods are suitable, sheep blood is recommended as a supplement, especially for throat cultures. Because *Haemophilus hemolyticus* fails to grow on sheep blood-supplemented agars, the number of beta-hemolytic colonies to be investigated as suspected streptococci will be reduced.

Selective agars such as phenylethyl alcohol (PEA) agar can be used for culture of steptococci from specimens expected to contain large numbers of gram-negative bacteria. Efforts to develop media for selective isolation of group A streptococci from throat specimens have included the incorporation of antibiotics that would inhibit normal oropharyngeal flora.[17,18,59,100,119] A commercially produced medium based on this principle has become available.[26] Selective media containing sulfamethoxazole and trimethoprim (SXT) must also contain sufficient thymidine to counteract the inhibitory effects of SXT (blockage of folate synthesis). Group A and B streptococci and enterococci are able to utilize exogenous thymidine and will grow on these media. Viridans streptococci and pneumococci tested by Coll and associates[27] were unable to utilize exogenous thymidine and were inhibited by SXT even in the presence of thymidine. The fact that thymidine levels vary between lots of basal media may explain the variable results obtained with SXT-containing media.

Determination of hemolysis:

Enzymes responsible for the beta-hemolysis produced by group A streptococci vary in their susceptibility to inhibition by oxygen. Thus anaerobic incubation has been recommended as a method of maximizing the detection of hemolytic strains. Beta-hemolysis may be obscured by the peroxide produced by streptococci growing in air or in the presence of increased CO_2. The interference of oxygen with the detection of beta-hemolysis can be overcome by a simple inoculation technique in which blood agar plates are stabbed in several places after streaking. Hemolytic reactions should be determined by examination of the areas immediately surrounding the stabs. Beta-hemolysis appears as complete clearing (the absence of red cells) of the medium. In the alpha reaction, usually accompanied by a greenish discoloration of the agar surrounding the colonies, blood cells are not completely lysed. Nonhemolytic (gamma-hemolytic) streptococci produce no reaction on blood agar. A fourth hemolytic reaction, alpha-prime or wide-zone alpha hemolysis, is characterized by a zone of complete hemolysis surrounding an area of incomplete hemolysis adjacent to the colony. It should be remembered that descriptions of hemolytic reactions were originally formulated as a result of microscopic study of subsurface colonies in pour plates. Although visual inspection of streaked and stabbed plates is usually sufficient for accurate determination of hemolytic reactions, areas around stabs can be examined microscopically under low power for unequivocal determinations.

Incubation:

If the streak-stab method of inoculation is used for blood agar plates, incubation at 35°C in ambient atmospheres is satisfactory for the cultivation of many streptococci, including group A and enterococci. Increased CO_2 tension is required for the growth of certain strains of *S. milleri*[82,113] and for pneumococci. Thus incubation of cultures in increased CO_2 is recommended to recover all types of streptococci.

Colonial Appearance:

Streptococci produce many different colony types on agar. Small, almost pinpoint colonies surrounded by zones of beta-hemolysis are characteristic of the minute beta-hemolytic streptococci. These organisms sometimes produce a distinct odor described as resembling that of caramel. Other streptococci form gray to whitish colonies that usually have a glistening appearance, although dry colonies also occur. Colonies can be further categorized by the hemolytic reaction produced. Group B streptococci tend to have smaller zones of beta-hemolysis than group A or large colony group C and G. The pneumococci form alpha-hemolytic colonies that may be mucoid or collapsed in the center giving the appearance of a button or nailhead. The enterococci form large (up to 1.5 mm in diameter) colonies. Occasionally, strains of group B streptococci and enterococci produce pigments (yellow to red).

Methods for Identification

Bacitracin and SXT susceptibility tests:

The bacitracin test can be used for presumptive identification of beta-hemolytic group A streptococci. A few colonies from a pure culture are streaked for confluent growth onto one-fourth of an agar plate containing trypticase-soy with 5% sheep blood medium. A bacitracin disk containing 0.04 U is placed on the streaked area and the plate is incubated overnight at 35°C. Any zone of inhibition around the disk is interpreted as a positive test for bacitracin susceptibility. SXT (23.75 μg sulfamethoxazole plus 1.25 μg trimethoprim) disks can be used in conjunction with bacitracin disks for more complete characterization. Plates are inoculated and incubated in the same manner as for bacitracin disks. Any zone of inhibition around the SXT disk is interpreted as a positive test for SXT susceptibility. Although exceptions occur, group A streptococci are bacitacin-susceptible and SXT-resistant; group B are resistant to both agents; and non-group A, B or D beta-hemolytic streptococci are resistant to bacitracin but susceptible to SXT.

PYR test:

This test is an assay for the presence of the enzyme, L-pyroglutamyl-peptide hydrolase, elaborated by group A streptococci and the majority of enterococci. Facklam and coworkers[50] concluded that the PYR test is more specific than, and equally as sensitive as, the bacitracin test for group A identification and comparable to the salt tolerance test for differentiation of enterococci and nonenterococcal streptococci. In the method described by Bosley et al.,[19] 0.2 mL of commercially prepared PYR broth (Todd-Hewett broth containing 0.01% L-pyrrolidonyl-beta-naphthylamide) is inoculated with a loopful of growth from a blood agar plate. After 4 h incubation at 35°C, one drop of PYR reagent (a solution of N, N-dimethylaminocinnamaldehyde) is added. In the presence of the enzyme, L-pyroglutamyl-peptide hydrolase, the PYR substrate is hydrolyzed to yield free beta-naphthylamine which reacts with the added PYR reagent to produce a deep red color within one minute. Any other color development, including orange, is considered a negative reaction. A variation of this test in which the substrate is placed on filter paper strips and only a 10 min incubation period is required is commercially available.[39] In another commercially available rapid test for this enzyme, the hydrolysis of a slightly different substrate results in the formation of a fluorescent product which is visualized with the aid of shortwave ultraviolet light.[120] It should be noted that the PYR test is not absolutely specific for *S. pyogenes* and enterococci. Some strains of aerococci,[50] staphylococci [96] and nutritionally variant streptococci[20] also produce this enzyme.

CAMP test:

The CAMP factor is a diffusable extracellular protein which acts synergistically with staphylococcal beta lysin to cause the lysis of red blood cells. The majority of group B streptococci produce this factor, which can be assayed in the CAMP test.[48] Single straight streaks of the streptococcus to be tested and a beta lysin-producing staphylococcal strain are made perpendicular to each other and 1-2 mm apart on a trypticase soy agar plate containing 5% sheep blood. After overnight incubation at 35°C, a distinct arrowhead-shaped zone of complete beta-hemolysis will appear in the area into which both staphylococcal beta lysin and group B streptococcal CAMP factor have diffused.

The CAMP test can also be performed with disks containing beta lysin[127] or clostridial alpha-toxin.[116]

Hippurate hydrolysis test:

Facklam and coworkers[37] found that 99.6% of 973 group B streptococci were able to hydrolyze hippurate. A small percentage of enterococci also have this ability. In the rapid test of Hwang and Ederer,[67] 0.4 mL of an aqueous solution of 1% sodium hippurate is inoculated with a loopful of growth from a blood agar plate. After 2 h incubation at 37°C, about 0.2 mL of ninhydrin solution (3.5% ninhydrin in a 1:1 mixture of acetone and butanol) is added to the suspension. After 10 min reincubation, a positive result caused by reaction of ninhydrin with the hippurate hydrolysis product, glycine, is visualized as the development of a deep purple color.

Bile esculin and salt tolerance tests:

Positive reactions in these two tests serve to presumptively identify enterococci. Group D streptococci are able to hydrolyze esculin in the presence of 40% bile but fail to grow in the presence of 6.5% NaCl.[41] The bile esculin test can be performed with bile esculin agar slants and the salt tolerance test with a broth medium, or both tests can be performed with plated agar media.[48] After receiving light inoculation and overnight incubation at 35°C, a positive bile esculin test appears as a blackening of the medium, while visible growth in salt-supplemented media is scored as a positive test.

Optochin and bile solubility tests:

These methods are widely used for identification of pneumococci. In the optochin disk test, suspected pneumococci are inoculated for heavy confluent growth onto a blood agar plate; an optochin (ethylhydrocupreine) disk is placed on the inoculated area and the plate is incubated overnight at 35°C in a CO_2 incubator or candle jar. Pneumococci will display inhibition zones greater than 14 mm in diameter with 6 mm optochin disks; zones greater than 16 mm will be observed if a 10 mm disk is used.[52] The lysis of pneumococcal cells in the presence of surface-active agents is demonstrated in the bile solubility test. In a direct plate version, a few drops of 10% sodium deoxycholate are placed directly onto a suspected colony. Pneumococcal colonies will dissolve after exposure to the detergent.[52]

Rapid VP test:

A rapid test for acetoin production by steptococci has been described by Bucher and von Graevenitz[23] for distinguishing minute beta-hemolytic group C and G streptococci (*S. milleri* or *S. anginosus*) from large colony-forming group C and G streptococci. The test will also distinguish group A minute beta-hemolytic isolates from *S. pyogenes*.[79] The large colony pyogenic group A, C and G streptococci fail to produce acetoin while the minute colony-forming strains are positive. The test is carried out by making a turbid suspension of cells in 0.2 mL of MR-VP broth, incubating the suspension at 37°C for 5 h, then adding 1 drop each of 0.5% creatine, alpha naphthol solution (0.8 g in 12 mL 95% ethanol) and 40% KOH, and shaking the suspension thoroughly. Development of a pink to red color within 15-30 min indicates a positive reaction. These methods can be used for presumptive identification of the various divisions of streptococci. Facklam and coworkers[41,47,48] have examined large numbers of streptococci using most of these methods. Although atypical strains are found occasionally, these simple tests offer a satisfactory alternative to serological or other more cumbersome methods. Reactions of the major divisions of clinically important streptococi and enterococci in the presumptive tests are summarized in Table 28:3. It is clearly not necessary to perform all tests on every isolate. Facklam and associates[50] have proposed the use of the CAMP, bile esculin and PYR tests as means for identification. With inclusion of the optochin or bile solubility test for pneumococci, this scheme could prove to be a simple protocol for presumptive identifications.

Commercially available identification systems:

In recent years a number of commercial systems for streptococcal identification have appeared. These products are probably most useful for identifying viridans streptococci or for differentiating species of enterococci, since most beta-hemolytic streptococci can be identified serologically or with presumptive tests. All of these commercial systems employ miniaturized biochemical tests for enzyme production and for the ability to metabolize various substrates. The manually operated systems[3,4,5,44,49,109] and one automated method[4,44] have been well described and evaluated in the literature. These systems may provide useful information when used to identify significant isolates or for epidemiological purposes.

Serological examinations:

Determination of the Lancefield group antigen of an isolate is in many cases sufficient for identification. Problems connected with reliance on serological reaction as the sole criterion for identification have been discussed under "Causative Organisms." Although fluorescent antibody staining is sometimes used for determination of Lancefield group antigen, serological grouping usually involves treatments designed to liberate the antigen from the cell. This extraction procedure is then followed by methods designed to detect the presence of the antigen. Once Lancefield antigen has been extracted from the cells, a precipitin test such as that used at the Centers for Disease Control[45] or agglutination reagents may be used for detection of the antigen. Before commercially prepared reagents for Lancefield grouping became available, a variety of other techniques were developed for serological examination of streptococci and a number of extraction methods have been described.[35,37,38,55,78,85,88,103,122] In recent years, commercially available reagents have been widely used for streptococcal grouping. Nitrous acid or enzyme solutions are used for antigen extraction. In some

Table 28:3. Reactions Displayed by Streptococci in Tests Used for Presumptive Identification.*

	Susceptibility to:		Hydrolysis of PYR	CAMP	Hydrolysis of hippurate	Bile esculin	Growth in 6.5% NaCl	Optochin susceptibility and bile susceptibility
	Bacitracin	SXT						
Group A (*S. pyogenes*)	+	−	+	−	−	−	−	−
Group B (*S. agalactiae*)	−†	−	−	+	+	−	+†	−
Large Colony Group C and G	−†	+	−	−	−	−	−	−
Group D Streptococci	−	+†	−	−	−	+	−	−
Enterococci	−	−	+†	−	−†	+	+	−
Pneumococci			−	−	−	−	−	+
Viridans Streptococci	−†	+	−	−	−†	−†	−	−
Minute Beta Hemolytic Streptococci	−		−		−			

* The information in the table is based on work by Facklam and others. See text for details of the tests mentioned and specific references. Symbols: + = positive; − = negative.

† Atypical results can occur occasionally

cases, the manufacturer recommends omission of the extraction step. Latex agglutination or coagglutination techniques are used for detection of antigen. Complete descriptions and instructions for use of these products are supplied by the manufacturers; the manufacturer's recommendations should be followed exactly when using a product. Products for the detection of group A,B,C,D,F and G Lancefield antigens are available, as well as reagents for detecting pneumococcal capsular antigens.

Products used for Lancefield grouping seem to work well with beta-hemolytic streptococci, but problems arise when nonhemolytic or alpha-reacting streptococci are examined. Hopfer and colleagues[66] found that enzymatic extraction of enterococci released antigens which crossreacted with group G latex agglutination reagents. Enzymatic extraction can also release material from certain viridans streptococci which crossreacts with group D antiserum and latex agglutination reagents.[46,108] The group D antigen is a teichoic acid, and compounds of this type are thought to be present in the cell walls of all gram-positive organisms. Thus crossreactions are not surprising. Facklam[42] has concluded that only group B and D reagents of commonly used antisera should be used for tests on nonhemolytic or alpha-reacting streptococci. This practice should separate nonhemolytic or alpha-reacting group B and group D streptococci and enterococci from viridans streptococci. It is the opinion of one of the authors (K.L.R.) however, that enterococci are best identified by presumptive tests and that group D streptococci (*S. bovis*) should be identfied by an extended series of physiological tests.

Serologic Tests

The assay of antibodies against streptococcal extracellular products or components of the streptococcal cell wall is used as an aid in diagnosing recent infection. These serological tests are employed when rheumatic fever or acute glomerulonephritis is suspected in the absence of a concurrent isolation of group A streptococci. Antibody levels reach a maximum within a few weeks after acute streptococcal infection. These maximum levels persist for about three months and occur coincidentally with the onset of rheumatic fever symptoms.[9]

Of the numerous antistreptococcal antibody tests which have been described, the three most suitable tests for routine use are the antistreptolysin O (ASO), antideoxyribonuclease B (ADN-B) and antihyaluronidase (AH) tests. The ASO and ADN-B tests are reproducible and employ commercially available reagents. The AH test is more efficient than the ASO for diagnosis of streptococcal pyoderma and acute glomerulonephritis.[75] Another commercially available test employs hemagglutination to detect antibodies to streptolysin O, deoxyribonuclease B, hyaluronidase, streptokinase and nicotinamide adenine dinucleotidase. This test is sensitive, but suffers from poor reproducibility and is probably best used only as a screening test.[9] Details on performance and interpretation of antistreptococcal antibody tests have been published.[14,75]

REFERENCES

1. Anonymous. Prevention of bacterial endocarditis. The Medical Letter 1986;28:22.
2. Anthony BF, Eisenstadt R, Carter J, Kim KS, Hobel CJ. Genital and intestinal carriage of group B streptococci during pregnancy. J Infect Dis 1981;143:761-6.
3. Appelbaum PC, Chaurushiya PC, Jacobs MR, Duffett A. Evaluation of the Rapid Strep system for species identification of streptococci. J Clin Microbiol 1984;19:588-91.
4. Appelbaum PC, Jacobs MR, Heald JI, et al. Comparative evaluation of the API 20S system and the Auto Microbic System Gram-Positive Identification card for species identification of streptococci. J Clin Microbiol 1984;19:164-8.
5. Appelbaum PC, Jacobs MR, Palko WM, Frauenhoffer EE, Duffett A. Accuracy and reproducibility of the IDS Rapid STR system for species identification of streptococci. J Clin Microbiol 1986;23:843-6.
6. Auckenthaler R, Hermans PE, Washington JA II. Group G streptococcal bacteremia: clinical study and review of the literature. Rev Infect Dis 1983;5:196-204.
7. Austrian R. Prevention of pneumococcal infection by immunization with capsular polysaccharides of *Streptococcus pneumoniae*: current status of polyvalent vaccines. J Infect Dis 1977;136(suppl):38-42.
8. Austrian R. Some observations on the pneumococcus and on the current status of pneumococcal disease and its prevention. Rev Infect Dis 1981;3(suppl):1-15.
9. Ayoub EM. Streptococcal antibody tests in rheumatic fever. Clin Immunol Newsletter 1982;3:107-11.
10. Ball LC, Parker MT. The cultural and biochemical characteristics of *Streptococcus milleri* strains isolated from human sources. J Hyg (Camb) 1979;82:63-78.
11. Bannatyne RM, Randall C. Ecology of 350 isolates of group F streptococcus. Am J Clin Pathol 1977;67:184-6.
12. Baumgarten A, von Graevenitz A, Greco T. Serological evidence for a causative role of non-group A hemolytic streptococci in pharyngitis. Zentral Bakt Hyg I Abt Orig A 1981;249:460-5.
13. Beachey EH, Simpson WA, Ofek I, Hasty DL, Dale JB, Whitnack E. Attachment of *Streptococcus pyogenes* to mammalian cells. Rev Infect Dis 1983;5(suppl 4):670-7.
14. Bisno AL. Rheumatic fever. In: Mandell GL, Douglas RG Jr, Bennett JE, eds. Principles and practice of infectious diseases. New York: John Wiley, 1979:1574-83.
15. Bisno AL. Acute rheumatic fever: Current concepts and controversies. In: Remington JS, Swartz MN, eds. Current clinical topics in infectious diseases; vol 5. New York: McGraw-Hill, 1984:316-41.
16. Bisno AL, Pearce IA, Wall HP, Moody MD, Stollerman GH. Contrasting epidemiology of acute rheumatic fever and acute glomerulonephritis. N Engl J Med 1970;283:561-5.
17. Black WA, Van Buskirk F. Gentamicin as a selective agent for the isolation of beta haemolytic streptococci. J Clin Pathol 1973;26:154-6.
18. Blanchette LP, Lawrence C. Group A streptococcus screening with neomycin blood agar. Am J Clin Pathol 1967;48:441-3.
19. Bosley GS, Facklam RR, Grossman D. Rapid identification of enterococci. J Clin Microbiol 1983;18:1275-7.
20. Bouvet A, Villeroy F, Cheng F, Lamesch C, Williamson R, Gutmann L. Characterization of nutritionally variant streptococci by biochemical tests and penicillin-binding proteins. J Clin Microbiol 1985;22:1030-4.

21. Brennan RO, Durack DT. The viridans streptococci in perspective. In: Remington JS, Swartz MN, eds. Current clinical topics in infectious diseases; vol 5. New York: McGraw-Hill, 1984:253-89.
22. Broome CV, Moellering RC, Watson BK. Clinical significance of Lancefield groups L-T streptococci isolated from blood and cerebrospinal fluids. J Infect Dis 1976;133:382-92.
23. Bucher C, von Graevenitz A. Differentiation in throat cultures of group C and G streptococci from *Streptococcus milleri* with identical antigens. Eur J Clin Microbiol 1984;3:44-5.
24. Burman LA, Norrby R, Trollfors B. Invasive pneumococcal infections: incidence, predisposing factors and prognosis. Rev Infect Dis 1985;7:133-42.
25. Campos JM, Charilaou CC. Evaluation of Detect-A-Strep and the Culturette Ten-Minute Strep ID kits for detection of group A streptococcal antigen in oropharyngeal swabs from children. J Clin Microbiol 1985;22:145-8.
26. Carlson JR, Merz WG, Hansen BE, Ruth S, Moore DG. Improved recovery of group A beta-hemolytic streptococci with a new selective medium. J Clin Microbiol 1985;21:307-9.
27. Coll PF, Ausina VR, Vernis JV, Mirelis BO, Prats GP. Exogenous thymidine and reversal of the inhibitory effect of sulfamethoxazole-trimethoprim on streptococci. Eur J Clin Microbiol 1984;3:424-6.
28. Collins MD, Jones D, Farrow JAE, Kilpper-Balz R, Schleifer KH. *Enterococcus avium* nom. rev., comb. nov.; *E. casseliflavus* nom. rev., comb. nov.; *E. durans* nom. rev., comb. nov.; *E. gallinarum* nom. rev., comb. nov.; and *E. malodoratus* sp. nov. Int J Syst Bacteriol 1984;34:220-3.
29. Colman G, Williams REO. Taxonomy of some human viridans streptococci. In: Wannamaker LW, Matsen JM, eds. Streptococci and streptococcal diseases; recognition, understanding and management. New York: Academic Press, 1972:281-99.
30. Cooksey RC, Thompson FS, Facklam RR. Physiological chracterization of nutritionally variant streptococci. J Clin Microbiol 1979;10:326-30.
31. Denny FW. Effect of treatment on streptococcal pharyngitis: is the issue really settled? Pediatr Infect Dis 1985;4:352-4.
32. Drow DL, Welch DF, Hensel D, Eisenach K, Long E, Slifkin M. Evaluation of the Phadebact CSF test for detection of the four most common causes of bacterial meningitis. J Clin Microbiol 1983;18:1358-61.
33. Duca E, Teodorovici GR, Radu C, et al. A new nephritogenic streptococcus. J Hyg (Camb) 1969;67:691-8.
34. Duma RJ, Weinberg AN, Medrek TF, Kunz LJ. Streptococcal infections. A bacteriologic and clinical study of streptococcal bacteremia. Medicine 1969;48:87-127.
35. Ederer GM, Herrman MM, Bruce R, Matsen JM, Chapman SS. Rapid extraction method with pronase B for grouping beta-hemolytic streptococci. Appl Microbiol 1972;23:285-8.
36. Edward EA, Coonrod JD. Coagglutination and counterimmunoelectrophoresis for detection of pneumococcal antigens in the sputum of pneumonia patients. J Clin Microbiol 1980;5:488-91.
37. El Kholy A, Facklam R, Sabre G, Rotta J. Serological identification of group A streptococci from throat scrapings before culture. J Clin Microbiol 1978;8:725-8.
38. El Kholy A, Wannamaker LW, Krause RM. Simplified extraction procedure for serological groupings of beta-hemolytic streptococci. Appl Microbiol 1974;28:863-9.
39. Ellner PD, Williams DA, Hosmer ME, Cohenford MA. Preliminary evaluation of a rapid colorimetric method for the presumptive identification of group A streptococci and enterococci. J Clin Microbiol 1985;22:880-1.
40. Facklam RR. Recognition of group D streptococcal species of human origin by biochemical and physiological tests. Appl Microbiol 1972;23:1131-9.
41. Facklam RR. Comparison of several laboratory media for presumptive identification of enterococci and group D streptococci. Appl Microbiol 1973;26:138-45.
42. Facklam RR. Physiological differentiation of viridans streptococci. J Clin Microbiol 1977;5:184-201.

43. Facklam RR. The major differences in the American and British *Streptococcus* taxonomy schemes with special reference to *Streptococcus milleri*. Eur J Clin Microbiol 1984; 3:91-3.
44. Facklam R, Bosley GS, Rhoden D, Franklin AR, Weaver N, Schulman R. Comparative evaluation of the API 20S and AutoMicrobic Gram-Positive Identification systems for non-beta-hemolytic streptococci and aerococci. J Clin Microbiol 1985;21:535-41.
45. Facklam RR, Carey RB. Streptococci and aerococci. In: Lennette EH, Balows A, Hausler WJ Jr, Shadomy HJ, eds. Manual of clinical microbiology, 4th ed. Washington, DC: American Society for Microbiology, 1985:154-75.
46. Facklam RR, Cooksey RC, Wortham EC. Evaluation of commercial latex agglutination reagents for grouping streptococci. J Clin Microbiol 1979;10:641-6.
47. Facklam RR, Padula JF, Thacker LG, Wortham EC, Sconyers BJ. Presumptive identification of group A, B and D streptococci. Appl Microbiol 1974;27:107-13.
48. Facklam RR, Padula JF, Wortham EC, Cooksey RC, Rountree HA. Presumptive identification of group A, B and D streptococci on agar plate media. J Clin Microbiol 1979;9:665-72.
49. Facklam RR, Rhoden DL, Smith PB. Evaluation of the Rapid Strep system for the identification of clinical isolates of *Streptococcus* species. J Clin Microbiol 1984;20:894-8.
50. Facklam RR, Thacker LG, Fox B, Eriquez L. Presumptive identification of streptococci with a new test system. J Clin Microbiol 1982;15:897-90.
51. Farrow JAE, Collins MD. Taxonomic studies on streptococci of serological groups C, G and L and possibly related taxa. Syst Appl Microbiol 1984;5:483-93.
52. Finegold SM, Martin WJ. Diagnostic microbiology. 6th ed. St. Louis: C.V. Mosby, 1982:184-5.
53. Fischer G, Horton RE, Edelman R. From the National Institute of Allergy and Infectious Disease: summary of the National Institutes of Health workshop on group B streptococcal infection. J Infect Dis 1983;148:163-6.
54. Forrer CB, Ellner PD. Distribution of hemolytic streptococci in respiratory specimens. J Clin Microbiol 1979;10:69-71.
55. Fuller AT. The formamide method for the extraction of polysaccharides from hemolytic streptococci. J Exp Pathol 1938;19:103-9.
56. Gardner SE, Mason EO Jr, Yow MD. Community acquisition of group B streptococcus by infants of colonized mothers. Pediatrics 1980;66:873-5.
57. Gerber GJ, Farmer WC, Fulkerson LL. Beta-hemolytic streptococcal pneumonia following influenza. JAMA 1978;240:242-3.
58. Ghaey K, Tolpin M, Schauf V, et al. Penicillin prophylaxis and the neonatal microbial flora. J Infect Dis 1985;152:1070-3.
59. Gunn BA, Ohashi DK, Gaydos CA, Holt ES. Selective and enhanced recovery of group A and B streptococci from throat cultures with sheep blood agar containing sulfamethoxazole and trimethoprim. J Clin Microbiol 1977;5:650-5.
60. Hendley JO, Sande MA, Stewart PM, Gwaltney JM. Spread of *Streptococcus pneumoniae* in families. I. Carriage rates and distribution of types. J Infect Dis 1975;132:55-61.
61. Henrichsen J, Ferrieri P, Jelinkova J, Kohler W, Maxted WR. Nomenclature of antigens of group B streptococci. Int J Syst Bacteriol 1984;34:500.
62. Hermans PE, Washington JA II. Polymicrobial bacteremia. Ann Intern Med 1970;73:387-92.
63. Hoeprich PD. Bacterial pneumonias. In: Hoeprich PD, ed. Infectious diseases. Philadelphia: Harper and Row, 1983:347-60.
64. Holmberg H, Danielsson D, Hardie J, Krook A, Whiley R. Cross reactions between alpha-streptococci and omniserum, a polyvalent pneumococcal serum, demonstrated by direct immunofluorescence, immunoelectroosmophoresis and latex agglutination. J Clin Microbiol 1985;21:745-8.
65. Holmberg H, Holme T, Krook A, Olsson T, Sjoberg L, Sjogren A. Detection of C polysaccharide in *Streptococcus pneumoniae* in the sputa of pneumonia patients by an enzyme-linked immunosorbent assay. J Clin Microbiol 1985;22:111-15.

66. Hopfer RL, Pinzon R, Wenglar M, Rolston KVI. Enzyme release of antigens from *Streptococcus faecalis* and *Listeria monocytogenes* cross-reactive with Lancefield group G typing reagents. J Clin Microbiol 1985;22:677-9.
67. Hwang M, Ederer GM. Rapid hippurate hydrolysis method for presumptive identification of group B streptococci. J Clin Microbiol 1975;1:114-15.
68. Ingram DL, Pearson AW, Occhiuti AR. Detection of bacterial antigens in body fluids with the Wellcogen *Haemophilus influenzae b, Streptococcus pneumoniae* and *Neisseria meningitidis* (ACYW135) latex agglutination tests. J Clin Microbiol 1983;18:1119-21.
69. Ingram DL, Suggs DM, Pearson AW. Detection of group B streptococcal antigen in early onset and late onset group B streptococcal disease with the Wellcogen Strep B latex agglutination test. J Clin Microbiol 1982;16:656-8.
70. Jones DE, Kanarek KS, Lim DV. Group B streptococcal colonization patterns in mothers and their infants. J Clin Microbiol 1984;20:438-40.
71. Kaplan EL. The group A streptococcal upper respiratory tract carrier state: an enigma. J Pediatr 1980;97:337-45.
72. Kenny GE. Counterimmunoelectrophoresis for the diagnosis of pneumococcal respiratory and other infections. In: Coonrod JD, Kunz LJ, Ferraro MJ, eds. The direct detection of microorganisms in clinical samples. New York: Academic Press, 1983:105-111.
73. Kiani D, Quinn EL, Burch KH, Madhaven T, Saravolatz LD, Neblett TR. The increasing importance of polymicrobial bacteremia. JAMA 1979;242:1044-7.
74. Kilpper-Balz R, Williams BL, Lutticken R, Schleifer KH. Relatedness of "*Streptococcus milleri*" with *Streptococcus anginosus* and *Streptococcus constellatus*. Syst Appl Microbiol 1984;5:494-500.
75. Klein GC. Immune response to streptococcal infection (antistreptolysin O, antideoxyribonuclease B). In: Rose NR, Friedman H, eds. Manual of clinical immunology. 2nd ed. Washington, DC: American Society for Microbiology, 1980:431-40.
76. Klein RS, Catalano MT, Edberg SC, Casey JI, Steigbigel NH. *Streptococcus bovis* septicemia and carcinoma of the colon. Ann Intern Med 1979;91:560-2.
77. Lam K, Bayer AS. Serious infections due to group G streptococci. Am J Med 1983;75:561-70.
78. Lancefield RC. Serological differentiation of human and other groups of hemolytic streptococci. J Exp Med 1933;57:571-95.
79. Lawrence J, Yajko DM, Hadley WK. Incidence and characterization of beta-hemolytic *Streptococcus milleri* and differentiation from *S. pyogenes* (group A), *S. equisimilis* (Group C) and large-colony group G streptococci. J Clin Microbiol 1985;22:772-7.
80. Lerner PI, Gopalakrishna KV, Wolinsky E, McHenry MC, Tan JS, Rosenthal M. Group B streptococcus (*S. agalactiae*) bacteremia in adults: analysis of 32 cases and review of the literature. Medicine 1977;56:457-73.
81. Libertin CR, Hermans PE, Washington JA. Beta-hemolytic group F streptococcal bacteremia: a study and review of the literature. Rev Infect Dis 1985;7:498-503.
82. Liu P. Carbon dioxide requirement of group F and minute colony G hemolytic streptococci. J Bacteriol 1954;68:282-8.
83. Loesche WJ, Rowan J, Straffon LH, Loos PJ. Association of *Streptococcus mutans* with human dental decay. Infect Immun 1975;11:1252-60.
84. Long PH, Bliss EA. Studies upon minute hemolytic streptococci. The isolation and cultural characteristics of minute beta hemolytic streptococci. J Exp Med 1934;60:619-31.
85. Maxted WR. Preparation of streptococcal extracts for Lancefield grouping. Lancet 1948;2:255-6.
86. McCormick JB, Kay D, Hayes P, Feldman R. Epidemic streptococcal sore throat following a community picnic. JAMA 1976;236:1039-41.
87. McCusker JJ, McCoy EL, Young CL, Alamares R, Hirsch LS. Comparison of Directigen Group A Strep Test with a traditional culture technique for detection of group A beta-hemolytic streptococci. J Clin Microbiol 1984;20:824-5.
88. Medrek TF, Barnes EM. The influence of the growth medium on the demonstration of a group D antigen in faecal streptococci. J Gen Microbiol 1962;28:701-9.

89. Melo JC, Raff MJ. Brain abscess due to *Streptococcus MG-intermedius (Streptococcus milleri)*. J Clin Microbiol 1978;7:529-32.
90. Merrill CW, Gwaltney JM Jr, Hendley JW, et al. Rapid identification of pneumococci. Gram stain vs. the quellung reaction. N Engl J Med 1973;288:510-12.
91. Moellering RC Jr, Watson BK, Kunz LJ. Endocarditis due to group D streptococci. Am J Med 1974;57:239-50.
92. Mohr DN, Feist DJ, Washington JA II, Hermans PE. Infections due to group C streptococci in man. Am J Med 1979;66:450-6.
93. Moody MD, Siegel AC, Pittman B, Winter CC. Fluorescent-antibody identification of group A streptococci from throat swabs. Am J Public Health 1963;53:1083-92.
94. Murray HW, Gross KC, Masur H, Roberts RB. Serious infections caused by *Streptococcus milleri*. Am J Med 1978;64:759-63.
95. Murray HW, Roberts RB. *Streptococcus bovis* bacteremia and underlying gastrointestinal disease. Arch Intern Med 1978;138:1097-9.
96. Oberhofer TR. Value of the L-pyrrolidonyl-β-naphthylamide hydrolysis test for identification of select gram-positive cocci. Diag Microbiol Infect Dis 1986;4:43-7.
97. Paredes A, Wong P, Mason EO Jr, Taber LH, Barrett FF. Nosocomial transmission of group B streptococci in a newborn nursery. Pediatrics 1976;59:679-82.
98. Parker MT, Ball LC. Streptococci and aerococci associated with systemic infection in man. J Med Microbiol 1976;9:275-302.
99. Patterson MJ, Hafeez AEB. Group B streptococci in human disease. Bacteriol Rev 1976;40:774-92.
100. Petts DN. Colistin-oxolinic acid-blood agar: a new selective medium for streptococci. J Clin Microbiol 1984;19:4-7.
101. Poole PM, Wilson G. Infection with minute-colony-forming β-haemolytic streptococci. J Clin Pathol 1976;29:740-5.
102. Rammelkamp CH, Denny FW, Wannamaker LW. Studies on the epidemiology of rheumatic fever in the armed services. In: Thomas L, ed. Rheumatic fever: a symposium. Minneapolis: University of Minnesota Press, 1952:72-83.
103. Rantz LA, Randall E. Use of autoclaved extracts of hemolytic streptococci for serological grouping. Stanford Med Bull 1955;13:290-1.
104. Reimer LG, Reller LB. Growth of nutritionally variant streptococci on common laboratory and 10 commercial blood culture media. J Clin Microbiol 1981;14:329-32.
105. Roberts RB. Viridans and beta-hemolytic (nongroup A,B and D) streptococci. In: Mandell GL, Douglas RG Jr, Bennett JE, eds. Principles and practice of infectious diseases. 2nd ed. New York: John Wiley, 1985:1162-72.
106. Roberts RB, Krieger AG, Schiller NL, Gross KC. Viridans streptococcal endocarditis: the role of various species, including pyridoxal-dependent streptococci. Rev Infect Dis 1979;1:955-65.
107. Romero R, Wilkinson HW. Identification of group B streptococci by immunofluorescence staining. Appl Microbiol 1974;28:199-204.
108. Ruoff KL, Ferraro MJ, Holden J, Kunz LJ. Identification of *Streptococcus bovis* and *Streptococcus salivarius* in clinical laboratories. J Clin Microbiol 1984;20:223-6.
109. Ruoff KL, Kunz LJ. Use of the Rapid STREP system for identification of viridans streptococcal species. J Clin Microbiol 1983;18:1128-40.
110. Ruoff KL, Kunz LJ, Ferraro MJ. Occurrence of *Streptococcus milleri* among beta-hemolytic streptococci isolated from clinical specimens. J Clin Microbiol 1985;22:149-51.
111. Schleifer KH, Kilpper-Balz R. Transfer of *Streptococcus faecalis* and *Streptococcus faecium* to the genus *Enterococcus* nom. rev. as *Enterococcus faecalis* comb. nov. and *Enterococcus faecium* comb. nov. Int J Syst Bacteriol 1984;34:31-4.
112. Shlaes DM, Lerner PI, Wolinsky E, Gopalakrishna KV. Infections due to Lancefield group F and related streptococci (*S. milleri, S. anginosus*). Medicine 1981;60:197-207.
113. Sisson PR, Ingham HR, Selkon JB. A study of carbon dioxide-dependent strains of *Streptococcus milleri*. J Med Microbiol 1978;11:111-16.

114. Slifkin M, Freedel D, Gil DM. Direct serogrouping of group B streptococci from urogenital and gastric swabs with nitrous acid extraction and the Phadebact streptococcus test. Am J Clin Pathol 1982;78:850-3.
115. Slifkin M, Gil GM. Evaluation of the Culturette Brand Ten-Minute Group A Strep ID technique. J Clin Microbiol 1984;20:12-14.
116. Smith JA, Ngui-Yen JH. Evaluation of a clostridial alpha-toxin disk test for rapid presumptive identification of group B streptococci. J Clin Microbiol 1980;12:18-21.
117. Stryker WS, Fraser DW, Facklam RR. Foodborne outbreak of group G streptococcal pharyngitis. Am J Epidemiol 1982;116:533-40.
118. Venezia RA, Ryan A, Alward S, Kostun WA. Evaluation of a rapid method for the detection of streptococcal group A antigen directly from throat swabs. J Clin Microbiol 1985;21:395-8.
119. Vincent WF, Gibbons WE, Gaafar HA. Selective medium for the isolation of streptococci from clinical specimens. Appl Microbiol 1971;22:942-3.
120. Wasilauskas BL, Hampton KD. Evaluation of the Strep-A-Fluor identification method for group A streptococci. J Clin Microbiol 1984;20:1205-6.
121. Watsky KL, Kollisch N, Densen P. Group G streptococcal bacteremia. Arch Intern Med 1985;145:58-61.
122. Watson BK, Moellering RC Jr, Kunz LJ. Identification of streptococci: use of lysozyme and *Streptomyces albus* filtrate in the preparation of extracts for Lancefield grouping. J Clin Microbiol 1975;1:274-8.
123. Webb BJ, Edwards MS, Baker CJ. Comparison of slide coagglutination test and countercurrent immunoelectrophoresis for detection of group B streptococcal antigen in cerebrospinal fluid from infants with meningitis. J Clin Microbiol 1980;11:263-5.
124. Welborn PP, Hadley WK, Newbrun E, Yajko DM. Characterization of strains of viridans streptococci by deoxyribonucleic acid hybridization and physiological tests. Int J Syst Bacteriol 1983;33:293-8.
125. Wellstood S. Evaluation of Phadebact and Streptex Kits for rapid grouping of streptococci directly from blood cultures. J Clin Microbiol 1982;15:226-30.
126. Wicher K, Kalinka C, Mlodozeniec P, Rose N. Fluorescent antibody technic used for identification and typing of *Streptococcus pneumoniae*. Am J Clin Pathol 1982;77:72-7.
127. Wilkinson HW. CAMP-disk test for presumptive identification of group B streptococci. J Clin Microbiol 1977;6:42-5.
128. Wilkinson HW. Analysis of group B streptococcal types associated with disease in human infants and adults. J Clin Microbiol 1978;7:176-9.

CHAPTER 29

SYPHILIS

Sheila A. Lukehart, Ph.D.

INTRODUCTION

The first clear descriptions of syphilis were recorded in the 15th century when an epidemic spread over Europe and Asia. Although this well-described epidemic led to the hypothesis that the disease was introduced to Europe from the New World by Columbus, earlier biblical and Asian writings contain descriptions of skin diseases consistent with syphilis. The early manifestations of the disease were quite severe by contemporary standards and the disease was termed "the great pox," in contrast to the other epidemic disease, smallpox. The sexual mode of transmission, as well as the primary and secondary manifestations, were recognized early; the late complications were recognized centuries later.

CAUSATIVE AGENT

Syphilis and the nonvenereal treponematoses (yaws, bejel and pinta) are caused by very closely related organisms belonging to the family *Spirochaetaceae*, order *Spirochaetales*. The genus *Treponema* (Table 29:1) includes 2 species pathogenic for humans, *Treponema pallidum* (3 subspecies) and *Treponema carateum*, as well as a number of avirulent species which are part of the normal flora of the oral and genital mucosal surfaces and of the gastrointestinal tract.

The pathogenic treponemes are spiral organisms (Fig. 29:1) 0.2 μm in diameter and 7-20 μm in length, having a characteristic corkscrew motility. All of the pathogenic treponemes are considered to be morphologically and, to date, antigenically identical. Historically, they have been speciated on the basis of the epidemiological and clinical features of the diseases they produce. DNA homology studies have demonstrated virtually complete

Table 29:1. Genus *Treponema*

Pathogens:	
Treponema pallidum, subspecies *pallidum*	Venereal syphilis
Treponema pallidum, subspecies *pertenue*	Yaws
Treponema pallidum, subspecies *endemicum*	Bejel, endemic syphilis
Treponema carateum	Pinta
Treponema paraluiscuniculi	Rabbit pathogen
Nonpathogens:	
Treponema denticola	Oral cavity
Treponema phagedenis	Genital mucosa
Treponema refringens	Genital mucosa
Treponema vincentii	Oral cavity
Treponema scoliodontum	Oral cavity
Treponema minutum	Genital mucosa

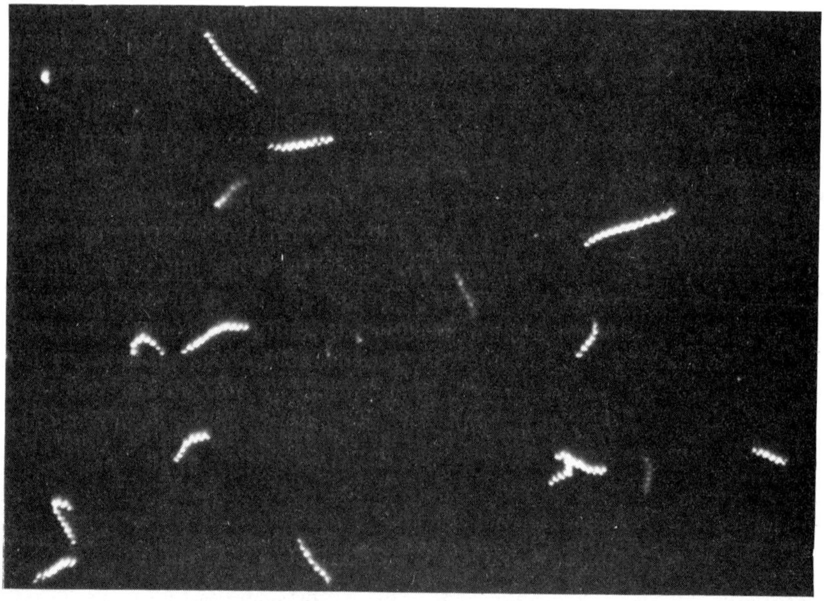

FIGURE 1. *Treponema pallidum* subspecies *pallidum* as viewed by darkfield microscopy. Original magnification 160×.

identity between the causative agents of venereal syphilis and yaws;[26] consequently, these organisms, with the causative agent of bejel, have been reclassified as subspecies of *T. pallidum*. The pathogenic treponemes cannot be cultivated continuously in vitro, although limited multiplication has been achieved in a tissue culture system.[13] Organisms are harvested from tissue of infected rabbits for laboratory investigation or for use in certain diagnostic tests. Because their survival in vitro is limited, little is known of the metabolism or physiology of these bacteria.

The cultivable nonpathogenic treponemes are morphologically similar to *T. pallidum* and may cause confusion in the microscopic examination of lesion material. Although the nonpathogens tested show essentially no DNA homology with *T. pallidum*,[25,32] there is considerable antigenic crossreactivity between the pathogenic and nonpathogenic treponemes, and antibodies raised against normal flora in uninfected persons may react in "specific" treponemal serological tests.

EPIDEMIOLOGY, PUBLIC HEALTH SIGNIFICANCE AND CONTROL

Syphilis is a disease with worldwide distribution. Though accurate prevalence data are lacking for many parts of the developing world, seropositivity rates in pregnant women in certain African regions range from 10-30%. In addition to adult morbidity, congenital infection is a major cause of prematurity, stillbirth, infant mortality and neonatal death in developing countries.[39]

Until recent decades, syphilis was a common disease even in developed countries. Autopsy studies in the United States in the early 20th century revealed a prevalence of 5-10%, [41,47] with rates as high as 25% in certain socioeconomic groups.[34] Education and control efforts initiated by Thomas Parran, coupled with the introduction of highly efficacious penicillin therapy, resulted in a dramatic decline in the incidence of infectious (primary and secondary) syphilis in the United States from the mid-1940s until the mid-1950s (Fig. 29:2). Since that time, the incidence has alternately risen and fallen, with the last dramatic increase between 1977 and 1982. Provisional 1986 figures show 67,750 new cases of syphilis, of which 27,200 were infectious. As for most sexually transmitted diseases, the peak incidence of infection is in young adults, 15-35 years of age.

In developed countries, the populations most affected by syphilis have changed dramatically in the past two decades, and syphilis is now a disease which disproportionally burdens the homosexual and bisexual population. In the United States, the percentage of white male patients with early syphilis who named a male sexual contact rose from 38% in 1969 to 70% in 1979.[12] Early epidemiological studies of patients with acquired immunodeficiency syndrome reflected this trend: 68% of homosexual AIDS patients had a history of past syphilis, compared to 6% of heterosexual AIDS patients.[16]

The heterosexual population, however, is also at risk for syphilis. Syphilis may be transmitted from a pregnant woman to her fetus, and, contrary to earlier hypotheses, there is now clear evidence of fetal infection as early as nine weeks gestation.[17] A 76% increase in early syphilis in women of

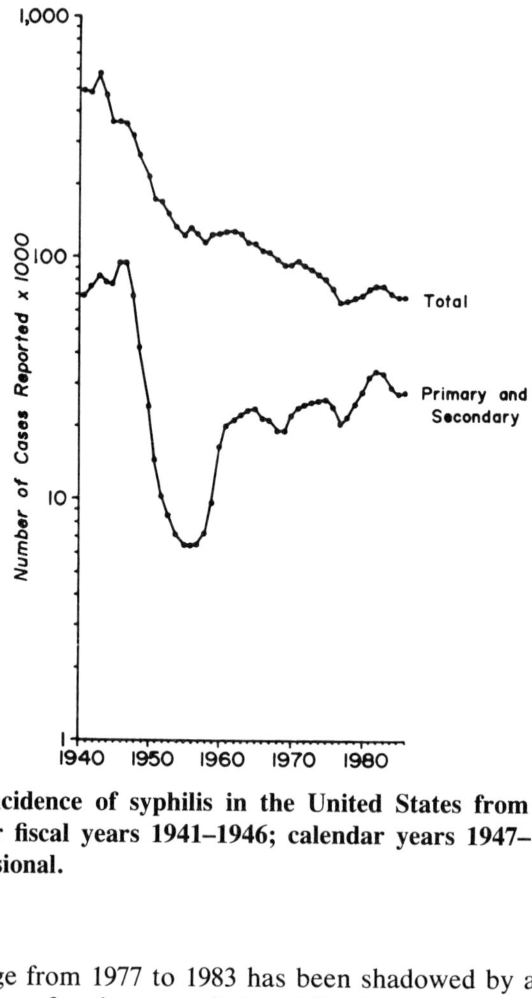

FIGURE 2. Incidence of syphilis in the United States from 1941 to 1986. Figures are for fiscal years 1941–1946; calendar years 1947–1986. Data for 1986 are provisional.

childbearing age from 1977 to 1983 has been shadowed by a dramatic rise in reported cases of early congenital syphilis, from 108 cases in 1978 to 268 cases in 1985, an increase of 150%.

Contact tracing, serological screening and epidemiological treatment are important components of control. Of all reported cases of early syphilis in 1983, 47% were identified as a direct result of contact tracing or serological screening. Interviews of patients with early syphilis disclose an average of 1.98 sexual contacts at risk per patient, and approximately 50% of contacts become infected. Widespread serological screening (premarital, prenatal, hospital admission) has been conducted in the United States, with over 45 million tests performed annually. The cost of premarital and hospital admission testing per new case diagnosed is very high, and the wisdom of such policies in low prevalence populations is being debated. Prenatal screening, however, is a major tool in the prevention of congenital syphilis;

it is mandated by law in most states and has been shown to be cost-effective even in populations with very low prevalence.[44]

DISEASE MANIFESTATIONS AND THERAPY

Clinical Course

Syphilis is a chronic, systemic infection characterized by periods of active disease, interrupted by months or decades of latency. Transmission occurs by direct contact of skin or mucosal surfaces with an infectious lesion. The organism multiplies at the site of inoculation and, within minutes or hours, gains access to the circulation and is seeded to many tissues. Following an incubation period which averages 4-6 weeks, a single primary lesion (chancre) appears at the site of inoculation; initially a small indurated papule, the chancre quickly enlarges and ulcerates. Only 25% of patients will have multiple primary lesions. Because the mode of transmission is sexual, the chancre is usually located in the genital, anal or oral regions. The chancre is infectious and *T. pallidum* can be identified by darkfield or fluorescence microscopy in exudative material. Accompanying manifestations may include firm, nontender regional (usually inguinal) lymphadenopathy. The chancre persists for several weeks or months, then heals spontaneously with little or no scarring.

The secondary manifestations, which appear several months following infection, may include skin rash, mucosal lesions, condylomata lata, malaise, headaches, alopecia and transient liver or kidney dysfunction. Skin lesions are the most common manifestation and usually consist of nonpruritic macules or papules on trunk and extremities, with a characteristic predilection for the palms and soles. The rash, mucous membrane lesions and condylomata lata are infectious, and *T. pallidum* may be identified by microscopic examination of lesion material. At the time of appearance of the rash, approximately 15% of patients have persistent or healing primary chancres. The secondary manifestations resolve spontaneously after a period of weeks to months, but may recur during the first year in 25% of patients.

The subsequent period of asymptomatic infection (latency) may persist for years or decades. In two-thirds of untreated patients, the latent stage will continue for life and no further evidence of disease will appear, despite the presence of persistent infection. In the preantibiotic era, tertiary or late syphilis developed in 30% of untreated patients. Tertiary syphilis may include symptomatic or asymptomatic involvement of the central nervous system (CNS), cardiovascular disease (aortitis, aneurysm), or gummatous destruction of skin, cartilage, bone or other tissues.

Pathogenesis

The pathogenesis of treponemal infection is poorly understood. Organisms appear to be located primarily in the extracellular spaces during early infection, although intracellular organisms have been described.[2,22,45,46] The ability of *T. pallidum* to reside intracellularly may contribute to the success of the bacterium in evading the host's immune response during the periods of lesion healing and longterm latency. The organism is not known to elaborate any toxins or to have any cytotoxic capacity; thus, the tissue destruction observed during active syphilis has been ascribed by some to the host's immune response to the bacterial antigens. The histologic picture of early and late lesions (intense lymphocyte, macrophage and plasma cell infiltration) is consistent with this hypothesis.

Therapy

Penicillin is the drug of choice for treatment of syphilis and resistance to this drug has not been documented. Because of the long generation time of *T. pallidum* (33 hours), the benzathine form of penicillin, which achieves prolonged levels of penicillinemia, is recommended. The optimal dose and duration of antimicrobial therapy have not been rigorously examined and the current recommendations (Table 29:2) are based on limited therapeutic trials. Published reports indicate a recurrence or treatment failure rate of approximately 5% following benzathine penicillin therapy for secondary syphilis.[4,42] For these reasons, certain public health officials recommend increased dosages and durations of therapy for early syphilis.

Alternative antimicrobial therapies are supported even less well by clinical trials. Tetracycline is the only recommended alternative drug (except for erythromycin in penicillin-allergic pregnant women). The efficacy of the tetracycline regime has not been carefully examined (particularly for neurosyphilis) and patient compliance is frequently poor. Some of the third-generation cephalosporins show promise as alternative therapies.[19]

SPECIAL CONSIDERATIONS IN DIAGNOSIS

Because of its protean manifestations and wide organ involvement, syphilis is a disease which can be extremely difficult to diagnose. One of the most studied, yet least understood, aspects of infection is central nervous system involvement. The infection may be asymptomatic or dramatic, causing blindness, paralysis and insanity in its most virulent form. Investigations in the preantibiotic era revealed that invasion of the central nervous system, when it occurred, took place in the first weeks or months of infection. Cerebrospinal fluid (CSF) abnormalities were observed in 15-26% of patients with secondary syphilis,[6,27,30] and *T. pallidum* could be identified by mi-

Table 29:2. Recommended Therapy for Syphilis

Stage	Recommended	Alternative
Early (Primary, Secondary, Early Latent)	Benzathine penicillin G 2.4 MU, intramuscularly	Tetracycline 500 mg four times daily × 15 days
Late Latent or latent of uncertain duration	Benzathine penicillin G 2.4 MU, intramuscularly per week for 3 weeks (7.2 MU total dose)	Tetracycline 500 mg four times daily × 30 days
*Neurosyphilis (symptomatic or asymptomatic)	Aqueous crystalline penicillin G, 12-24 MU IV daily × 10 days; followed by benzathine penicillin G, 2.4 MU IM weekly for 3 weeks OR Aqueous procaine penicillin G 2.4 MU IM daily *plus* probenecid 500 mg PO four times daily, both for 10 days; followed by benzathine penicillin G 2.4 MU IM weekly for 3 weeks OR Benzathine penicillin G 2.4 MU IM weekly for 3 weeks	Tetracycline 500 mg four times daily × 30 days
Cardiovascular or late benign	Benzathine penicillin G 2.4 MU IM weekly for three weeks	Tetracycline 500 mg four times daily × 30 days
Syphilis in pregnancy	Treat according to stage	†Erythromycin 500 mg four times daily × 15 or 30 days
Contact to person with early syphilis	Benzathine penicillin G, 2.4 MU, intramuscularly	As for early syphilis

* Benzathine penicillin G does not achieve treponemacidal levels in the cerebrospinal fluid and has given inferior results for treatment of neurosyphilis. For penicillin-allergic patients, tetracycline is recommended though there are no controlled studies to support its efficacy. Doxycycline has higher theoretical efficacy for neurosyphilis because of better CSF penetration, but has not been examined carefully.

† Failure of erythromycin to prevent congenital syphilis has been repeatedly documented in the literature. Penicillin allergy should be confirmed by skin test before alternative regimens are used. Some experts recommend hospitalization and desentization of penicillin-allergic women in order to permit penicillin therapy[50,52]. All infants born to women treated during pregnancy with erythromycin must be treated with penicillin at birth.

croscopy or animal inoculation even in patients without obvious CSF pathology.[6] The risk of progression to symptomatic neurosyphilis was roughly proportional to the severity of the CSF abnormalities during early disease.[31] Despite these observations, evaluation of patients for CNS involvement is rarely performed, even in late latent syphilis (where it is currently recommended) unless the patient exhibits signs or symptoms.

When CSF examination is done, interpretation of the findings may be problematic. Increased cell or protein concentrations are nonspecific indicators of CNS inflammation, and the only specific test for neurosyphilis, the CSF-VDRL, is notoriously insensitive, even in symptomatic patients. Perhaps more disturbing is the fact that benzathine penicillin, which is recommended for treatment of syphilis, does not penetrate the blood-brain barrier in measurable quantities,[9,29,37] and therapy with this drug is almost certainly not adequate for patients with CNS infection. This fact may indicate the reason for the 5% treatment failure rate: treponemes which are sequestered in the CNS may be protected by their location from the antibacterial effects of the drug and may subsequently serve as a source of organisms for relapse or CNS progression. Numerous case reports can be found in the literature documenting failure of benzathine penicillin to cure CNS infection in patients with asymptomatic neurosyphilis.[15,48] Although no changes in therapy or evaluation of patients with early syphilis have been recommended by the Centers for Disease Control (CDC), clinicians should consider these issues, particularly when dealing with patients with apparent treatment failure or relapse.

STANDARD DIAGNOSTIC CRITERIA

The diagnosis of syphilis is based on sexual history, clinical manifestations, demonstration of the causative agent and serological testing. No single diagnostic method is sufficiently sensitive and specific for all stages of disease and each stage has different diagnostic requirements.

History

A history of exposure to syphilis is clearly helpful in guiding the diagnosis. However, a patient's historical report may be unreliable and a negative history should not deter the clinician from pursuing the diagnosis of syphilis in a patient with evidence of infection.

Clinical Presentation

Diagnosis based on clinical manifestations alone may also be unreliable. Syphilis has been called "the great imitator" and its varied clinical manifestations can resemble many other infectious or noninfectious diseases. Syphilis must be considered in the differential diagnosis of widely disparate clinical presentations that include skin rashes, headaches, visual or hearing abnormalities, neurologic abnormalities, dementia, alopecia and liver or kidney dysfunction.

Syphilis is responsible for 20% of genital ulcer disease in the United

States and Europe, but must be considered in the differential diagnosis of all genital ulcerations. The most common manifestation of the primary stage is the chancre, which is characteristically a painless, well-circumscribed, indurated ulcer. Many primary chancres, however, have an atypical appearance and may be mistaken for other causes of genital ulceration, such as herpes and chancroid. The accuracy of a morphological diagnosis of syphilis in studies of penile ulcerations in sexually transmitted diseases clinics is only 42-78%;[5,11] in settings where syphilis is seen less frequently, the accuracy would be even lower.

The rash of secondary syphilis may be so subtle as to go unrecognized by the patient or the clinician; it may resemble other dermatologic conditions such as eczema, pityriasis rosea, tinea versicolor and psoriasis. Condylomata lata, a manifestation of the secondary stage, may be mistaken for genital warts. In latent syphilis, there are no clinical manifestations to aid in diagnosis and few, if any, clinical findings are pathognomonic for tertiary syphilis.

Demonstration of the Causative Agent

The microscopic demonstration of *T. pallidum* in lesion material provides a specific method for diagnosis of patients with early active (primary, secondary) disease. Because *T. pallidum* stains poorly with routine bacteriologic stains, it must be identified with specialized microscopy. Two methods are currently available: darkfield microscopy and immunofluorescence staining.

In darkfield microscopy, a special condenser is placed on the microscope to bend the light at oblique angles so that only those rays reflected by the object on the slide enter the microscope objective. The lack of direct light entering the objective results in a black or "dark" field where only those cells, particles or bacteria that reflect the light are visible. Detailed descriptions of the darkfield microscopic technique can be found in other texts.[21,49] Darkfield microscopy is both rapid and inexpensive, and because the examination can be done in the clinic, results are available promptly. There are several disadvantages: (1) differentiation of *T. pallidum* from nonpathogenic commensal spirochetes is very difficult and requires both a darkfield condenser and the expertise of a highly trained microscopist, rarely available except in specialized clinics; (2) an actively motile organism must be observed for accurate identification and the poor survival of *T. pallidum* outside the host dictates immediate examination of specimens, so that transport of specimens is not possible; (3) Self-treatment with topical antibacterial agents by patients may make it impossible to detect motile organisms and (4) red blood cells and other debris commonly found in specimens are highly refractile and may obscure *T. pallidum*.

An alternate method for detection of *T. pallidum* in lesion material is the direct fluorescent antibody test for *T. pallidum* (DFA-TP). In this test, the organism is identified in fixed smears by reaction with fluorescein-tagged polyvalent anti-*T. pallidum* globulin. Crossreactivity with commensal spirochetes is minimized by prior absorption of the polyvalent antiserum with *T. phagedenis* biotype Reiter. This test can be performed on transported specimens by central laboratories, since motility is not required. Sensitivity of 86% and 100% specificity have been demonstrated for the DFA-TP versus 74% and 97%, respectively for darkfield microscopy.[8] The DFA-TP can be adapted for examination of biopsy, autopsy or placental tissues. Despite the obvious advantages of this test, it has not become widely used. Specific methodology for performing the DFA-TP can be found in "Laboratory Methods for Diagnosis of Sexually Transmitted Diseases."[21]

Serological Tests

Serological diagnosis of syphilis is based upon a two-tiered system in which nontreponemal tests are used initially for screening and quantitation, followed by more specific treponemal tests for confirmation. The nontreponemal tests, which detect antibody to a cardiolipin-lecithin-cholesterol mixture, are rapid and inexpensive; therefore, they are used for routine screening. The treponemal tests depend upon reactivity with pathogenic *T. pallidum* in an effort to measure more "specific" antibodies.

Nontreponemal tests:

The most commonly used nontreponemal tests are the Venereal Disease Research Laboratory (VDRL) and rapid plasma reagin (RPR) tests, followed by the unheated serum reagin (USR) and the reagin screen test (RST). These tests detect the presence of anti-cardiolipin IgM and IgG antibodies called "reagin" by flocculation of the test antigen. (This "reagin" is not to be confused with allergy-associated IgE antibody, called reaginic antibody.) The VDRL is the only serological test recommended for use on cerebrospinal fluid. In the VDRL test, flocculation of the antigen is determined by microscopic examination of the serum-antigen mixture on a glass slide. The disadvantages of the VDRL test include the requirements for preparing fresh antigen suspension daily, for microscopic examination and for heating the serum prior to testing. Details of the specific methodology for performing qualitative and quantitative VDRL tests may be found in the "Manual of Tests for Syphilis."[49]

The RPR card test also uses a cardiolipin-lecithin-cholesterol antigen, but is performed on coated, disposable cards. Flocculation may be visualized macroscopically due to the inclusion of charcoal particles in the antigen suspension. The advantages of the RPR are several: it does not require heating of serum prior to testing, results are determined macroscopically and the antigen suspension is stabilized. Unlike the VDRL, the RPR is easy to perform in a clinic or office setting. Because of ease of use, the RPR is now the most commonly performed screening test for syphilis. Detailed methodology for performing the qualitative and quantitative RPR tests may be found in "Laboratory Methods for the Diagnosis of Sexually Transmitted Diseases."[21]

The USR also has the advantage of a stabilized antigen suspension and does not require heating of sera prior to testing.

The sensitivities and specificities of the commonly used nontreponemal tests are comparable and vary with stage of disease (Table 29:3). VDRL and RPR antibody generally appears during the primary stage and the reactivity rate depends upon the duration of symptoms. For example, a patient with a primary lesion of two days' duration is likely to be seronegative, while a patient with a healing lesion of 6 weeks' duration is more likely to be seropositive. It is important that the clinician be aware that primary syphilis may be present in the absence of reactive serology and that nonreactive serology alone should not exclude syphilis in a patient with genital ulceration. Nontreponemal tests are very sensitive during the secondary stage and are usually reactive in high titer (> 16 dils). Rarely, a very high-titered serum may appear nonreactive when tested undiluted, showing a prozone phenomenon. Testing of serum dilutions will give a positive result. In latent and tertiary syphilis, the nontreponemal tests may be nonreactive in approximately 25% of patients; the reason for this absence of antibody reactivity is not clear, but there is no evidence that this indicates spontaneous cure.

Because cardiolipin is a normal lipid constituent of mammalian tissues, anti-cardiolipin antibody may be produced in the absence of treponemal infection, resulting in a "Biological False Positive" (BFP) reaction. BFP reactions may be either transient (lasting several weeks or months) or chronic: common causes are recent viral infections, immunizations, drug addiction, malaria or other chronic infections, rheumatoid arthritis, systemic lupus erythematosus and other autoimmune conditions, or aging. The rate

Table 29:3 Reactivity of Serologic Tests in Untreated Syphilis*

	Stage of Disease			
	Primary	Secondary	Latent	Late
VDRL, RPR	59–87†	100	73–91	37–94
FTA-ABS	86–100	99–100	96–99	96–100
MHA-TP	64–87	96–100	96–100	94–100

* Modified with permission from: Jaffe H. "Management of the reactive serology." In: Holmes KK, Mardh PA, Sparling PF, Wiesner PJ, eds. *Sexually transmitted diseases*. New York: McGraw-Hill, 1984:314.

† Percent reactive.

of BFP reactivity in a young adult population is thought to be 1% or less; in geriatric populations, it may be 5-10%. When false positive tests occur, they are usually, but not always, of low titer (< 8 dils).

All sera which are reactive in nontreponemal tests should be tested quantitatively to determine antibody titer. A significant (4-fold) rise in titer indicates active disease, while a 4-fold decrease in titer following therapy indicates efficacy of the therapeutic regimen. Either the VDRL or RPR can be used quantitatively; however, titer comparisons should always employ the same test for both specimens.

Treponemal tests:

The currently used treponemal tests include the fluorescent treponemal antibody-absorption (FTA-ABS) test and the hemagglutination tests (microhemagglutination assay for *Treponema pallidum*, MHA-TP; hemagglutination treponemal test for syphilis, HATTS). In the FTA-ABS, antibody is detected by fluorescein-tagged anti-human IgG following reaction of the patient's serum with whole *T. pallidum* fixed to a microscope slide. The demonstration of brightly fluorescing *T. pallidum* on the slide when viewed with a fluorescence microscope indicates the presence of anti-treponemal antibodies. In the MHA-TP and HATTS tests, anti-treponemal antibody is detected by its ability to agglutinate erythrocytes coated with *T. pallidum* antigen. The FTA-ABS is more labor-intensive and expensive than the hemagglutination tests, but has the advantage of being more sensitive in the early primary stage of disease (Table 29:3). All treponemal tests are equally sensitive in the secondary stage and beyond. Treponemal tests are not used quantitatively and remain reactive following therapy. Detailed methodology for performing FTA-ABS and hemagglutination tests can be found in "Laboratory Methods for the Diagnosis of Sexually Transmitted Diseases."[21]

Despite the fact that treponemal tests measure antibody against *T. pallidum*, they are not necessarily more specific than nontreponemal tests in all situations and, therefore, are not appropriate as screening tests. Most persons produce antibodies against the nonpathogenic treponemes; these antibodies crossreact with *T. pallidum* and may cause false-positive reactivity in treponemal tests. Both the FTA-ABS and the hemagglutination tests minimize this possibility by dilution of the patient's serum in "sorbent" prepared from cultures of nonpathogenic *T. phagedenis* biotype Reiter. Crossreactive antibodies are either diluted or absorbed so that false positivity is eliminated in most cases. This approach is not 100% effective, however, and in a population with a low prevalence of syphilis, the predictive value of a reactive treponemal test is low. Treponemal tests are used appropriately and have a high positive predictive value in the following situations: (1) as a confirmation test for a reactive nontreponemal test; (2) in VDRL-nonreactive patients with historical evidence of latent syphilis or clinical evidence of tertiary syphilis; (3) in VDRL-nonreactive patients with suspect early lesions. It should be noted that both nontreponemal and treponemal tests will be reactive in persons with nonvenereal treponemal diseases (yaws, pinta, bejel).

USE OF DIAGNOSTIC TESTS FOR SYPHILIS

Screening

Serological screening of persons without historical or clinical evidence of syphilis should be performed at regular intervals only in persons at high risk for acquiring disease (male and female prostitutes, homosexual men with multiple partners) and in persons with other sexually transmitted diseases. Prenatal screening should be performed on all pregnant women at their first prenatal visit, preferably in the first trimester, and repeated during the third trimester in women at high risk for acquiring sexually transmitted diseases. The cost-effectiveness of premarital and hospital admission screening is debatable.

A nontreponemal test should be used for screening and reactive results confirmed with a treponemal test. To decrease the chance of misdiagnosis due to laboratory error, a second serum sample should be tested from those persons with initially reactive results, especially from those for whom a reactive result appears unlikely. Reactive serological tests on pregnant women should be confirmed promptly so that therapy can be initiated.

Contacts

Sera from persons identified as contacts of patients with early syphilis should be examined with a nontreponemal test; this result will establish a baseline value for evaluating status following therapy. Epidemiologic therapy is indicated for all contacts, regardless of serological status.

Patients with Lesions

Darkfield microscopic examination of exudate from moist lesions (ulcer, rash or condylomata lata) is the most rapid and inexpensive method for establishing a definitive diagnosis of syphilis. If microscopic examination is positive, serological confirmation is not necessary for initiation of therapy, but serum should be collected prior to therapy for quantitative testing. If darkfield examination is negative or not available, serological testing is needed to establish a diagnosis. Primary syphilis can exist in the absence of microscopic or serologic evidence, therefore, negative tests should be repeated (after 1-2 days for darkfield microscopy, 1-2 weeks for serologic tests, no alternative diagnosis). Serologic tests are reactive in virtually all patients with secondary syphilis.

Asymptomatic Patients

Patients with either latent or asymptomatic late syphilis are identified by serologic testing. Evaluation of these patients should include lumbar puncture (cerebrospinal fluid for cells, protein, VDRL) to rule out neurologic involvement. All patients with CSF abnormalities should be treated for neurosyphilis.

Symptomatic Tertiary Syphilis

Any patient with signs or symptoms compatible with tertiary syphilis should have serological testing. Because the nontreponemal tests may not be reactive in such patients, treponemal tests should be specifically requested. If there is serological evidence of syphilis, lumbar puncture should be performed for CSF examination. All patients with CSF abnormalities should be treated for neurosyphilis.

Patients with Past Syphilis

Treponemal tests are likely to remain reactive even many years following effective therapy and are not helpful in evaluating patients with a history of syphilis. In the absence of symptoms and signs, a diagnosis of active syphilis can definitely be made in such patients only by demonstrating a significant rise in nontreponemal antibody titer. If historical titers are not available, a presumptive diagnosis may be made on the basis of a current high titer (> 8 dils).

Follow-up Evaluation

Follow-up quantitative nontreponemal tests are recommended to demonstrate efficacy of therapy. Patients should have follow-up serologic testing at 3, 6, 9 and 12 months post-therapy; patients with syphilis of more than 1 year's duration should be tested up to 24 months. Follow-up testing should always employ the same test used on the initial specimen.

The nontreponemal antibody titer should fall after effective therapy and most patients with early active syphilis will become seronegative within the first 1-2 years. Patients with syphilis of longer duration will show less dramatic reductions in titer and may not become seronegative. Approximately 50-60% of patients with treated late latent syphilis remain seropositive in low titer indefinitely.[14] Failure of an initially high-titered serum to decrease 4-fold within 1 year or a definitive (4-fold) increase in titer indicates active infection (either treatment failure, relapse or reinfection) and such patients should be evaluated for neurosyphilis prior to retreatment.

Patients treated for neurosyphilis should be followed with regular quantitative nontreponemal tests and repeated lumbar punctures for a minimum of 3 years. Effective therapy will first be indicated by decrease in cell concentration, then protein concentration in the CSF and finally by a decrease in the CSF-VDRL titer. CSF parameters may take many months or several years to return to normal.

NEW METHODS FOR DIAGNOSIS

The recent development of molecular technologies has permitted the identification of important antigenic molecules of *T. pallidum* and the investigation of the host's immune response to those antigens. Tools used in these investigations may also be applied to the diagnosis of syphilis and promising new tests are being developed.

Identification of *T. pallidum*

Three new approaches to *T. pallidum* detection have been explored. Norgard et al.[33] described the detection of *T. pallidum* dried on filter paper, using specific monoclonal antibodies, radiolabeled rabbit anti-mouse IgG and autoradiography. The sensitivity of this dot blot test after a 2-4 day autoradiography period was 500-1000 organisms and the method was specific for *T. pallidum*. Antibodies with the highest sensitivity were those which recognized the major 47,000-48,000 dalton antigen of *T. pallidum*. This detection method used rabbit-propagated *T. pallidum* and has not been tested with clinical specimens.

Another new filter paper-based identification method involves detection of *T. pallidum* DNA in lesion material, using a radiolabeled DNA probe constructed from a cloned *T. pallidum* gene.[36] The molecule, 4D, encoded by this gene has been shown to be a surface antigen of *T. pallidum*. Preliminary field studies of the DNA probe are promising, but the sensitivity and specificity are not as high as for darkfield microscopy or the monoclonal antibody slide test.

A third method for detection of *T. pallidum* involves the microscopic identification of the organism with a fluorescein-tagged monoclonal antibody.[20,24] The antibody, H9-1, is specific for the 47,000-48,000 dalton antigen of pathogenic treponemes and shows no crossreactivity with commensal spirochetes, *Leptospira* or *Borrelia*.[20] Exudate from a suspect lesion is collected on a microscope slide as for darkfield microscopy, then air-dried and fixed with acetone. The time required for staining and examining the slide is 30-40 min; and theoretically, a single treponeme should be detectable on the slide. In a clinical trial of patients with genital ulceration, this method was shown to be 100% sensitive and specific.[20]

All of these antigen detection methods have distinct advantages over existing methods. Specimens for these new tests can be transported readily to a laboratory, precluding the need for specialized equipment and technical expertise in the clinic or physician's office, thus making the test more widely available than is darkfield microscopy. Transportation to a laboratory, however, delays evaluation of the specimen and does not permit the immediate treatment of persons with suspicious lesions, unless the diagnosis can be made on other grounds. It is unlikely, therefore, that any of these tests will replace darkfield microscopy where it is available, but new tests may provide readily available *T. pallidum* detection tests for the vast majority of clinicians who lack access to specialized microscopy.

Serological Testing

A number of new serodiagnostic tests have been developed based on ELISA[10,23,35,43] and radioimmunoassay[3,28,51] techniques. These tests, however, employ preparations of whole *T. pallidum* or components of the nonpathogenic Reiter treponeme as antigen. Despite favorable initial sensitivity and specificity data, these tests have the same inherent limitations as existing treponemal tests because of antibody to crossreacting treponemal antigens.

The recent characterization of pathogen-specific antigenic determinants of *T. pallidum* has also permitted development of other new serologic tests. Hensel and coworkers [18] used a purified 17,000 dalton treponemal antigen in an immunoblotting assay to detect antibodies in patients with various stages of syphilis. This test was reactive in 130 sera from seropositive patients with treated and untreated syphilis and nonreactive in 30 nonsyphilitic sera. The test was not used to examine VDRL-negative sera from patients with early primary disease, and it is technically cumbersome.

Alderete and coworkers[1] developed an ELISA assay in which fibronectin is bound to an ELISA plate and used to capture three *T. pallidum* antigens from a suspension of detergent-solubilized bacteria. These antigens are then used for binding and detection of antibodies in patients' sera. The test has been shown to be reactive in 38 patients with various stages of syphilis and in 22 patients with yaws; however, sera from VDRL-negative patients with early primary lesions were not examined. Antisera raised against the nonpathogenic Reiter treponeme and sera from patients with chronic diseases commonly associated with BFP reactions were nonreactive in this test.

Radolf and coworkers[38] described the first use of a cloned *T. pallidum* antigen, 4D, for serodiagnosis in an ELISA assay. Sera from 105 treated and untreated syphilis patients were examined. The test was reactive in 81% of patients with primary syphilis (compared to 96% with the VDRL),

100% of patients with secondary and early latent syphilis, 84% of patients with late latent disease and 57% of patients with tertiary disease. Sera from 172 nonsyphilitic control persons and 20 BFP reactors were uniformly nonreactive. This same antigen was re-evaluated by radioimmunoassay[7] and demonstrated 55% sensitivity in primary syphilis (compared to 83% for FTA-ABS and 88% for MHA-TP). It gave false-positive results in fewer than 3% of normal sera. A cloned 37 Kd *T. pallidum* antigen has also been evaluated[40] in an RIA procedure, with 76% sensitivity in primary syphilis and 88% in patients of all stages. This test was reactive in 5% of normals and 9.5% of BFP reactors.

Thcse studics indicate the potential for improving serodiagnostic tests by using well-characterized antigens. Studies have not yet, however, addressed two of the most troublesome issues in serodiagnosis: (1) the evaluation of patients with early primary infection who are still nonreactive in current tests, and (2) the evaluation of suspected infection in patients who are seropositive because of past syphilis. Unless newly developed tests can address these issues in a significant way, the increased cost of new "high-tech" tests may preclude their widespread use. Over 45 million serologic tests for syphilis are performed in the United States each year, largely for screening (premarital, prenatal, hospital admissions, blood banking) and more expensive tests would be unlikely to be used unless they provided distinct advantages over the existing inexpensive cardiolipin tests. New tests may provide alternatives to current confirmation tests, however, offering increased specificity.

REFERENCES

1. Alderete JF, Freeman-Shade L, Baseman JB. Immunodiagnostic test for detection of serum antibody to *Treponema pallidum* (Syphilis): fibronectin as a capture vehicle for treponemal adhesins. J Immunol Meth 1985;84:365-73.
2. Azar HA, Pham TD, Kurban AK. An electron microscopic study of a syphilitic chancre. Arch Pathol 1970;90:143-50.
3. Baughn RE, Musher DM. Radioimmunoassays for the detection of antibodies to treponemal polypeptide antigens in serum. J Clin Microbiol 1985;21:922-8.
4. Brown ST. Treatment of secondary syphilis. J Amer Vener Dis Assoc 1976;3:136-42.
5. Chapel TA, Brown WJ, Jeffries C, Stewart JA. How reliable is the morphological diagnosis of penile ulcerations? Sex Transm Dis 1977;4:150-2.
6. Chesney AM, Kemp JE. Incidence of *Spirochaeta pallida* in cerebrospinal fluid during early stage of syphilis. JAMA 1924;22:1725-8.
7. Coates SR, Sheridan PJ, Hansen DS, Laird WJ, Erlich HA. Serospecificity of a cloned protease-resistant *Treponema pallidum*-specific antigen expressed in *Escherichia coli*. J Clin Microbiol 1986;23:460-4.
8. Daniels KC, Ferneyhough HS. Specific direct fluorescent antibody detection of *Treponema pallidum*. Health Lab Sci 1977;14:164-71.
9. Dunlop EMC, Al-Egaily SS, Houang ET. Penicillin levels in blood and CSF achieved by treatment of syphilis. JAMA 1979;241:2538-46.

10. Farshy CE, Hunter EF, Larsen SA, Cerny EH. Double-conjugate enzyme-linked immunosorbent assay for immunoglobulins G and M against *Treponema pallidum*. J Clin Microbiol 1984;20:1109-13.
11. Fast MV, Lourdes J, D'Costa J, et al. The clinical diagnosis of genital ulcer disease in men in the tropics. Sex Transm Dis 1984;11:72-6.
12. Fichtner RR, Aral SO, Blount JH, Zaidi AA, Reynolds GH, Darrow WW. Syphilis in the United States: 1967-1978. Sex Transm Dis 1983;10:77-80.
13. Fieldsteel AH, Cox DL, Moeckli RA. Cultivation of virulent *Treponema pallidum* in tissue culture. Infect Immun 1981;32:908-15.
14. Fiumara NJ. Serologic responses to treatment of 128 patients with late latent syphilis. Sex Transm Dis 1979;6:243-6.
15. Green BM, Miller NR, Bynum TE. Failure of penicillin G benzathine in the treatment of neurosyphilis. Arch Intern Med 1980;140:1117-18.
16. Guinan ME, Thomas PA, Pinsky PF, et al. Heterosexual and homosexual patients with the acquired immunodeficiency syndrome. Ann Intern Med 1984;100:213-18.
17. Harter CA, Benirschke K. Fetal syphilis in the first trimester. Am J Obstet Gynecol 1976;124:705-11.
18. Hensel U, Wellensiek HJ, Bhakdi S. Sodium dodecyl sulfate-polyacrylamide gel electrophoresis immunoblotting as a serological tool in the diagnosis of syphilitic infection. J Clin Microbiol 1985;21:82-7.
19. Hook EW III, Baker-Zander SA, Moskovitz BL, Lukehart SA, Handsfield HH. Ceftriaxone therapy for asymptomatic neurosyphilis. Sex Transm Dis 1986;13:185-8.
20. Hook EW III, Roddy RE, Lukehart SA, Hom J, Holmes KK, Tam MR. Detection of *Treponema pallidum* in lesion exudate with a pathogen-specific monoclonal antibody. J Clin Microbiol 1985;22:241-4.
21. Larsen SA, Hunter EF, McGrew BE. Syphilis. In: Wentworth BB, Judson FN, eds. Laboratory methods for the diagnosis of sexually transmitted diseases. Wahington, DC: American Public Health Association, 1984:1-42.
22. Lauderdale V, Goldman JN. Serial ultrathin sectioning demonstrating the intracellularity of *Treponema pallidum* . Br J Vener Dis 1972;48:87-96.
23. Lindenschmidt EG, Laufs R, Muller F. Microenzyme-linked immunosorbent assay for the detection of specific IgM antibodies in human syphilis. Br J Vener Dis 1983;59:151-6.
24. Lukehart SA, Tam MR, Hom J, Baker-Zander SA, Holmes KK, Nowinski RC. Characterization of monoclonal antibodies to *Treponema pallidum*. J Immunol 1985;134:585-92.
25. Miao R, Fieldsteel AH. Genetics of *Treponema*: Relationship between *Treponema pallidum* and five cultivable treponemes. J Bacteriol 1978;133:101-7.
26. Miao RM, Fieldsteel AH. Genetic relationship between *Treponema pallidum* and *Treponema pertenue*, two noncultivable human pathogens. J Bacteriol 1980;141:427-9.
27. Mills CH. Routine examination of the cerebrospinal fluid on syphilis: its value in regard to more accurate knowledge, prognosis and treatment. Br Med J 1927;2:527-32.
28. Miller JM, Donowho EW, Trent DW, Moody EE. A solid-phase radioimmunoassay for the detection of antibodies to *Treponema pallidum*. Sex Transm Dis 1979;6:43-9.
29. Mohr JA, Griffits W, Jackson R, Saadah H, Bird P, Riddle J. Neurosyphilis and penicillin levels in cerebrospinal fluid. JAMA 1976:236:2208-8.
30. Moore JE. Asymptomatic neurosyphilis V. A comparison of early and late symptomatic neurosyphilis. Arch Dermatol Syph 1928;18:99-108.
31. Moore JE, Hopkins HH. Asymptomatic neurosyphilis. JAMA 1930;95:1637-41.
32. Nath K. Restriction analysis of DNA from *Treponema pallidum*, the causative agent of syphilis. Mol Gen Genet 1983;191:126-31.
33. Norgard MV, Selland CK, Kettman JR, Miller JN. Sensitivity and specificity of monoclonal antibodies directed against antigenic determinants of *Treponema pallidum* Nichols in the diagnosis of syphilis. J Clin Microbiol 1984;20:711-17.
34. Olansky S, Simpson L, Schuman SH. Untreated syphilis in the male Negro: Environmental factors in the Tuskegee study. Public Health Rep 1954;69:691-8.

35. Pederson NS, Peterson CS, Vejtorp M, Axelson NH. Serodiagnosis of syphilis by an enzyme-linked immunosorbent assay for IgG antibodies against the Reiter treponeme flagellum. Scand J Immunol 1982;15:341-8.
36. Perine PL. Use of DNA probes for diagnosis of treponemal diseases. In: Leive L, ed. Microbiology 86. Washington, DC: American Society for Microbiology, 1986.
37. Polnikorn N, Witoonpanich R, Vorachit M, Vejjajiva S, Vejjajiva A. Penicillin concentrations in cerebrospinal fluid after different treatment regimens for syphilis. Br J Vener Dis 1980;56:363-7.
38. Radolf JD, Lernhardt E, Fehniger TE, Lovett MA. Serodiagnosis of syphilis by enzyme-linked immunosorbent assay with purified recombinant *Treponema pallidum* antigen 4D. J Infect Dis 1986;153:1023-7.
39. Ratnam AV, Din SN, Hira SK, et al. Syphilis in pregnant women in Zambia. Br J Vener Dis 1982;58:355-8.
40. Rodgers GC, Laird WJ, Coates SR, Mack DH, Huston M, Sninsky JJ. Serological characterization and gene localization of an *Escherichia coli*-expressed 37-kilodalton *Treponema pallidum* antigen. Infect Immun 1986;53:16-25.
41. Rosahn PD. Autopsy studies in syphilis. J Vener Dis Inform 1947;(suppl)21:1-67.
42. Schroeter AL, Lucas JB, Price EV, Falcone VH. Treatment for early syphilis and reactivity of serologic tests. JAMA 1972;221:471-6.
43. Stevens RW, Schmitt ME. Evaluation of an enzyme-linked immunosorbent assay for treponemal antibody. J Clin Microbiol 1985;21:399-402.
44. Stray-Pedersen B. Economic evaluation of maternal screening to prevent congenital syphilis. Sex Trans Dis 1983;10:167-72.
45. Sykes JA, Miller JN. Intracellular location of *Treponema pallidum* (Nichols Strain) in the rabbit testis. Infect Immun 1971;4:307-14.
46. Sykes JA, Miller JN, Kalan AJ. *Treponema pallidum* within cells of a primary chancre from a human female. Br J Vener Dis 1974;50:40-4.
47. Symmers D. Anatomic lesions in late acquired syphilis: A study of 314 cases based on the analysis of 4,880 necropsies at Bellevue Hospital. JAMA 1916;66:1457-62.
48. Tramont EC. Persistence of *Treponema pallidum* following penicillin G therapy. JAMA 1976;236:2206-7.
49. United States Public Health Service. Manual of Tests for Syphilis. Atlanta, GA: National Communicable Disease Center Venereal Disease Program, 1969; publication no. 411.
50. Wendel GD, Stark BJ, Jamison RB, Molina RD, Sullivan TJ. Penicillin allergy and desensitization in serious infections during pregnancy. N Engl J Med 1985;312:1229-32.
51. Zeltzer PM, Pepose JS, Bishop NH, Miller JN. Microassay for immunoglobulin G antibodies to *Treponema pallidum* with radioiodinated protein A from *Staphylococcus aureus*: immunoglobulin G response in experimental syphilis in rabbits. Infect Immun 1978;21:163-70.
52. Ziaya PR, Hankins GDV, Gilstrap LC, Halsey AB. Intravenous penicillin desensitization and treatment during pregnancy. JAMA 1986;256:2561-2.

CHAPTER 30

TUBERCULOSIS AND OTHER MYCOBACTERIOSES

Cora E. Musial, Ph.D. and Glenn D. Roberts, Ph.D.

INTRODUCTION

The genus *Mycobacterium* includes the etiologic agents of tuberculosis, leprosy and nontuberculous mycobacterioses. Tuberculosis and leprosy are of global importance and are considered as public health priorities in many developing countries by the World Health Organization. It is estimated that 1500 million people are infected with the tubercle bacillus, 20 million have positive sputum cultures and are capable of transmitting the disease, 3-5 million new cases occur each year and there are 600,000 deaths per year. It is also estimated that approximately 35 million people have leprosy, most of whom are living in central Africa and certain regions of Asia.[46] Disseminated nontuberculous disease is being reported with greater frequency in immunosuppressed patients, including a high prevalence among those with the acquired immune deficiency syndrome (AIDS).

Tuberculosis, caused by *Mycobacterium tuberculosis* and *M. bovis*, has, for the most part, been controlled in developed countries. An improved standard of living and adequate chemotherapy has resulted in a reduction in the number of infections caused by *M. tuberculosis*, just as *M. bovis* infections have been controlled through the pasteurization of milk and tuberculin testing of dairy cows. However, immigrants, migratory farm workers (some from other countries), American Indians, Eskimos and the increasing population of elderly people are all potential sources of tuberculosis and contribute to the continuing number of cases in the United States. With an increasing number of immunosuppressed patients with malignancies and AIDS, more disseminated nontuberculous mycobacterioses can be expected, contributing to the importance of the mycobacteria in clinical and laboratory practice.

CAUSATIVE ORGANISMS

The mycobacteria are aerobic, nonsporeforming, nonmotile, slightly curved or straight bacilli, 0.2-0.6 by 1.0-10.0 μm. They have a high cell wall lipid content which causes the organism to be resistant to staining with basic dyes; therfore, they do not stain well with Gram's method. If methods are used which promote uptake of dyes, the organisms are not easily decolorized even in acidified organic solvents; therefore, the mycobacteria are described as acidfast as well as alcoholfast. Even when they are stained by acidfast methods, these organisms may appear beaded or granular and during growth on culture media some of the organisms may lose their acidfastness.

Most of the mycobacteria grow slowly and require 2-6 weeks for detection on special media at specific temperatures. The rapidly growing species require less than 5 days after subculture on simple media incubated at 20-40°C for growth to appear. Initial recovery from a clinical specimen may require longer.

The mycobacteria are found in soil, water, food and animals. All can potentially cause disease in humans. However, many species are saprophytes which rarely cause disease.

CLINICAL MANIFESTATIONS AND EPIDEMIOLOGY

The mycobacteria categorized in Table 30:1 are considered medically important in that they may be found in clinical specimens. The clinical laboratory must have the capability to recover and identify these species.

M. tuberculosis probably causes most of the human mycobacterioses in the United States. Infection with this organism is acquired by inhalation of droplet nuclei containing tubercle bacilli aerosolized by infected individuals through coughing or sneezing. These nuclei are small enough (1-10 μm) to pass the mucociliary mechanisms of the respiratory tract and penetrate into alveoli. In nonimmune individuals, the bacilli form a nodule or tubercle in the lung parenchyma. Cells from the host's immune system contribute to granuloma formation at the primary site of infection, which is followed by tissue destruction (caseous necrosis) and cavity formation. This infection can spread to other parts of the host's lung or be disseminated to others through respiratory secretions. The bacilli are also phagocytized by alveolar macrophages and carried to lymph nodes where the bacteria multiply and may eventually go into the bloodstream to all parts of the body.

Since the mid 1950s, the number of cases of tuberculosis and number of deaths from the disease in the United States have declined. Prior to that time, over 100,000 new active cases were reported annually. In 1984, however, only 22,255 cases of tuberculosis were reported to the Centers for Disease Control (CDC) to yield a rate of 9.4 cases/100,000 persons,

Table 30:1. Distinctive Properties of Cultivable Mycobacteria Encountered in Clinical Specimens*†

Group	Complex‡	Species	Clinical Significance§	Growth rate ‖ at 45°C	37°C	31°C	24°C	Colony type: Usual colony morphology¶	Pigmentation**	Niacin	Susceptibility to T2H†† (5 μg/ml)	Nitrate reduction
		M. ulcerans	1	–	–	S	–	R	N	–	–	–
	TB	*M. tuberculosis*	1	–	S	S	–	R	N(0)	+(95)	–	+(97)
		M. bovis	1	–	S		–	Rt	N(0)	–(4)	+	–(9)
(I)§§ Photochromogens		*M. marinum*	2		∓	M	M	S/SR	P(100)	∓(21)	–	–(0)
		M. kansasii	2		S	S	S	SR/S	P(96)	–(4)	–	+(99)
		M. simiae	3–2	–	S			S	P(90)	±(63)	–	–(28)
		M. asiaticum		–	S		S		P(86)	–(0)	–	–(5)
(II) Scotochromogens	*M. scrofulaceum*	*M. scrofulaceum*	3–2		S	S	S	S	S(97)	–(0)	–	–(5)
		M. szulgai	1		S	S	S	S or R	S/P(93)	–(0)	–	+(100)
		M. gordonae	4		S		S	S	S(99)	–(0)	–	–(1)
		M. flavescens	4		M		M	S	S¶¶(100)	–(0)	–	+(92)
		M. xenopi	3	S	S			Sf	S(21)	–(0)	–	–(7)
(III) Nonchromogens	*M. avium*	*M. avium-intracellulare* complex	2	–/+	S		±	St/R	N(87)	–(0)	–	–(4)
		M. gastri	4		S		S	S/SR/R	N(100)	–(0)	–	–(0)
		M. malmoense	1		S	S	S	S	N(88)	–(0)	–	–(1)
		M. haemophilum	1	–	–	S***	S	R	N	–	–	–
		M. nonchromogenicum	4		S		S	SR	N	–	–	+
	M. terrae	*M. terrae*	4		S		S	SR	N(93)	–(1)	–	±(67)
		M. triviale	4		M		S	R	N(100)	–(0)	–	+(89)
(IV) Rapid Growers	*M. fortuitum*	*M. fortuitum*	4–3	–	R		R	Sf/Rf	N(100)	∓	–	+(100)
		M. chelonae	4–3	–	R		R	S/R	N(100)	∓	–	–(1)
		M. phlei	4	R	R		R	R	S			+
		M. smegmatis	4	R	R		R	R/S	N			+
		M. vaccae	4		R		R	S	S			+

(Continued)

Table 30:1. *Continued*

Species	Semiquan-titative catalase (mm)	68°C catalase	Tween hydrolysis	Tellurite reduction	Tolerance to 5% NaCl	Iron Uptake	Arylsul-fatase, 3 days	Mac Conkey agar	Urease‡‡	Pyrazina-midase 4 days	Agglu-tination tests available
M. ulcerans	<45	+	−		−		−		V	−	
M. tuberculosis	<45(89)	−(1)	±(68)	∓(36)	−(0)	−	−(0)	−	±(64)	+	
M. bovis	<45(69)	−(2)	−(21)		−(0)	−	−(0)	−	±(50)	−	
M. marinum	<45(98)	−(30)	+(97)	∓(39)	−(0)	−	∓‖‖(41)	−	+(83)	+	+
M. kansasii	>45(93)	+(91)	+(99)	∓(31)	−(0)	−	−(0)	−	∓(49)	−	+
M. simiae	>45(93)	+(95)	−(9)	+(82)	−(0)	−	−(0)		±(69)	+	+
M. asiaticum	>45(95)	+(95)	+(95)	−(20)	−(0)	−	−(0)		−(10)	−	
M. scrofulaceum	>45(84)	+(94)	−(2)	±(64)	−(0)	−	V(0)	−	V(31)	±	+
M. szulgai	>45(98)	+(93)	∓(49)	±(53)	−(0)	−	V(0)	−	+(72)	+	+
M. gordonae	>45(90)	+(96)	+(100)	−(29)	−(0)	−	V(0)	−	V(31)	∓	+
M. flavescens	>45(94)	+(100)	+(100)	∓(44)	±(62)	−	−(0)	−	+(72)	+	
M. xenopi	>45(85)	±(31)	−(12)	±(65)	−(0)	−	±(36)	−	−(0)	V	+
M. avium-inracellulare complex	<45(98)	±(60)	−(2)	+(81)	−(0)	−	−(1)	∓	−(2)	+	+
M. gastri	<45(100)	−(11)	+(100)	±(50)	−(0)	−	−(0)	−	∓(44)	−	
M. malmoense	<45(99)	±(66)	+(99)	+(74)	−(0)	−	−(0)		−(9)	+	
M. haemophilum	<45	−	−	−	−	−	−	−	−	+	
M. nonchromogenicum	>45	+	+	−	−	−	−	V	−	V	
M. terrae	>45(93)	+(92)	+(99)	∓(46)	−(2)	−	−(2)	V	−(13)	V	
M. triviale	>45(100)	+(100)	+(100)	−(25)	+(100)	−	±(56)	−	∓(33)	V	
M. fortuitum	>45(93)	+(90)	∓(43)	+(92)	+(85)	+	+(97)	+	+(70)	+	+
M. chelonae	>45(92)	±(53)	∓(39)	+(89)	V†††	−	+(95)	+	+(89)	+	+
M. phlei	>45	+	+	+	+	+	−	−			
M. smegmatis	>45	+	+	+	+	+	−	−			
M. vaccae	>45	+	+	+	V	+	−	−			

* From references 13, 50.

† Plus and minus signs indicate the presence or absence, respectively, of the feature; blank spaces indicate either that the information is not currently available or that the property is unimportant.

V = variable; ± = usually present; ∓ = usually absent; Percent of CDC-tested strains positive in each test is given in parentheses and test result is based on these percentages [13].

‡ For most clinical laboratories, designation to the complex is usually sufficient.
§ Potential clinical significance: 1 = present only as pathogens; 2 = present usually as pathogens; 3 = presently commonly as nonpathogens; 4 = present usually as nonpathogens.
‖ S = Slow; M = Moderate; R = Rapid.
¶ R = Rough; S = Smooth; SR = Intermediate in roughness; t = thin or transparent; f = filamentous extensions.
** P = Photochromogenic; S = Scotochromogenic; N = Nonchromogenic. Note: *M. szulgai* is scotochromogenic at 37°C and photochromogenic at 24°C.
†† T2H = Thiophene-2-carboxylic acid hydrazide.
‡‡ Urease test was performed by the method of Steadham 1979.
§§ Refers to the Runyon group.
‖‖ Arylsulfatase, 14 days, is +.
¶¶ Young cultures may be nonchromogenic or possess only pale pigment which may intensify with age.
*** Requires hemin as growth factor.
††† *M. chelonae* subsp. *chelonae* is −; *M. chelonae* subsp. *abscessus* is +.

continuing a downward trend from past years. Even with the current rate of decline, however, it appears that the disease will probably not be eliminated before the year 2100, if then. It should be noted that over 20,000 new cases and 1,800 deaths still occur yearly. Hundreds of cases still occur in children, most of whom are less than 5 years of age, and this serves as evidence that tuberculosis is still a prevalent infection.[5] Also, during 1978 to 1981, many cases were found among the influx of Southeast Asian refugees. Case rates are highest for persons over 65 years of age and for males of darkskinned races, followed by darkskinned females, then white males and females.[4]

Mycobacteria other than *M. tuberculosis*, including *M. kansasii* and *M. avium-intracellulare* complex, can cause pulmonary disease, but person-to-person spread is not believed to occur. Rather, these organisms are most likely acquired from natural sources in the environment, but the mechanisms of pulmonary infection and the fate of the mycobacteria after inhalation remain obscure. In addition to lung involvement, a wide variety of tissues, especially the lymph nodes, skin, soft tissues, bones, joints and tendons of the skeletal system, may be affected. Pneumoconiosis, chronic obstructive pulmonary disease and healed tuberculosis are common predisposing factors in the pathogenesis of lung disease caused by nontuberculous mycobacteria. Life-threatening disseminated disease is usually associated with immunosuppression in patients such as those with AIDS and irreversible hematologic disorders, but rarely found in previously healthy people.[64]

M. leprae, the etiologic agent of Hansen's disease or leprosy, cannot be cultured in vitro. The clinical diagnosis is confirmed by histopathologic examination of skin lesions, or in some instances, of lymph nodes and bone marrow, for the presence of acidfast bacilli (AFB).

THERAPY

Multiple drugs must be given in combination when treating mycobacterioses to avoid emergence of resistant organisms. Drug resistance during antituberculous chemotherapy does occur and the settings associated with a high rate of drug-resistant organisms are: tuberculosis in Asians and hispanic patients, patients having previous treatment, patients with positive sputum cultures after three months of therapy and patients with exposure to drug-resistant tuberculosis. To treat uncomplicated pulmonary tuberculosis, isoniazid and rifampin are administered for 9 months, with streptomycin or ethambutol added for the first 2-8 weeks. In studies using such a regimen for 6 months, the isoniazid and rifampin can be given twice weekly instead of daily after the first month, a less expensive treatment more apt to ensure patient compliance.[65] For treatment of tuberculosis involving children, organs other than the lungs, certain patient characteristics, concurrent disease or adverse drug reactions, refer to the American Thoracic Society (ATS) recommendations.[2]

Treatment of mycobacterioses caused by other mycobacteria may be difficult because these organisms generally exhibit greater drug resistance. *M. kansasii*, however, is highly susceptible to rifampin and therapy should always include rifampin and one or two other drugs such as isoniazid and ethambutol or streptomycin for 18-24 months. *M. avium-intracellulare* complex is resistant to most of the antituberculous drugs. Multiple drugs may be effective and some investigators suggest the use of four or more chosen from among isoniazid, rifampin, ethambutol, ethionamide and either streptomycin, capreomycin or kanamycin. In AIDS patients with disseminated disease, clofazimine and ansamycin are being used. Surgical resection has been recommended for local disease. *M. fortuitum* and *M. chelonae* are resistant to the common antituberculous drugs. They are often found in extrapulmonary sites, especially in areas of soft tissue injury and drainage, and debridement or excision are recommended. Treatment with multiple drugs may be attempted when chemotherapy is warranted but the response is unpredictable. In some cases, antibiotics such as amikacin, doxycycline and sulfonamides have been reported to be effective. It should be noted that concurrent infections with both *M. tuberculosis* and other mycobacteria occur.[2]

Isoniazid is the drug of choice for use in preventive therapy of tuberculin skin test reactors because of its high potency and low toxicity. For specific recommendations on preventive therapy, refer to recommendations of the ATS.[2]

PUBLIC HEALTH SIGNIFICANCE

Even with the advent of effective chemotherapy for tuberculosis, public health authorities must still follow nonhospitalized patients with active disease to continually assess the patient's compliance with chemotherapy and to monitor its efficacy. This is particularly important for immigrant cases and infections in younger patients, since many are caused by multiply resistant strains. Public health authorities must evaluate case contacts and administer preventive therapy to new skin test converters. Authorities should have surveillance programs for monitoring populations of migratory agricultural laborers, which have spread tuberculosis in the United States.[29] Finally, public health laboratories must maintain a level of proficiency that provides accurate recovery, identification and drug susceptibility testing of the mycobacteria and serve as reference and referral centers for other laboratories.

DIAGNOSTIC PROCEDURES

Levels of Laboratory Service

Some laboratories may not have the facilities to work safely with mycobacteria. Others may not receive a sufficient volume of specimens containing mycobacteria to maintain proficiency. Therefore, as illustrated in Table 30:2, the College of American Pathologists (CAP) and the ATS have suggested varying levels of proficiency for laboratories working with mycobacteria.[14,49,50]

Safety Procedures in the Mycobacteriology Laboratory

It is necessary to implement and enforce safety procedures specific to the mycobacteriology laboratory because of the nature of the organism and its mode of transmission. Personnel should have an initial chest X-ray, yearly skin tests and preferably wear a mask, gloves, gown, cap and shoe coverings when working. A separate room under negative pressure and equipped with a class I or class IIA biologic safety cabinet should be used. All work involving cultures, such as making smears, inoculating cultures and adding reagents to biochemical tests, must be done in the biologic safety cabinet. Towels soaked with phenolic disinfectant can be used to cover the work surfaces, to line discard pans and to wipe the edges of culture tubes to prevent dripping. The cabinet and work area should be cleaned with disinfectant before and after work and an ultraviolet light should irradiate the work area when it is not in use. To prevent aerosols, sealed centrifuge cups, electric induction incinerators (not bunsen burners) and splashproof discard containers should be used. To prevent splattering of material from inoculating loops, wires or spades before flaming, a bottle containing sand and either 95% ethyl alcohol or a 5% phenol solution can be used for wiping the implement before sterilization. Finally, tuberculocidal germicides with the correct contact time must be utilized.

Collection of Specimens

Optimal recovery of mycobacteria from clinical specimens is dependent on good specimen collection, appropriate temporary specimen storage and proper processing prior to culturing. Because certain specimens such as those from respiratory sources are contaminated with other microorganisms, all specimens should be refrigerated to inhibit growth of contaminating organisms if prompt processing is not possible. A routine culture for other bacteria should be performed to determine if decontamination is necessary and, if so, for what period of time. If a routine culture is not done, a portion of the specimen should be inoculated onto the surface of a blood agar plate,

Table 30:2. Suggestions for Limiting the Extent or Level of Service Offered by Clinical Laboratories*

Extent of services (College of American Pathologists)	Levels of laboratory service for mycobacterial diseases (American Thoracic Society)†
Extent 1 No mycobacteriological procedures performed.	
Extent 2 Acidfast stain of exudates, effusions, and body fluids, etc., with inoculation and referral of cultures to reference laboratories for further identification.	*Level I* a. Collect adequate clinical specimens. b. Transport specimens to a higher-level laboratory for isolation and identification. c. May prepare and examine smears for presumptive diagnosis or as a means of monitoring the progress of diagnosed patients on chemotherapy or both.
Extent 3 Isolation of mycobacteria; identification of *M. tuberculosis* and preliminary identification of the nontuberculous forms as photochromogens, scotochromogens, nonchromogens, and rapid growers; drug susceptibility testing may or may not be performed.	*Level II* Perform functions of Level I laboratories, including preparation of smears, and a. Process specimens as necessary for culture on standard egg-based media or egg- and agar-based media. b. Identify *M. tuberculosis*. c. May perform drug susceptibility studies of *M. tuberculosis*. d. Retain mycobacterial cultures for additional or repeat tests; 6 months is recommended.
Extent 4 Definitive identification of mycobacteria isolated to the extent required to establish a correct clinical diagnosis and to aid in the selection of safe and effective therapy; drug susceptibility testing may or may not be performed.	*Level III* Perform all functions of Level I and II laboratories, and a. Identify all *Mycobacterium* species from clinical specimens; cultures with known reaction patterns for growth and biochemical activities should be tested routinely with clinical isolates for quality control. b. Should perform drug susceptibility studies of mycobacteria. c. May conduct research and provide training.

* From reference 50.
† For the complete text of levels of service with applicable references, see reference 14.

the plate incubated at 35°C overnight and read prior to processing a mycobacterial culture.

Sputum:

An early morning specimen (5-10 mL) produced by a deep cough, or an expectorated sputum induced by a heated, aqueous, sterile aerosol of 10% glycerin and 15% NaCl (or of 10% NaCl) should be collected in a sterile container 3-5 times over a period of several days. If possible, the patient should rinse his/her mouth with water (not mouthwash) prior to collection and care should be taken not to introduce saliva or nasal secretions into the specimen. Induced sputum specimens should be labeled as such since they can be mistaken for saliva. Twenty-four hour sputum specimens are not acceptable and should not be collected.

Gastric washings:

Swallowed sputum can be obtained from patients who cannot produce sputum, small children and those too ill to expectorate by collection of gastric contents. The specimen should be collected early in the morning and at least 8 hours after the ingestion of food. Gastric contents are aspirated from the patient's stomach via an inserted tube connected to a syringe and placed in a sterile container. Lavage fluid (20-30 mL sterile distilled water) is then inserted through the tube or swallowed, then aspirated and added to the original specimen. If the specimen will not be processed within 4 hours, approximately 100 mg of powdered sodium bicarbonate or another alkaline buffer salt should be added to neutralize gastric acids.

Urine:

An early morning clean-voided or clean-catch midstream specimen is collected in a sterile container. If possible, the entire volume of urine should be collected, or a minimum of 15 mL. A specimen may be collected through an indwelling catheter by direct aspiration of the catheter with a sterile needle and syringe. A pooled 24-h specimen is not acceptable.

Feces:

Although previously used years ago to diagnose gastrointestinal tuberculosis, feces have not been routinely cultured for mycobacteria until recently when needed to assist in detecting *M. avium-intracellulare* complex infection in AIDS patients. This organism is commonly recovered in large numbers from the feces before other specimens are positive. A recommended procedure is to make a thin smear of stool for an acidfast stain and culture the stool only if AFB are seen. To culture the specimen, a small amount of stool is emulsified in 5 mL of Dubos albumin broth, incubated at 35°C overnight and processed as if it were a contaminated specimen such as sputum. If immediate processing is not possible, the specimen should be frozen at -20°C.[11] Requests to culture feces for mycobacteria from other types of patients are rare and usually unwarranted.

Tissues, fluids and exudates:

Tissue is collected aseptically in a sterile bottle containing sterile distilled water or saline and homogenized in broth (nutrient or Dubos) using a tissue grinder or homogenizer. As with feces, if immediate processing is not possible, freeze the tissue. Specimens (amount needed for culture) such as cerebrospinal fluid (2 mL), abdominal (peritoneal, paracentesis, dialysis, bile) and chest (pleural, thoracentesis, empyema) fluids (10-15 mL), exudates (transudates, drainages, ulcers) (3-5 mL), and pericardial, synovial (joint) fluids and others (2-3 mL) are collected aseptically and placed in a sterile container. Body fluids should be diluted in saline or buffer before centrifugation to aid in sedimenting the mycobacteria, which are relatively buoyant (specific gravity near unity) due to the high lipid content of their cell walls.

Blood:

Blood from AIDS patients may contain circulating mycobacteria. The most practical system for isolating them appears to be the Isolator lysis-centrifugation system (E.I. duPont de Nemours). Another method used by many laboratories is the BACTEC system (Johnston Laboratories), which provides an automated radiometric method for detection. An alternative method used by some includes processing the blood specimen using the Isolator followed by inoculating a BACTEC blood culture medium. Currently, Johnston Laboratories is evaluating a specific blood culture medium for recovery of mycobacteria.

Processing of Clinical Specimens

Most specimens containing mycobacteria are contaminated with other microorganisms making decontamination necessary. The procedures employed rely on the fact that mycobacteria are more resistant to the treatment than are the other organisms. Procedures must be adhered to strictly to prevent a reduction in the number of mycobacteria since they are also susceptible to the agents. All work is performed in a biologic safety cabinet. Tubes containing processed specimens are centrifuged in safety cups sealed with domed lids. The high lipid content of their cell walls gives mycobacteria greater buoyancy in liquids, requiring greater forces during centrifugation. Centrifugation at a minimum of 2000 X g for 15-30 min is required. The most currently accepted decontamination reagents are N-acetyl-L-cysteine-sodium hydroxide, sodium hydroxide or Zephiran-trisodium phosphate. A procedure using oxalic acid has been reported to be useful for decontamination of specimens containing *Pseudomonas aeruginosa* and other gram-negative bacteria. A procedure using cetylpyridinium chloride can be used for decontamination during transit for sputum specimens in transport for up to 24 h. Specimens must then be subjected to one of the other decontamination procedures.

See Chapter 45, "Media, Reagents and Stains," for the formulations for all media and reagents described in the following procedures.

N-acetyl-L-cysteine (NALC)-sodium hydroxide procedure:

NALC is a mucolytic agent and NaOH serves as the decontaminant.

1. Centrifuge specimens greater than 10 mL volume for 30 min, pour off the supernatant fluid and resuspend the sediment in 2-5 mL M/15 sterile phosphate buffer, pH 6.8[56] or sterile water. If the specimen is mucoid, add 50-100 mg of NALC and centrifuge.
2. Treat resuspended sediment and specimens up to 10 mL as follows. Place the specimen in a 50-mL conical, screwcapped centrifuge tube, add an equal volume of NALC-4% NaOH, vortex for 15-30 s trying not to cause much frothing of the specimen since excessive aeration will inactivate the NALC.
3. Let stand at room temperature for 15 min, fill the tube to 50 mL with buffer, mix and centrifuge at a minimum of 2000-2500 X g for 15-20 min.
4. Pour off the supernatant fluid into a splashproof discard can containing 5% phenol or another disinfectant solution. Wipe the lip of the tube to prevent contamination of its exterior.
5. With an applicator stick or a sterile 3 mm diameter bacteriologic loop, smear some of the sediment over a 2 cm^2 area on a glass microscope slide. If the amount of sediment is very small, add 1 mL sterile 0.2% bovine albumin solution, pH 6.8 first and then make smears. If a swab is received for processing, place it in a centrifuge tube with 2 mL NALC-NaOH and 2 mL distilled water or saline, mix, allow to digest for 15 min, remove swab and finish processing as for other specimens.

Sodium hydroxide procedure:

NaOH, 2% may be substituted for the NALC-NaOH solution in the procedure if specimens are processed shortly after collection. A maximum of 4% NaOH can be used, but treatment time should not be increased. At Mayo Clinic, an equal volume of 2% NaOH is added to the specimen, which is then vortexed for 15-30 s and allowed to react for varying times: sputum, induced sputum and urine containing gram-positive bacteria - 20 min; bronchial washings, gastric washings and urine - 15 min; specimens known to contain gram-negative bacteria - 25 min. No decontamination treatment is required for uncontaminated tissue, cerebrospinal and other body fluids. When decontamination is completed, the specimen is neutralized with 1.25N hydrochloric acid containing bromcresol purple. As acid is added, the suspension appears blue and then becomes yellow. A few drops of 2% NaOH are then added until the suspension again becomes and remains blue, indicating neutralization of the acid. The tube must be agitated to ensure uniform coloration. Specimens are centrifuged and all but 0.5 mL of supernatant fluid is discarded.

Zephiran-trisodium phosphate procedure:

1. An equal volume of Zephiran-trisodium phosphate is added to the specimen in a screwcapped container and vigorously mixed for 30 min on a mechanical shaker.
2. The mixture is allowed to stand for an additional 30 min, centrifuged and the supernatant fluid discarded.
3. The sediment is resuspended in 20 mL of Neutralizing Buffer[23] (Difco Laboratories) and centrifuged again for 20 min. Most of this supernatant fluid is discarded and the remaining suspension is used to inoculate media. The buffer contains phospholipid to neutralize the benzalkonium chloride in the digestant, which may inhibit mycobacterial growth on some media.

Oxalic acid procedure:

Sometimes specimens containing *Pseudomonas* species are not satisfactorily decontaminated with these procedures. The oxalic acid procedure[6] is reported to be better than procedures employing alkali for inactivation. An equal amount of 5% oxalic acid is mixed with the specimen, allowed to react for 30 min, 0.85% sodium chloride solution is added, the mixture centrifuged, supernatant fluid decanted and sediment neutralized to pH 7 with 4% NaOH.

Microscopic Methods

Because of the high lipid content of their cell walls, mycobacteria are able to retain dye even after being subjected to acid-alcohol, i.e., they are acidfast. This property allows microscopy to be used as a presumptive test in the laboratory diagnosis of mycobacterial disease, regardless of whether Ziehl-Neelsen, Kinyoun or fluorochrome staining procedures are used. The presence of fluorescence in the fluorochrome procedure is indicative of acidfastness. Acidfast smear results are used to aid in rapidly establishing a tentative diagnosis in conjunction with clinical findings, to determine appropriate dilution of inocula for direct drug susceptibility testing and to monitor efficacy of therapy, e.g., to determine whether a hospitalized patient may be discharged. However, smear and culture results do not always correlate. Mycobacteria may no longer be viable due to chemotherapy or the decontamination procedure, resulting in a positive smear and a negative culture. Conversely, a smear may be negative but the culture positive, due to the small number of mycobacteria present, i.e., the insensitivity of the smear. False-positive and false-negative results may be due to the staining procedure itself. Inadequate destaining and poor contrast between stain and counterstain may make recognition of mycobacteria difficult. Smears which are too thick may detach from the slide. Acidfast organisms not originally in a specimen may be added by tap water, contaminated stain bottles, cross contamination of specimens or smears and contaminated immersion oil on a lens used to view a positive smear, then used to view a subsequent smear without cleaning. Therefore, care must be taken when making and viewing smears. New slides must be used; slides should be kept separate from one another; washing of slides with filtered water during the staining procedure must be gentle.

Preparation of smears:

Prepare a smear by taking a portion of mucopurulent material directly from a specimen or sediment of a processed specimen using a 3 mm diameter inoculating loop or a sterile applicator stick and spread it onto a 2 cm^2 area of a new, clean, glass microscope slide. Air-dry and heat-fix the smear by placing the slide on an electric warmer for 2 h at 65-75°C or passing it quickly through a flame two separate times. Sputum specimens which will not be used for culture can be treated with household bleach (5-6% sodium hypochlorite) to kill viable bacteria. Equal amounts of sputum and bleach should be placed in a 50 mL centrifuge tube, shaken, allowed to react for 10-30 min, filled with water, mixed and centrifuged. Smears are made from the sediment.[24] The sensitivity of the smear can be increased by concentrating the sodium hypochlorite-treated sputum specimen by filtration through a polycarbonate filter with a pore size of 0.45 μm.[48]

Fluorescence Microscopy:

Acidfast bacilli will stain with the fluorochrome auramine O and fluoresce brightly. Such stains can be scanned easily and rapidly with a 25 X objective.

Auramine-rhodamine staining procedure of Truant:[55]

1. Flood heat-fixed smear with auramine O-rhodamine B reagent for 15 min at room temperature.
2. Rinse with distilled water and drain.
3. Decolorize with acid-alcohol for 2 min.
4. Rinse with distilled water and drain.
5. Flood slide with potassium permanganate counterstain for 2 min.
6. Rinse with distilled water, drain and air-dry.
7. Examine with fluorescence microscope using 25 X or 40 X objective to detect yellow-orange fluorescing bacteria.

A fluorescence microscope with a light source which emits light in the blue visible or ultraviolet range is used. Barrier filters are used to select specific wavelengths of light which cause the dye molecules to be excited and fluoresce. The Zeiss BG-12 or Corning 5113 excitation filters and Corning OG-1 barrier filter can be used. Using a dry darkfield condenser allows a larger field of vision (most fluorescence work is done with oil on the condenser) and, therefore, a lower total magnification for scanning the smear. A method using blue-light microscopy has been described[36] and reported[35] as successful in detecting acidfast bacilli in clinical specimens. A microscope with a quartz-halogen lamp and a combination of exciter and barrier filters is used.

Brightfield microscopy:

Acidfast bacilli are detected because of their contrast with non-acidfast organisms, if any, and the background. Either the Ziehl-Neelsen or Kinyoun procedure can be used.[38] The Kinyoun procedure is preferable to the Ziehl-Neelsen, because the latter requires constant application of heat while staining with carbolfuchsin and constant monitoring to ensure that slides do not dry during heating. The higher concentrations of carbolfuchsin and phenol in the Kinyoun procedure allows for penetration of the stain into the mycobacterial cell wall without application of heat.

Ziehl-Neelsen procedure:

1. Flood slides with carbolfuchsin and heat slowly to steaming; maintain for 4-5 min.
2. Wash with water and decolorize with acid-alcohol until no further stain can be rinsed off.
3. Counterstain with methylene blue for 20-30 s.
4. Rinse, drain and dry by blotting.
5. Examine, using brightfield microscopy with an oil immersion objective at 800-1000 X magnification, for red-staining bacteria against a blue background.

Kinyoun procedure:

1. Cover slide with a strip of filter paper and flood with carbolfuchsin for 5 min at room temperature.
2. Remove filter paper and rinse with water. Decolorize slide with acid-alcohol until no further stain can be rinsed off.
3. Counterstain with methylene blue for 1 min.
4. Rinse, drain and dry by blotting.
5. Examine, using brightfield microscopy with an oil immersion objective at 800-1000 X magnification, for red-staining bacteria against a blue background.

Quantitation and Reporting of smears:

Quantitation and reporting is based on observations made at 800-1000 X magnification. Smears are reported as follows:[47]

Number of Acidfast Bacilli Seen	Report
0	Negative for AFB (-)
1-2/300 fields	Number seen (±)
1-9/100 fields	Number/100 fields (1+)
1-9/10 fields	Number/10 fields (2+)
1-9/field	Number/field (3+)
>9/field	>9/field (4+)

To approximate the number of bacilli observed at other magnifications: at 650X, divide the count by 2; at 450X, divide the count by 4; and at 250X, divide the count by 10. For example, if 8 AFB per 10 fields are seen at 450X, the count at 1000X would be 2 AFB per 10 fields. If only 1-2 AFB are seen on the entire slide, the report should state the number seen and the slide categorized as ±, since it is sometimes difficult to distinguish bacteria from artifacts. In this case, an additional specimen should be requested.

Primary Isolation and Culture

Culture media should be both selective and nonselective because, although most mycobacteria survive the liquefaction and decontamination processes, some of the cells may be injured and the total population may be reduced. A nonselective, inspissated egg medium such as Lowenstein-Jensen, ATS or Petragnani, should be used for primary isolation. These media contain potato flour, glycerol and fresh whole eggs and/or fresh egg yolks. Petragnani medium also contains whole milk and Lowenstein-Jensen medium contains salts. All three have malachite green (0.02-0.05 g/100 mL). Lowenstein-Jensen medium is usually preferred since mycobacteria are often inhibited by the higher concentration of malachite green in the Petragnani medium, and the ATS medium is less selective due to its low concentration of malachite green. Media, such as Middlebrook 7H10 or 7H11 agars made with or without antibiotics, can be used as primary recovery media. They consist of defined salts, vitamins, cofactors, oleic acid, albumin, catalase, glycerol and 0.0025 g/100 mL malachite green. Middlebrook 7H10 medium also contains dextrose while Middlebrook 7H11 medium also has 0.1% casein hydrolysate to improve the recovery of isoniazid-resistant strains of *M. tuberculosis* . Cycloheximide, lincomycin and naladixic acid are added to Middlebrook 7H10 (Mycobactosel, Baltimore Biological Laboratory Microbiology Systems) and carbenicillin, amphotericin B, polymyxin B and trimethoprim lactate to Middlebrook 7H11 to make these media selective. Antimicrobics can also be added to Lowenstein-Jensen medium, however, antimicrobial drugs in any medium may affect the growth of mycobacteria.[50]

Lowenstein-Jensen medium is thought by some to yield more positive results, but the transparent Middlebrook agar perhaps allows for better recovery of mycobacteria, due to earlier recognition of growth, typical colony morphology and contaminants.[41] Dubos albumin broth or Middlebrook 7H9 broth can be inoculated with several drops of sediment from a processed body fluid or 1 mL of sterile body fluid may be inoculated directly into 5 mL of broth.

To inoculate solid medium, place 0.5 mL of undiluted sediment on one plate each of Middlebrook 7H10 and 7H11 agar. Inoculate two slants of egg medium with 0.25 mL of sediment each. If desired, a 1:10 dilution of the sediment may be used in addition to inoculation of undiluted sediment, since dilution may aid in obtaining isolated colonies, allow colonial morphology to be seen more clearly and lessen the effect of substances in the inoculum potentially toxic to mycobacteria.

Plates are placed inverted into polyethylene CO_2-permeable bags and sealed. Tubes are placed in a horizontal position on a slant until the sediment has been absorbed; then they are incubated in a vertical position with caps loosened. Incubation is at 35-37°C in an atmosphere of 5-10% CO_2 for the first three weeks followed by tightening of caps on the tubes and incubation of tubes and plates at 35-37°C in an atmosphere of ambient air for an additional 5 weeks. All specimens with positive acidfast smears and negative cultures at the end of 8 weeks are incubated for an additional 8 weeks. A duplicate set of media for cultures of skin lesions and environmental samples are incubated at 30°C for enhancing recovery of *M. marinum, M. ulcerans* and some rapid growers. Specimens from skin lesions should also be inoculated onto blood agar, chocolate agar, Middlebrook 7H10 agar with hemolyzed sheep erythrocytes or Lowenstein-Jensen containing 1% ferric ammonium citrate, and incubated at both 20°C and 32°C for detection of *M. haemophilum* which requires hemin for growth.

All cultures are examined for the presence of mycobacteria, aerobic actinomycetes and fungi. Young cultures (0-4 weeks) should be examined twice weekly. Older cultures (4-8 weeks) should be examined weekly.

Preliminary Methods for Identification

The mycobacteria commonly associated with human infection can be identified by a few simple biochemical tests after being grouped by their growth rate and photoreactivity. When growth is observed on solid media, a Kinyoun stain should be done to confirm acidfastness and to check for the presence of contaminating organisms. A tube containing 5.0 mL of Middlebrook 7H9 broth with ADC (Albumin-Dextrose-Catalase) enrichment is inoculated with colonies and 0.2 mL of this suspension is used to inoculate 2 tubes of Middlebrook 7H10 medium for the induction of pigment formation. One tube is wrapped in black paper and both are incubated with caps loosened at 35-37°C in an atmosphere of 5-10% CO_2. After sufficient growth

FIGURE 30:1. Tests for the Identification of Acid-Fast Bacilli.*

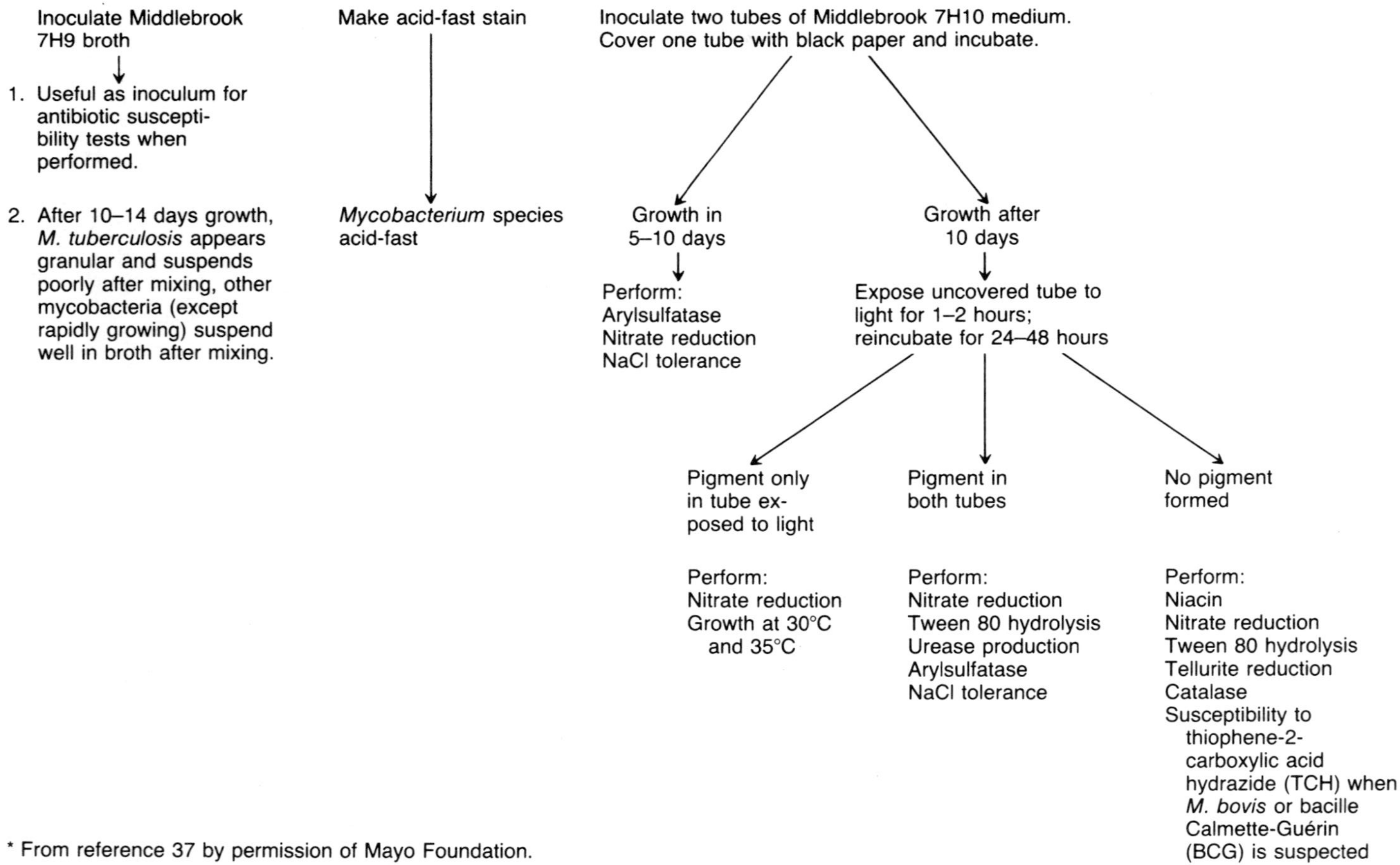

* From reference 37 by permission of Mayo Foundation.

appears, expose the uncovered tube to light for 30-60 min. Reincubate the uncovered tube for an additional 24 h and check for yellow pigmentation of colonies. Unwrap the covered tube and examine the culture for pigmentation. If growth remains a buff color when compared to the uncovered (yellow) culture, the organism is considered photochromogenic. If both tubes show pigmentation, the organism is considered scotochromogenic. If both tubes remain nonpigmented, the organism is considered nonchromogenic. If a subculture shows visible evidence of growth within 5-10 days, the organism is considered a rapid grower. Figure 30:1[37] presents a scheme for interpreting preliminary reactions of growth rate and pigmentation in respect to selection of biochemical tests for identification of the isolate. Methods for identification of mycobacteria commonly encountered in clinical specimens follow.

Rapidly growing mycobacteria: These organisms usually exhibit white to buff colored colonies that are creamy in appearance. See Figure 30:2[37] for tests for identification.

Photochromogenic mycobacteria: Tests useful for identifying these mycobacteria, which develop a yellow to yellow-orange pigmentation only after exposure to visible light, are found in Figure 30:3.[37]

Scotochromogenic mycobacteria: Tests useful for identifying these mycobacteria, which produce yellow to orange pigment in the presence or absence of light are found in Figure 30:4.[37]

Nonchromogenic mycobacteria: Tests to be used for identifying these mycobacteria are found in Figure 30:5.[37] Of the organisms in this group, *M. avium-intracellulare* complex may sometimes produce a slight yellow pigment, as will some older cultures of this species. *M. terrae* complex, *M. gastri* and *M. triviale* are usually not thought to be clinically significant. Colonies of these three species are usually smooth, dome-shaped and suspend easily to give a homogeneous suspension in Middlebrook 7H9 broth.

Table 30:3[38] describes characteristics used in the presumptive identification of mycobacteria, including growth rate, pigment production and colonial morphology on agar and features in broth. In many instances, the previously mentioned characteristics can allow the laboratory to provide the physician with some idea of the identity of an organism or can rule out certain species, i.e., *M. tuberculosis*. In addition, the selection of certain biochemical confirmation tests may be influenced by the tentative identification of an organism. Additional test information for the definitive identification of these organisms may be found in Table 30:1.

FIGURE 30:2. Identification of Rapidly Growing Mycobacteria of Clinical Significance.*

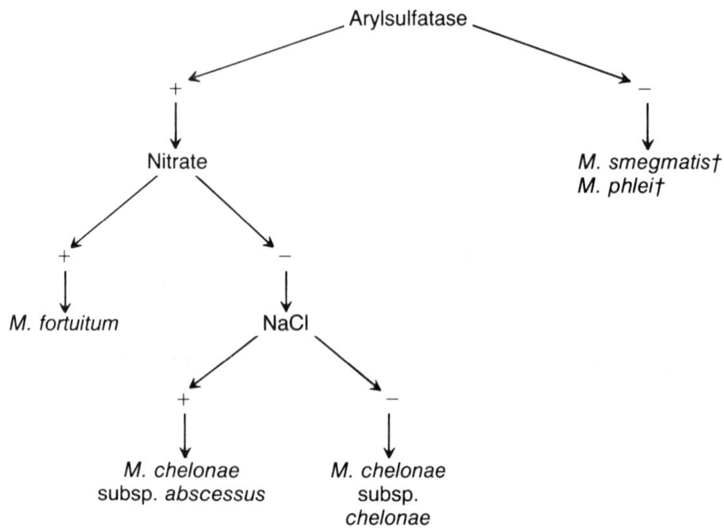

* From reference 37 by permission of Mayo Foundation.
† Require additional biochemical testing for differentiation.

Methods for Definitive Identification

Biochemical tests must be performed to establish the definitive identity of mycobacteria. Usually, only a few tests are necessary, but results of a single test should never be used solely as the basis for identifying an isolate. It should be remembered that individual strains may sometimes give an atypical test result and biochemical variation among isolates within a species is to be expected. Test procedures commonly used for the definitive identification of clinically important mycobacteria follow.

Nitrate reduction:[58]

Some species of mycobacteria produce the enzyme, nitrate reductase, which catalyzes the reduction of nitrates to nitrites. This test is performed to detect the presence of nitrate reductase.

1. Emulsify 1 loopful of a freshly grown culture in 3-5 drops of sterile distilled water in a sterile screwcapped test tube.
2. Add 2 mL sodium nitrate phosphate buffer, shake and incubate for 2 h at 37°C.

FIGURE 30:3. Identification of Common Photochromogenic Mycobacteria.*

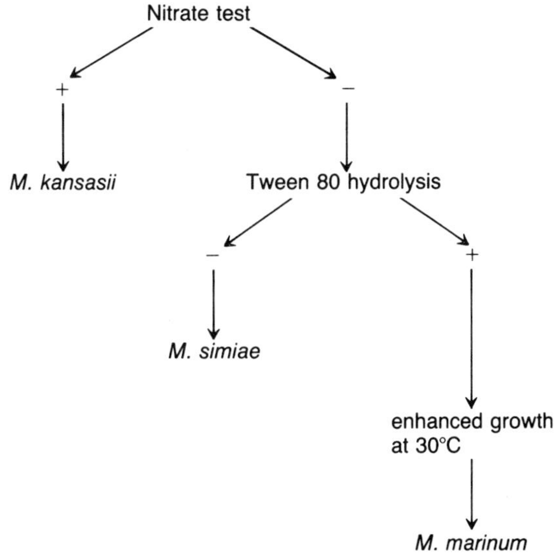

* From reference 37 by permission of Mayo Foundation.

3. Add one drop of hydrochloric acid solution, 2 drops of sulfanilic acid solution and 2 drops of N-naphthylethylenediamine dihydrochoride solution.
4. Observe for the presence of a red color. If a red color develops, the test is positive and the organism has produced nitrate reductase.
5. If no color develops, the test must be confirmed by adding a small amount of zinc dust. The development of a red color then indicates that the test result is negative. If no color change develops, the test result is positive due to complete reduction of nitrate to ammonia.
6. Use *M. kansasii* as a positive control and *M. avium-intracellulare* complex as a negative control.

Disk method:

An alternative method involves use of a reagent-impregnated paper disk.[37]

1. A loopful of freshly growing culture is inoculated into a tube containing nitrate solution.
2. Incubate the tube in a water bath at 37°C for 45 min.
3. Use plastic forceps to add a reagent-impregnated paper disk. Observe

FIGURE 30:4. Identification of Common Scotochromogenic Mycobacteria.*

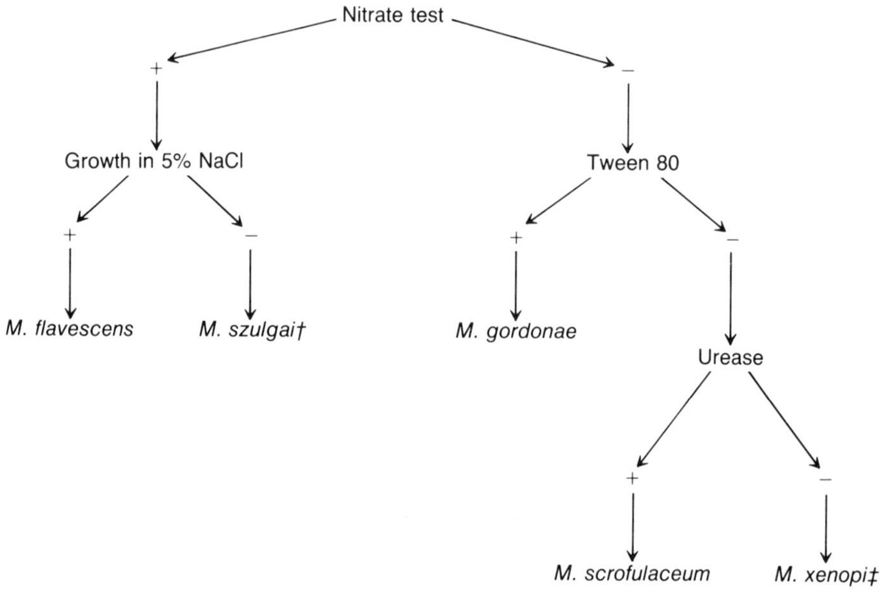

* From reference 37 by permission of Mayo Foundation.
† *M. szulgai* may be photochromogenic at 25°C and scotochromogenic at 35°C; arylsulfatase test is sometimes positive.
‡ *M. xenopi* has the ability to grow at 42°C; arylsulfatase test is sometimes positive.

for the development of a pink color within 30 s, indicating a positive test. The lack of a color change indicates a negative test.

4. Use the controls specified for the standard test.

Strip method:

Commercially available nitrate test strips (Difco Laboratories) can also be used, but the positive control must be strongly positive for test results to be reliable. If the strip test is negative or if the positive control is not strongly positive, the test must be repeated using one of the other two methods. Performance of the test is as follows.

1. Make a very turbid suspension of a freshly growing culture in 1 mL of sterile saline in a 13 X 100 mL sterile, screwcapped tube.
2. Insert a nitrate test strip without touching the bottom or sides of the tube.

FIGURE 30:5. Identification of Common Nonchromogenic Mycobacteria.*

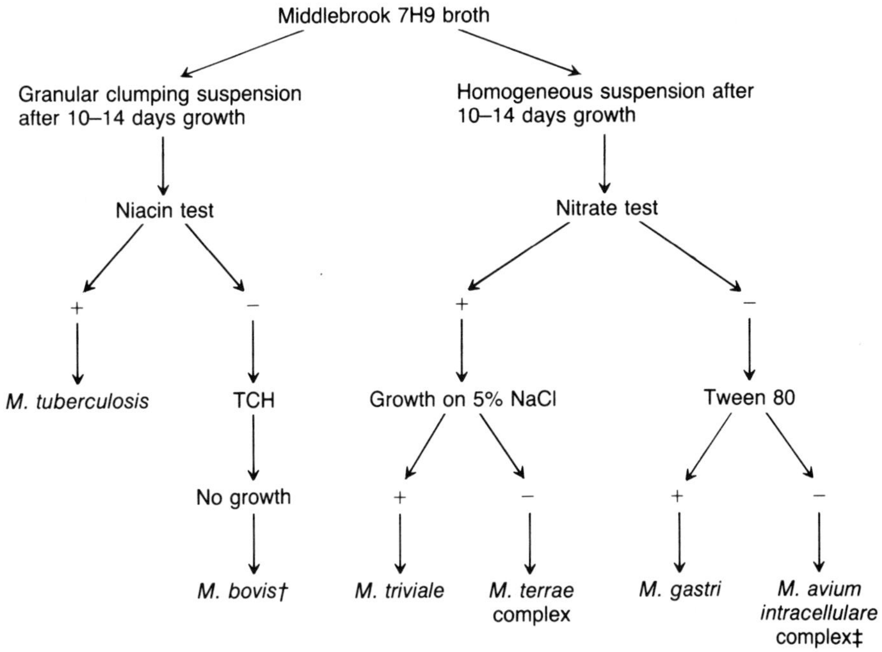

* From reference 37 by permission of Mayo Foundation.
† *fM. bovis* is sometimes positive for niacin.
‡ Tellurite is often positive with *M. avium-intracellulare* complex.

3. Cap the tube tightly and incubate upright in a water bath for 2 h at 37°C. Gently shake without tilting after the first hour.
4. After 2 h, tilt the tube to wet the entire strip and allow to stand for 10 min with the strip covered by the liquid.
5. Observe the top of the strip for a blue color change (positive reaction). No color change is a negative reaction.

Niacin production:

Because *M. tuberculosis* produces large amounts of free niacin but is unable to convert it to niacin ribonucleotide, accumulation of water-soluble niacin in an egg-base medium occurs. An aqueous extract of the medium around growing colonies is made and can be tested for niacin. This test is performed to distinguish *M. tuberculosis* from other slowly growing non-chromogenic mycobacteria.[22,42] A 3 to 4 week-old culture actively growing

Table 30:3. Features Useful for Making a Presumptive Identification of Mycobacteria*

Organism	Growth rate (days)	Pigment production in		Colonial morphology on Middlebrook 7H10 agar	Features of suspension in Middlebrook 7H9 broth
		light	dark		
Mycobacterium avium-intracellulare complex	10–21	Buff to yellow	Buff to yellow	Colonies are thin, transparent, glistening or matte, smooth, entire and rounded; some colonies rough and wrinkled	Uniformly homogeneous suspension
Mycobacterium bovis	25–90	Colorless to buff	Colorless to buff	Colonies are small, thin, often nonpigmented, raised, rough, later wrinkled and dry; some colonies inhibited on this medium	Heterogeneous; fine granular suspension
Mycobacterium chelonae	3–7	Buff	Buff	Colonies are rounded, smooth, matte, periphery entire or scalloped, no branching filaments; some colonies are rough and wrinkled	Heterogeneous; coarsely granular suspension
Mycobacterium fortuitum	3–7	Buff	Buff	Colonies are circular, convex, wrinkled or matte; branching filaments on periphery are obvious.	Heterogeneous; coarsely granular suspension
Mycobacterium gastri	10–21	Colorless to buff	Colorless to buff	Colonies are round, smooth, convex and glistening; often resembles *M. avium-intracellulare* complex	Uniformly homogeneous suspension
Mycobacterium gordonae	10–25	Yellow to orange	Yellow to orange	Colonies are round, smooth, convex, yellow to orange and glistening	Uniformly homogeneous yellow suspension
Mycobacterium haemophilum	14–28	Buff to gray	Buff to gray	Colonies are grayish-white, smooth to rough	Usually homogeneous suspension
Mycobacterium kansasii	10–21	Yellow	Buff	Colonies are raised and smooth; some are rough and wrinkled; carotene crystals numerous after exposure to light	Usually heterogeneous, finely granular suspension; some isolates give a uniformly homogeneous suspension
Mycobacterium marinum	5–14	Yellow	Buff	Colonies are round, smooth; some may be wrinkled	Uniformly homogeneous suspension
Mycobacterium scrofulaceum	10–14	Yellow	Yellow	Colonies are smooth, moist, yellow and round	Uniformly yellow and homogeneous

Mycobacterium simiae	7–14	Yellow	Buff	Colonies are smooth, domed and slightly pigmented	Heterogeneous; coarsely granular suspension
Mycobacterium smegmatis	3–7	Buff to yellow	Buff to yellow	Colonies are raised, rough, wrinkled and have scalloped edges	Heterogeneous; finely granular suspension
Mycobacterium szulgai	14–28	Yellow to orange	Buff at 25°C; yellow at 37°C	Colonies are smooth to rough; periphery somewhat irregular	Heterogeneous; finely granular suspension
Mycobacterium terrae	10–21	Buff	Buff	Colonies are round, smooth, glistening and sometimes colorless	Uniformly homogeneous suspension
Mycobacterium tuberculosis	12–28	Buff	Buff	Colonies are flat, rough, spreading with irregular periphery	Uniformly heterogeneous; coarsely granular suspension
Mycobacterium xenopi complex	28–42	Yellow	Yellow	Colonies are small, domed, yellow, smooth or rough; at 45°C, resemble a miniature "birds nest"	Uniformly homogeneous suspension

* From reference 38 by permission of Mayo Foundation.

on an egg-base medium, or other agar medium which has been supplemented with 0.1-0.5% asparagine, is suitable. A heavy growth is necessary for the test.

1. Add 1.0 mL sterile water or saline to the culture slant.
2. Scrape colonies from the surface of the slant to allow the liquid to be in direct contact with the medium for 15-30 min.
3. Remove 0.5 mL of the liquid to a glass tube.
4. Add 0.5 mL of a 4% solution of aniline in 95% ethanol and 0.5 mL of a 10% aqueous solution of cyanogen bromide.
5. Observe for the presence of a yellow color within 1-2 min. The presence of a yellow color indicates the presence of free niacin. A colorless test indicates a lack of niacin and is interpreted as being negative.
6. Use *M. tuberculosis* as a positive control and *M. avium-intracellulare* complex as a negative control.
7. Tubes containing the test suspensions should be discarded in an alkaline disinfectant (10% NaOH) to neutralize the cyanogen bromide.

Strip method:

A commercially available paper strip test for niacin production (Difco Laboratories; Remel) may also be used.

1. Add 1 mL sterile distilled water to the surface of a slant having a large number of colonies. The surface is lightly penetrated with a wire to allow niacin in the medium to solubilize in the water.
2. After 15 min, transfer 0.6 mL of the water to a 12 X 75 mm screwcapped tube and add a niacin test strip.
3. Cap the tube tightly and incubate at room temperature, with occasional mixing. After 20 min, if the liquid is yellow, the test is positive. No color development indicates a negative test.

Tween 80 hydrolysis:[19,62]

The usually nonpathogenic, slowly growing scotochromogenic and nonphotochromogenic mycobacteria produce a lipase that hydrolyzes Tween 80 (polysorbate 80 or polyoxyethylene sorbitan monooleate). When the Tween 80 in the test substrate is hydrolyzed, it releases a complexed neutral red from the substrate, resulting in a change in color of the substrate. The change is due to hydrolysis of the Tween 80, not to a change in pH.

1. Prepare the substrate containing phosphate buffer, Tween 80 and neutral red, dispense in 2.0 mL amounts into 16 X 125 mm screwcapped tubes and autoclave.
2. Inoculate a loopful of an actively growing culture into the substrate.
3. Cap the tube tightly and incubate for 10 days at 35-37°C.
4. Observe for a color change from amber to pink or red within 5 days,

indicative of a positive test. A color change between 5 and 10 days is an equivocal result. No color change is considered a negative test.

5. Use *M. kansasii* as a positive control and *M. avium-intracellulare* complex as a negative one.

A commercially available test reagent (TB Hydrolysis Reagent, Difco Laboratories) can be used in the procedure. Two drops of reagent are added to 1 mL distilled water in a sterile 13 X 100 mm screwcapped tube to make the substrate used in the test. The remainder of the procedure is performed as for the standard test.

Arylsulfatase production:[59]

The enzyme arylsulfatase splits the tripotassium salt of phenolphthalein disulfate into free phenolphthalein and the remaining salts. When sodium bicarbonate is added, it reacts with the free phenolphthalein to form a red diazo reaction. The 3-day procedure is helpful in differentiating clinically significant, rapidly growing mycobacteria, while the 14-day test may aid in distinguishing some of the slowly growing mycobacteria.

1. Inoculate a loopful of an actively growing culture into 3 mL of sterile Middlebrook 7H9 broth containing glycerol and phenolphthalein disulfate tripotassium salt in a 16 X 125 mm screwcapped tube.
2. Incubate for 3 or 14 days at 35-37°C.
3. Add 4-5 drops of sodium bicarbonate solution to each tube. A color change to pink or purple is indicative of free phenolphthalein and therefore the presence of arylsulfatase, a positive test. No color change is indicative of a negative test.
4. Use *M. fortuitum* as a positive control and *M. avium-intracellulare* complex as a negative control.

Dubos broth many be substituted for Middlebrook 7H9. The test can also be done with an unenriched agar base medium (Wayne Arylsulfatase Agar, Baltimore Biological Laboratory) which is inoculated with 1 drop of a suspension of the organism to be tested, incubated and read after the addition of 1 mL sodium bicarbonate solution.

Catalase tests:

Catalase is an enzyme produced by all mycobacteria except some isoniazid-resistant isolates of *M. tuberculosis*. It is an enzyme which splits hydrogen peroxide into water and oxygen, the oxygen being visible as bubbles during the reaction. The relative activity of the enzyme is measured semiquantitatively and after heating (as a measure of heat stability). The semiquantitative method is useful for separating species that produce large from those producing small amounts of catalase. Heat-labile catalase is inactivated at 68°C as shown for *M. tuberculosis, M. bovis* and *M. gastri*.

Semiquantitative catalase test:[25]

1. Prepare a dense suspension of the test organism in 1 mL distilled water and inoculate the entire surface of a Lowenstein-Jensen medium deep.
2. Incubate the tube in an upright position with cap loosened for 2 weeks at 35-37°C.
3. Add 1 mL of Tween 80-hydrogen peroxide solution and allow the reaction to proceed for 5 min at room temperature.
4. Measure the height of the column of bubbles produced and report as < 45 mm or >45 mm.
5. Use *M. fortuitum* as a positive control and *M. tuberculosis* as a negative control.

Catalase inactivation at 68°C:[26]

1. Suspend a loopful of growth from an actively growing culture in 0.5 mL of M/15 phosphate buffer, pH 7.0 in a 16 X 125 mm screwcapped tube.
2. Place the tube in a 68°C water bath for 20 min.
3. Cool to room temperature and add 0.5 mL of the Tween 80- hydrogen peroxide solution. The presence of bubbles indicates a positive test. A tube should be held for 20 min before being reported as negative.
4. Use the same organisms for controls as used in the semiquantitative test.

Sodium chloride tolerance:[17]

All rapidly growing mycobacteria except *M. chelonae* subsp. *chelonae* and other unnamed subspecies have the ability to grow in the presence of 5% NaCl. All slowly growing mycobacteria except *M. triviale* cannot tolerate this increased salt concentration and fail to grow.

1. Inoculate the entire surface of a Lowenstein-Jensen medium slant containing 5% NaCl (Difco Laboratories) with 0.1 mL of a slightly turbid suspension of an actively growing culture of the test organism in sterile distilled water. Inoculate a Lowenstein-Jensen slant without added NaCl with 0.1 mL of the same suspension.
2. Incubate the slants for 2-3 weeks at 35-37°C and observe for growth. Growth on both media is recorded as a positive test and growth on only NaCl-free medium as a negative test.
3. Use *M. fortuitum* as a positive control and *M. avium-intracellulare* complex as a negative control.

Urease production:

Urease hydrolyzes urea into ammonia and carbon dioxide with a resulting shift to an alkaline pH. When a urease-producing organism is grown on a medium containing urea and a phenol red indicator, the shift to an alkaline pH causes the indicator to change from orange to pink. Certain species of mycobacteria produce urease, which is helpful in differentiating between species. A broth[54] or disk[34] method may be used. A simplified broth method has also been developed.[51]

Broth method:

1. Dispense 4 mL of a urea-containing substrate into a 16 X 125 mm screwcapped tube.
2. Inoculate with a loopful of growth from an actively growing culture.
3. Incubate for 3 days at 35-37°C and observe for a color change to pink or red, indicating a positive test. The absence of color change is indicative of a negative test.

Disk method:

1. Emulsify several colonies in 0.5 mL distilled water and add one urea disk (Difco Laboratories).
2. Incubate for 4 h in a 37°C water bath and examine for a red color, indicative of a positive test.
3. Use *M. kansasii* as a positive control and *M. avium-intracellulare* complex as a negative one.

Tellurite reduction:[20]

Rapidly growing mycobacteria and some isolates of *M. avium-intracellulare* complex produce tellurite reductase which reduces colorless potassium tellurite to black metallic tellurite within 3-4 days, unlike other nonchromogenic, slower growing mycobacterial species.

1. Emulsify isolated colonies from an actively growing culture into 5 mL of tellurite test medium to yield a slightly turbid suspension.
2. Incubate for 7 days at 35-37°C in the absence of an increased (5-10%) CO_2 atmosphere.
3. Add 2 drops of the potassium tellurite test reagent to the 7-day old culture and incubate for an additional 9 days.
4. Examine the tube daily for the presence of a black sediment indicative of a positive test. The pigment of scotochromogenic organisms may mask the true color of the reaction, in which case a heavy brown precipitate is noted. The absence of a color change is indicative of a negative test.
5. Use *M. avium-intracellulare* complex as a positive control and *M. kansasii* as a negative control.

Thiophene-2-carboxylic acid hydrazide (TCH) susceptibility:[57]

TCH susceptibility is a trait used to identify *M. bovis*, since TCH selectively inhibits the growth of *M. bovis* but not that of other mycobacteria, including *M. tuberculosis*.

1. Prepare a suspension with a turbidity of a McFarland No. 0.5 barium sulfate standard in Middlebrook 7H9 broth from an actively growing culture and dilute it 1:100 and 1:10,000 with sterile Middlebrook 7H9 broth or saline.
2. Place 3 drops of the 1:100 dilution on a plate of Middlebrook 7H10 medium containing 1.0 μg/mL TCH and on one with medium containing 5.0 μg/mL TCH. Inoculate a medium without TCH to serve as a control.
3. Repeat this procedure using the 1:10,000 dilution.
4. Tilt the plates to evenly distribute the suspension over the surface of the plate and incubate in sealed polyethylene bags at 35-37°C in an atmosphere of 5-10% CO_2.
5. Read when colonies can be counted. Organisms are considered susceptible to TCH if growth on TCH-containing medium is less than 1% of growth on control medium. The absence of growth on the media containing either 1 μg/mL or 5 μg/mL of TCH is considered a positive test and is characterisitic of *M. bovis*; however, occasionally an isoniazid-resistant strain of *M. tuberculosis* will fail to grow on the TCH-containing media.
6. Use *M. bovis* as a positive control and *M. tuberculosis* as a negative one.

Pyrazinamidase:

The rate at which pyrazinamide is degraded by pyrazinamidase to free pyrazinoic acid is the basis for this test.[60] The presence or absence of this enzyme is often helpful when used with results of other biochemical tests.

1. Heavily inoculate 2 tubes of pyrazinamidase medium with the growth from a 2-3 week old culture.
2. Incubate the tubes at 35-37°C.
3. After 4 days, add 1 mL of freshly prepared ferrous ammonium sulfate solution to one of the tubes.
4. Refrigerate the tube for 4 h and examine against a white background for a pink band in the agar, indicative of a positive test. If the test is positive, the remaining tube may be discarded.
5. If the 4-day test is negative, remove the other tube from the incubator after 7 days and test as was done after 4 days. *M. tuberculosis, M. avium-intracellulare* complex and *M. marinum* are positive at 4 days whereas *M. bovis* and *M. kansasii* are negative. *M. bovis* usually remains negative at 7 days while many strains of *M. kansasii* become positive.
6. Use *M. avium-intracellulare* complex as a positive control and a tube of uninoculated medium as a negative control.

Iron uptake:[61]

Rapidly growing mycobacteria with the exception of *M. chelonae* have the ability to take up soluble iron salts from the medium and produce a rusty-brown color in the presence of ferric ammonium citrate.

1. Inoculate a Lowenstein-Jensen slant with 1 drop of a slightly turbid suspension of the test organism and incubate at 35-37°C until growth appears.
2. Add 1 drop of 20% aqueous ferric ammonium citrate for each 1 mL of medium and reincubate the culture for a maximum of 21 days. A positive test is indicated by the development of a rusty-brown color in the colonies and a change in the color of the medium to a light tan.
3. The test can also be performed by preparing Lowenstein-Jensen slants containing 2.5% ferric ammonium citrate. Inoculation of the medium and interpretation of the test are the same, but the slant is incubated at 28°C for the 21 days. Also, in this method, colonies of the unnamed subspecies of *M. chelonae* will be tan and the edge of the slant will appear a rusty-brown color.[45]
4. Use *M. fortuitum* as a positive control and *M. chelonae* as a negative control.

Radiometric Detection of Mycobacteria

An automated technique for detection of $^{14}CO_2$ liberated by bacteria during decarboxylation of ^{14}C-labeled substrates in medium was reported in 1969.[10] This method of detecting the presence of bacteria by actually detecting a metabolic product has recently been applied to detection of mycobacterial growth.[8,31] Mycobacteria in clinical specimens are detected more rapidly than by conventional culture methods when using the BACTEC system (Johnston Laboratories) to radiometrically monitor growth.[15,33,39] Direct susceptibility testing of mycobacteria can also be performed with the BACTEC system. In the study by Roberts et al,[39] the average detection times for BACTEC- positive cultures from acidfast smear-positive specimens were 8.3 days for *M. tuberculosis* and 5.2 days for other mycobacteria. By conventional methods, detection times were 19.4 and 17.8 days, respectively. These times do not include time required for identification, done by conventional methods (Table 30:4).

For the BACTEC procedure, a portion (0.5 mL) of a decontaminated specimen is inoculated into a vial containing 4 mL of Middlebrook 7H12 medium consisting of Middlebrook 7H9 broth base with ^{14}C-labeled palmitic acid (Johnston Laboratories). An antibiotic supplement (PANTA, Johnston Laboratories) of polymyxin B, amphotericin B, naladixic acid, trimethoprim and azlocillin reconstituted with polyoxyethylene stearate (POES) is also added to the vial. PANTA helps inhibit nonmycobacterial contamination and POES is a growth-promoting substance for many mycobacteria, especially *M. tuberculosis* and *M. bovis*. If microorganisms are present, they will utilize the ^{14}C-labeled substrate and produce $^{14}CO_2$ which is released into the atmosphere above the medium in the vial. A sample of this atmosphere is analyzed for radioactivity in the BACTEC instrument during each reading for the quantity of labeled CO_2 present. This quantity of $^{14}CO_2$

Table 30:4. Detection Times for Mycobacteria Recovered in the BACTEC® System*

Number of Isolates	Species	Mean†	Median†	Range†
64	*M. avium-intracellulare* complex	7.9	7.0	2–21
31	*M. tuberculosis*	14.0	14.0	2–43
7	*M. kansasii*	6.5	7.0	2–28
6	*M. fortuitum*	10.8	7.0	7–28

* From the Mayo Clinic Mycobacteriology Laboratory. Routine use of BACTEC® system began March, 1986. Data collected from March-September, 1986.
† Stated in days. Times do not include time for identification of the isolate.

is reported as the Growth Index (GI) The GI is directly proportional to the rate and amount of growth in the vial. After each reading, fresh 5% CO_2 in air is added back to the vial.

At Mayo Clinic, an auramine-rhodamine acidfast stain is made directly from specimens needing no decontamination, and after decontamination and concentration of specimens that are subjected to these procedures. The specimen is then inoculated into a BACTEC bottle (vial 12B) containing the medium described, and onto the surface of a biplate containing Middlebrook 7H11 with polymyxin B, trimethoprim lactate, carbenicillin and Middlebrook 7H10 medium. The BACTEC bottle is incubated at 35-37°C in an ambient air atmosphere for 6 weeks, read twice a week for the first 3 weeks and once a week for the remaining 3 weeks. The biplate is incubated in an inverted position in a polyethylene bag at 35-37°C in an atmosphere of 5-10% CO_2 and examined twice a week for 8 weeks.

When the Growth Index is ≥10, an auramine-rhodamine stained smear is examined. If the bottle contains bacteria in the presence or absence of mycobacteria, 0.2 mL from the vial is inoculated onto a blood agar plate, which is incubated at 35-37°C in an atmosphere of 5-10% CO_2 overnight. If growth occurs on this plate, the original decontaminated specimen (kept at 4°C for 2 weeks) is retreated for 25 min and 0.2 mL is inoculated onto a blood agar plate and incubated as before. If positive, no further attempt to isolate mycobacteria is made; if negative, the retreated specimen is inoculated into a new BACTEC vial. If the auramine-rhodamine stained smear from a vial with a GI ≥10 is positive for AFB and the culture is not contaminated with other bacteria, 0.2 mL from the vial is inoculated onto each side of a new biplate.

When sufficient growth is present on a biplate, a Kinyoun stained smear is examined to determine if a pure culture of mycobacteria is present. This growth is used to inoculate a tube of Middlebrook 7H9 broth for susceptibility testing and appropriate biochemical tests selected on the basis of the growth rate and colonial morphology.

Radiometric Identification of Mycobacteria

Vials are read daily. When the GI is ≥50, 1 mL is inoculated into a BACTEC NAP(*p*-nitro-α-acetyl-amino-β-hydroxy-propiophenone) differentiation test (Johnston Laboratories) and read daily for 2-5 days. If the GI is >100, a dilution of the vial is made according to the manufacturer's instructions and a portion of the dilution inoculated into a NAP test vial and read as before.

The original vial or dilution vial is used as a control for the NAP test and also read daily. *M. tuberculosis* and *M. bovis* are sensitive to NAP. Inhibition of their growth is indicated by a decreasing daily GI reading. Other mycobacterial species are not significantly inhibited by NAP so they will continue to grow and exhibit increased GI readings. The NAP test is a rapid and accurate test to differentiate the *M. tuberculosis-M. bovis* group from other mycobacteria.[27,32]

Rapid Methods for Identification

Subculture and subsequent biochemical testing of mycobacterial isolates for species identification is slow. Several weeks may pass from the time growth is initially detected to final identification of the isolate. Since the selection of antimycobacterial drugs for therapy is usually based on the identification of the organism, rapid identification methods would aid in optimizing drug selection. Of the relatively few methods available, gas-liquid chromotography (GLC) has proved to be a useful tool.

Gas-liquid chromotography:

Anderson demonstrated the uniqueness and complexity of the mycobacterial cell-wall lipids[1] and by using this property, studies have attempted to differentiate mycobacterial species by column chromatography, infrared spectroscopy, thin-layer chromatography and gas-liquid chromatography. Gas-liquid methods to rapidly identify mycobacteria from clinical specimens have been developed.[52,53] Mycobacterial lipids are saponified in methanolic NaOH, treated with boron trifluoride in methanol, extracted in a mixture of chloroform-hexane and the resulting hydrolysis products are analyzed by GLC.[37,38]

1. One loopful (1 mm) of organism (no agar) from the primary recovery medium is added to a 6 X 50 mm glass Durham tube containing 0.05 mL NaOH in absolute methanol (0.5 mol/L).
2. The tube is plugged with a 200 μL polypropylene centrifuge tube and incubated at 70°C for 30 min in a dry heating block.
3. The mixture is cooled and 0.1 mL 14% (wt/vol) boron trifluoride methanol is added and the tube incubated at 70°C for 5 min.
4. After cooling, 0.05 mL saturated NaCl solution is added, followed by

the addition of 0.2 mL chloroform-hexane (1:4, vol/vol) and mixing on a shaker for 5 min.

5. Centrifuge at 1000 X g for 5 min and transfer the upper phase to another 16 X 50 mm glass tube.
6. Evaporate to dryness in a water bath at 50-60°C under a stream of nitrogen or air.
7. Reconstitute with 20 μL chloroform and inject 2 μL into the chromatograph.
8. A glass column 16 ft in length (ca. 1.82 m) with an internal diameter of 2 mm, packed with 3% OV-17 on 100-200 mesh Supelcoport (Supelco, Inc.) is used. The injector port and detector temperatures are kept at 275°C and 315°C, respectively. The column oven is held at 170°C for 2 min after injection and is then raised 6°C/min to a final temperature of 300°C, which is maintained for 15 min. Zero-grade helium (Union Carbide, Linde Division) is used as carrier gas at a flow rate of approximately 17mL/min. Detector attenuation is 1×10^{-10} AmV.
9. Standards of fatty acids having carbon chains ranging from $C^{13:0}$ - C^{22} and C^{24} in addition to myristyl laurate, myristyl palmitate, palmityl palmitate and stearyl stearate are included with each series of sample testing. Chromatograms are read by comparing the retention times of mycobacterial components to those of the standards.

Figure 30:6[53] represents a chromatogram typical of *M. tuberculosis*. Organisms are characterized according to the decision tree presented in Figure 30:7.[53] When an organism is grouped into the *M. avium-intracellulare* complex, *M. gastri* and *M. scrofulaceum* category, tellurite, urease and catalase inactivation at 68°C tests are performed to distinguish the 3 species. *M. bovis* is distinguished from *M. tuberculosis* by the niacin test and susceptibility to TCH, while *M. xenopi* is distinguished by its ability to grow at 45°C and its characteristic yellow pigment. *M. fortuitum* and *M. chelonae* are differentiated by the nitrate test and NaCl tolerance. Most other species can be identified by GLC alone. Currently, GLC using a capillary column method is being evaluated at Mayo Clinic and separation of the species appears to be superior to separation with a glass column.

Nucleic Acid Probes for Detection and Identification

Specific DNA probes to the ribosomal RNA of mycobacteria have been developed (Gen-Probe). They include a genus level probe which detects all clinically significant *Mycobacterium* species; a probe which detects *M. tuberculosis, M. bovis, M. bovis* BCG, *M. africanum* and *M. microti*; a *M. avium* species-specific probe; and a *M. intracellulare* species-specific probe. An assay for culture confirmation has been developed which can be completed in 2 h. Plans for extended use of DNA probes are currently under development.

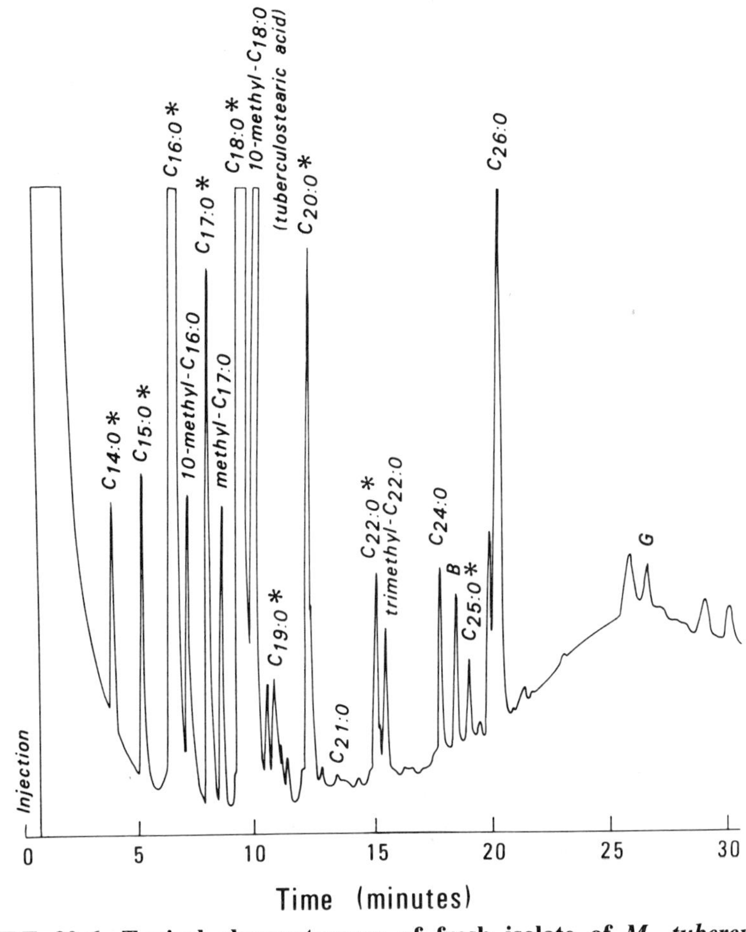

FIGURE 30:6. Typical chromatogram of fresh isolate of *M. tuberculosis*. Identity of each peak was determined by mass spectroscopy. Peaks marked with an asterisk are present in all mycobacterial species. From Tisdall et al. 1979.

Serotyping

Because of the complex relationships between the antigens of different mycobacterial species, serologic procedures have not been very successful for use in identification and when they are used, provide information below the species level only. Also, typing is possible only if growth on agar medium is smooth and stable cell suspensions can be prepared. W. B. Schaefer extensively studied agglutination-adsorption serotyping reactions for identification and classification of nontuberculous mycobacteria. The

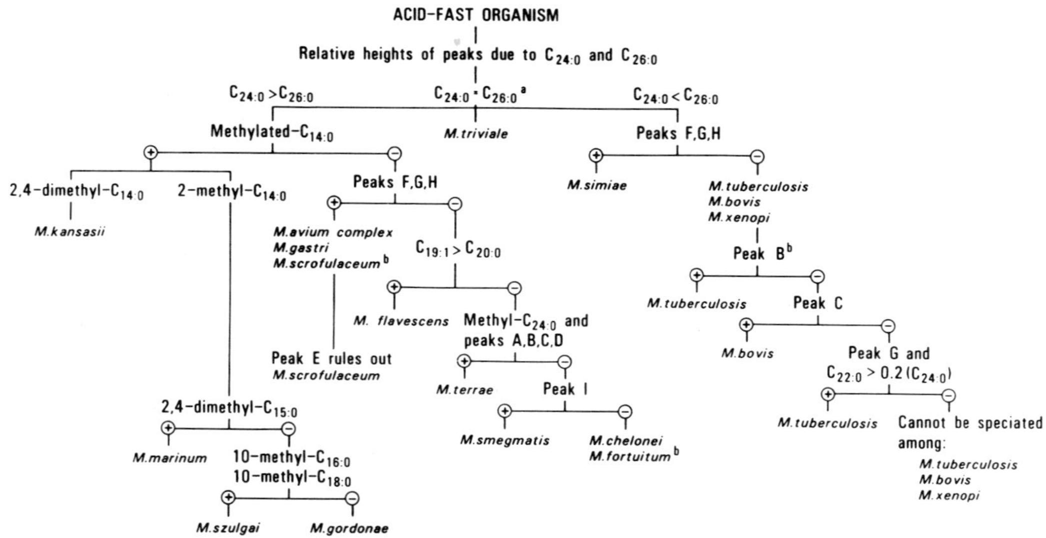

[a] $0.8 \leq C_{24:0}/C_{26:0} \leq 1.2$

[b] Not all cultures can be speciated past this step

FIGURE 30:7. Identification of mycobacteria by gas-liquid chromatography. From Tisdall et al. 1979.

methods used are described in a review.[43] Because antisera are not commercially available and these methods are fairly time-consuming, numerous other methods such as lipid analysis by thin-layer chromatography, slide agglutination, micromethod agglutination and fluorescent antibody techniques have been attempted and described.[12] Serotyping has been limited primarily to *M. avium, M. intracellulare* and *M. scrofulaceum* complex and has been used mainly to study the epidemiology of this group. In a recent report on *M. avium* complex infections in immunocompromised patients,[18] 77% of the isolates from disseminated cases were serovar 4, suggesting the possibility of a common source. Since members of the *M. avium-intracellulare* complex cannot be distinguished on the basis of cultural and biochemical tests, serotyping is useful in epidemiological studies.

Phage Typing

There are 12 typing phages for *M. tuberculosis*. Sensitivity or lack of it to these phages categorizes the bacterium into 1 of 4 phage types. The surface-lawn technique and the soft agar overlay method are the two standardized procedures used. Phage typing of *M. bovis, M. kansasii* and *M. xenopi* has been reported; however, a phage typing scheme for *M. avium-intracellulare* complex strains has yet to be developed. Of the rapidly growing species, *M. phlei* can be tentatively identified by its phage sensitivity, as can *M. smegmatis*, but other characteristics are more reliable for determining the species of the rapidly growing mycobacteria. Phage typing may, however, have some utility for determining the subspecies of rapidly growing species.[7]

Serologic Diagnosis

A test for the serologic diagnosis of tuberculosis is needed because results of tuberculin skin tests may be unreliable and recovery and identification of the etiologic agent is time-consuming.[66] There is also a need for tests indicating disease activity and prognosis because of the chronic nature of tuberculosis.[28] Several investigators have demonstrated serum antibodies to tuberculin antigens using complement fixation, hemagglutination, agglutination and precipitation in gel. More recently, the enzyme-linked immunosorbent assay (ELISA) technique has been used to detect antibody to PPD, mycobacterial glycolipids, antigen 5 and other antigens of *M. tuberculosis*. The sensitivity and specificity of the ELISA test may be enhanced by using purified antigens such as antigen 5, as shown by Daniel and coworkers.[9] In work by Zeiss and colleagues,[67] a study of an ELISA using PPD as antigen was shown to be more helpful than smear and culture for diagnosis of pulmonary tuberculosis. In this study, the ELISA and first smear were found to complement each other and together offered a rapid indication of which patients required more extensive evaluation. Zeiss[66] suggests other research areas in the serology of tuberculosis, including detection of secretory IgA specific for tuberculosis antigen. Also, in those patients with active disease and a negative IgG serologic test, most of the antibody may be part of immune complexes, making it necessary to be able to detect free tuberculosis antigen. Finally, better methods, such as cloning techniques, are needed for obtaining purified antigens.

Quality Control

A program of quality control and proficiency testing is essential for the mycobacteriology laboratory. Positive and negative control smears must be run with each set of patient slides to assure proper performance of staining and examination procedures. Growth and other media used in biochemical and susceptibility tests should be inoculated with appropriate stock cultures for performance testing. Appropriate positive and negative control organisms should be inoculated with each biochemical test on clinical isolates to ensure validity of results. Susceptibility testing media should be tested with susceptible and resistant strains. Finally, each laboratory should be enrolled in at least one proficiency testing program as a check of overall performance.

EVALUATION OF LABORATORY RESULTS

M. tuberculosis is the most common mycobacterial pathogen currently isolated in the United States today. However, the nontuberculous mycobacteria or mycobacteria other than the tubercle bacillus (MOTT bacilli) have been recognized with greater frequency as the number of tuberculosis cases declines. *M. kansasii* and *M. avium-intracellulare* complex cause most of the MOTT-related disease. These MOTT bacilli were formerly classified in numbered groups proposed by Runyon,[40] which are no longer used but frequently cited; they are still usually classified by the group terms listed in Table 30:1.

Factors determining the significance of a clinical mycobacterial isolate include the quantity of growth, repeated recovery of the organism, tissue site of origin of the isolate, species isolated and the presence of host risk factors.[63] It should be noted here that tubercular meningitis, uncommon in the United States, may be difficult to diagnose. Positivity of acidfast smear from cerebrospinal fluid (CSF) ranges from 10-90%[16,30] with most cases having negative smears. Higher yields may be obtained by centrifuging 10-20 mL of CSF and preparing a thick smear by layering several successive drops of sediment on a slide.[30] Culture positivity ranges from 38-88%[30] and it may take 6 weeks for cultures to become positive.[44] Many are still negative.

Experience in the literature varies with the individual reports presented. In a recent review of mycobacterial meningitis,[21] 4 of 21 patients had positive CSF smears and mycobacteria were isolated from 20 of the 21 patients. One patient's CSF was smear-positive and culture-negative.

Central nervous system (CNS) tuberculosis has recently been reported in patients with AIDS and AIDS-related complex;[3] all but one of the patients were also intravenous drug abusers. In view of this report and a predicted rise in the number of AIDS cases, the ability to diagnose CNS tuberculosis may become increasingly important. Finally, cultures of all clinical isolates should be held for at least 6 months after final identification and susceptibility reports have been completed, in the event that additional drug and other testing is required.

REFERENCES

1. Anderson RJ. The chemistry of the lipids of the tubercle bacillus. Yale J Biol Med 1943;15:311-45.
2. Bailey WC, Albert RK, Davidson PT, et al. Treatment of tuberculosis and other mycobacterial diseases. American Thoracic Society - Medical Section of the American Lung Association, 1982. Am Rev Respir Dis 1983;127:790-6.
3. Bishburg E, Sunderam G, Reichman LB, Kapila R. Central nervous system tuberculosis with the acquired immunodeficiency syndrome and its related complex. Ann Intern Med 1986;105:210-13.
4. Centers for Disease Control. Annual summary, 1983. Morbid Mortal Weekly Rep 1984;32:62-5.
5. Centers for Disease Control. Tuberculosis - United States, 1984. Morbid Mortal Weekly Rep 1985;34:299-307.
6. Corper HJ, Uyei N. Oxalic acid as a reagent for isolating tubercle bacilli and a study of the growth of acid-fast nonpathogens on different mediums with their reactions to chemical reagents. J Lab Clin Med 1930;15:348-69.
7. Crawford JC, Bates JH. Phage typing of mycobacteria. In: Kubica GP, Wayne LG, eds. The mycobacteria: a sourcebook. New York: Marcel Dekker, 1984:123-32.
8. Cummings DM, Ristroph D, Camargo EE, Larson SM, Wagner HN Jr. Radiometric detection of the metabolic activity of *Mycobacterium tuberculosis*. J Nucl Med 1975;16:1189-91.
9. Daniel TM, Debanne SM, Vanderkupp F. Enzyme linked immunosorbent assay using *Mycobacterium tuberculosis* antigen 5 and PPD for the serodiagnosis of tuberculosis. Chest 1985;88:388-92.
10. Deland FH, Wagner HN Jr. Early detection of bacterial growth with carbon-14 labelled glucose. Radiology 1969;92:154-5.
11. Finegold SM, Baron EJ, eds. Diagnostic microbiology. St. Louis: CV Mosby, 1986:594-631.
12. Good RC, Beam RE. Seroagglutination. In: Kubica GP, Wayne LG, eds. The mycobacteria: a sourcebook. New York: Marcel Dekker, 1984:105-22.
13. Good RC, Silcox VA, Kilburn JO, Plikaytis BD. Identification and drug susceptibility test results for *Mycobacterium* spp. Clin Microbiol Newsletter 1985;7:133-5.
14. Hawkins JE, Good RC, Kubica GP, et al. Levels of laboratory services for mycobacterial diseases. Am Rev Respir Dis 1983;128:213.

15. Horstmeier CD, DeYoung DR, Doerr KA, Roberts GD. A comparison of a radiometric method and conventional media for recovery of mycobacteria in clinical specimens [Abstract]. Annual Meeting of the American Society for Microbiology. Washington, DC: American Society for Microbiology, 1982:302.
16. Karandanis D, Schulman JA. Recent survey of infectious meningitis in adults: review of laboratory findings in bacterial, tuberculous and aseptic meningitis. South Med J 1976;69:449-57.
17. Kestle DG, Abbott VD, Kubica GP. Differential identification of mycobacteria. II. Subgroups of groups II and III (Runyon) with different clinical significance. Am Rev Respir Dis 1967;95:1041-52.
18. Kiehn TE, Edwards FF, Brannon P, et al. Infections caused by *Mycobacterium avium* complex in immunocompromised patients: diagnosis by blood culture and fecal examination, antimicrobial susceptibility tests, and morphological and seroagglutination characteristics. J Clin Microbiol 1985;21:168-73.
19. Kilburn JO, O'Donnell KF, Silcox VA, David HL. Preparation of a stable mycobacterial Tween hydrolysis test substrate. Appl Microbiol 1973;26:826.
20. Kilburn JO, Silcox VA, Kubica GP. Differential identification of mycobacteria. V. The tellurite reduction test. Am Rev Respir Dis 1969;99:94-100.
21. Klein NC, Damsker B, Hirschman SZ. Mycobacterial meningitis: restrospective analysis from 1970 to 1983. Am J Med 1985;79:29-34.
22. Konno K. New chemical method to differentiate human-type tubercle bacilli from other mycobacteria. Science 1956;124:985.
23. Krasnow I, Kidd GC. The effect of a buffer wash of sputum sediments digested with Zephiran trisodium phosphate on the recovery of acid-fast bacilli. Am J Clin Pathol 1965;44:238-40.
24. Krasnow I, Wayne LG. Comparison of methods for tuberculosis bacteriology. Appl Microbiol 1969;18:915-17.
25. Kubica GP, Jones WD Jr, Abbott VD, Beam RE, Kilburn JO, Cater JC Jr. Differential identification of mycobacteria. I. Tests on catalase activity. Am Rev Respir Dis 1966;94:400-5.
26. Kubica GP, Pool GL. Studies on the catalase activity of acid-fast bacilli. I. An attempt to subgroup these organisms on the basis of their catalase activities at different temperatures and pH. Am Rev Respir Dis 1960;81:387-91.
27. Laszlo A, Handzel V. Radiometric diagnosis of mycobacteria. Eur J Clin Microbiol 1986;5:152-5.
28. Lind A, Ridell M. Immunologically based diagnostic tests: humoral antibody methods. In: Kubica GP, Wayne LG, eds. The mycobacteria: a sourcebook. New York: Marcel Dekker, 1984:221-48.
29. Lowell AM. Tuberculosis - its social and economic impact and some thoughts on epidemiology. In: Kubica GP, Wayne LG, eds. The mycobacteria: a sourcebook. New York: Marcel Dekker, 1984:1021-55.
30. Meyers BR. Tuberculous meningitis. Med Clin N Am 1982;66:755-62.
31. Middlebrook G, Reggiardo Z, Tigertt WD. Automatable radiometric detection of growth of *Mycobacterium tuberculosis* in selective media. Am Rev Respir Dis 1977;115:1066-9.
32. Morgan MA, Doerr KA, Hempel HO, Goodman NL, Roberts GD. Evaluation of the *p*-nitro-α-acetylamino-β-hydroxypropiophenone differential test for identification of *Mycobacterium tuberculosis* complex. J Clin Microbiol 1985;21:634-5.
33. Morgan MA, Horstmeier CD, DeYoung DR, Roberts GD. Comparison of a radiometric method (BACTEC) and conventional culture media for recovery of mycobacteria from smear-negative specimens. J Clin Microbiol 1983;18:384-8.
34. Murphy DB, Hawkins JE. Use of urease test disks in the identification of mycobacteria. J Clin Microbiol 1975;1:465-8.
35. Pollock HM, Wieman EJ. Smear results in the diagnosis of mycobacterioses using blue-light fluorescence microscopy. J Clin Microbiol 1977;5:329-31.
36. Richards OW, Miller DK. An efficient method for the identification of *M. tuberculosis* with a simple fluorescence microscope. Am J Clin Pathol 1941;11:1-8.

37. Roberts GD. Mayo Clinic mycobacteriology laboratory procedure manual. Rochester, MN: Mayo Foundation, 1985.
38. Roberts GD. Mycobacteria and nocardia. In: Washington JA II, ed. Laboratory procedures in clinical microbiology. New York: Springer-Verlag, 1985:379-418.
39. Roberts GD, Goodman NL, Heifets L, et al. Evaluation of the BACTEC radiometric method for recovery of mycobacteria and drug susceptibility testing of *Mycobacterium tuberculosis* from acid-fast smear-positive specimens. J Clin Microbiol 1983;18:689-96.
40. Runyon EH. Anonymous mycobacteria in human disease. Med Clin N Am 1959;43:273-90.
41. Runyon EH. Identification of acid-fast pathogens utilizing colony characteristics. 3rd ed. Salt Lake City: Veterans Administration, 1972.
42. Runyon EH, Selin MJ, Harris HW. Distinguishing mycobacteria by the niacin test. Am Rev Tuberc Pulm Dis 1959;79:663-5.
43. Schaefer WB. Serological identification of atypical mycobacteria. In: Bergan T, Norris JR, eds. Methods in microbiology; vol 13. London: Academic Press, 1979:323-43.
44. Scully RE, Mark EJ, McNeely BU. Case records of the Massachusetts General Hospital, Case 2-1982. N Engl J Med 1982;306:91-7.
45. Silcox VA, Good RC, Floyd MM. Identification of clinically significant *Mycobacterium fortuitum* complex isolates. J Clin Microbiol 1981;14:686-91.
46. Smith DW. Mycobacteria. In: Braude AI, Davis CE, Fierer J, eds. Infectious disease and medical microbiology. Philadelphia: WB Saunders, 1984:364-71.
47. Smithwick RW. Laboratory manual for acid-fast microscopy. 2nd ed. Atlanta: Centers for Disease Control, 1976.
48. Smithwick RW, Stratigos CB. Acid-fast microscopy on polycarbonate membrane filter sputum sediments. J Clin Microbiol 1981;13:1109-13.
49. Sommers HM. Mycobacterial proficiency testing in the quality evaluation programs of the College of American Pathologists, 1972. Am J Clin Pathol 1974;61:980-9.
50. Sommers HM, Good RC. *Mycobacterium*. In: Lennette EH, Balows A, Hausler WJ Jr, Shadomy HJ, eds. Manual of clinical microbiology. 4th ed. Washington, DC: American Society for Microbiology, 1985:216-48.
51. Steadham JE. Reliable urease test for identification of mycobacteria. J Clin Microbiol 1979;10:134-7.
52. Tisdall PA, DeYoung DR, Roberts GD, Anhalt JP. Identification of clinical isolates of mycobacteria with gas-liquid chromatography: a 10-month follow-up study. J Clin Microbiol 1982;16:400-2.
53. Tisdall PA, Roberts GD, Anhalt JP. Identification of clinical isolates of mycobacteria with gas-liquid chromatography alone. J Clin Microbiol 1979;10:506-14.
54. Toda T, Hagihara Y, Takeya K. A simple urease test for the classification of mycobacteria. Am Rev Respir Dis 1960;83:756-61.
55. Truant JP, Brett WA, Thomas W Jr. Fluorescence microscopy of tubercle bacilli stained with auramine and rhodamine. Henry Ford Hosp Med Bull 1962;10:287-96.
56. Vestal AL. Procedures for the isolation and identification of mycobacteria. Atlanta: Centers for Disease Control, 1975; US Public Health Service Publ. 76-8230.
57. Vestal AL, Kubica GP. Differential identification of mycobacteria. III. Use of thiacetazone, thiophen-2-carboxylic acid hydrazide and triphenyltetrazolium chloride. Scand J Respir Dis 1967;48:142-8.
58. Virtanen S. A study of nitrate reduction by mycobacteria. Acta Tuberc Scand 1960;48(suppl):1-119.
59. Wayne LG. Recognition of *Mycobacterium fortuitum* by means of the three-day phenolphthalein sulfatase test. Am J Clin Pathol 1961;36:185-7.
60. Wayne LG. Simple pyrazinamidase and urease tests for routine identification of mycobacteria. Am Rev Respir Dis 1974;109:147-51.
61. Wayne LG, Doubek JR. Diagnostic key to mycobacteria encountered in clinical laboratories. Appl Microbiol 1968;16:925-31.

62. Wayne LG, Doubek JR, Russell RL. Tests employing Tween 80 as substrate. Am Rev Respir Dis 1964;90:588-97.
63. Wolinsky E. When is an infection disease? Rev Infect Dis 1981;3:1025-7.
64. Wolinsky E. Nontuberculous mycobacteria and associated diseases. In: Kubica GP, Wayne LG, eds. The mycobacteria: a sourcebook. New York: Marcel Dekker, 1984:1141-207.
65. Youmans GP. Tuberculosis. In: Youmans GP, Paterson PY, Sommers HM, eds. The biologic and clinical basis of infectious diseases. Philadelphia: WB Saunders, 1985:348-67.
66. Zeiss CR. Serologic diagnosis of tuberculosis. Clin Microbiol Newsletter 1986;8:112-13.
67. Zeiss CR, Kalish SB, Erlich KS, et al. IgG antibody to purified protein derivative by enzyme-linked immunosorbent assay in the diagnosis of pulmonary tuberculosis. Am Rev Respir Dis 1984;130:845-8.

CHAPTER 31

TULAREMIA

Michael Gelfand, M.D.

INTRODUCTION

Tularemia is an acute, febrile, granulomatous, infectious zoonosis caused by *Francisella tularensis*. The disease has been called "rabbit fever," "deerfly fever" and "plague-like illness of ground squirrels."[7] The causative organism was isolated on coagulated egg medium in 1912 by McCoy and named *Bacterium tularense*, after Tulare County, California, the site of discovery. The current name, *Francisella*, was given in honor of Dr. Edward Francis, a lifelong student of tularemia, who was a major contributor to our understanding of this disease.[9]

CAUSATIVE ORGANISM

F. tularensis is a small (0.2 X 0.7 μm), nonmotile, nonencapsulated, nonsporulating, pleomorphic, bipolar staining, gram-negative rod. The organism frequently stains poorly and is a strict aerobe. An enriched medium is required for propagation. The organism withstands dessication and low temperatures well and is extremely infectious.[13]

CLINICAL MANIFESTATIONS

The clinical picture of tularemia in humans varies according to the route of infection, the infecting dose and the biotype of the infecting organism (A or B). The incubation period is 3-5 days (range: 1-14). The most common form of infection, ulceroglandular tularemia (80% of reported cases), presents with an indolent ulcer at the entry site and painful regional lymphadenopathy. Rabbit-associated cases usually have hand or finger lesion(s), while approximately 80% of tick-associated infections have a primary lesion on the legs, trunk or genitalia. The ulcer may not be apparent, resulting in a glandular form of the disease.

The remaining 20% of tularemia cases are distributed among the typhoidal, pneumonic, oculoglandular and oropharyngeal forms.[6] Pericarditis, peritonitis, meningitis and osteomyelitis are rarely reported. Rhabdomyolysis, hepatitis and renal failure have been described recently.[7] Nonspecific findings of fever, chills, malaise, fatigue, headache, myalgias and prostration are common to all forms of tularemia. Rash has been reported in up to 20% of the cases with papular and vesicopapular eruptions, erythema nodosum and erythema multiforme being most common.

THERAPY

Streptomycin is the drug of choice and is usually given in a dose of 15-20 mg/kg/day for 10-14 days. Gentamicin (5 mg/kg/day) may be an acceptable alternative to streptomycin.[11] The therapeutic value of other aminoglycosides is unknown. Tetracycline and chloramphenicol are also active, but clinical relapses are more common with these drugs than with streptomycin. Erythromycin has been used with success in a few recently reported cases.[14] Penicillin G, ampicillin, cephalothin and sulfa drugs are not active against *F. tularensis* and are ineffective in treatment of the disease. Some of the third generation cephalosporins are very active in vitro, but no clinical experience has been reported so far.[1] Susceptibility testing is unnecessary in routine practice. The mortality of appropriately treated tularemia has been less than 1% in recent years.

EPIDEMIOLOGY

Tularemia is a disease of wild animals, perpetuated primarily by their ectoparasites. Man is only incidentally infected. Infection in humans follows the handling of infected animals, bites by blood-sucking arthropods, ingestion of improperly cooked meat or contaminated water and inhalation of airborne organisms. Recently there have been reports of a number of cases of tularemia resulting from bites or scratches by cats whose mouth parts had been contaminated by eating infected animals.[8] In the United States the most important reservoir hosts are rabbits, hares and muskrats. Vectorborne tularemia is transmitted primarily by ticks and deer flies. Many other wild mammals, domestic animals, birds, amphibians, fish and invertebrates have been infected. *F. tularensis* has been recovered from mud and water from streams and wells. Most human cases are sporadic, but clusters and epidemics of various sizes have been reported. The largest numbers of cases in the United States have been reported from Arkansas, Missouri, Texas,

Utah and Tennessee. Tickborne cases predominate in the spring and summer months, while rabbit-associated cases increase in the winter months.

PUBLIC HEALTH SIGNIFICANCE, PREVENTION AND CONTROL

The incidence of human tularemia in the United States has declined steadily since 1939 to levels of 0.6-1.3/1,000,000 population; however, the disease is still responsible for appreciable morbidity in some parts of the world and among certain occupational groups. Critical at-risk groups in the United States are hunters and their families, fur processors, microbiology laboratory workers and outdoor enthusiasts. Inanimate objects contaminated with *Francisella* have been implicated in transmission to man.[7] The risk of person-to-person transmission is minimal and infected patients need not be isolated. To minimize the risk of tularemia, people should avoid contact with wild animals or tick-infested areas.

Tularemia is among the leading causes of laboratory-acquired infections. Bacteriology personnel attempting isolation or working with *F. tularensis* should be protected with masks and surgical gloves and all work should be performed in a biological safety cabinet.

Inactivated tularemia vaccines are not effective. Live, attenuated vaccine modifies the severity of the disease but does not provide complete protection. The incidence of typhoidal tularemia, but not of the ulceroglandular form, was drastically reduced in laboratory personnel immunized with live attenuated vaccine.[4] Immunity is cell-mediated and longlasting. Humoral immunity plays little or no role. Laboratory workers frequently exposed to *F. tularensis* and other occupationally exposed individuals are candidates for immunization. The vaccine is available by consultation with the Centers for Disease Control. Immunity following natural infection is incomplete. Repeated episodes of cutaneous route reinfection have been reported, including four episodes of ulceroglandular tularemia in Dr. Edward Francis. *F. tularensis* is quite susceptible to disinfection. It can be killed with heating to 56°C or with detergent.

DIAGNOSTIC PROCEDURES

Microscopic Methods

Biopsy of various organs may reveal microabscesses and/or granulomas and giant cells, and may resemble a tuberculous or fungal infection. Conventional microscopic examination of dye-stained clinical specimens is unproductive. The organisms are very small, occur singly or in clumps, both intracellularly and extracellularly and have a hint of bipolar staining.

Direct or indirect fluorescent antibody tests are rapid and specific for identification of *F. tularensis* in smears of exudates, tissue impressions and tissue sections. Materials for fluorescent-antibody staining are available commercially.

Primary Isolation and Culture

Blood, sputum (if pneumonia is present) and scrapings from skin ulcers or conjunctival lesions should be taken prior to administration of antibiotics. *F. tularensis* is rarely recovered from blood except early in infection and in untreated fulminant disease. Fluctuant lymph nodes should be aspirated and cultured. Suspected sources of infection, such as animal carcasses, water or ticks can readily be cultured.

Cystine glucose blood agar (CGBA) is the medium of choice. It is available commercially or can be prepared in the laboratory, but is rarely available for routine use in an average clinical laboratory. Commercially available chocolate agars with supplements containing cysteine or cystine also may be satisfactory for growth but often require a prolonged incubation period (7-10 days).[5,13] On either medium, growth appears as small (1 mm), smooth, gray, opaque colonies adhering to the surface of the media (Figure 31:1, see color plate). A small zone of partial hemolysis usually surrounds the colonies on CGBA.[13]

Thayer-Martin medium and other selective, antibiotic-containing media have been successfully employed for the isolation of *F. tularensis* from clinical specimens containing mixed flora (sputum, throat swabs).[2] Occasional isolates of *F. tularensis* have been fortuitously recovered on charcoal yeast extract agar employed for isolation of *Legionella* species.[14] The growth of *F. tularensis* in blood cultures is slow, and may fail to be detected in a radiometric system (BACTEC). Acridine orange stains and routine blind subcultures on supplemented chocolate agar are useful.[5]

F. tularensis can be isolated readily by the subcutaneous inoculation of specimens into mice, hamsters, rabbits or guinea pigs. Pure cultures can be obtained from the spleen of a sacrificed animal by subinoculation onto suitable bacteriologic media. Animal inoculation should be attempted only if adequate isolation facilities are available for housing highly infectious animals. Animal inoculation is not required nor recommended for the routine identification of *F. tularensis* isolates.[13]

Methods for Identification

Smooth gray colonies that appear on recommended media in 24-96 h at 37°C are suggestive of *F. tularensis*. A Gram stain of the growth usually reveals closely aligned but individual, minute, gram-negative, bipolar-staining organisms. Characteristic morphology is more readily observed in

Giemsa-stained preparations. Poor or absent growth on blood-containing media without cystine is an additional useful marker.[14] Important differential criteria for the identification of *F. tularensis* are: absence of growth on ordinary media and little or no growth on blood-enriched media that lack added cysteine or cystine, relatively slow colonial growth on special media, distinctive cellular morphology (small size, in particular) and staining properties, specific fluorescent antibody reaction and slide agglutination with specific antiserum.[13] *F. tularensis* produces acid but not gas from glucose, maltose, mannose and fructose. Biochemical characterization, however, is neither necessary nor recommended for identification.

Serological confirmation is routinely and rapidly accomplished by slide agglutination. All strains of *F. tularensis* agglutinate with specific antiserum. Commercially available concentrated antigen can be used undiluted to prepare a positive control; the negative control should show no clumping. Crossreactions are rare and are characterized by slow and incomplete clumping.

Markers of Epidemiology

There are two recognized biovars or subspecies: *F. tularensis* var. (biovar) *tularensis* (type A) and *F. tularensis* var. (biovar) *palaearctica* (type B). Type A is found only in North America. It is highly virulent for rabbits and man, ferments glycerol and is citrulline ureidase-positive. Type A is most often associated with disease transmitted by rabbits and ticks. Type B is found in most countries of the Northern Hemisphere. It is less virulent than Type A and produces a mild, often subclinical disease in humans. Type B is citrulline ureidase-negative, does not ferment glycerol and has been isolated most often from aquatic animals (beavers, muskrats, voles) and natural running water. Both Type A and B can be tickborne and coexist in the same ecosystem.[10] The two subspecies are indistinguishable antigenically.

Serologic Tests

Blood specimens for serological tests should be taken as soon as tularemia is suspected and 2-3 weeks later for convalescent titers.

A tube agglutination, or microagglutination test, is the most useful procedure for demonstrating the presence of, or rise in, antibody titer. Precipitin, hemagglutination, complement fixation and enzyme-linked immunosorbent assay (ELISA) tests for detection of serum antibodies have also been described. The ELISA is very promising because of high sensitivity but is not commercially available.[12]

The agglutination test with patient serum is standard. Agglutination titers are usually negative in the first week of illness and are positive in 50-70% of the patients after two weeks of illness. A 4-fold rise in titer is diagnostic of infection; a single convalescent titer of 1:160 or greater is diagnostic of past or current infection. The titers may remain elevated at diagnostic levels for many years after the acute episode. Low-titered crossreactions can occur with antigen of *Brucella* species; therefore, a control with a *Brucella* antigen should be included. Crossreacting antibodies usually do not show as high a titer as the specific tularemia titer during an active infection.

The tularemia skin test is more sensitive than the agglutination test during the early acute illness and remains positive longer after acute infections.[3] The antigen, however, is not commercially available.

The cell-mediated immunity can also be measured by a whole-blood lymphocyte stimulation test. The test is very sensitive and specific in early tularemia, but is time-consuming and, therefore, impractical for clinical diagnostic purposes.

CLINICAL SIGNIFICANCE OF LABORATORY TESTS

Isolation of *F. tularensis*, or demonstration of a specific 4-fold rise in titer confirms a diagnosis of tularemia. Demonstration of a single high titer (>1:160) in an appropriate clinical setting is highly suggestive.

REFERENCES

1. Baker CN, Hollis DG, Thornsberry C. Antimicrobial susceptibility testing of *Francisella tularensis* with a modified Mueller-Hinton broth. J Clin Microbiol 1985;22:212-15.
2. Berdal BP, Soderlund E. Cultivation and isolation of *Francisella tularensis* on selective chocolate agar, as used routinely for the isolation of gonococci. Acta Pathol Microbiol Scand 1977;85:108-9.
3. Buchanan TM, Brooks GF, Brachman PS. The tularemia skin test. Ann Intern Med 1971;74:336-43.
4. Burke DS. Immunization against tularemia: analysis of the effectiveness of live *Francisella tularensis* vaccine in prevention of laboratory-acquired tularemia. J Infect Dis 1977;135:55-60.
5. Centers for Disease Control. Tularemia pneumonia-Tennessee. Morbid Mortal Weekly Rep 1983;32:262-9.
6. Dienst FT. Tularemia: a perusal of three hundred thirty-nine cases. J Louisiana State Med Soc 1963;115:114-27.
7. Evans ME, Gregory DW, Schaffner W, McGee ZA. Tularemia: a 30-year experience with 88 cases. Medicine 1985;64:251-69.
8. Evans ME, McGee ZA, Hunter PT, Schaffner W. Tularemia and the tomcat. JAMA 1981;246:1343.
9. Francis E. Tularemia. JAMA 1925;84:1243-50.
10. Markowitz LE, Hynes NA, Crus DP, et al. Tick-borne tularemia: an outbreak of lymphadenopathy in children. JAMA 1985;254:2922-5.
11. Mason WL, Eigelsbach HT, Little SF, Bates JH. Treatment of tularemia, including pulmonary tularemia with gentamicin. Am Rev Respir Dis 1980;121:39-45.

12. Viljanen MK, Nurmi T. Salminen A. Enzyme-linked immunosorbent assay (ELISA) with bacterial sonicate antigen for IgM, IgA and IgG antibodies to *Francisella tularensis*: comparison with bacterial agglutination test and ELISA with lipopolysaccharide antigen. J Infect Dis 1983;148:715-20.
13. Weaver RE, Hollis DG, Bottone EJ. Gram-negative fermentative bacteria and *Francisella tularensis*. In: Lennette EH, Balows A, Hauser WJ Jr, Shadomy HJ, eds. Manual of clinical microbiology. Washington, DC: American Society for Microbiology, 1985:316-19.
14. Westerman EL, McDonald J. Tularemia pneumonia mimicking Legionnaires' disease: isolation of organism on CYE agar and successful treatment with erythromycin. South Med J 1983;76:1169-70.

CHAPTER 32

VAGINOSIS, CHANCROID AND GRANULOMA INGUINALE

Carol A. Spiegel, Ph.D.

BACTERIAL VAGINOSIS

INTRODUCTION

The clinical syndrome now known as bacterial vaginosis (BV) was first described by Gardner and Dukes in 1955.[7] It has also been known as nonspecific vaginitis, *Haemophilus* vaginitis, *Gardnerella*-associated vaginosis and anaerobic vaginosis.

CAUSATIVE ORGANISMS

No single species has been identified as the etiologic agent of BV. When Gardner and Dukes described the syndrome, they also identified *Gardnerella vaginalis* (formerly known as *Haemophilus vaginalis* and *Corynebacterium vaginale*) as the etiologic agent. Subsequent studies using a selective, differential medium for isolation of *G. vaginalis* showed that the organism is present in almost all women with BV, but it is also present in >50% of women without vaginosis.[19]

Other recent studies have shown an association of BV with a mixed anaerobic flora. The organisms include *Bacteroides bivius, B. disiens*, black-pigmented *Bacteroides*, peptostreptococci, *Mobiluncus curtisii* and *M. mulieris*.[15,17,18] Few or no facultative lactobacilli (the predominant organism in the normal vagina) are present. The anaerobes, with the possible exception of *Mobiluncus* spp., may be present as part of the endogenous vaginal flora. Although the pathogenesis of this syndrome has not yet been defined, it is thought to be a result of this inversion in the quantities of organisms which make up the endogenous flora, i.e., the usually predominant lactobacilli are replaced by *G. vaginalis* and the anaerobic bacteria, usually minor components of the endogenous flora.

The prevalence of vaginal colonization by *Mycoplasma hominis* is increased in BV as is the prevalence of serum antibody to this agent.[9] However, response to appropriate therapy with metronidazole does not predict eradication of *M. hominis* from the vagina.

CLINICAL MANIFESTATIONS

BV is a very common, generally mild syndrome, usually characterized by an increased vaginal discharge. The patient may notice a "fishy" odor from this discharge, especially immediately after intercourse. Vaginal irritation may occur. The presence of symptoms, however, does not correspond well with a clinical diagnosis of BV. In one study, 54% of women with BV had no symptoms while 32% of normal women were symptomatic.[1] A clinical diagnosis of BV is made by examining the vaginal discharge and detecting at least three of the following four characteristics: (1) thin, homogeneous, adherent discharge, (2) pH greater than 4.5, (3) clue cells and (4) a fishy odor on addition of 10% KOH.[1]

THERAPY[3]

The drug of choice for BV is metronidazole (500 mg by mouth twice a day for 7 days). Approximately 12% of patients so treated will have a recurrence of the syndrome in the subsequent 6 weeks. An alternate mode of therapy is ampicillin or amoxicillin (500 mg by mouth 4 times a day for 7 days). The recurrence rate is 40-60% in patients so treated, but it may be used when metronidazole is contraindicated, as in pregnancy. There is currently no indication that treatment of male partners affects the recurrence rate in the female. Sulfa creams, often used in the past to treat this syndrome, are not effective.

EPIDEMIOLOGY

The epidemiology of BV has not been well studied and sexual transmission has not been proven. Piot et al[10] determined the biotype of *G. vaginalis* in females with BV and their asymptomatic male partners. They found that the same biotype was present in both the female and her partner for 24 h following intercourse. The anaerobic flora of the male urethra is difficult to determine and no good studies have been published.

Sexual transmission of BV has been implied by anecdotal reports of women who report the onset of symptoms just after changing sexual partners.

However, unpublished clinical trials have shown that treatment of the male partner with metronidazole does not prevent reinfection of the female.

PUBLIC HEALTH SIGNIFICANCE, PREVENTION AND CONTROL

In one report of the prevalence of bacterial vaginosis in a university student health population, 20% of the women attending the women's clinic for any reason had a clinical diagnosis of BV.[1] Half of these were asymptomatic. In a sexually transmitted disease clinic where a greater percentage of the women are attending because of vaginal symptoms, the prevalence is even higher.

BV, itself, usually causes very mild symptoms, but because of its high prevalence it is of public health significance. In addition, many of the organisms associated with BV are associated with anaerobic pelvic inflammatory disease and postpartum endometritis. In addition, there is accumulating evidence that women with BV in the third trimester of pregnancy are at increased risk of premature rupture of membranes, thus also putting the fetus at risk.

BV may or may not represent a "sexually transmitted" disease. Sexual activity may not transmit the agents but rather alter the environment to allow an inversion of the flora; or this inversion may occur independent of sexual activity but be associated with it only temporally. These are major questions that need to be answered before adequate prevention and control measures can be designed.

DIAGNOSTIC PROCEDURES

These tests, listed under Clinical Manifestations as characteristic of BV, may be performed in the clinic rather than in the clinical laboratory.

(1) Abnormal Discharge: The discharge is described as thin, homogeneous and adherent.

(2) pH: The pH of vaginal fluid is tested using nitrazine paper. A pH of greater than 4.5 is considered abnormal.

(3)Clue Cells: A suspension of vaginal fluid in saline is examined for the presence of squamous epithelial cells covered with coccobacillary organisms such that the cell border is obliterated. (Fig. 32:1. See color plate.)

(4) Amine Odor Test: When 10% potassium hydroxide is added to vaginal fluid on a slide or in a tube, a "fishy" amine odor is detected.

Other tests may be performed in the clinical laboratory.

Direct Gram Stain

A direct Gram stain of vaginal fluid can be used to detect the inversion of flora.[16] Large gram-positive rods are the *Lactobacillus* morphotype. (Fig. 32:2A. See color plate.) When these are seen alone, or in combination with small gram-variable rods (the *Gardnerella* morphotype) (Fig. 32:2B. See color plate.), but with no other morphotypes, the smear is interpreted as normal. When a more mixed flora is present, including not only the *Gardnerella* morphotype but also other gram-negative and gram-positive bacteria, such as curved rods, gram-negative rods, fusiforms and gram-positive cocci, and when the *Lactobacillus* morphotype is present only in low numbers (0-5 per oil immersion field), the smear is interpreted as consistent with BV. (Fig. 32:2C. See color plate.)

Gas-Liquid Chromatography

The inversion in the flora can also be detected by this method.[15] *Lactobacillus* spp., which are lactic acid-producing organisms, predominate in the normal vagina. During BV they are replaced by *Bacteroides* spp. (succinate producers), butyrate-producing *Peptostreptococcus* spp. (acetate and butyrate producers), *Mobiluncus* spp. (acetate and succinate producers) and other anaerobic organisms. An increase in the concentration of *G. vaginalis* (an acetate producer) also occurs. This change in the flora is reflected by a change in the vaginal acids, which can be detected by gas-liquid chromatography.

Thin Layer Chromatography

The fishy odor associated with BV, detected upon addition of 10% potassium hydroxide to vaginal fluid, is due to the presence of amines which volatilize at an alkaline pH.[4] Putrescine and cadaverine are the two most prevalent amines in BV. These can be detected and identified by thin layer chromatography, which is more sensitive than the Amine Odor Test.

CLINICAL SIGNIFICANCE OF LABORATORY TESTS

BV is not diagnosed by culture of a particular pathogen but by clinic or laboratory detection of specific signs of the syndrome. The clinical diagnosis takes considerable expertise. The amine odor can be subtle, and it takes training to appropriately identify clue cells and the characteristic homogeneous discharge. The clinical diagnosis relies on the presence of three of four signs to provide acceptable specificity. For instance, the presence of menstrual blood or semen in the vaginal fluid will increase the pH which would lead to a false diagnosis of BV if it were the only criterion required.

Several laboratory tests have been described for diagnosis of BV. Thin-layer chromatography is sensitive and specific but is not cost- and time-effective. Gas-liquid chromatography would be a reasonable test if the instrumentation (a gas chromatograph with a flame ionization detector) were available. The direct Gram stain is the most cost- and time-effective laboratory test available, but one must be aware of its limitations. Adequate training in slide interpretation is necessary. Some Gram stains will be atypical. For instance, gram-positive cocci in chains or clusters may predominate. In such circumstances, a diagnosis other than BV should be considered.

Culture is not recommended as a diagnostic tool. The prevalence of *G. vaginalis* in women without BV obviates its usefulness as a diagnostic test or as a test of cure. Anaerobic bacteria are also part of the endogenous flora and so culture for them is not contributory. *Mobiluncus* spp. can be detected microscopically in about 50% of the cases of BV. If improved methods for their detection indicate a significantly greater prevalence in BV than in the healthy state, growth of *Mobiluncus* or their detection by some other method may provide a diagnostic test in the future.

CHANCROID

INTRODUCTION

Chancroid (soft chancre) was so named by Brasseau in 1852 to differentiate it from the hard chancre of syphilis. It is one of the "classic" sexually transmitted diseases.

CAUSATIVE ORGANISM

Chancroid is caused by *Haemophilus ducreyi*, first described by Ducrey in 1888. *H. ducreyi* is a gram-negative, rod-shaped, fastidious organism which requires X factor (hemin), serum and additional nutritional supplements to grow. In addition, 1-5% CO_2, a temperature of 33°C and an atmosphere saturated with moisture are required. It has been suggested that because *H. ducreyi* shows minimal DNA homology (0-6%) with other members of the genus, it be removed from the genus *Haemophilus*.[2]

CLINICAL MANIFESTATIONS[11]

In males, chancroid is characterized by the presence of one or more painful, irregular, nonindurated, often foul-smelling ulcers. These are typically located on the penis. Characteristic lesions are undermined and have a necrotic irregular base covered by a gray-yellow exudate. Some lesions resemble furuncles and others superficial ulcers. In women, ulcers are usually more numerous, less painful and tend to occur on the cervix and near the anus. About 40% of patients have uni- or bilateral lymphadenopathy. Without appropriate therapy, the lesions will suppurate and buboes will form. The ulcerative lesions of chancroid, syphilis, herpes simplex and granuloma inguinale cannot accurately be distinguished on physical examination.

THERAPY

Therapeutic regimens for the treatment of chancroid have been reviewed by Schmid.[13] Although resistance to sulfonamides is common, *H. ducreyi* is susceptible to the combination of trimethoprim and sulfamethoxazole, except for strains with high-level resistance to trimethoprim. Such strains have begun to appear in Thailand. Single-dose therapy with ceftriaxone was at least 94% effective: single-dose therapy with cefotaxime was less effective, presumably because of its shorter half-life. Penicillin and ampicillin are not effective therapeutic agents because *H. ducreyi* contains a plasmid which codes for beta-lactamase. One would predict then that treatment with clavulanic acid, a beta-lactamase inhibitor, and amoxicillin would be effective. Two small studies which have examined this issue reported cures in over 95% of cases.

In three studies evaluating thiamphenicol (each using a different treatment regimen), cure was achieved in at least 89% of cases. The quinolones and roxithromycin are active in vitro, but clinical trials are needed for these agents.

The Centers for Disease Control (CDC) recommends erythromycin (500 mg by mouth 4 times a day for 7 days) or ceftriaxone (250 mg intramuscularly in a single dose).[3] Alternate therapies include trimethoprim-sulfamethoxazole and amoxicillin-clavulanic acid.

EPIDEMIOLOGY

Chancroid is endemic in parts of the world such as East, Central and South Africa where it is the most common cause of genital ulcers. In the United States, the number of cases of chancroid peaked at 5000 in 1947 and then declined. Since 1981, the number of cases has increased due to outbreaks in California, Florida, New York, Boston, Pennsylvania and Texas. Epidemics have most often occurred in hispanic and black communities where prostitutes have played an important role in transmission.

PUBLIC HEALTH SIGNIFICANCE, PREVENTION AND CONTROL

Chancroid is currently endemic in Florida and New York. Other recent epidemics have been terminated because of intensive surveillance, contact tracing, treatment of symptomatic and asymptomatic sexual partners and treatment of symptomatic and asymptomatic prostitutes. The role of asymptomatic carriers in disease transmission needs definition. Based on our current understanding of the transmission of chancroid, control measures should be aimed at prostitutes. The role of military personnel returning from endemic areas such as Singapore should also be considered.

DIAGNOSTIC PROCEDURES

Because the agent of a genital ulcer cannot be accurately determined from the appearance of the lesion, laboratory testing plays an important role both in diagnosis and control.

Rapid Methodology

No direct detection methods are commercially available at this time; however, research on two immunological procedures has recently been published.[12] An indirect fluorescent method using monoclonal antibodies to outer membrane proteins was used to detect *H. ducreyi* in samples from patients with genital ulcers during chancroid outbreaks in Orlando, Florida and New York City. A dot immunobinding method was also evaluated. In this method, the patient's serum antibody which has been bound to *H. ducreyi* outer membranes is detected with immunoperoxidase-labeled antihuman globulin. This latter method detected 55 and 83%, respectively, of patients in Orlando and New York with a clinical diagnosis of chancroid. These methods offer much promise as future diagnostic tests.

Primary Isolation and Culture

Two media are recommended for primary isolation of *H. ducreyi*,[6] enriched gonococcal (GcHbS) and enriched Mueller-Hinton agars (MHHb). In a study comparing these two media for primary isolation of *H. ducreyi* from 111 patients with genital ulcers, 41% were culture-positive on both media, 7% on MHHb only and 20% on GcHbS only. An additional 7 patients were culture-positive when resampled 48 h later. When culture-negative patients who had either antimicrobial therapy prior to culture, spontaneous remission of their ulcers or a diagnosis of syphilis were eliminated, culture was >90% sensitive.

Both media should be incubated at 33-35°C in a water-saturated environment containing 1-5% CO_2. A candle jar containing moist toweling works well. Typical yellow-gray, irregular, adherent colonies which can be pushed over the agar surface usually appear after 48 h of incubation. Cultures should be held 5 days before being called negative. On Gram stain, small gram-negative rods in long parallel rows resembling a school of fish are seen. Organisms demonstrating this colonial and Gram stain morphology which require X (hemin) but not V (NAD) factor can be identified as *H. ducreyi*.

CLINICAL SIGNIFICANCE OF LABORATORY TESTS

A positive culture for *H. ducreyi* is diagnostic for chancroid. The patient, whether symptomatic or not, should be treated, as should all known sexual partners.

GRANULOMA INGUINALE[8,14]

INTRODUCTION

The first written description of granuloma inguinale was made in 1882 by K. McLeod, a surgeon in Calcutta, India. McLeod called it serpiginous ulceration of the groin. It has also been called the lupoid form of the so-called groin ulceration, ulcerating granuloma of the pudenda, granuloma inguinale tropicum, Donovanosis and granuloma venereum.

CAUSATIVE ORGANISM

The etiologic agent of granuloma inguinale is *Calymmatobacterium granulomatis*, formerly called *Donovania granulomatis*. It has been grown in the yolk sac of living chick embryos and in complex artificial media, but no medium is readily available for its cultivation. The organism is encapsulated, nonmotile and has a corrugated surface structure when visualized by electron microscopy. These characteristics suggest a relationship to members of the genus *Klebsiella*.

CLINICAL MANIFESTATIONS

The disease is characterized by formation of a firm papule which may (1) erode to form a beefy red ulcer which bleeds profusely, (2) be raised and verrucous with or without an ulcer, (3) become necrotic or (4) present as a band-like scar around the infected area. Disease is not associated with lymphadenopathy unless the lesions become secondarily infected. Lesions are usually located on the genitalia but may be found elsewhere, especially in the oral cavity, where they may be confused with actinomycosis.[5] This is thought to be spread by autoinoculation.

THERAPY

In the preantibiotic era, lesions were removed surgically, often only to recur. Patients usually respond well to oxy- or chlortetracycline, the drugs of choice, given 2 g/day by mouth for 10-14 days. Alternate therapeutic agents include trimethoprim-sulfamethoxazole, chloramphenicol and streptomycin. Penicillin is not effective.

EPIDEMIOLOGY

Granuloma inguinale is endemic in parts of India, southern China, islands of the South Pacific, northern Australia, the west coast of Africa, Guinea, Brazil and the West Indies. It is predominantly a disease of dark-skinned people, rarely occurring in Caucasians. The epidemiology is poorly understood. It is considered a sexually transmitted disease because it is most prevalent during the years of greatest sexual activity and because lesions most commonly occur on the genitalia. Infection is transmitted in only 12-52% of cases of known exposure, suggesting either that the organism is transmitted poorly or that resistance to infection is high. The average incubation period is thought to be about 17 days but a very broad range of times has been reported.

PUBLIC HEALTH SIGNIFICANCE, PREVENTION AND CONTROL

Although it was much more common in the black population of the southern United States 40-50 years ago, granuloma inguinale is now rare in the U.S. Because it is not a reportable disease, the actual prevalence is unknown. The reservoir is also unknown, although the organism may be part of the fecal flora. Current control measures are limited to treatment of those with documented disease.

DIAGNOSTIC PROCEDURES

A Wright or Giemsa stain of material which has been collected by scraping the lesion is examined. The organisms, so called Donovan bodies, are seen within mononuclear cells (macrophages). They are blue, rod-shaped (1.0-1.5 by 0.5-0.7 μm) organisms, often with a surrounding pink capsule. Vacuolization of the cytoplasm is common and accumulations of dark blue chromatin occur at the poles of the cells. A smaller coccoid or diplococcal form resembling a closed safety pin may occur.

CLINICAL SIGNIFICANCE OF LABORATORY TESTS

The presence of Donovan bodies is diagnostic and the patient should be treated.

REFERENCES

1. Amsel R, Totten PA, Spiegel CA, Chen KCS, Eschenbach D, Holmes KK. Nonspecific vaginitis: Diagnostic criteria and microbial and epidemiologic associations. Am J Med 1983;74:14-22.
2. Casin I, Grimont F, Grimont PAD, Sanson-Le Pors M-J. Lack of deoxyribonucleic acid relatedness between *Haemophilus ducreyi* and other *Haemophilus* species. Int J Syst Bacteriol 1985;35:23-5.
3. Centers for Disease Control. STD treatment guidelines. Morbid Mortal Weekly Rep 1985;34S:75-108.
4. Chen KCS, Culbertson NJ, Knapp JS, Kenny GE, Holmes KK. Rapid method for simultaneous detection of arginine dihydrolase system and amino acid decarboxylases in microorganisms. J Clin Microbiol 1982;16:909-19.
5. Coovadia YM, Steinberg JL, Kharsany A. Granuloma inguinale (donovanosis) of the oral cavity. S Afr Med J 1985;68:815-17.
6. Dylewski J, Nsanze H, Maitha G, Ronald A. Laboratory diagnosis of *Haemophilus ducreyi*: Sensitivity of culture media. Diag Microbiol Infect Dis 1986;4:241-5.
7. Gardner HL, Dukes CD. *Hemophilus vaginalis* vaginitis. Am J Obstet Gynecol 1955;69:962-76.
8. Kampmeier RH. Granuloma inguinale. Sex Trans Dis 1984;11:318-21.
9. Paavonen J, Miettinen A, Stevens CE, Chen KCS, Holmes KK. *Mycoplasma hominis* in nonspecific vaginitis. Sex Trans Dis 1983;10:271-5.
10. Piot P, van Dyck E, Peeters M, Hale J, Totten PA, Holmes KK. Biotypes of *Gardnerella vaginalis*. J Clin Microbiol 1984;20:677-9.
11. Ronald AR, Plummer FA. Chancroid and *Haemophilus ducreyi*. Ann Intern Med 1985;102:705-7.
12. Schalla WO, Sanders LL, Schmid GP, Tam MR, Morse SA. Use of dot-immunobinding and immunofluorescence assays to investigate clinically suspected cases of chancroid. J Infect Dis 1986;153:879-87.
13. Schmid GP. The treatment of chancroid. JAMA 1986;255:1757-62.
14. Sehgal VN, Prasad ALS. Donovanosis. Int J Dermatol 1986;25:8-16.
15. Spiegel CA, Amsel R, Eschenbach DA, Schoenknecht FD, Holmes KK. Anaerobic bacteria in nonspecific vaginitis. N Engl J Med 1980;303:601-7.
16. Spiegel CA, Amsel R, Holmes KK. Diagnosis of bacterial vaginosis by direct Gram stain of vaginal fluid. J Clin Microbiol 1983;18:170-7.
17. Spiegel CA, Eschenbach DA, Amsel R, Holmes KK. Curved anaerobic bacteria in bacterial (nonspecific) vaginosis and their response to antimicrobial therapy. J Infect Dis 1983;148:817-22.
18. Spiegel CA, Roberts M. *Mobiluncus* gen. nov., *Mobiluncus curtisii* subspecies *curtisii* sp. nov., *Mobiluncus curtisii* subspecies *holmesii* subsp. nov., and *Mobiluncus mulieris* sp. nov., curved rods from the human vagina. Int J Syst Bacteriol 1984;34:177-84.
19. Totten PA, Amsel R, Hale J, Piot P, Holmes KK. Selective differential human blood bilayer media for isolation of *Gardnerella (Haemophilus) vaginalis*. J Clin Microbiol 1982;15:141-7.

CHAPTER 33

VIBRIO INFECTIONS

David L. Tison, Ph.D.

INTRODUCTION

References in the ancient medical literature describing clinical features similar to epidemic or Asiatic cholera can be found dating back to the time of Hippocrates. Authentic descriptions of cholera as a disease entity originated from the early 1500s. Accurate documentation of the epidemiology of cholera began in ernest with the onset of the first documented cholera pandemic in 1817. During this pandemic (1817-1823), cholera spread from Bengal and India east to China, Indonesia and Japan and west to southeastern Europe. The second cholera pandemic beginning in 1829 saw the global spread of this disease. Cholera spread from Bengal and India to China, Persia and Russia. From these areas the scourge of cholera spread throughout Europe, Arabia, East and North Africa and in 1832 reached the shores of North America, where it quickly spread to Central and South America. We are currently in the midst of the seventh cholera pandemic. Cholera was reported from 37 countries in 1982 with 54,856 cases worldwide.[7]

An infectious etiology was suspected for cholera by many pioneering bacteriologists. The work of Neale, Boehm, Henle, Snow, Budd, Pacini, Macnamara and finally Koch and his colleagues established a bacterial etiology for cholera. The organism was described by Pacini in 1854 and named *Vibrio cholera*, which was subsequently amended to *V. cholerae*. It is interesting to note that it was Koch, through his culture and isolation of organisms from intestinal lesions, who was ultimately successful in establishing the bacterial etiology. While Roux and colleagues, following the methods of Pasteur in attempting to reproduce the disease in animals, failed to identify the agent of cholera.[15]

Other *Vibrio* species infecting humans have been described relatively recently. *Vibrio parahaemolyticus* was first recognized as a human pathogen in 1950 when a foodborne outbreak of gastroenteritis occurred in Japan.[10] Other *Vibrio* species associated with gastroenteritis or soft tissue infections have been described since then.

CAUSATIVE ORGANISMS

V. cholerae strains typically associated with Asiatic or epidemic cholera are of the O1 serovar and toxigenic (produce cholera toxin). Serovars of *V. cholerae* other than the O1 have been referred to as non-cholera or nonagglutinating (NAG) vibrios. The majority of non-O1 *V. cholerae* strains do not produce cholera toxin (are nontoxigenic). Non-O1 *V. cholerae* strains most commonly cause gastroenteritis (aquired from consuming shellfish) or wound infections due to exposure to brackish water.[9,13]

V. parahaemolyticus is most commonly a cause of gastroenteritis but has also been isolated from wounds. *V. alginolyticus*, most frequently found in cases of wound infection and external otitis, was previously classified as biogroup 2 of *V. parahaemolyticus*. A particularly virulent organism, *V. vulnificus*, causes rapidly progressing wound infections or a primary septicemia which is frequently fatal. *V. vulnificus* has been referred to in the literature as "the lactose-positive, Lac+ or L+ vibrio," was designated as Centers for Disease Control (CDC) group EF-3, and was originally described as *Beneckea vulnifica*.[17]

Other *Vibrio* species encountered less frequently include *V. mimicus* (formerly classified as sucrose-negative *V. cholerae*), *V. fluvialis* (initially described as the Group F vibrio and designated as CDC group EF-6), *V. furnissii* (formerly classified as biogroup 2 of *V. fluvialis*), *V. hollisae* (designated as CDC group EF-13) and *V. damsela* (previously CDC group EF-5). *Vibrio* species isolated from single cases of human infections include *V. metschnikovii* (formerly CDC Enteric group 16) and *V. cincinnatiensis*. Other *Vibrio* species formerly found only in the environment have recently been implicated in human infection. A summary of pathogenic *Vibrio* species and the diseases they cause is shown in Table 33:1.

CLINICAL MANIFESTATIONS

Epidemic or Asiatic cholera continues to be a significant public health problem affecting tens of thousands of people worldwide each year. Cholera is characterized by voluminous loss of fluids due to the action of cholera toxin in the small bowel. Cholera toxin is an oligomeric protein (mol wt 84,000) composed of an A unit (mol wt 30,000) and five B units (mol wt 10,000). One B unit binds to the ganglioside G_{M1} receptor on the membrane of intestinal epithelial cells while the A_1 subunit activates adenylate cyclase, producing increased levels of cyclic AMP and hypersecretion of water and

Table 33:1. Diseases Caused by Pathogenic *Vibrio* Species

Organism	Primary disease	Other diseases
V. cholerae O1	Cholera	Wound infections
V. cholerae non O1	Gastroenteritis	Wound infections
V. mimicus	Gastroenteritis	Wound infections
V. parahaemolyticus	Gastroenteritis	Wound infections
V. fluvialis	Gastroenteritis	None reported
V. furnissii	Gastroenteritis	None reported
V. hollisae	Gastroenteritis	None reported
V. vulnificus	Septicemia or wound infections	Pneumonia* endometritis*
V. alginolyticus	Wound infections	External otitis
V. damsela	Wound infections	None reported
V. cincinnatiensis	Meningitis*	None reported
V. metschnikovii	Cholecystitis with septicemia*	None reported

* A single case of this type of infection has been reported in the literature.

electrolytes.[8] The outpouring of electrolytes and water produces copious purging, resulting in the severe dehydration associated with the classical clinical presentation of cholera. The initial symptoms of cholera are an increase in peristalsis followed by loose stools, which progress to the watery, mucus-flecked, "rice water" stools characteristic of cholera. Vomiting may occur in the early stages of the disease. There is little abdominal pain although muscle cramping may result from dehydration and electrolyte imbalance. Dehydration, hypovolemic shock, hypoglycemia and metabolic acidosis must all be managed in patients with cholera to prevent death.

The ability to produce cholera toxin is almost exclusively limited to the O1 serovar of *V. cholerae*, although rare strains of non-O1 serovars which carry the cholera toxin gene have been identified.[11] Toxigenic non-O1 *V. cholerae* may produce clinical illness indistinguishable from classical cholera, although these strains are not associated with epidemic cholera. Nontoxigenic *V. cholerae* may also produce gastroenteritis, presumably through the action of toxins other than cholera toxin.[13] Wound or soft tissue infections may also be caused by *V. cholerae*, predominantly by nontoxigenic, non-O1 serovars.[9]

Vibrio mimicus produces gastroenteritis and wound infections identical to non-O1 *V. cholerae* infections. Rare strains have been identified which possess the cholera toxin gene. *V. mimicus* also has somatic antigens in common with a number of non-O1 serovars of *V. cholerae*.

V. parahaemolyticus gastroenteritis is the most common *Vibrio* infection in developed countries. Outbreaks associated with the consumption of contaminated seafood have been documented throughout the world. Symptoms include watery and sometimes bloody diarrhea, abdominal cramps, nausea, vomiting, headache, low-grade fever and chills. Many cases are less severe and the illness is selflimited with a duration of 2-3 days.[2] Extraintestinal infections caused by *V. parahaemolyticus* have also been reported, most of which have been wound or soft tissue infections.

Gastroenteritis caused by *V. hollisae, V. fluvialis* or *V. furnissii* is rare in developed countries. Large numbers of fecal leukocytes and erythrocytes have been present in documented cases. Diarrhea caused by these organisms is generally selflimited with a duration of 1-2 days. Cholera toxin is not produced by these species although other enterotoxins have been identified.

V. vulnificus is a particularly virulent species which causes two distinct clinical presentations. Primary septicemias caused by *V. vulnificus* are frequently associated with consumption of raw oysters[2] while wound or soft tissue infections develop after exposure to sea water. Primary *V. vulnificus* sepsis is a life-threatening infection with a fatality rate near 50%.[2] Many patients have preexisting liver disease which presumably predisposes these individuals to *V. vulnificus* infection, due to increased availability of serum iron. The initial symptom is malaise, which rapidly progresses to fever, chills and prostration. Many patients develop hypotension that may lead to death. The course of the disease progresses at a dramatic rate with less than 24 hours between initial symptoms and intractable hypotension. Frequently, metastatic cutaneous lesions develop, progressing from erythematous or ecchymotic areas to bullae or vesicles which develop into necrotic ulcers. Autopsy findings reveal signs of gram-negative shock, hemorrhage and necrosis of involved muscles and skin. *V. vulnificus* is frequently isolated from the blood and cutaneous lesions of these patients.[17]

Wound infections caused by *V. vulnificus* may be severe but the mortality rate is low compared to that of primary sepsis. Swelling and erythema occur initially, followed by the rapid development of bullae or vesicles, leading to tissue necrosis. Symptoms are usually fever and chills, and in some cases, severe pain. Extensive debridement is often necessary and amputation has been required in some cases.

Wound or soft tissue infections are the primary clinical presentation of *V. alginolyticus* and *V. damsela*. Infections caused by *V. alginolyticus* most commonly involve the external ear, whereas *V. damsela* typically causes purulent wound infections.[17] *V. metschnikovii* has been isolated from a single case of cholecystitis and *V. cincinnatiensis* from a single case of meningitis.

THERAPY

Fluid replacement is the primary therapy for classical cholera as well as for gastroenteritis caused by other *Vibrio* species, especially those which produce cholera toxin. Volumes of isotonic polyelectrolyte solution in excess of one liter per hour for 24 hours or longer may be required to replace the large quantities of water and electrolytes lost during the acute phase of the disease. Antimicrobial therapy may shorten the duration of diarrhea and thereby reduce fluid losses; tetracycline is the drug of choice. Antimicrobial therapy should be reserved for cases in which rehydration therapy alone may not be adequate, since plasmid-mediated antibiotic resistance in *V. cholerae* has been documented. Oral or intravenous fluid and electrolyte replacement remain essential to prevent acidosis and electrolyte imbalances in those patients receiving antibiotics.

Antimicrobial therapy is critical in the treatment of *V. vulnificus* infections, particularly sepsis. Early administration of an aminoglycoside or tetracycline before the onset of hypotension appears to be critical. In vitro antimicrobial susceptibility tests indicate that *V. vulnificus* is susceptible to most antimicrobials used against gram-negative bacteria.[18] However, animal studies indicate that tetracycline may be most effective in vivo.[17] Debridement is generally required in addition to antimicrobial therapy for successful treatment of wound infections. Tetracyclines are also appropriate for treatment of wound infections caused by other *Vibrio* species.

EPIDEMIOLOGY

Endemic areas around the Bay of Bengal have historically been the origin of cholera pandemics. Importation of cholera from endemic areas has been assumed to be the source of cholera in nonendemic areas, particularly when cholera has been identified in developed countries. However, endemic foci of cholera have recently been identified in the United States and Mexico.[3] Asymptomatic carriers of the cholera vibrio may also be an important source of the organism in nonendemic areas. Air travel has recently become a significant mode of transmission, that is, of rapid transport of infected individuals.

The association of cholera and environmental conditions was recognized by Macnamara and described in his classical treatise on cholera, published in 1876. *V. cholerae* persists in the environment when warm water temperature and moderate salinity favor proliferation. Koch, in 1885, attributed the periodicity of epidemics to an acquired immunity lasting 3-4 years. In 1893 Koch described two main types of epidemics; (a) an explosive type, apt to end as abruptly as it started, and (b) a protracted type which commenced slowly and followed an insidiously prolonged course.[15]

Fecal-oral transmission of cholera has been recognized since early investigations of the disease in the mid-1800s. Waterborne infections due to feces-contaminated drinking water are most common in developing countries. Foodborne infections primarily associated with the consumption of raw or undercooked shellfish are more common in developed countries.

Outbreaks of *V. parahaemolyticus* gastroenteritis have occurred throughout the world since the first documented epidemic in Japan in 1950 in which there were 20 fatalities among the 272 affected individuals.[10] Contaminated seafood is the usual vehicle in cases of *V. parahaemolyticus* gastroenteritis.

Non-O1 *V. cholerae, V. mimicus*, and *V. fluvialis* have also been isolated during cholera outbreaks in Asia.[17] Little is known about the epidemiology of these or other *Vibrio* spp. infections, however.

Vibrio infections in the U.S. generally occur sporadically as individual cases, particularly as wound infections. Clusters of cases of *V. cholerae* and of *V. parahaemolyticus* gastroenteritis have been documented recently in geographically diverse areas.[2]

PUBLIC HEALTH SIGNIFICANCE, PREVENTION AND CONTROL

Snow's classic work published in 1855, in which he documented drinking water from a specific London pump as the point source of a cholera outbreak, laid the ground work for cholera control measures practiced today. Control of cholera is centered in three principal areas: (a) improved sanitation, (b) public health education and (c) epidemiologic surveillance. Sanitation efforts should be aimed at eliminating contamination not only of drinking water supplies but also of shellfish harvesting areas. Educational programs should include campaigns during the off-season to teach methods of prophylaxis that aid in prevention of gastrointestinal diseases. These include handwashing, boiling drinking water, thoroughly cooking food, proper cleansing of utensils and control of flies. Emphasis should be placed on the need for early reporting of suspected cases and on the importance of rapid suppression of outbreaks. Surveillance programs must include attempts to forecast seasonal outbreaks in endemic areas. This may include environmental monitoring in shellfish harvesting areas. Mechanisms for the rapid identification of acute cases as well as carriers must also be available and the ability to rapidly disseminate this information.

A killed, whole cell vaccine is available which is effective in stimulating partial protection of short duration, lasting up to 6 months. Active immunization is of no value in epidemic control or in the management of case contacts. Vaccination is not normally recommended.[4] Contacts should be monitored for 5 days following exposure. Chemoprophylaxis of household contacts with tetracycline or furazolidone is recommended.[4]

These control measures are also appropriate for the control of epidemic gastroenteritis caused by other *Vibrio* species. Seasonal monitoring of the incidence of *Vibrio* species in shellfish harvesting areas of endemic areas may be appropriate.

DIAGNOSTIC PROCEDURES

Microscopic Methods

Direct examination of stools for curved, rod-shaped bacteria characteristic of vibrios may be useful in epidemic situations but is not helpful in nonepidemic ones. The pleomorphic nature of these bacteria and the morphologic similarity of *Vibrio* and *Campylobacter* renders microscopy on stools in nonepidemic situations of little use and possibly misleading.

Primary Isolation and Culture

Stool specimens should be collected early in the course of illness, ideally within the first 24 hours and before the administration of antimicrobial agents. Rectal swabs are acceptable specimens in the acute phase of illness, although they are not desirable from convalescent patients nor for identifying carriers. Vomitus may also be collected for culture.[7] Usual specimen collection procedures should be used for extraintestinal sources.

Inoculation of bacteriologic culture media should be done as soon as possible after specimen collection. Liquid, "rice-water" stools may be transported at room temperature, since *Vibrio* species maintain viability in this alkaline fluid. Formed stools or rectal swabs should be transported in Cary-Blair medium without refrigeration. Special care should be taken to prevent drying of the specimen, since *Vibrio* species are very susceptible to drying. Buffered glycerol-saline, commonly used as an enteric transport medium, is unsatisfactory even for short periods.[7]

Routine primary isolation media are generally sufficient for isolation of *Vibrio* species, which will grow well on nonselective media such as blood agar and on selective media such as MacConkey agar. More inhibitory, selective media may fail to support the growth of these organisms. Enrichments and/or specific selective media may be used for isolation, particularly when clusters of related cases are suspected. Alkaline peptone broth may be used for enrichment of *Vibrio* in feces. Incubate inoculated broth for 6-8 h at 35°C, then subculture from the surface of the broth to a nonselective medium (blood or gelatin agar) and to selective media such as MacConkey or thiosulfate-citrate-bile salts-sucrose (TCBS) agar and incubate overnight at 35°C. Subculture after overnight incubation (12-18 h) has also proved successful, although subculture at an earlier interval is recommended. The inclusion of TCBS agar in the routine media inoculated for enteric pathogens failed to improve the isolation rate of *Vibrio* species from sporadic cases in an endemic area of the U.S.[7]

Methods for Identification

Primary isolation media should be screened for oxidase-positive colonies characteristic of *Vibrio, Aeromonas* and *Plesiomonas*. These genera are strongly oxidase-positive, as are the oxidase-positive *Pseudomonas* species, using either the dimethyl or the tetramethyl oxidase reagents. *Enterobacteriaceae* are easily differentiated since they are oxidase-negative. *Vibrio* spp. may or may not be hemolytic on blood agar and are lactose nonfermenters on MacConkey agar. Vibrios can be differentiated on TCBS agar according to their ability to ferment sucrose. Sucrose-fermenting species such as *V. cholerae* and *V. alginolyticus* produce yellow colonies, whereas sucrose-negative species such as *V. parahaemolyticus* and *V. vulnificus* appear as green colonies. Oxidase testing should be done with growth from a nonselective medium since false-negative reactions may occur with growth from selective media. Several methods for screening primary plates for oxidase-positive organisms are described by Farmer et al.[7] Genera of the *Vibrionaceae* can be differentiated from *Pseudomonas* species by testing for fermentative versus oxidative metabolism. Vibrio are oxidase-positive and fermentative (as are *Aeromonas* and *Plesiomonas): Pseudomonas* are typically oxidase-positive but are oxidative, while *Enterobacteriaceae* are oxidase-negative and fermentative (Table 33:2). Triple sugar iron (TSI) or Kliger iron agar (KIA) slants can be used to test for fermentative metabolism. KIA is most useful for screening since all pathogenic *Vibrio* species produce an alkaline slant over an acid butt (K/A). Oxidase activity may be tested with growth from alkaline slants of KIA or TSI. *V. furnissii* and *V. damsela* will produce gas in these media whereas all other pathogenic *Vibrio* species are anaerogenic.

Vibrio can be differentiated from *Aeromonas* and *Plesiomonas* strains by the inhibition of growth by the pteridine compound referred to as O/129 or the vibriostatic reagent.[17] Reactions useful in differentiating between genera of the *Vibrionaceae* are given in Table 33:3.

Vibrio can be speciated using biochemical tests commonly used to identify *Enterobacteriaceae*. It is important to note that organisms of the genus *Vibrio* have an absolute requirement for Na^+. *V. cholerae* and *V. mimicus* will grow well in the presence of the trace amounts of Na^+ available in bacteriologic media. All other pathogenic *Vibrio* species require supplementation of the media with a minimum of about 0.5% NaCl; 1% NaCl is recommended for reliable reactions. Media which require NaCl supplementation include Moeller decarboxylase medium, peptone, methyl red/Voges-

Table 33:2. Characteristics Generally Useful in Differentiating the Genus *Vibrio* from *Pseudomonas* and the *Enterobateriaceae*

	Vibrio	*Pseudomonas*	*Enterobacteriaceae*
Fermentative metabolism	+	−	+
Oxidase	+	+	−
Growth stimulated by NaCl	+	−	−

Table 33:3. Characteristics Generally Useful in Differentiating the Pathogenic *Vibrio* Species from *Aeromonas* and *Plesiomonas*

	Vibrio	*Aeromonas*	*Plesiomonas*
Growth stimulated by NaCl	+	−	−
Gelatinase	+	+	−
Lysine decarboxylase	V*	−	+
Sensitivity to O/129 (150 μg)	+	−	V

* Variable reaction

Proskauer, gelatin and nitrate broths. The ability to grow in 1% peptone or nutrient broth with 0 to 10% NaCl can be used to differentiate among pathogenic *Vibrio* species. *V. cholerae* and *V. mimicus* will grow in media without added NaCl but the growth is stimulated by the addition of 0.5-1%. Typical biochemical reactions are produced with overnight incubation at 35°C in an ambient air atmosphere. Characteristics of pathogenic *Vibrio* species are given in Tables 33:4 and 33:5.

Reliable identifications can also be made using commercial kit systems designed for identification of *Enterobacteriaceae*. The API 20E (Analytab Products) system has been evaluated and found to be useful, although modifed diluent composition and incubation conditions increased the reliability of results.[12] Data bases used for identifications with commercial systems may provide misleading results when attempting to identify pathogenic *Vibrio* species. It is recommended that biochemical reactions generated by kit identification systems be used in combination with supplemental tests and reference charts. Excellent reference charts and information on identification of pathogenic *Vibrio* species can be found in the literature.[1,7]

Markers of Epidemiology

V. cholerae O1 responsible for cholera pandemics up to the turn of this century were nonhemolytic, but O1 strains isolated from pilgrims journeying to Mecca who were quarantined at El Tor, Egypt, were found to be hemolytic. Subsequent study of hemolytic, or El Tor, strains have identified other distinguishing characteristics. El Tor strains, in addition to producing hemolysis of sheep erythrocytes, produce acetoin (Voges-Proskauer positive), agglutinate chicken erythrocytes and are resistant to polymyxin B. Classical strains of *V. cholerae* O1 produce the opposite reactions. Classical and El Tor strains also have specific phage types. These characteristics have been used to follow the spread of *V. cholerae* O1 for epidemiological purposes. Cholera outbreaks in the Eastern Hemisphere since 1973 have been caused by nonhemolytic El Tor strains. An increased incidence of

Table 33.4 Characteristics of Lysine Decarboxylase-Positive, Pathogenic *Vibrio* Species

	V. cholerae	*V. mimicus*	*V. parahaemolyticus*	*V. vulnificus*	*V. alginolyticus*	*V. cincinnatiensis*
Oxidase	+*	+	+	+	+	+
Indole	+	+	+	+	+/−	−
Voges-Proskauer	+/−†	−	−	−	+	+
Simmons citrate	+/−	+/−	+	+	+/−	+
Lysine decarboxylase	+	+	+	+	+	+
Ornithine decarboxylase	+	+	+	+	+/−	−
Arginine dihydrolase	−‡	−	−	−	−	−
Fermentation of:						
Sucrose	+	−	−	−	+	+
Lactose	(+)§	(+)	−	+	−	−
L-arabinose	−	−	+	−	−	+
D-mannitol	+	+	+	+/−	+	−
Maltose	+	+	+	+	+	ND‖
D-cellobiose	−	−	−	+	−	+
Salicin	−	−	−	+	−	+
Gas from glucose	−	−	−	−	−	−
Nitrate to nitrite	+	+	+	+	+	+
Gelatinase	+	+	+	+	+	−
Growth in:						
0% NaCl	+	+	−	−	−	−
3% NaCl	+	+	+	+	+	+
6% NaCl	−	−	+	+/−	+	+
10% NaCl	−	−	−	−	+	−

* + = greater than 90% of strains positive
† +/− = variable reaction, predominant reaction is shown as numerator
‡ − = greater than 90% of strains negative
§ (+) = positive reaction delayed >3 days
‖ ND = no data

classical strains has recently been reported in Bangladesh. Endemic cholera in the U.S. has been caused by hemolytic strains of *V. cholerae* O1.

Strains of *V. parahaemolyticus* causing gastroenteritis have been found to produce a heat-stable hemolysin which is active against human erythrocytes when tested on Wagatsuma medium. This reaction is known as the Kanagawa phenomenon; it has been found in greater than 95% of clinical isolates and less than 1% of isolates from environmental sources.[16] Recent clinical isolates of *V. parahaemolyticus* in the U.S. have been found to be urease-positive in contrast to strains found in the past.[7]

No distinctions between *V. vulnificus* strains isolated from clinical or environmental sources have been identfied.[18] A biovar found in an eel pathogen in Japan appears to be phenotypically distinct from strains isolated from human infections.[17]

Toxigenicity Tests

Cholera toxin is a heat-labile enterotoxin genetically very similar to the heat-labile enterotoxin of *Escherichia coli*.[14] Assay methods include cyto-

Table 33.5 Characteristics of Arginine Dihydrolase-Positive or Decarboxylase-Negative, Pathogenic *Vibrio* Species

	V. fluvialis	*V. furnissii*	*V. damsela*	*V. hollisae*	*V. metschnikovii*
Oxidase	+*	+	+	+	−†
Indole	−	−/+‡	−	−	−/+
Voges-Proskauer	−	−	+	−	+
Simmons citrate	+	+	−	−	+
Lysine decarboxylase	−	−	+/−	−	−/+
Ornithine decarboxylase	−	−	−	−	−
Arginine dihydrolase	+	+	+	−	+/−
Fermentation of:					
Sucrose	+	+	−	−	+
Lactose	−	−	−	−	+/−
L-arabinose	+	+	−	+	−
D-mannitol	+	+	−	−	+
Maltose	+	+	+	−	+
Cellobiose	−/+	−/+	−	−	−
Salicin	−	−	−	−	−
Gas from glucose	−	+	+	−	−
Nitrate to nitrite	+	+	+	+	−
Gelatinase	+	+	−	−	+
Growth in:					
0% NaCl	−	−	−	−	−
3% NaCl	+	+	+	+	+
6% NaCl	+	+	+	+	+
10% NaCl	−	−	−	−	−

* + = greater than 90% of strains positive
† − = greater than 90% of strains negative
‡ −/+ = variable reaction, predominant reaction is shown as numerator

toxicity, animal skin permeability and intestinal fluid accumulation, immunological and genetic assays for the detection of the cholera toxin gene. Toxins other than cholera toxin have been identified from many of the pathogenic *Vibrio* species. Specific information on methods for detection of enterotoxins may be found in the review by Wachsmuth.[19]

Serologic Tests

The O1 serovar of *V. cholerae* can be further divided into subgroups based upon antigenic determinants. These subgroups are designated Ogawa, Inaba and Hikojima. Several different serotyping schemes for *V. cholerae* have been described.[5,7] Greater than 60 serovars of *V. cholerae* have been identified, based on somatic or O antigenic determinants. All O serovars have a common flagellar or H antigen. Antisera for identifying the O1 serovar is available from commercial sources and may be useful in clinical laboratories.[6] Identification of non-O1 serovars is of value for epidemiologic purposes and should be done by a reference laboratory. A serotyping scheme for *V. parahaemolyticus* has also been developed for use in reference laboratories for epidemiologic purposes.[7]

CLINICAL SIGNIFICANCE OF LABORATORY TESTS

V. cholerae remains the pathogenic *Vibrio* species of most significance worldwide. Identification of endemic foci of O1 *V. cholerae* in areas other than the Indian subcontinent, including the U.S. Gulf Coast, along with the natural occurrence of other pathogenic *Vibrio* species in coastal regions, emphasizes the need for clinical laboratories to maintain procedures for the isolation and identification of these bacteria. Non-O1 serovars of *V. cholerae* are increasingly recognized as agents of gastroenteritis and wound infections. Clusters of *V. parahaemolyticus* gastroenteritis continue to occur in the U.S. and elsewhere. The devastating consequences of *V. vulnificus* infections and the natural distribution in U.S. coastal waters are well documented.

The ability of clinical microbiology laboratories to identify *Vibrio* to the species level is important, since this information may guide physicians as to the potential clinical course of the infection. The recognition of gram-negative bacilli which are fermentative, oxidase-positive and show enhanced growth in media supplemented with NaCl is the key to recognizing pathogenic *Vibrio* species. Screening primary plates for oxidase-positive colonies is the single most important factor in recognizing these organisms, since they grow on bacteriologic media commonly used for the primary isolation of pathogenic bacteria from clinical specimens. Supplementation of biochemical test media with NaCl is also important to insure reliable reactions.

REFERENCES

1. Baumann PA, Furniss AL, Lee JV. Genus *Vibrio*. In: Kreig NR, Holt JG, eds. Bergey's manual of systematic bacteriology; vol 1. Baltimore: Williams and Wilkins, 1985:518-38.
2. Blake PA, Weaver RE, Hollis DG. Diseases of humans (other than cholera) caused by marine vibrios. Ann Rev Microbiol 1980;34:341-67.
3. Blake PA, Allegra DT, Snyder JD, et al. Cholera -- A possible endemic foci in the United States. N Engl J Med 1980;302:305-9.
4. Benenson AS, ed. Control of communicable diseases in man. 14th ed. Washington, DC: American Public Health Association, 1985:75-9.
5. Brenner DJ, Davis BR, Kudok Y, et al. Serological comparison of two collections of *Vibrio cholerae* non-O1. J Clin Microbiol 1982;16:319-23.
6. Donovan TJ, Lee JV. Quality of antisera used in the diagnosis of cholera. Lancet 1982;2:866.
7. Farmer JJ III, Hickman-Brenner FW, Kelly MT. *Vibrio*. In: Lennette EH, Balows A, Hausler WJ Jr, Shadomy HJ, eds. Manual of clinical microbiology. Washington, DC: American Society for Microbiology, 1985:282-308.
8. Field M. Modes of action of enterotoxins of *Vibrio cholerae* and *Escherichia coli*. Rev Infect Dis 1979;1:918-25.

9. Hughes JM, Hollis DG, Gangarosa EJ, Weaver RE. Non-cholera vibrio infections in the United States: clinical, epidemiologic and laboratory features. Ann Intern Med 1978;88:602-6.
10. Joseph SW, Kaper JB, Colwell RR. *Vibrio parahaemolyticus* and related vibrios. CRC Crit Rev Microbiol 1982;10:77-124.
11. Kaper JB, Moseley SL, Falkow S. Molecular characterization of environmental and non-toxigenic strains of *Vibrio cholerae*. Infect Immun 1981;32:661-7.
12. MacDonell MT, Singleton FL, Hood MA. Diluent composition for use of API 20E in characterizing marine and estuarine bacteria. Appl Environ Microbiol 1982;44:423-7.
13. Morris JG Jr, Wilson R, Davis BR, et al. Non-group 1 *Vibrio cholerae* gastroenteritis in the United States: clinical, epidemiologic and laboratory characteristics of sporadic cases. Ann Intern Med 1981;94:656-8.
14. Moseley SL, Falkow S. Nucleotide sequence homology between the heat-labile enterotoxin gene of *Escherichia coli* and *Vibrio cholerae* deoxyribonucleic acid. J Bacteriol 1980;144:444-6.
15. Pollitzer R. Cholera. Geneva: World Health Organization, 1959.
16. Sakazaki R, Tamura K, Kato T, Obara Y, Yamai S, Hobo K. Studies on the enteropathogenic facultatively halophilic bacteria, *Vibrio parahaemolyticus*. III. Enteropathogenicity. Jap J Med Sci Biol 1968;21:325-31.
17. Tison DL, Kelly MT. *Vibrio* species of medical importance. Diag Microbiol Infect Dis 1984;2:263-76.
18. Tison DL, Kelly MT. Virulence of *Vibrio vulnificus* strains from marine environments. Appl Environ Microbiol 1986;51:1004-6.
19. Wachsmuth IK. Laboratory detection of enterotoxins. In: Ellner P, ed. Infectious diarrheal diseases: current concepts and laboratory procedures. New York: Marcel Dekker, 1984:93-115.

Section 3: Antimicrobial Susceptibility Testing

CHAPTER 34

CONVENTIONAL PROCEDURES FOR ANTIMICROBIAL SUSCEPTIBILITY TESTING

Peter C. Fuchs, M.D., Ph.D.

INTRODUCTION

Antimicrobial agents have been available for treating infectious diseases for nearly half a century. It was apparent from the earliest days of antimicrobial chemotherapy that not all microorganisms were susceptible to any single agent. Although certain organisms were consistently susceptible to specific antimicrobial agents (e.g., *Streptococcus pyogenes* to penicillin), there were many (e.g., staphylococci) whose susceptibility varied from strain to strain and for which some means for predicting therapeutic response was needed. From this need have developed the modern antimicrobial susceptibility tests.

The first antimicrobial susceptibility test was described by Alexander Fleming in his original report on penicillin in 1929.[8] In this agar diffusion method penicillin was added to a trough cut out of agar and bacterial isolates were inoculated perpendicular to the trough. Diffusion of the antibiotic into the adjacent agar inhibited susceptible isolates in the vicinity of the trough. By modern standards, this was a crude test. The first significant susceptibility test to be developed was the broth dilution test described by Rammelkamp and Maxon in 1942.[25] Although modern versions of this test are better standardized and occasionally used in specific circumstances, the method is impractical for testing routine clinical isolates against multiple antimicrobials. The introduction of the agar disk diffusion method two years later led to the development of a more practical approach.[14,35] Over the next 20 years, numerous modifications and changes were suggested for the disk diffusion test, but it was not until the landmark paper of Bauer, Kirby, Sherris and Turck that the procedure was standardized and placed on solid footing.[4] All known variables were standardized and the zone diameters of bacterial inhibition were measured. By correlation with minimal inhibitory concentrations (MICs) determined by broth dilution, inhibitory zone diameters were interpretively categorized as susceptible, intermediate or resistant. This became the standard method used by most clinical laboratories in the United States and is the basis of the current standardized disk diffusion method promulgated by the National Commitee for Clinical Laboratory Standards (NCCLS).[16]

Although the disk diffusion test performed satisfactorily in most clinical situations, the fact that the interpretive criteria of this test are based on correlations with MICs spurred the development of practical dilution testing methods. A microdilution method was described in 1966[15] and later a similar method shown to produce results comparable to the standard broth dilution method.[9] Numerous improvements and refinements over the next decade have resulted in the introduction of commercially prepared frozen[3] and dried[12] microdilution systems, of which there are now many. The microdilution test is currently included as a standardized method in the NCCLS document on dilution methods for aerobic bacteria[17] together with the standard broth dilution and agar dilution methods. It should be noted, that despite the increasing popularity of microdilution test systems, there are no data to date that show any clinical superiority of these systems over the disk diffusion test.

Agar dilution is another satisfactory and proven method of susceptibility testing.[36] This method offers economic advantages for large volume laboratories, but is usually not practical for smaller laboratories.

The role of the antimicrobial susceptibility test is one of aiding the selection of an appropriate antimicrobial agent for treating a specific infection. It is important to realize, however, that the susceptibility test is not the only factor that needs to be considered in this selection. Other factors that are important include: 1) the nature of the causative organism and infection; 2) the immune status of the host; 3) possible interaction of the antibiotic with other drugs the patient may be receiving; 4) the pharmacokinetics of the antibiotic in relation to the site of infection; 5) conditions of the patient that may be contraindications to use of the drug; and 6) past experience with treating comparable infections. Because of such considerations, an antimicrobial agent other than the one most effective by in vitro testing is sometimes selected for therapy. However, in most situations, susceptibility test results play an important role in the selection process.

Since antimicrobial susceptibility tests play a sometimes crucial role in the treatment of patients, it is essential that the test results be as accurate and reliable as possible. Numerous factors besides organism susceptibility can affect the results of any susceptibility testing system.[7] Consequently, it is essential that these variables be controlled such that the only variable measured by the test system is microbial susceptibility.

Quality assurance, including routine testing of reference strains with stable, known susceptibilities, is an important feature. It is also strongly recommended that laboratories participate in proficiency testing surveys that include antimicrobial susceptibility testing, such as those provided by several state laboratories and the College of American Pathologists Survey Program.

Other significant factors affecting the value of antimicrobial susceptibility testing are the selection of microbes and antimicrobials to be tested. There is no reason to routinely test microorganisms whose susceptibility profiles are constant and totally predictable. For example, *S. pyogenes* isolated from the pharynx is always susceptible to penicillin, the drug of choice-hence there is no value in testing this. An exception would be the patient allergic to penicillin for whom tetracycline or erythromycin is being considered for treatment. Since some *S. pyogenes* are resistant to these drugs, susceptibility testing could be justified. Thus, antimicrobial susceptibility testing is indicated for those pathogens whose susceptibility cannot be predicted from their identity. This would include such common pathogens as staphylococci, enterococci, *Enterobacteriaceae* and pseudomonads. An important corollary is the assumption that the true pathogen has been isolated. From specimens that are readily contaminated (e.g., wounds, sputums and urines), it is sometimes difficult to recognize the true pathogen(s) when mixtures of organisms are grown. Such problems can often be avoided by ascertaining that an appropriate specimen has been properly procured.

The antimicrobial agents appropriate for testing by a particular laboratory are determined by 1) the organisms in question and 2) the antimicrobial agents available to the physician. Because of the nature of susceptibility testing, it is usually impractical to utilize a different set of antibiotics for each species of bacterium tested. A practical compromise is to utilize two different groups of antibiotics: one for gram-positive and one for gram-negative isolates; and to report those appropriate for the specific organism. For example, first and second generation cephalosporins may be included in the set of antimicrobial agents for gram-negative microorganisms, but would not be reported if the organism tested was *Pseudomonas aeruginosa*. Patient clientele is also an important determinant. For example, hospital laboratories should be testing a higher proportion of parenteral antimicrobial agents, whereas outpatient laboratories should test a predominance of oral agents. Furthermore, with increasing numbers of hospitals utilizing closed formularies, it is prudent for the laboratories to test those therapeutic equivalents on their respective hospital formularies. This is a potential difficulty for laboratories using commercial systems in which the antibiotics tested are already predetermined. A third factor that can affect selection of antimicrobials for testing is high prevalence of multiresistant organisms. If, for example, a hospital has an endemic *Klebsiella* strain that is resistant to most of the drugs on a standard panel of antibiotics, it may be necessary to incorporate other drugs in the panel to find any to which the organism is susceptible.

Table 34:1 lists sample panels of antimicrobials for gram-positive and gram-negative bacteria. The actual panel selected by a given laboratory should be determined by careful consideration of the above factors and after consultation with the clinical staff.

DISK DIFFUSION SUSCEPTIBILITY TESTING[4,16]

In the disk diffusion susceptibility test, the organism is inoculated on Mueller-Hinton agar and antibiotic-containing paper disks are placed on the surface of the agar. During the 16-18 h incubation period, the antimicrobial agents diffuse from their respective disks into the surrounding agar and produce circular zones of growth inhibition that are roughly proportional to the degree of susceptibility. Based on previous comparisons with MICs, the measured zone diameter of growth inhibition around each disk is translated into one of four categories of susceptibility: susceptible, intermediate, moderately susceptible or resistant. The disk diffusion test is practical, relatively easy to perform and a reliable method for determining antimicrobial susceptibility of bacteria that grow rapidly aerobically. With a few exceptions, it is of little or no value for detecting susceptibility of slow-growing and/or fastidious organisms. Also, in those uncommon situations in which knowledge of the actual MIC is important to therapeutic decisions, the disk diffusion test must yield to one of the dilution methods.

Materials

1. Mueller-Hinton agar (MHA): Because of the significant lot-to-lot variation in MHA, it is recommended that only those lots that have been tested and found to meet the acceptance limits of the NCCLS (M6-P) be used.[18]
2. Broth: A clear broth that supports the growth of usual bacterial pathogens, such as Mueller-Hinton broth is acceptable.
3. Antimicrobial impregnated filter paper disks for disk diffusion testing are available commercially. Disks should be stored at -20°C or less. A working supply (one week) may be refrigerated (4-8°C). All containers should contain active dessicant and be allowed to equilibrate with room temperature before opening to minimize condensation.
4. Flat bottom petri dishes with internal diameters of 14 cm or 9 cm may be used, depending upon the number of antimicrobials being tested.

Table 34:1. Sample Antimicrobial Panels for Gram-Positive and Gram-Negative Bacteria—(excluding urinary tract specific antimicrobials)

Drug	Alternates*	Report for:
	GRAM-POSITIVE PANEL	
Amoxicillin/ Clavulanate		Staphylococci
Ampicillin		Enterococci
Cephalothin	Cefazolin	Staphylococci† Streptococci
Chloramphenicol		Staphylococci, Streptococci
Clindamycin		Staphylococci, Streptococci
Erythromycin		Staphylococci, Streptococci
Gentamicin	Amikacin, Kanamycin Netilmicin, Tobramycin	Staphylococci
Oxacillin	Nafcillin, Methicillin	Staphylococci
Penicillin†		Staphylococci, Streptococci, Enterococci
Tetracycline		Staphylococci, Streptococci
Trimethoprim/ sulfamethoxazole		Staphylococci
Vancomycin		Staphylococci, Enterococci, Streptococci
	GRAM-NEGATIVE PANEL	
Drug	Alternates*	Report for:
Amikacin		Enterics, Pseudomonads
Ampicillin		Enterics
Cefamandole	Cefonicid, Cefuroxime	Enterics
Cefazolin	Cephalothin	Enterics
Cefotaxime	Cefoperazone, Ceftazidime, Ceftizoxime, Ceftriaxone, Moxalactam	Enterics, Pseudomonads
Cefoxitin	Cefotetan	Enterics
Chloramphenicol		Enterics
Gentamicin	Netilmicin, Tobramycin	Enterics, Pseudomonads
Mezlocillin	Piperacillin	Enterics, Pseudomonads
Tetracycline		Enterics
Ticarcillin	Carbenicillin	Enterics, Pseudomonads
Trimethoprim/ sulfamethoxazole		Enterics, Pseudomonads
	OPTIONAL CONSIDERATIONS	
	Azlocillin	Pseudomonads
	Aztreonam	Enterics, Pseudomonads
	Imipenem	Enterics, Pseudomonads
	Kanamycin	Enterics
	Amoxicillin/clavulanate	Enterics
	Ticarcillin/clavulanate	Enterics, Pseudomonads

* "Alternates" Refer to drugs of similar spectrum that could be tested—it does *not* imply that the results of testing one drug are applicable to the others.

† Staphylococci resistant to oxacillin or other penicillinase-resistant penicillins should be considered resistant to the cephalosporins, regardless of cephalosporin susceptibility test results.

5. Sterile nontoxic swabs on applicator sticks.
6. MacFarland 0.5 turbidity standard. Add 0.5 mL of 0.048 M barium chloride to 99.5 mL of 0.36 N sulfuric acid. Aliquot 5 mL into a screwcapped tube of the same size used in procedure. Store in dark at room temperature. Vortex prior to use.

Medium Preparation

The MHA should be prepared from dehydrated base according to the manufacturer's instructions. After autoclaving, the medium is cooled to 45-50°C in a water bath. Sufficient medium to achieve a uniform depth of 4 mm is poured into petri dishes placed on a flat surface. This will require approximately 60 and 25 mL for 14 and 9 cm plates respectively. These may be safely stored at refrigerator temperature for one week or longer if held in properly sealed containers which prevent excess loss of moisture. The pH of the medium should be checked and should be 7.3 + 0.1.

Test Procedure

1. The inoculum is prepared by touching the tops of 4 to 5 colonies of the same morphological type with a wire loop and suspending them in a tube containing 4-5 mL of broth. Incubate at 35°C for 2-8 h until the turbidity reaches or exceeds that of a 0.5 MacFarland standard. If this standard is exceeded, the suspension should be diluted with broth until it is visually comparable to the 0.5 MacFarland standard. An alternate method for preparing the inoculum is the preparation of direct saline or broth suspension of colonies from an 18 to 24 h nonselective agar plate, with immediate adjustment of turbidity to match the 0.5 MacFarland standard. This is the method of choice for organisms that grow poorly in broth, e.g., *Streptococcus pneumoniae* and *Haemophilus influenzae*, or to maximize the recognition of heteroresistant subpopulations of bacteria such as those in methicillin-resistant *Staphylococcus aureus*.
2. Within 15 min of inoculum standardization, dip a sterile nontoxic swab into the inoculum, and remove excess inoculum by rotating the swab against the inside wall of the tube with firm pressure. Inoculate the entire surface of a MHA plate evenly in three directions approximately 60 degrees from each other. Replace the lid and allow to dry for 3 to 5 min. An alternate agar overlay method of inoculation of common rapid growing pathogens has also been shown to be acceptable.[2]
3. Place the appropriate antibiotic-impregnated disks on the agar surface, either individually with sterile forceps or with a dispenser. Press each disk down gently with sterile forceps or needle to assure good contact with the agar surface. The disks should be distributed such that each

is at least 24 mm (center to center) from its nearest neighbor and 12 mm from the edge of the plate.

4. Within 15 min of placing the disks on the agar, invert the plates and incubate them at 35°C in air (i.e., no added CO_2).
5. After 16-18 h incubation, measure to the nearest mm the zone diameter of growth inhibition (determined by the unaided eye) around each disk (including the disk diameter) with calipers, ruler or a template held on the back of the plate, with reflected light against a dark nonreflective background.
6. Interpret the zone diameters for each antimicrobial agent as susceptible, intermediate, moderately susceptible or resistant as shown in Table 34:2. Definitions of these categories are as follows:
   A. Susceptible: The microorganism is susceptible to the antimicrobial agent at levels achieved in blood and tissues with the standard recommended doses of that drug.
   B. Intermediate: The result is indeterminate, i.e., neither susceptible nor resistant. Use of drugs in this category should not be considered unless MICs are determined. It should not be considered the same as moderately susceptible.
   C. Moderately susceptible: The organism is susceptible to levels achieved by greater than usual doses of the antimicrobial agent (but still nontoxic levels). Used primarily for beta-lactams.
   D. Resistant: The microorganism is resistant to achievable nontoxic blood levels of the antimicrobial agent.

Exceptions

1. Incomplete inhibition of growth may occur around trimethoprim and sulfonamide disks if antagonists such as thymidine or thymine are present. Usually there is a clear ring of heavy growth within which is a haze of reduced growth. If the growth within the ring is equal to or less than 20% that of surrounding growth, the diameter of this ring should be measured. Likewise, with *Proteus mirabilis* and *P. vulgaris*, swarming may occur into the areas of inhibited growth around certain drugs, but this can be ignored if a well-demarcated zone of inhibition is present.
2. For testing *H. influenzae*, the MHA should be supplemented with 1% hemoglobin or 5% lysed horse blood plus a supplement containing V and X factors. The alternate (direct) method of inoculum standardization should be employed. The ampicillin zone diameter breakpoints are different from those of other organisms (see Table 34:2).
3. For testing *Neisseria gonorrhoeae*, the disk diffusion test is currently valid only for testing susceptibility to penicillin. Instead of MHA, the medium for testing *N. gonorrhoeae* should be GC agar base supple-

Table 34:2. Zone Diameter Interpretive Standards and Approximate Minimum Inhibitory Concentration (MIC) Correlates*

Antimicrobial Agent	Disk Content	Zone Diameter, nearest whole mm: Resistant	Intermediate[b]	Moderately Susceptible[b]	Susceptible	Approximate MIC Correlates[a]: Resistant	Susceptible
Amikacin[c]	30μg	≤14	15–16	—	≥17	≥ 32μg/mL	≤ 16μg/mL
Ampicillin[d] when testing gram-negative enteric organisms	10μg	≤11	12–13	—	≥14	≥ 32μg/mL	≤ 8μg/mL
when testing staphylococci[e]	10μg	≤28	—	—	≥29	β-lactamase[e]	≤0.25μg/mL
when testing *Haemophilus* species[f]	10μg	≤19	—	—	≥20	≥ 4μg/mL	≤ 2μg/mL
when testing enterococci[g,h]	10μg	≤16	—	≥17[h]	—	≥ 16μg/mL	—
when testing non-enterococcal streptococci and *Listeria monocytogenes*[g,h]	10μg	≤21	—	22–29	≥30	≥ 4μg/mL	≤0.12μg/mL
Augmentin when testing *Haemophilus* & staphylococci[e,f]	20/10μg	≤19	—	—	≥20	—	≤ 4/2μg/mL
when testing other organisms	20/10μg	≤13	14–17	—	≥18	≥32/16μg/mL	≤ 8/4μg/mL
Azlocillin when testing *Pseudomonas*[e]	75μg	≤14	15–17	—	≥18	≥ 256μg/mL	≥ 64μg/mL
Aztreonam	30μg	≤15	—	16–21	≥22	≥ 32μg/mL	≤ 8μg/mL
Carbenicillin when testing the *Enterobacteriaceae*[e]	100μg	≤17	18–22	—	≥23	≥ 32μg/mL	≤ 16μg/mL
when testing *Pseudomonas*	100μg	≤13	14–16	—	≥17	≥ 512μg/mL	≤ 128μg/mL
Cefamandole[j]	30μg	≤14	15–17	—	≥18	≥ 32μg/mL	≤ 8μg/mL
Cefazolin[j]	30μg	≤14	15–17	—	≥18	≥ 32μg/mL	≤ 8μg/mL
Cefonicid[j]	30μg	≤14	15–17	—	≥18	≥ 32μg/mL	≤ 8μg/mL
Cefoperazone[j]	75μg	≤15	—	16–20	≥21	≥ 64μg/mL	≤ 16μg/mL
Ceftotaxime[j]	30μg	≤14	—	15–22	≥23	≥ 64μg/mL	≤ 8μg/mL
Cefoxitin[j]	30μg	≤14	15–17	—	≥18	≥ 32μg/mL	≤ 8μg/mL

Ceftazidime[j]	30μg	≤14	15–17	—	≥18	≥ 32μg/mL	≤ 8μg/mL
Ceftizoxime when testing, urinary isolates of *P. aeruginosa*	30μg	≤10	—	≥11	—	≥ 64μg/mL	—
when testing other organisms	30μg	≤14	—	15–19	≥20	≥ 32μg/mL	≤ 8μg/mL
Ceftriaxone	30μg	≤13	—	14–20	≥21	≥ 64μg/mL	≤ 8μg/mL
Cefuroxime[j]	30μg	≤14	15–17	—	≥18	≥ 32μg/mL	≤ 8μg/mL
Cephalothin[j]	30μg	≤14	15–17	—	≥18	≥ 32μg/mL	≤ 8μg/mL
Chloramphenicol	30μg	≤12	13–17	—	≥18	≥ 25μg/mL	≤12.5μg/mL
Cinoxacin[k]	100μg	≤14	15–18	—	≥19	≥ 64μg/mL	≤ 16μg/mL
Clindamycin[l]	2μg	≤14	15–16	—	≥17	≥ 2μg/mL	≤ 1μg/mL
Doxycycline[m]	30μg	≤12	13–15	—	≥16	≥ 16μg/mL	≤ 4μg/mL
Erythromycin	15μg	≤13	14–17	—	≥18	≥ 8μg/mL	≤ 2μg/mL
Gentamicin[c]	10μg	≤12	13–14	—	≥15	≥ 8μg/mL	≤ 4μg/mL
Imipenem	10μg	≤13	14–15	—	≥16	≥ 16μg/mL	≤ 4μg/mL
Kanamycin	30μg	≤13	14–17	—	≥18	≥ 25μg/mL	≤ 6μg/mL
Methicillin when testing staphylococci[n]	5μg	≤ 9	10–13	—	≥14	—	≤ 3μg/mL
Mezlocillin[e]	75μg	≤12	13–15	—	≥16	≥ 256μg/mL	≤ 64μg/mL
Minocycline[m]	30μg	≤14	15–18	—	≥19	≥ 16μg/mL	≤ 4μg/mL
Moxalactam[j]	30μg	≤14	—	15–22	≥23	≥ 64μg/mL	≤ 8μg/mL
Nafcillin when testing staphylococci[n]	1μg	≤10	11–12	—	≥13	—	≤ 1μg/mL
Nalidixic Acid[k]	30μg	≤13	14–18	—	≥19	≥ 32μg/mL	≤ 8μg/mL
Netilmicin[c]	30μg	≤12	13–14	—	≥15	≥ 32μg/mL	≤ 12μg/mL
Nitrofurantoin[k]	300μg	≤14	15–16	—	≥17	≥ 100μg/mL	≤ 25μg/mL
Norfloxacin	10μg	≤12	13–16	—	≥17	≥ 16μg/mL	≤ 4μg/mL
Oxacillin when testing staphylococci[n]	1μg	≤10	11–12	—	≥13	—	≤ 1μg/mL
when testing pneumococci for penicillin G susceptibility	1μg	≤19	—	—	≥20	—	≤0.06μg/mL

(Continued)

Table 34:2. Zone Diameter Interpretive Standards and Approximate Minimum Inhibitory Concentration (MIC) Correlates* (Continued)

Antimicrobial Agent	Disk Content	Zone Diameter, nearest whole mm: Resistant	Intermediate[b]	Moderately Susceptible[b]	Susceptible	Approximate MIC Correlates[a]: Resistant	Susceptible
Penicillin G when testing staphylococci[e]	10 units	≤28	—	—	≥29	β-lactamase[e]	≤ 0.1μg/mL
when testing *N. gonorrhoeae*	10 units	≤19	—	—	≥20	β-lactamase	≤ 0.1μg/mL
when testing enterococci[g,h]	10 units	≤14	—	≥15[h]	—	≥ 16μg/mL	—
when testing non-enterococcal streptococci and *L. monocytogenes*[g,h]	10 units	≤19	—	20–27	≥28	≥ 4μg/mL	≤0.12μg/mL
Piperacillin[e]	100μg	≤14	15–17	—	≥18	≥ 256μg/mL	≤ 64μg/mL
Streptomycin	10μg	≤11	12–14	—	≥15	—	—
Sulfonamides[k,o]	250 or 300μg	≤12	13–16	—	≥17	≥ 350μg/mL	≤ 100μg/mL
Tetracycline[m]	30μg	≤14	15–18	—	≥19	≥ 16μg/mL	≤ 4μg/mL
Ticarcillin[e]	75μg	≤11	12–14	—	≥15	≥ 128μg/mL	≤ 64μg/mL
Tobramycin[c]	10μg	≤12	13–14	—	≥15	≥ 8μg/mL	≤ 4μg/mL
Trimethoprim[k,o]	5μg	≤10	11–15	—	≥16	≥ 16μg/mL	≤ 4μg/mL
Trimethoprim-sulfamethoxazole[o]	1.25/23.75μg	≤10	11–15	—	≥16	≥8/152μg/mL	≤2/38μg/mL
Vancomycin	30μg	≤ 9	10–11	—	≥12	—	≤ 5μg/mL

a. These correlates are not meant for use as breakpoints for susceptibility categorization with dilution MIC tests as described in NCCLS M7-T. Use M7-T for categorization with dilution tests.

b. The category "intermediate" should be reported. It generally indicates that the test result is equivocal (see 2.3.2.). When designated in this table, a "moderately susceptible" result should be reported to indicate susceptibility under certain conditions (see 2.3.2.2). Other β-lactams are currently being considered for definition of a moderately susceptible category.

and aztreonam are recently studied beta-lactams having a separate diagnostic disk and a wider spectrum of antimicrobial activity, especially against gram-negative bacilli than do other previously approved cephalosporins. Therefore, the 30 μg cephalothin disk cannot be used as the class representative for these drugs even through cefazolin is considered a "first generation" drug. The cephalothin disk should only be used for testing susceptibility to cephalothin, cefaclor, cefadroxil, cephalexin, cephapirin, and cephradine. Cefazolin, cefamandole (or cefonicid or cefuroxime or

c. The zone sizes obtained with aminoglycosides, particularly when testing *P. aeruginosa*, are very medium-dependent because of variations in divalent cation content. These interpretive standards are to be used only with Mueller-Hinton medium that has yielded zone diameters within the correct range shown in Table 34:3 when performance tests were done with *P. aeruginosa* ATCC® 27853. Organisms in the intermediate category may be either susceptible or resistant when tested by dilution methods and should therefore more properly be classified as "indeterminant" in their susceptibility.

d. Class disk for ampicillin, amoxicillin, bacampicillin, cyclacillin, and hetacillin.

e. Resistant strains of *S. aureus* produce β-lactamase and the testing of the 10 unit penicillin disk is preferred. Penicillin G SHOULD be used to test the susceptibility of all penicillinase-sensitive penicillins, such as ampicillin, amoxicillin, azlocillin, bacampicillin, hetacillin, carbenicillin, mezlocillin, piperacillin, and ticarcillin. Results may also be applied to phenoxymethyl penicillin or phenethicillin.

f. For testing *Haemophilus* use Mueller-Hinton agar supplemented with 1% hemoglobin (or 5% horse blood) and 1% IsoVitaleX (BBL), Supplement XV (Difco) or an equivalent synthetic supplement. Adjust pH to 7.2. Prepare the inoculum by suspending growth from a 24-hour chocolate agar plate in Mueller-Hinton broth to the density of a turbidity standard (see 4.1.3). The vast majority of ampicillin-resistant strains of *Haemophilus* produce detectable β-lactamase.

g. For enterococci, other *Streptococcus* spp. and non-penicillinase-producing pencillin-sensitive organisms, and *Listeria monocytogenes*, the former intermediate interpetation should be reported as "Moderately Susceptible." Results in this category include *enterococci* and *Listeria* which for blood or serious invasive tissue infections require high dosage of penicillin or ampicillin, often combined with an aminoglycoside (gentamicin) for improved therapeutic response and bactericidal action.

h. For streptococci, staphylococci, and other penicillin-sensitive organisms, "SUSCEPTIBLE" results should be regarded as "VERY SUSCEPTIBLE." Enterococci strains (*S. faecalis, S. faecium, and S. durans*) producing zones ≥30mm for ampicillin or ≥28mm for penicillin are quite unusual and the streptococcal speciation procedures should be reexamined.

j. Cefazolin, cefamandole, cefonicid, cefuroxime, cefoxitin, cefotaxime, moxalactam, ceftizoxime, ceftazidime, ceftriaxone, cefoperazone, ceforanide), cefoxitin, cefoperazone, cefotaxime (or aztreonam or ceftazidime or ceftizoxime or ceftriaxone or moxalactam) should be tested separately against the enteric bacilli (see Table 34:1). *S. aureus* exhibiting resistance to one of the penicillinase-resistant penicillins (MRSA) MUST be reported as resistant to cephalosporin-like antimicrobial agents, regardless of in vitro disk test results, because most cases of documented MRSA infection have responded poorly to cephalosporin chemotherapy. Methicillin-resistant, coagulase-negative *Staphylococcus* spp. also appear not to respond well to cephalosporin treatment.

k. Susceptibility data for cinoxacin, nalidixic acid, nitrofurantoin, norfloxacin, sulfonamides, and trimethoprim apply only to organisms isolated from urinary tract infections.

l. The clindamycin disk is used for testing susceptibility to both clindamycin and lincomycin.

m. Tetracycline is the class disk for all tetracyclines, and the results can be applied to chlortetracycline, demeclocycline, doxycycline, methacycline, minocycline, and oxytetracycline. However, certain organisms may be more susceptible to doxycycline and minocycline than to tetracycline. (See footnote I, Table 34:1.)

n. Of the antistaphylococcal, β-lactamase resistant penicillins, either oxacilin, nafcillin, or methacillin may be tested, and results can be applied to the other two of these drugs and to cloxacillin and dicloxacillin. Oxacillin is preferred due to more resistance to degradation in storage and its application to pneumococcal testing (methicillin also usable) and because it is more likely to detect heteroresistant strains more easily. Do not use nafcillin on blood-containing media. Cloxacillin disks SHOULD NOT be used because they may not detect methicillin-resistant *S. aureus*. When an intermediate result is obtained with staphylococci, the strains should be further investigated to determine if they are heteroresistant.

o. The sulfisoxazole disk can be used for any of the commercially available sulfonamides. Blood-containing media, except media containing lysed horse blood, are NOT satisfactory for testing sulfonamides. The Mueller-Hinton agar should be as thymidine-free as possible for sulfonamide and/or trimethoprim testing. (See footnote, Table 34:3.)

* From M2-A3, *Performance Standards for Antimicrobial Disk Susceptibility Tests, Third Edition; Approved Standard* Published December 1984 NCCLS VOL. 4 NO. 16.

mented with X and V factors without hemoglobin. The alternate (direct) method for inoculum standardization should be used. The incubation atmosphere should be supplemented with 3-10% CO_2. Resistant isolates, whether penicillinase-producers or not, will have zones of inhibition equal to or less than 19 mm.

4. For testing *S. pneumoniae* susceptibility to penicillin, the MHA should be supplemented with 5% sheep blood. The alternate (direct) method for inoculum standardization should be used. A 1.0 μg oxacillin or 5 μg methicillin (not penicillin) disk should be used. Penicillin-susceptible isolates will have inhibitory zone diameters of 20 mm or more, whereas resistant (MIC greater than 1 μg/mL) and relatively resistant (MIC 0.12-1.0 μg/mL) will have diameters of 19 mm or less. This test is not satisfactory for distinguishing penicillin-resistant from relatively resistant strains of *S. pneumoniae*.
5. Methicillin-resistant staphylococci (MRS) continue to present problems in detection. For best detection of these heteroresistant strains, it is recommended that the alternate (direct) method of inoculum standardization and the oxacillin 1 μg disk be used. The presence of tiny colonies or a faint film of growth within otherwise clear zones of inhibition around the disks of penicillinase-resistant penicillins or cephalosporins should alert one to the possibility of MRS. Also, most MRS are resistant to multiple other non-beta-lactam antimicrobial agents.

Quality Assurance

Control strains should be routinely tested as a check that all components of the test system are functioning properly. Standard control strains include: *Escherichia coli* (ATCC 25922), *S. aureus* (ATCC 25923) and *P. aeruginosa* (ATCC 27853). If amoxicillin/clavulanate or ticarcillin/clavulanate is being tested, *E. coli* (ATCC 35218) should also be included as a control. The acceptable ranges of zone diameters for each antimicrobial with these control strains are listed in Table 34:3. When the zone diameters fall outside these limits, the reason should be ascertained, appropriate remedial action taken and the tests repeated.

Control strain testing should be done each day of susceptibility testing, unless the conditions for less frequent (weekly) testing are met.[11,16] These conditions are met if: 1) there is documentation that all control strains were tested for at least 30 consecutive test days; 2) for each drug-organism combination, no more than 3 of the 30 consecutive tests had zone diameters outside the limits listed in Table 34:3; and 3) for each drug-organism combination, none of the 6 zone size ranges (obtained from grouping the 30 test results in 6 groups of 5 consecutive tests each) were larger than the allowable range for precision listed in Table 34:4. When a problem is detected with the weekly monitoring system, a return to daily monitoring is required until there is documented resolution of the problem.

BROTH DILUTION ANTIMICROBIAL SUSCEPTIBILITY TESTING[17]

The broth dilution susceptibility test allows the determination of the MIC of an antimicrobial agent. This is accomplished by preparing a series of varying concentrations of antimicrobial agents (usually twofold serial dilutions) in broth, inoculating them with the appropriate inoculum of test organisms, and after overnight incubation identifying the lowest concentration of each drug permitting no visible growth.

The standard broth dilution method (BD) involves tubes of broth containing antimicrobial agents, whereas the more practical microdilution method (MD) places the antimicrobials in microtiter tray wells. The MD method is currently as practical as the disk diffusion test. Many steps of the MD method lend themselves to varying degrees of automation, a feature capitalized upon by a number of commercial entities.

In addition to providing MICs, the broth dilution methods enable antimicrobial susceptibility testing of many fastidious and slower growing pathogens which cannot be tested satisfactorily by disk diffusion. Also, it is the first step in the determination of minimal bactericidal concentration (MBC). Whereas blood may be added to MHA in the disk diffusion test to enhance the growth of certain organisms, the addition of whole blood to broth dilution tests is not advisable because the endpoints are difficult to detect. Serum, lysed blood or blood digests can be added for strains requiring such for growth.

Materials

1. Mueller-Hinton Broth (MHB).
2. Magnesium stock solution of 10 mg Mg^{++}/mL (8.36 g of $MgCl_2 \cdot 6\ H_2O$ in 100 mL deionized distilled water). Sterilize by filtration.
3. Calcium stock solution of 10 mg Ca^{++}/mL (3.68 g of $CaCl_2 \cdot 2\ H_2O$ in 100 mL deionized distilled water). Sterilize by filtration.
4. 13 X 100 mm sterile test tubes (BD) or microdilution trays (MD) with round or conical bottom wells and a filling apparatus.
5. Standardized or reference antimicrobial powders-obtainable from the appropriate drug manufacturer or United States Pharmacopea.

Medium and Antimicrobial Preparation

Since MHB is normally deficient in CA^{++} and Mg^{++} cations, and since this deficiency results in falsely low MICs of aminoglycosides (for *P.*

Table 34:3. Control Limits for Monitoring Antimicrobial Disk Susceptibility Tests - Zone Diameter (mm) Limits for Individual Tests on Mueller-Hinton Medium[a] without Blood or Other Supplements*

Antimicrobial Agent	Disk Content	*E. coli* (ATCC® 25922)	*S. aureus* (ATCC® 25923)	*P. aeruginosa* (ATCC® 27853)	*E. coli* (ATCC® 35218)
Amikacin	30μg	19–26	20–26	18–26	—
Ampicillin	10μg	16–22	27–35	—	—
Augmentin	20/10μg	19–25	28–36	—	18–22
Azlocillin	75μg	—	—	24–30	—
Aztreonam[c]	30μg	28–36	—	23–29	—
Carbenicillin	100μg	23–29	—	18–24	—
Cefamandole[c]	30μg	26–32	26–34	—	—
Cefazolin	30μg	23–29	29–35	—	—
Cefonicid	30μg	25–29	22–28	—	—
Cefoperazone	75μg	28–34	24–33	23–29	—
Cefotaxime	30μg	29–35	25–31	18–22	—
Cefotetan[c]	30μg	28–34	17–23	—	—
Cefoxitin	30μg	23–29	23–29	—	—
Ceftazidime	30μg	25–32	16–20	22–29	—
Ceftizoxime	30μg	30–36	27–35	12–17	—
Ceftriaxone[c]	30μg	29–35	22–28	17–23	—
Cefuroxime	30μg	20–26	27–35	—	—
Cephalothin	30μg	17–22	29–37	—	—
Chloramphenicol	30μg	21–27	19–26	—	—
Cinoxacin	100/μg	26–32	—	—	—
Clindamycin	2μg	—	24–30	—	—
Doxycycline	30μg	18–24	23–29	—	—
Erythromycin	15μg	—	22–30	—	—

Gentamicin	10μg	19–26	19–27	16–21	—
Imipenem[c]	10μg	26–32	—	20–28	—
Kanamycin	30μg	17–25	19–26	—	—
Methicillin[b]	5μg	—	17–22	—	—
Mezlocillin	75μg	23–29	—	19–25	—
Minocycline	30μg	19–25	25–30	—	—
Moxalactam	30μg	28–35	18–24	17–25	—
Nafcillin[b]	1μg	—	16–22	—	—
Nalidixic Acid	30μg	22–28	—	—	—
Netilmicin	30μg	22–30	22–31	17–23	—
Nitrofurantoin	300μg	20–25	18–22	—	—
Norfloxacin[c]	10μg	28–35	17–28	22–29	—
Oxacillin[b]	1μg	—	18–24	—	—
Penicillin G	10 units	—	26–37	—	—
Piperacillin	100μg	24–30	—	25–33	—
Streptomycin	10μg	12–20	14–22	—	—
Sulfisoxazole	250μg or 300μg	18–26	24–34	—	—
Tetracycline	30μg	18–25	19–28	—	—
Ticarcillin[c]	75μg	24–30	—	22–28	—
Tobramycin	10μg	18–26	19–29	19–25	—
Trimethoprim[c]	5μg	21–28	19–26	—	—
Trimethoprim-sulfamethoxazole[a]	1.25/23.75μg	24–32	24–32	—	—
Vancomycin	30μg	—	15–19	—	—

a. To determine whether the Mueller-Hinton medium has sufficiently low levels of thymine and thymidine, a *Streptococcus faecalis* (ATCC® 29212) may be tested with trimethoprim-sulfamethoxazole disks. An inhibition zone of ≥24 mm which is essentially free of fine colonies indicates a sufficiently low level of thymine and thymidine.

b. Several laboratories have reported difficulties with these quality control parameters, therefore, the parameters are currently being re-evaluated, and revised figures, if any, will be published in the future supplements.

c. Consider as tentative for twelve months after publication of this document.

* From M2-A3, *Performance Standards for Antimicrobial Disk Susceptibility Tests, Third Edition; Approved Standard* Published December 1984 NCCLS VOL. 4 NO. 16.

Table 34:4. Maximum Zone Diameter Range[a] That Should be Observed in a Series of Five Consecutive Control Test Results[b]*

Antimicrobial Agent	Disk Content	*E. coli* (ATCC® 25922)	*S. aureus* (ATCC® 25923)	*P. aeruginosa* (ATCC® 27853)	*E. coli* (ATCC® 35218)
Amikacin	30µg	6	6	6	—
Ampicillin	10µg	6	8	—	—
Augmentin	20/10µg	9	8	—	9
Azlocillin	75µg	—	—	8	—
Aztreonam	30µg	10	—	10	—
Carbenicillin	100µg	10	—	8	—
Cefamandole	30µg	8	8	—	—
Cefazolin	30µg	8	8	—	—
Cefonicid	30µg	8	8	—	—
Cefoperazone	75µg	10	10	—	—
Cefotaxime	30µg	10	10	—	—
Cefotetan	30µg	8	8	—	—
Cefoxitin	30µg	8	8	—	—
Ceftazidime	30µg	8	8	8	—
Ceftizoxime	30µg	10	10	8	—
Ceftriaxone	30µg	10	10	10	—
Cefuroxime	30µg	8	8	—	—
Cephalothin	30µg	8	8	—	—
Chloramphenicol	30µg	10	10	—	—
Cinoxacin	100µg	9	—	—	—
Clindamycin	2µg	—	6	—	—
Doxycycline	30µg	8	8	—	—
Erythromycin	15µg	—	9	—	—

Gentamicin	10μg	6	6	6	—
Imipenem	10μg	6	—	6	—
Kanamycin	30μg	9	9	—	—
Methicillin	5μg	—	9	—	—
Mezlocillin	75μg	8	—	8	—
Minocycline	30μg	9	9	—	—
Moxalactam	30μg	10	10	10	—
Nafcillin	1μg	—	6	—	—
Nalidixic Acid	30μg	10	—	—	—
Netilmicin	30μg	6	6	6	—
Nitrofurantoin	300μg	6	6	—	—
Norfloxacin	10μg	9	9	9	—
Oxacillin	1μg	—	6	—	—
Penicillin G	10 units	—	8	—	—
Piperacillin	100μg	8	—	8	—
Streptomycin	10μg	8	8	—	—
Sulfisoxazole	250μg or 300μg	9	9	—	—
Tetracycline	30μg	9	9	—	—
Ticarcillin	75μg	8	—	8	—
Tobramycin	10μg	6	6	6	—
Trimethoprim	5μg	10	10	—	—
Trimethoprim-sulfamethoxazole	1.25/23.75μg	10	10	—	—
Vancomycin	30μg	—	6	—	—

a. Zone Diameter Range is defined as the largest minus the smallest zone diameter in a group of five consecutive control test results.
b. Maximum zone diameter ranges have been calculated using formulae for determining control charts for ranges (ASTM Manual on Quality Control of Materials, Special Technical Publication 15-C, American Society for Testing and Materials, Philadelphia, Pa., 1951). Performance within these limits indicates that test precision is sufficient to ensure that the probability of major interpretative error (R ⇌ S) is less than 1%.
*From M2-A3, *Performance Standards for Antimicrobial Disk Susceptibility Tests, Third Edition; Approved Standard* Published December 1984 NCCLS VOL. 4 NO. 16.

aeruginosa) and tetracycline, it is important to supplement the MHB with these cations. Cation supplemented MHB (CSMHB) is described in Chapter 45, ''Media, Reagents and Stains.''

Stock solutions of each antimicrobial agent are prepared at 10 times the highest concentration to be tested, using the appropriate solvents and diluents as outlined by the NCCLS.[17] These may be stored in tightly sealed vials or ampules at -20°C, or preferrably, at -60°C or less, for at least 6 months.

To prepare drug solutions for testing,[7,15] add 1.0 mL of stock solution to 9.0 mL of CSMHB (or multiples thereof) for preparation of the highest test concentration. This first working solution serves as the source for the next three dilutions: 1.0 mL to 1.0, 3.0 and 7.0 mL of CSMHB, respectively. The lowest concentration solution of these serves as the source for the next three dilutions, etc., until the full range of concentrations has been achieved. These solutions are then dispensed in 1.0 mL volumes in tubes (BD) or in 0.1 mL or 0.05 mL volume in the wells of microtiter trays (MD) - depending on method of inoculation. MD trays may be stored for 4 weeks at -20°C or less, and for even longer (6-8 weeks) at -60°C or less. Do not use a self-defrosting freezer.

Test Procedure

1. Prepare a suspension of the organism to be tested equal to a 0.5 MacFarland standard by either the standard or alternate (direct) method for disk diffusion testing. Based on the expected colony count of this suspension (1×10^8 colony forming units (CFU) per mL) and the method of inoculation, this suspension should be diluted sufficiently to achieve a final concentration in all inoculated tubes or wells of approximately 5×10^5 CFU/mL. If, for example in BD, a 1.0 mL inoculum is added to each tube containing CSMHB with antibiotic, the inoculum concentration should be 1×10^6 CFU/mL - a 1:100 dilution of the original standardized suspension. For MD, if the inoculator delivers 5 μL to each well containing 0.1 mL, a final concentration of 5×10^5 CFU/mL is achieved by diluting the original standardized suspension 1:10 with distilled water.
2. Inoculate each tube or well within 15 min of inoculum standardization and dilution. For BD add 1.0 mL of inoculum to the growth control tube (no antimicrobial) and each antimicrobial-containing tube in the dilution series. For commercial MD systems, follow the inoculation instructions of the manufacturer. For in-house prepared MD trays, use an inoculating device that delivers a small but reliable quantity of inoculum (5 μL or less) to wells containing 100 μL of broth, or pipettes that deliver 50 μL of inoculum to wells containing 50 μL of broth.

MD trays should be sealed, covered with an empty MD tray or incubated in humidified chambers.

3. Incubate the tubes or trays at 35°C in air with no supplemented CO_2 for 16 to 20 h.
4. Examine tubes or wells with the unaided eye for the presence or absence of growth and compare with the growth in the control tube or well. The lowest concentration with no visible growth is the endpoint and MIC.
5. Refer to Table 34:5 for interpretive categorization of the MIC results for each drug as susceptible, moderately susceptible or resistant.[17] Ideally, both the MIC and interpretive category should be provided in the susceptibility report.

Exceptions

1. For testing strains of *Haemophilus* spp., the CSMHB should be further supplemented with lysed horse blood (2-3%) and nicotinamide adenine dinucleotide (NAD) (10 μg/mL). Incubation should be for 24 h at 35°C in air.
2. For testing *Listeria monocytogenes* and streptococci, the CSMHB should be supplemented with laked horse blood. Some streptococcal strains may require supplemental atmospheric CO_2 for growth, but this should not be used unless needed.
3. For testing *N. meningitidis*, incubate at 35°C for 24 h with supplemental CO_2.
4. To enhance the detection of staphylococci resistant to penicillinase-resistant penicillins, oxacillin is the test drug of choice. The CSMHB should be supplemented with 2% NaCl.[1,34] The alternate (direct) method of inoculum standardization should be used. Incubate in air at 30-35°C for 24 h.
5. Rapid growing mycobacteria such as *M. fortuitum* and *M. chelonei* may be tested by this system. The inoculum is prepared from an overnight growth in MHB + 0.02% Tween 80 adjusted to a 0.5 MacFarland standard. After inoculating CSMHB with antimicrobials, incubate at 35°C for 72 h.

Quality Assurance

In order to assure high quality performance of the test system, routine testing of stable control organisms with susceptibility endpoints in the mid-range of most antibiotic series is strongly recommended. Recommended strains that best meet these criteria are: *E. coli* (ATCC 25922) *P. aeruginosa* (ATCC 27853), *S. aureus* (ATCC 29213), *S. faecalis* (ATCC 29212) and *E.*

Table 34:5. MIC Interpretive Standards (μg/mL) of Three Categories of Susceptibility*

Antimicrobial Agent	Susceptible	Moderately Susceptible[a]	Resistant
Amikacin[b]	≤16	32	≥64
Amoxicillin–clavulanic acid			
when testing *Haemophilus* and staphylococci[c,d,g]	≤4/2	—	≥8/4
when testing other organisms	≤8/4	16/8	≥32/16
Ampicillin[e]			
when testing *Enterobacteriaceae*	≤8	16	≥32
when testing staphylococci[c]	≤0.25	—	≥0.5
when testing *Haemophilus* species[d]	≤2.0	—	≥4.0
when testing enterococci[f]	—	≤8.0	≥16
when testing non-enterococcal streptococci and other gram positives[f]	≤0.12	0.25–2.0	≥4.0
Azlocillin when testing *Pseudomonas*	≤64	—	≥128
Aztreonam	≤8	16	≥32
Carbenicillin			
when testing *Enterobacteriaceae*	≤16	32	≥64
when testing *Pseudomonas*	≤128	—	≥256
Cefamandole[g]	≤8	16	≥32
Cefazolin[g]	≤8	16	≥32
Cefonicid[g]	≤8	16	≥32
Cefoperazone[g]	≤16	32	≥64
Ceforanide[g]	≤8	16	≥32
Cefotaxime[g]	≤8	16–32	≥64
Cefotetan[g]	≤16	32	≥64
Cefoxitin[g]	≤8	16	≥32
Ceftazidime[g]	≤8	16	≥32
Ceftizoxime[g]			
when testing organisms other than urinary tract isolates of *P. aeruginosa*	≤8	16–32	≥64
Ceftriaxone[g]	≤8	16–32	≥64

Cefuroxime[g]	≤8	16	≥32
Cephalothin[g]	≤8	16	≥32
Chloramphenicol	≤8	16	≥32
Clindamycin[h]	≤0.5	1–4	≥8.0
Doxycycline[j]	≤4	8	≥16
Erythromycin[h]	≤0.5	1–4	≥8.0
Gentamicin[b]	≤4	8	≥16
Imipenem	≤4	8	≥16
Kanamycin[b]	≤16	32	≥64
Methicillin			
when testing staphylococci[k]	≤8	—	≥16
Mexlocillin[l]	≤16	32–64	≥128
Minocycline[h]	≤4	8	≥16
Moxalactam	≤8	16–32	≥64
Nafcillin			
when testing staphylococci[k]	≤2	—	≥4.0
Netilmicin[b]	≤4	8–16	≥32
Oxacillin			
when testing staphylococci[k]	≤2	—	≥4.0
Penicillin G			
when testing staphylococci[c,f]	≤0.12	—	≥0.25
when testing *N. gonorrhoeae*[d]	≤0.12	0.25–2.0	≥4.0
when testing enterococci[f]	—	≤8	≥16
when testing non-enterococcal streptococci[f]	≤0.12	0.25–2.0	≥4.0
when testing pneumococci	≤0.06	0.12–1.0	≥2.0
Piperacillin[l]	≤16	32–64	≥128
Rifampin	≤2	4	≥8
Tetracycline[j]	≤4	8	≥16
Ticarcillin[c]	≤16	32–64	≥128

Table 34:5. MIC Interpretive Standards (μg/mL) of Three Categories of Susceptibility* (Continued)

Antimicrobial Agent	Susceptible	Moderately Susceptible[a]	Resistant
Ticarcillin–clavulanic acid[g]	≤16	32–64	≥128
Tobramycin[b]	≤4	8	≥16
Trimethoprim-sulfamethoxazole[m]	≤2/38	—	≥4/76
Vancomycin	≤4	8–16	≥32
Urinary Tract Antimicrobial Agents			
Ceftizoxime			
when testing gram-negative bacilli including *P. aeruginosa*	≤128	—	≥256
Cinoxacin[n]	≤16	—	≥32
Nalidixic acid[n]	≤16	—	≥32
Nitrofurantoin[n]	≤64	—	≥128
Norfloxacin[n]	≤4	8	≥16
Sulfonamides[n]	≤256	—	≥512
Trimethoprim[n]	≤8	—	≥16
Trimethoprim/suflamethoxazole[m]	≤2/38	4/76–8/152	≥16/304

a. When designated in this table, a ''moderately susceptible'' result should be reported to indicate susceptibility under certain conditions (see 1.7.2) for example, when an antimicrobial agent is concentrated in the urine or when maximum dosing, as indicated in the package insert, is used for systemic infections. In the past, we used the ''conditionally susceptible'' category for strains susceptible to urine concentration; if adequate data are presented to support its use, it can be included in future supplemental tables.

b. The MICs obtained with aminoglycosides, particularly when testing *P. aeruginosa,* are very medium-dependent because of variations in divalent cation content. These interpretive standards are to be used only with Mueller-Hinton agar that has yielded gentamicin zone diameters within the correct range when performance tests were done with *P. aeruginosa* ATCC® 27853 by the M2-A3 method. Cation-supplemented Mueller-Hinton broths will yield similar MIC results.

that MICs obtained with first-generation cephalosporins will be the same. (See Table 34:1 for other drug groupings with a similar spectrum of activity.) Antimicrobial agents listed in the spectrum classes in Table 34:1 have been placed there because of qualitative similarities in their spectrum of activity using applicable MIC breakpoints, i.e., if an organism is susceptible to one of these drugs, it is likely to be susceptible to the others at the breakpoints shown in this table. It does not imply, however, that the MICs will be the same.

S. aureus strains exhibiting heteroresistance to one of the penicillinase-resistant penicillins (MRSA) must be reported as resistant to cephalosporins and other newer β-lactams such as amoxicillin-clavulanic acid, imipenem, and tricarcillin-calvulanic acid, regardless of the in-vitro test results. This is primarily because in most cases of documented MRSA infection, the patient has responded poorly to the cephalosporin therapy or convincing clinical data have yet to be

These values are listed for concentrations used in a $\log_2$ dilution scheme. Some investigators have suggested that concentrations halfway between these intervals are more appropriate for testing aminoglycosides and for breakpoints (like 6, 12, or 24 μg/mL, depending upon the drug).

c. Resistant strains of *S. aureus* produce β-lactamase and the testing of penicillin instead of ampicillin is preferred. Pencillin G should be used to test the susceptibility of all staphylococci to all penicillinase-sensitive penicillins, such as ampicillin, amoxicillin, azlocillin, bacampicillin, hetacillin, carbenicillin, mezlocillin, piperacillin, and ticarcillin. Results may also be applied to phenoxymethyl penicillin, or phenethicillin. Only one category of susceptibility is appropriate for penicillinase-negative staphylococci. A penicillin MIC of ≤0.03 μg/mL usually implies lack of β-lactamase production and MICs of ≥0.25 μg/mL should be considered resistant; staphylococci with MICs between these values may or may not produce the enzyme.

d. When testing *Haemophilus* or *Neisseria* use media modifications. Interpretive criteria may also be applicable to *Branhamella catarrhalis*.

e. Class representative for ampicillin, amoxicillin, bacampicillin, cyclacillin, and hetacillin.

f. For streptococci, staphylococci, and other penicillin-sensitive organisms, "Susceptible" results should be regarded as "Very Susceptible." Enterococcal strains (*S. faecalis, S. faecium,* and *S. durans*) having MICs of ≤0.5 μg/mL for ampicillin or for pencillin G are quite unusual and the streptococcal speciation procedures should be reexamined. Moderately susceptible range MICs are more common with enterococci, some strains of other *Streptococcus* spp. and *Listeria*. Results in this interpretive category for these organisms, when isolated from blood or serious invasive tissue infections, require high dosage of penicillin G or ampicillin, often combined with an aminoglycoside (gentamicin) for improved therapeutic response and bactericidal action.

g. Aztreonam, cefotetan, ceftazadime, ceftriaxone, and imipenem are widely studied β-lactams that have a generally wider spectrum of antimicrobial activity, especially against gram-negative bacilli, when compared to previously approved β-lactams like cephalothin. Although cephalothin can be used as the class representative for first-generation cephalosporins (cephalothin, cefaclor, cefadroxil, cephalexin, cephapirin, cefazolin, and cephradine), it cannot be used as the class representative for other cephalosporins. This does not imply derived confirming clinical efficacy (clavulanic acid combinations and imipenem). Methicillin-resistant, coagulase-negative *Staphylococcus* spp. also appear not to respond well to these drugs, but fewer data are available than with MRSA.

h. Moderately susceptible category designates organisms most likely to require parenteral administration of the macrolide or lincomycin.

j. Tetracycline is the representative for all tetracyclines and the results can be applied to chlortetracycline, demeclocycline, doxycycline, methacycline, minocycline, and oxytetracycline. However, certain organisms may be more susceptible to doxycycline and minocycline than to tetracycline.

k. Interpretive guidelines imply the use of CSMHB containing 2% NaCl. Of the antistaphylococcal, β-lactamase-resistant penicillins, either oxacillin or methicillin may be tested, and results can be applied to the other PRP drugs, nafcillin, cloxacillin, and dicloxacillin. Oxacillin is preferred due to more resistance to degradation in storage and because it is more likely to detect heteroresistant strains. Do not use nafcillin with blood-containing media. Cloxacillin should not be used because it may not detect methicillin-resistant *S. aureus*.

l. Unlike most of the antimicrobial agents listed here, in which the susceptible-moderately susceptible breakpoint correlates with the susceptible disk breakpoint, the *Pseudomonas*-active acylamino penicillins (mezlocillin and piperacillin) have breakpoints that correlate with the moderately susceptible (intermediate)—resistant breakpoints of the disk test. The criteria for other drugs in this spectrum class and the carboxypenicillins are specific for testing either *Pseudomonas* only or *Enterobacteriaceae* (see table listings).

m. Trimethoprim–sulfamethoxazole can also be used for certain systemic infections. Strains causing this infection should be susceptible at ≤2/38 μg/mL, but best responses have been observed for strains with MICs ≤0.5/9.5 μg/mL.

n. Susceptibility data for cinoxacin, nalidixic acid, nitrofurantoin, norfloxacin, sulfonamides, and trimethorprim apply only to organisms isolated from urinary tract infections. Sulfisoxazole can be used for any of the commercially available sulfonamides. Blood-containing media, except media containing lysed horse blood, are not satisfactory for testing sulfonamides. The Mueller-Hinton medium should be as thymidine-free as possible for sulfonamide and/or trimethoprim testing.

* From M2-A3, *Performance Standards for Antimicrobial Disk Susceptibility Tests, Third Edition; Approved Standard* Published December 1984 NCCLS VOL. 4 NO. 16.

coli (ATCC 35218), the last for amoxicillin/clavulanate and ticarcillin/clavulanate. The two *E. coli* and the *P. aeruginosa* strains are the same as those used for quality assurance of the disk diffusion susceptibility test. Appropriate control strains should be run on each test day unless the conditions for weekly testing have been met. These are essentially the same as for disk diffusion susceptibility testing.

AGAR DILUTION ANTIMICROBIAL SUSCEPTIBILITY TESTING[7,17,36]

The basic principles of agar dilution are the same as those of broth dilution. Because up to 37 organisms can be tested on a single series of plates, agar dilution offers an economic advantage for large volume laboratories. It also has the advantage that blood, as well as other supplements, can be added to the medium, and that quality control strains can be tested on the same medium used for test organisms. The potential weaknesses of agar dilution are: 1) it does not lend itself to the performance of MBC testing; 2) swarming *Proteus* spp. can overrun some antibiotic plates unless precautions are taken; 3) since breakpoint concentrations rather than serial twofold dilutions of each drug are usually tested, there is less MIC precision than with broth dilution; and 4) some antibiotics (e.g., some beta-lactams and tetracycline) have a shorter shelf life in agar than in broth.

Materials

1. MHA.
2. Suitable broth (e.g., MHB or trypticase soy broth).
3. Standardized or reference antimicrobial powder.
4. Replicating device.
5. 90 mm square or round petri dishes.

Medium and Antimicrobial Preparation

Antimicrobial solutions should be prepared as stock solutions and stored in the manner described for broth dilution.

MHA should be prepared from dehydrated base according to the manufacturer's instructions. After autoclaving, the MHA should be allowed to cool to 48-50°C and held at that temperature in a water bath. Any desired supplements (e.g., defibrinated sheep, horse or rabbit blood, X and V factors, hemoglobin, etc.) should be added at this time. If blood is chocolatized, the medium must be cooled to 48-50°C before adding the antibiotic solution.

Appropriate dilutions of antibiotic solutions are then added to the molten

MHA at a ratio of 1 mL antibiotic solution to 9 mL of MHA. Thus the concentration of antibiotic in solution should be ten times the desired concentration in agar. Mix thoroughly, and pour the mixture rapidly to a depth of 3 to 4 mm into a petri dish on a flat level surface. Allow the agar to solidify at room temperature. If not used immediately, these plates should be stored at 4-8°C in sealed plastic bags. Most antibiotics are stable under these conditions for up to four weeks, but some (e.g., tetracyclines, cefaclor, ampicillin, methicillin, clavulanate and imipenem) are less stable and control strains should be run routinely.

Test Procedure

1. Prepare a suspension of the test organism with turbidity equivalent to a 0.5 MacFarland standard, using either the standard or alternate (direct) method described for disk diffusion testing. Dilute the suspension 1:10 to achieve an inoculum concentration of 1 X 10^7 CFU/mL.
2. Dispense an aliquot of each suspension to a well of the seed block of a Steers replicator[29] or comparable device.
3. With the replicating device, apply an inoculum (1 to 2 μL) of each organism to the surface of each antimicrobial plate and one MHA plate without antimicrobial agents. This will result in the desired inoculum of 10^4 CFU/spot.
4. Allow the plates to sit bottom side down at room temperature until the inocula are absorbed into the agar. Then invert the plates and incubate them at 35°C for 16-20 h in air.
5. Examine plates for the presence or absence of growth. The lowest concentration of each antimicrobial that inhibits growth (ignore single colony or faint inoculum haze) is considered the MIC.
6. The interpretive categories for the MICs of each drug are listed in Table 34:5, and should be included with the MIC in the susceptibility report.

Exceptions

1. When swarming *Proteus* spp. are among the organisms being tested, action must be taken to prevent their swarming - such as pressing glass cylinders into the agar around the inocula containing *Proteus* spp. or increasing the agar content of the medium.
2. When testing *N. gonorrhoeae*, the antibiotic-containing medium should be DST agar[17] or Proteose #3 agar[10] supplemented with 1% hemoglobin and 1% Kellogg supplement.[37] After inoculation, the plates should be incubated at 35°C in 5-10% CO_2 for 24 h.
3. For testing *N. meningitidis*, the MHA plates should be incubated in 5-10% CO_2 at 35°C for 24 h.

4. For streptococci, the MHA should be supplemented with 5% sheep blood.
5. To enhance the detection of methicillin-resistant (heteroresistant) staphylococci, the MHA should be supplemented with 4% NaCl. Growth on plates containing oxacillin (6 μg/mL) incubated for 24 h at 35°C indicate resistance.[34] Methicillin (10 μg/mL) or nafcillin (6 μg/mL) may be used as alternatives.

Quality Assurance

Because of the greater lability of certain antibiotics in agar, appropriate quality control strains should be tested each day of susceptibility testing. The recommended strains are the same as for broth dilution.

β-LACTAMASE TESTS

The production of β-lactamase by *H. influenzae, N. gonorrhoeae* and staphylococci correlates well with resistance to penicillin and ampicillin as determined by both standard in vitro susceptibility tests and clinical experience. Because some tests for β-lactamase provide results in a matter of minutes in contrast to overnight incubation for conventional susceptibility tests, these more rapid tests play an important role in providing timely and relevant information to the clinician.

There are at least three types of β-lactamase tests that produce rapid results: the iodometric method,[5] the acidometric method[33] and the chromogenic cephalosporin (nitrocefin) method.[21] These three methods are equally sensitive and specific for detecting β-lactamase production by the three organisms listed above, but the nitrocefin method is more sensitive with gram-negative bacilli. Because of its ease of performance and reagent stability, the nitrocefin test[21] has generally superceded the other methods in most clinical laboratories.

Nitrocefin Test[21]

Dissolve 10 mg of nitrocefin in 1 mL of dimethylsulfoxide (DMSO) and dilute to 20 mL in phosphate buffer, pH 7.0. This solution will contain 500 μg/mL of nitrocefin, have a yellow color and be stable at 4-8°C for 8 weeks or more.

Prepare a heavy suspension of the organism to be tested in a small volume (50-100 μL) of the nitrocefin solution in a small tube or microtiter tray well. After thorough mixing, observe for a color change from yellow to red for up to one hour. Most *H. influenzae* and *N. gonorrhoeae* that produce β-lactamase will produce a color change within five minutes, but some staphylococci may take up to an hour. Staphylococci often produce the color change more quickly if they have been preinduced by growth in subinhibitory concentrations of a β-lactamase-inducer such as oxacillin - e.g., colonies at the edge of the zone of inhibition around an oxacillin disk.

There are a number of modifications of this test, including performing the test directly on agar plates with *H. influenzae* and *N. gonorrhoeae*. However, the color change is not always as easy to detect on agar. Also, commercial systems using nitrocefin are available, e.g., cefinase (Baltimore Biological Laboratories).

MINIMAL BACTERICIDAL CONCENTRATION (MBC)

In broth dilution susceptibility testing, the MIC is defined as the lowest concentration of drug with no grossly visible growth. However, if this tube or well is subcultured onto an agar plate, substantial bacterial growth may occur - indicating that, although the drug inhibited growth at that concentration, it did not kill the organism. When all the tubes or wells with no visible growth are subcultured, the lowest concentration with 99.9% or more reduction of the initial bacterial population is referred to as the MBC. The determination of MBCs remains a controversial test for two major reasons:

1. The clinical relevance of in vitro MBC testing has yet to be unequivocally demonstrated. Although it is generally accepted that bactericidal activity of antimicrobial agents is important for immunocompromised hosts with infections and in certain types of infection such as bacterial endocarditis, meningitis and osteomyelitis, the evidence that MBC determination plays a useful role in antibiotic selection is not well established.
2. The test for determining MBCs has not been standardized. There are numerous variables in the test which can significantly affect the endpoint. These include: 1) growth phase of the bacteria in the inoculum;[13,32] 2) media that vary in pH, concentration of divalent cations, salt, phosphates and proteins; 3) presence or absence of serum in the medium;[24,26] 4) degree of contact between antimicrobial and test microbe;[32] 5) volume of medium transferred for counting survivors;[22] and 6) all the factors that can affect the broth dilution method for MIC determination.[7]

Although no universally accepted standardized method exists for MBC determination currently, the NCCLS Subcommittee for Bactericidal Activity Testing Parameters has published a proposed standard (M26-P),[19] which should be a major step in this direction.

Test Procedure

1. The basic procedure for the broth dilution susceptibility test should be followed with the following modifications:
   a. Use 13 X 100 mm glass tubes with 2 mL of antibiotic-containing CSMHB of each dilution and one tube containing no antibiotic.
   b. Use the standard method for inoculum standardization to turbidity equal to 0.5 MacFarland standard.
   c. Inoculate 0.1 mL of a 1:20 dilution of the standardized suspension into each tube with a pipetter. Release the inocula beneath the broth surface. Mix by flushing several times without creating bubbles or splashing sides of tube.
   d. Perform a colony count of the inoculum by preparing a 1:1000 dilution (0.1 mL of inoculated growth control broth in 100 mL of sterile water) and spreading 0.1 mL over the surface of a blood agar plate. The number of colonies present after incubation times 10^4 equals the colony count of the inoculated tubes of broth.
   e. After 20 h incubation at 35°C, mix each suspension gently and repeat mixing at 24 h.
2. At 24 h, remove 0.01 mL of each culture without visible growth with a calibrated pipetter and streak onto a blood agar plate.
3. After overnight incubation at 35°C, count the number of colonies on each plate.
4. The endpoint (MBC) is the lowest concentration subculture that yields colony counts equal to or less than the so-called rejection value.[22] The rejection value is a function of the original colony count of the inoculum and the Poisson distribution model. Tables providing rejection values for various inoculum concentrations have been published.[22]

Comments:

For most organisms tested against bactericidal antibiotics such as the β-lactams and aminoglycosides, the MBC will be the same or within 2 $\log_2$ concentration of the MIC. Several types of deviations from this may occur:

1. Persisters. Occasionally about 0.1% of the inoculated bacteria will survive all concentrations of the drug tested when the MIC is quite low. A similar number of bacteria will usually be present on all subculture plates. Retesting these persisters results in the same phenomenon. The lowest concentration at which a stable number of bacteria persist is probably a valid endpoint.
2. Eagle phenomenon. This is a paradoxical phenomenon in which the number of survivors increases as the drug concentration increases beyond the apparent MBC. The explanation for this phenomenon is uncertain, but the apparent MBC is probably a valid endpoint.
3. Tolerance. This refers to the survivial of bacteria in numbers greater

than the rejection value in the presence of a bactericidal drug at concentrations equal to or greater than 32 times higher than the MIC. Delayed killing can often be observed if subcultures are performed after 48 to 72 h of incubation.

Another method of testing for bactericidal activity is the so-called time-kill method that is rarely used in clinical laboratories, but it may, in fact, have better clinical correlation.[6]

SERUM BACTERICIDAL TEST

In principle, the serum bactericidal test (SBT) is essentially the same as the broth dilution bactericidal test. However, instead of testing known dilutions (concentrations) of antibiotics, the SBT tests serial dilutions of sera of patients receiving antibiotics. The indication for the test are the same as for MBC determination. However, there are several theoretical advantages of the SBT, since it provides a measure of some of the in vivo variables that influence the effectiveness of antimicrobial therapy. These include such variables as drug interaction with other drugs, absorption and excretion of drugs, effect of active metabolites of antibiotics, serum protein-binding of the antibiotic, etc. As with MBC determination, published data correlating the SBT with clinical response are conflicting. This is undoubtedly for the same reason - viz., lack of technical standardization of the SBT.[23] This issue is also being addressed by the NCCLS Subcommittee for the Serum Bactericidal Test and a proposed standard (M21-P) has been published.[20] Once a standardized procedure is accepted, evaluation of its clinical relevance will be more feasible and meaningful. The procedure outlined is based on some of the better controlled studies.[20,22,24,26,27,28,30,31]

Test Procedure

1. Using sterile technique, collect timed serum specimens from the patient corresponding to expected peaks and trough levels of antibiotic. Peak levels should be chosen 30 min after completion of an IV infusion, 60 min after an IM injection or 90 min after an oral dose of the drug; trough levels should be drawn within 15 min prior to the next dose.
2. Immediately transport the specimen to the laboratory, centrifuge and aseptically remove the serum. If the test is not being done within two hours, freeze the serum.
3. The test medium should be a combination of CSMHB and pooled normal human serum at a final 1:1 ratio. The CSMHB must meet the quality assurance standards for broth dilution testing. The pooled human serum (from healthy human volunteers or commercial source) should be screened and shown to be free of: HBsAg, HIV antibody,

β-lactamase activity and other antimicrobial activity. The serum should be adjusted to a pH of 7.3 + 0.1 at 25°C (using 0.1 N HC1 or NaOH as appropriate) and filtered using a 0.80 and a 0.45 μm filter.

4. Using 13 X 100 mm glass tubes numbered 1 to 10, add 1.0 mL of patient's serum to tubes 1 and 2, and 1.0 mL of pooled serum to tubes 2 thru 10. Make serial twofold dilutions beginning with tube 2 and ending with tube 9, using a separate pipette for each step and vortexing each newly diluted mixture. Remove 1.0 mL from tube 9 and discard. Add 1.0 mL of CSMHB to each tube 1 thru 10 to achieve a final volume of 2.0 mL in each tube.
5. Prepare a standardized suspension of the patient's isolate, equivalent to a 0.5 MacFarland standard as described for disk diffusion testing. Use a 1:20 dilution of this suspension in broth for the inoculum.
6. Inoculate each tube with 0.1 mL of inoculum with a calibrated pipetter and release the inocula beneath the surface of the medium. Mix by flushing without creating bubbles or splashing the walls of the tube.
7. Perform a colony count of the inoculum as described for MBC determination.
8. Incubate and subculture as described for MBC determination.
9. The endpoint is the highest serum dilution that yields colony counts equal to or less than the rejection value,[22] which is determined by the same method as for the MBC.

Comment:

The same phenomena of persisters, Eagle effect and tolerance that occur with MBC determination are encountered occasionally with SBTs.

In addition to growth control (tube 10), quality assurance of the test system can be accomplished by performing MBC determinations of the patient's drug with appropriate standard reference strains (see broth dilution) with and without pooled serum. The MBCs of many antimicrobials against these strains have been published.[26]

Macrodilution methods are generally preferable to microdilution because of the greater reliability of procuring adequate subculture volumes.

REFERENCES

1. Barry AL, Badal RE. Reliability of the microdilution technic for detection of methicillin-resistant strains of *Staphylococcus aureus*. Am J Clin Pathol 1977;67:489-95.
2. Barry AL, Garcia F, Thrupp LD. An improved single-disc method for testing the antibiotic susceptibility of rapidly growing pathogens. Am J Clin Pathol 1970;53:149-58.
3. Barry AL, Jones RN, Gavan TL. Evaluation of the Micro-Media System for quantitative antimicrobial drug susceptibility testing: a collaborative study. Antimicrob Agents Chemother 1978;13:61-9.
4. Bauer AW, Kirby WMM, Sherris JC, Turck M. Antibiotic susceptibility testing by a standardized single disc method. Am J Clin Pathol 1966;45:493-6.

5. Catlin BW. Iodometric detection of *Haemophilus influenzae* beta-lactamase: rapid presumptive test for ampicillin resistance. Antimicrob Agents Chemother 1975;7:265-70.
6. Drake TA, Sande MA. Studies of the chemotherapy of endocarditis. Correlation of in vitro, animal model and clinical studies. Rev Infect Dis 1985;5(Suppl 2):345-53.
7. Ericsson HM, Sherris JC. Antibiotic sensitivity testing. Report of an international collaborative study. Acta Pathol Microbiol Scand 1971;217(Suppl):1-90.
8. Fleming A. On the antibacterial action of cultures of a penicillium, with special reference to their use in the isolation of *B. influenzae*. Br J Exp Pathol 1929;10:226-36.
9. Gavan TL, Town MA. A microdilution method for antibiotic susceptibility testing: An evaluation. Am J Clin Pathol 1970;53:880-5.
10. Jaffe HW, Biddle JW, Thornsberry C, et al. National gonorrhea therapy monitoring study: in vitro antibiotic susceptibility and its correlation with treatment results. N Engl J Med 1976;294:5-9.
11. Jones RN, Edson DC, Marymont JV. Evaluations of antimicrobial susceptibility test proficiency by the College of American Pathologists Survey Program. Am J Clin Pathol 1982;78:168-72.
12. Jones RN, Gavan TL, Barry AL. The evaluation of the Sensititre microdilution antibiotic susceptibility system against recent clinical isolates: a three laboratory collaborative study. J Clin Microbiol 1980;11:426-9.
13. Kim KS, Anthony BF. Importance of bacterial growth phase in determining minimal bactericidal concentrations of penicillin and methicillin. Antimicrob Agents Chemother 1981;19:1075-7.
14. Marley DC. A simple method for testing the sensitivity of wound bacteria to penicillin and sulfathiazole by use of impregnated blotting paper discs. J Pathol Bacteriol 1945;57:379-82.
15. Marymont JH, Wentz RM. Serial dilution antibiotic sensitivity testing with the microtitrator system. Am J Clin Pathol 1966;45:548-51.
16. National Committee for Clinical Laboratory Standards. Performance standards for antimicrobial disk susceptibility tests. Approved Standard M2-A3. Villanova, PA: National Committee for Clinical Laboratory Standards, 1984.
17. National Committee for Clinical Laboratory Standards. Standard methods for dilution antimicrobial susceptibility tests for bacteria which grow aerobically. Approved Standard M7-A. Villanova, PA: National Committee for Clinical Laboratory Standards, 1985.
18. National Committee for Clinical Laboratory Standards. Evaluating production lots of dehydrated Mueller-Hinton agar. M6-P. Villanova, PA: National Committee for Clinical Laboratory Standards, 1986.
19. National Committee for Clinical Laboratory Standards. Methods for determining bactericidal activity of antimicrobial agents. M-26P. Villanova, PA: National Committee for Clinical Laboratory Standards, 1987.
20. National Committee for Clinical Laboratory Standards. Methodology for the serum bactericidal test. M-21P. Villanova, PA: National Committee for Clinical Laboratory Standards, 1987.
21. O'Callaghan CH, Morris A, Kirby SM, Shingler AH. Novel method for detection of β-lactamase by using a chromogenic cephalosporin substrate. Antimicrob Agents Chemother 1972;1:283-8.
22. Pearson RD, Steigbigel RT, Davis HT, Chapman SW. Method for reliable determination of minimal lethal antibiotic concentrations. Antimicrob Agents Chemother 1980;18:699-708.
23. Pien FD, Vosti KL. Variation in performance of the serum bactericidal test. Antimicrob Agents Chemother 1974;6:330-3.
24. Pien FD, Williams RD, Vosti KL. Comparison of broth and human serum as the diluent in the serum bactericidal test. Antimicrob Agents Chemother 1975;7:113-14.
25. Rammelkamp CH, Maxon T. Resistance of *Staphylococcus aureus* to the action of penicillin. Proc Soc Exp Biol Med 1942;51:386-9.

26. Reimer LG, Stratton CW, Reller LB. Minimal inhibitory and bactericidal concentrations of 44 antimicrobial agents against three standard control strains in broth with and without human serum. Antimicrob Agents Chemother 1981;19:1050-5.
27. Reller LB, Stratton CW. Serum dilution test for bactericidal activity. II. Standardization and correlation with antimicrobial assays and susceptibility tests. J Infect Dis 1977;136:196-203.
28. Shanholtzer CJ, Peterson LR, Mohn ML, Moody JA, Gerding DN. MBCs for *Staphylococcus aureus* as determined by macrodilution and microdilution techniques. Antimicrob Agents Chemother 1984;26:214-19.
29. Steers E, Foltz E, Graves BS, Riden J. An inocula replicating apparatus for routine testing of bacterial susceptibility to antibiotics. Antibiot Chemother 1959;9:307-11.
30. Stratton CW, Reller LB. Serum dilution test for bactericidal activity. I. Selection of a physiologic diluent. J Infect Dis 1977;136:187-95.
31. Stratton CW, Weinstein MP, Reller LB. Correlation of serum bactericidal activity with antimicrobial agent level and minimal bactericidal concentration. J Infect Dis 1982;145:160-8.
32. Taylor PC, Schoenknecht FD, Sherris JC, Linner EC. Determination of minimum bactericidal concentrations of oxacillin for *Staphylococcus aureus*: influence and significance of technical factors. Antimicrob Agents Chemother 1983;23:142-50.
33. Thornsberry C, Kirven LA. Ampicillin resistance in *Haemophilus influenzae* as determined by a rapid test for beta-lactamase production. Antimicrob Agents Chemother 1974;6:653-4.
34. Thornsberry C, McDougal LK. Successful use of broth microdilution in susceptibility tests for methicillin-resistant (heteroresistant) staphylococci. J Clin Microbiol 1983;18:1084-91.
35. Vincent JC, Vincent HW. Filter paper disc modification of the Oxford cup penicillin determination. Proc Soc Exp Biol Med 1944;55:162-4.
36. Washington JA. The agar dilution technique. In: Balows A, ed. Current techniques for antibiotic susceptibility testing. Springfield, IL: Charles C. Thomas, 1974:54-62.
37. White LA, Kellogg DS Jr. *Neisseria gonorrhoeae* identification in direct smears by a fluorescent antibody-counterstain method. Appl Microbiol 1965;13:171-4.

CHAPTER 35

AUTOMATED AND INSTRUMENTED PROCEDURES FOR ANTIMICROBIAL SUSCEPTIBILITY TESTING

Steven D. Brown, Ph.D.

INTRODUCTION

Prior to the 1960s, there were relatively few successful attempts at bringing automated techniques to the clinical microbiology laboratory. First generation instruments, introduced in the late sixties and early seventies, met with only limited success and failed to achieve widespread acceptance. Since that time, mechanization within the microbiology laboratory has steadily grown to the point where machines now perform a wide variety of previously manual tasks. The clinical microbiologist is faced with the difficult problem of critically examining each available instrument and selecting one which is most appropriate for meeting the laboratory's specialized needs and requirements.

The performance of antimicrobial susceptibility tests has lent itself most readily to mechanization. Today, this is accomplished by monitoring optical or fluorometric changes of growth patterns in an antibiotic-containing medium compared with growth in an antibiotic-free control. Earlier attempts to monitor changes in growth by radiometry,[9] bioluminescence,[14] microcalorimetry [3] or electrical impedance[7] met with limited success.

Several automated or mechanized systems, approved by the Food and Drug Administration (FDA), are capable of producing either a category type of result (i.e., susceptible, intermediate or resistant) or a minimum inhibitory concentration (MIC) report. These results can be achieved within three hours of incubation with some instruments and are the result of truly innovative approaches to susceptibility testing. Other instruments are merely automated or mechanized approaches to more traditional susceptibility testing methodologies. In either case, these instruments have made a profound impact on the field of clinical microbiology and are likely to play an even more important role in the future.

In selecting an instrument best suited for an individual laboratory, a variety of factors must be carefully considered. The first parameter to be considered is the accuracy and reproducibility of the system. Clinical evaluations are available which analyze this aspect of performance. A second, and equally important, parameter to be considered is the mechanical reliability of the instrument. This information is more difficult to obtain. In most instances, all that can be accomplished is to contact a current user of the system and query them regarding the service record of the unit. Thirdly, the system must be versatile. It must be easily updated to accept newer developments in technology and computer software. Finally, the system must produce results which are justifiable financially. This parameter must include not only the cost of the instrument plus expendables, but also alterations in staffing and workflow which may be necessary to accomodate the system.

This chapter will only address the accuracy and reproducibility of each of the various systems. Parameters such as mechanical reliability, versatility and cost effectiveness must be analyzed in light of overall test volume and the specific needs of each individual laboratory.

INSTRUMENTATION OF AGAR AND MICRO-BROTH DILUTION PROCEDURES

Agar Dilution

In the late 1950s, Steers et al[31] developed a replicate plating device which provided for the simultaneous inoculation of up to 36 isolates onto a series of antibiotic-containing agar plates. The Cathra Replianalyzer System (MCT Diagnostics) adapted this technique by including a series of biochemical plates for the identification of the isolates and devising a computer program capable of analyzing and interpreting the data. Early evaluations of the instrument were promising.[5]

The system is based upon the manual recording of visible growth on a defined series of biochemical plates and a user-defined panel of antibiotic-containing agar plates. The system represents primarily a computer-assisted method of recording standardized agar dilution susceptibilities, and thus is limited to high-volume laboratories capable of using an agar dilution approach for routine susceptibilities. A smaller version of the same system is designed for small-volume laboratories and requires that each plate be read completely before proceeding to the next plate. In either case, the antibiotic-containing plates are not available commercially, a fact which limits the usefulness of the system to those institutions capable of preparing their own plates.

Micro-broth Dilution

Although microtitration methods for antimicrobial susceptibility testing have been available for some time,[33] their entry into the commercial marketplace did not occur until the 1970s. Since that time, broth microdilution techniques have provided an efficient and economical alternative to the more cumbersome dilutional procedures. The microtiter techniques have the advantages of less storage space, ease of use and standardization of media and drug preparations. Lyophilized trays have the additional advantages of extended shelf-life, room temperature storage and the ability to test antibiotics (e.g., imipenem) which cannot be stored at -20°C.

Commercially available automated dispensers, such as the MIC-2000 (Dynatech Laboratories), the Quick Spense System (Bellco Glass) and the Anderson-Pasco System (Pasco), allow for the "in-house" preparation of susceptibility trays (see Chapter 45 for addresses of manufacturers). On-site preparation of the trays has the distinct advantage of versatility; an essential feature when one considers the speed with which newer antibiotics are being introduced and the rapidity with which hospital formularies are revised.

The next step toward automation occurred when microdilution plates became commercially available and instruments were produced which assisted in recording the results. Within the last few years, there has been a veritable explosion in the number of manufacturers offering pre-prepared trays and instruments for the identification and antimicrobial susceptibility testing of rapidly growing organisms. The manufacturers which currently dominate the marketplace include: American Micro Scan (Touchscan, Autoscan-4 and Autoscan WalkAway systems), Becton Dickinson (Sceptor), Gibco Diagnositics (Sensititre), Beckman Micro Media Systems (Micro-Coder) and Difco Laboratories (Pasco MIC-ID). API Analytab Products currently markets a manual system for susceptibility testing (Unisept system) and promises to have its fully automated ALADIN system available in the near future. List prices range from around $7,000 for the simpler, manually operated systems to over $85,000 for the MicroScan WalkAway. Less expensive models require manual data entry via a lightpen, joystick or a specialized keyboard, whereas those at the other end of the spectrum are able to provide varying levels of automated reading and recording of data.

The Sensititre, Sceptor and API systems use lyophilized panels which can be stored at room temperatures and have an extended shelf life. The remaining systems utilize frozen trays which must be delivered and stored at -20°C. All systems require 16-24 hours of incubation with the exception of GIBCO's Sensititre system which is capable of producing reliable results[30] in 3-5 hours using fluorescent substrates. Other manufacturers are in the process of developing and evaluating methods for the production of reliable results in 6 hours or less.

All of the systems currently available claim to be capable of accurately identifying the majority of commonly encountered gram-negative organisms. Accuracy in identification generally ranges from 93-98%[1,2,4,39] although many of the newer systems are still awaiting comparative evaluations. Gram-negative identification systems are available separately, but are frequently combined with dilutions of antimicrobial agents, thus providing a susceptibility-identification panel. Biochemical panels for the identification and susceptibility testing of gram-positive aerobes, fastidious organisms and anaerobic isolates are currently available from only a small number of manufacturers.

Comparative studies have found the accuracy of the various microdilution susceptibility systems to be very good[12,15,20,37] and to correlate well with disk diffusion, agar dilution and in-house broth microdilution procedures.[36] Agreement between two or more systems is generally around 92-95% with less than 2% major discrepancies. Most authors agree that automated systems are reliable and represent valuable tools for the performance of susceptibility tests. In fact, it is widely speculated that commercially prepared, mechanically read panels offer a greater degree of reproducibility than is possible through in-house preparation and manual reading of similar trays.

The greatest drawback to the use of commercially available trays is the limited selection of antibiotics on any given test tray. Several manufacturers currently market a variety of trays with differing antibiotic combinations in an effort to match hospital formularies as closely as possible. Other manufacturers, such as GIBCO, will "custom make" susceptibility trays in order to meet the specific needs of individual clients. The manufacturers that provide custom made panels usually require a sizable minimum order, frequently leading to storage difficulties as well as problems with outdating of the trays.

A second drawback to commercially prepared trays is the long delay between the introduction of a new drug into the marketplace and its availability on the tray itself. Manufacturers vary widely in their ability to place a new antibiotic into their test systems. Delays of up to 2 years have been noted with certain manufacturers. Needless to say, this delay is generally unacceptable and limits the usefulness of a given susceptibility instrument or system.

The final dilemma pertaining to the use of commercial microdilution trays is that of quality control. Due to limitations of space on the tray, many of the commercial systems do not provide a full range of dilutions for each antibiotic tested. This factor makes it virtually impossible to achieve on-scale quantitative results for all antibiotics when using standard reference strains for quality control. Thus, only gross changes in antibiotic activity are detected. This feature may require the use of specific control organisms from the manufacturer in addition to the standard reference strains for quality control.

AUTOBAC

The Autobac system is a semiautomated approach to the identification and antimicrobial susceptibility testing of aerobic isolates. The system was originally developed by Pfizer Diagnostics but is now marketed by the Organon Teknika Corporation. This instrument utilizes photometric monitoring of growth in a specially designed, multi-chambered cuvette which contains a battery of user-selected antimicrobial agents. The technologist prepares a standardized inoculum of the organism in question, transfers the inoculum to the multi-chambered cuvette, then places the cuvette into a shaker/incubator. After 3-5 hours of incubation, the cuvette is manually transferred to the photometer unit which measures the amount of light scattered in each compartment of the compound cuvette. The degree of light scattering, known as the light-scattering index (LSI), can then be used to determine the amount of growth present. The internal computer uses the LSI to determine if the organism is susceptible, intermediate or resistant to each of the antibiotics in the test panel.

An extensive, collaborative investigation of the Autobac I revealed a 90% correlation between the system and conventional Bauer-Kirby test results.[35] The majority of the discrepancies appeared to be unique to certain drug-organism combinations (e.g., *Pseudomonas* versus kanamycin, *Enterobacter* versus ampicillin and cephalothin, etc.). Later reports uncovered additional discrepancies with certain drug-organism combinations.[6,22,32,38] Despite these peculiarities, the system has been quite reliable in providing rapid susceptibility testing results.

The system's capabilities were later expanded to include minimum inhibitory concentration (MIC) susceptibility reports in addition to the original S-I-R type of reporting. The MIC modification was made possible by testing two concentrations of each antibiotic and computer-assisted interpretation of the data. The MIC method was accurate and the results were equivalent to those obtained by more traditional methods.[29]

The Autobac Series II instrument provides identification of enteric and nonfermentative organisms as well as qualitative and quantitative susceptibility test results. The system also performs inexpensive screening of urine samples for the presence of significant bacteriuria. The predictive value of a negative screen has been shown to be 99%.[16]

Advantage Microbiology Center

The Advantage Microbiology Center is the latest modification of an instrument developed by Abbott Diagnostics and originally marketed as the MS-2 Microbiology System. In its present configuration, the unit can perform rapid (3-6 hour) automated susceptibility testing, gram-negative bacterial identification in 4-5 hours, urine screening for significant bacteriuria in 1-5 hours and yeast identification in approximately 24 hours. The instrument performs these functions by photometrically scanning the disposable cuvette at 5 minute intervals and recording colorimetric and/or turbidimetric changes as a result of microbial growth. The Advantage System differs from the Autobac in that it is slightly more automated, requiring fewer manual manipulations, and is capable of providing a clinically relevant type of MIC report (e.g., <4 μg/mL or >16 μg/mL) from a single antibiotic elution disk.

Susceptibility results are generated by comparing the kinetic growth potential of an organism with the growth of the organism in the presence of a single concentration of a given antibiotic. Computerized analysis of the resultant growth curve is used to extrapolate the MIC for the drug in question.

Published reports indicate 94% accuracy in the identification of *Enterobacteriaceae* when compared to conventional tube methodology[25] or the API 20E (Analytab Products).[11] The system accurately identifies 96% of all yeast isolates[8] and produces accurate susceptibility results with most nonfastidious, facultative aerobic organisms.[34] Evaluation of the urine screening capabilities indicate an overall accuracy of 84%[24] to 96%[13] in identifying significant bacteriuria.

The Advantage system is unique in that the instrument is easily adaptable for a variety of research applications. It has been used to perform synergism studies, mutagenicity studies, drug stability tests, Schlichter testing, serum bioassays of antimicrobic levels, studies of growth inhibitors and enhancers, etc. The flexibility and versatility of the instrument makes this system very desirable for those laboratories combining routine clinical microbiology with clinical research.

AutoMicrobic System (AMS)

The AutoMicrobic System (Vitek Systems) was the first microbiological instrument to utilize "space age" technology in that it was originally developed for use by the National Aeronautics and Space Administration. Although initially designed to detect, enumerate and identify organisms directly from clinical specimens (urine), the system has been expanded to include antibiotic susceptibility testing, yeast identification, anaerobe speciation, *Neisseria* identification and *Haemophilus* biotyping. The majority of these functions can be performed in less than 13 hours.

The heart of the system is a plastic test card, approximately the size of a credit card. The unit contains a series of small wells or microcuvettes. A measured volume of urine is placed into the card inoculator and the unit is placed into a diluting module. The instrument then automatically dilutes and dispenses the specimen into each of the microcuvettes of the test card. After inoculation, the card is placed in the incubator module which optically "reads" the card at predetermined time intervals for changes in growth. Once the card is placed into the incubation chamber, all reading functions are fully automated. Identification and susceptibility testing of rapidly growing organisms can frequently be accomplished in as little as 4 hours.

The AMS has been shown to have an accuracy of 97%[17] for the identification of *Enterobacteriaceae* and an accuracy of 96%[18] with non-fermentative organisms. Organisms obtained directly from blood culture bottles and incubated for 5 hours in the AMS were identified in 92% of the cases studied.[23] Identification accuracy for medically important yeasts was 96% when combined with morphological examination.[28]

Results of studies examining the accuracy of various susceptibility test cards have varied widely. Overall agreement with microdilution systems has ranged from a high of 96.2%[19] for *Pseudomonas aeruginosa*, to a low of 77.9%[26] for enterococci. Numerous investigators have found the overall accuracy to be >80% when compared to a variety of microdilution methods.[15,19,21,2,6] It is important to emphasize that many of the discrepancies noted were the result of problems with specific organism-antibiotic combinations.

The Vitek AMS is presently the only instrument on the market which is capable of enumeration and selective identification of organisms directly from a clinical specimen. This is accomplished through the use of a variety of nonconventional, selective media within the urine IDENTI-PAK card. This feature of the AMS system has been shown to have a quantitation accuracy of 99% and an identification accuracy of 95% after 1-13 hours of incubation.[27] Although the direct identification capabilities of the instrument are highly desirable, the total cost of the system limits its usefulness to high-volume laboratories. A smaller version of the system, the Vitek Jr., is now available for lower volume laboratories at a substantially reduced cost. The Vitek Jr., therefore, is capable of producing economically justifiable susceptibility results in a fraction of the time required for conventional testing.

A variety of epidemiology and data management software programs are available to enhance the usefulness of the system. However, the high cost of the system has placed the unit beyond the reach of most clinical laboratories.

CONCLUSION

The goal of all instrumented susceptibility systems should be to produce consistently reliable results, with decreased overall costs within a time frame which will be of value to the physician and the patient. Most instrumented procedures are effective in removing technologist variability as a cause of minor discrepancies in bacterial identification and susceptibility testing. It is also believed that automated instruments improve the overall efficiency and productivity of the microbiology laboratory and result in a more rapid turn around time for completed reports. These parameters are difficult to document and critically evaluate; they can be expected to vary widely from laboratory to laboratory.

The cost effectiveness of these instrumented procedures is a matter of continuing debate and is not easily determined. An instrument may provide a substantial cost savings at one institution, yet may actually increase overall costs at a second institution. Thus, it is imperative that each laboratory carefully evaluate the impact of an instrument before a purchase agreement is signed. This evaluation is far from easy. In many cases the increased cost to the laboratory is greatly outweighed by a decrease in the patients' overall length of stay as the result of rapidly reporting susceptibility results. Rapid reporting may also increase the utilization of specific antibiotic therapy rather than relying on the use of expensive, broad spectrum, emperic coverage.

The final aspect to be considered is the speed with which laboratory results are transmitted to the physician. There is little value in producing a 4- or 13-hour automated susceptibility report if there is no mechanism for rapidly conveying that information to the physician. All too frequently, the many advantages of automated procedures are not fully realized due to a failure to link the technologies for rapid procedures with the ability to rapidly transmit the resulting information.

Ultimately, the decision to automate, as well as the type of instrument to purchase, rests squarely with individual laboratories. One instrument which meets all of the needs of each and every laboratory has yet to be invented. Interlaboratory variables such as workload volume, extent of service, hours of coverage, the number and skill level of technologists, the availability of computer-assisted reporting and record-keeping functions and the accessibility of capital funding, all serve to complicate the decision making process. Each laboratory must decide which instrument will meet their greatest needs at a justifiable cost.

REFERENCES

1. Barry AL, Badal RE, Effinger LJ. Reproducibility of three microdilution systems for identification of *Enterobacteriaceae*, compared with API 20E and Micro-ID systems. Curr Microbiol 1979;3:21-5.
2. Barry AL, Badal RE, Effinger LJ. Identification of *Enterobacteriaceae* in frozen microdilution trays prepared by Micro-Media Systems. J Clin Microbiol 1979;10:492-6.
3. Binford JS, Binford LF, Alder P. A semi-automated microcalorimetric method of antibiotic sensitivity testing. Am J Clin Pathol 1973;59:86-94.
4. Borchardt KA, Gibson J. Comparison of enteric identification systems. Health Lab Sci 1977;14:5-10.
5. Brown SD, Washington JA II. Evaluation of the Repliscan system for identification of *Enterobacterieceae*. J Clin Microbiol 1978;8:695-9.
6. Cleary TJ, Maurer D. Methicillin-resistant *Staphylococcus aureus* susceptibility testing by an automated system, Autobac I. Antimicrob Agents Chemother 1978;13:837-41.
7. Colvin HJ, Sherris JC. Electrical impedance measurement in the reading and monitoring of broth dilution susceptibility tests. Antimicrob Agents Chemother 1977;12:61-6.
8. Cooper BH, Prowant S, Alexander B, Brunson DH. Collaborative evaluation of the Abbott yeast identification system. J Clin Microbiol 1984;19:853-6.

9. DeBlanc HJ, Charache P, Wagner HN, Jr. Automated radiometric measurement of antibiotic effect on bacterial growth. Antimicrob Agents Chemother 1972;2:360-6.
10. DeGirolami PC, Eichelberger KA, Salfity LC, Rizzo MF. Evaluation of the AutoSCAN-3, a device for reading microdilution trays. J Clin Microbiol 1983;18:1292-5.
11. DiPersio JR, Dyke JW, Vannest RD. Evaluation of the updated MS-2 bacterial identification system in comparison with the API 20E system. J Clin Microbiol 1983;18:128-35.
12. Gavan TL, Jones RN, Barry AL. Evaluation of the Sensititre system for quantitative antimicrobial drug susceptibility testing: A collaborative study. Antimicrob Agents Chemother 1980;17:464-9.
13. Godowski KC, Hodges WJ. Accuracy and effect upon clinical workload of the MS-2 urine screen and antibiotic susceptibility system. Lab Med 1981;12:758-64.
14. Gutekunst RR. Rapid procedures under development and evaluation: Bioluminescence and impedance measurement. In: Bondi A, Bartola JT, Prier JE, eds. The clinical laboratory as an aid in chemotherapy of infectious diseases. Baltimore: University Park Press, 1977:85-100.
15. Hansen SL, Freedy PK. Concurrent comparability of automated systems and commercially prepared microdilution trays for susceptibility testing. J Clin Microbiol 1983;17:878-86.
16. Heinz T, Pezzlo M, Thrupp L. Clinical and laboratory efficiency of rapidly screening urine cultures by nephelometry. Am J Clin Pathol 1982;77:305-11.
17. Isenberg HD, Gavan TL, Smith PB, et al. Collaborative investigation of the AutoMicrobic system *Enterobacteriaceae* biochemical card. J Clin Microbiol 1980;11:694-702.
18. Johnson JE, Brinkley AW. Identification of nonfermentative gram-negative bacilli using the Vitek AutoMicrobic System (AMS) Abstract. Annual Meeting of the American Society for Microbiology 1981; C122.
19. Johnson JE, Jorgensen JH, Crawford SA, Redding JS, Pruneda RC. Comparison of two automated instrument systems for rapid susceptibility testing of gram-negative bacilli. J Clin Microbiol 1983;18:1301-9.
20. Jones RN, Thornsberry C, Barry AL, et al. Evaluation of the Sceptor microdilution antibiotic susceptibility testing system: A collaborative investigation. J Clin Microbiol 1981;13:184-94.
21. Kelly MT, Latimer JM, Balfour LC. Comparison of three automated systems for antimicrobial susceptibility testing of gram-negative bacilli. J Clin Microbiol 1982;15:902-5.
22. Lampe MF, Aitken CL, Dennis PG, Forsythe PS, Patrick KE. Schoenknecht FD, Sherris JC. Relationship of early readings of minimal inhibitory concentrations to the results of overnight tests. Antimicrob Agents Chemother 1975;8:429-33.
23. Malloy PA, Ducate MJ, Schreckenberger PC. Comparison of four rapid methods for identification of *Enterobacteriaceae* from blood cultures. J Clin Microbiol 1983;17:493-9.
24. McCarthy LR, Gavan TL, Robson J, Corlett C. Evaluation of the MS-2 urine screening method for detection of bacteriuria. J Clin Microbiol 1982;16:250-2.
25. McCracken AW, Martin WJ, McCarthy LR, Schwab DA. Evaluation of the MS-2 system for rapid identification of *Enterobacteriaceae*. J Clin Microbiol 1980;12:684-9.
26. Morello JA, Graves MH. Evaluation of the Vitek AMS gram-positive susceptibility (GPS) card. Proceedings of Fourth Annual AMS User Group Symposium, 1982:1-7.
27. Nicholson DP, Koepke JA. The AutoMicrobic system for urines. J Clin Microbiol 1979;10:823-33.
28. Oblack DL, Rhodes JC, Martin WJ. Clinical evaluation of the AutoMicrobic system yeast biochemical card for rapid identification of medically important yeasts. J Clin Microbiol 1981;13:351-5.
29. Schoenknecht FD, Washington JA II, Gavan TL, Thornsberry C. Rapid determination of minimum inhibitory concentrations of antimicrobial agents by the Autobac method: a collaborative study. Antimicrob Agents Chemother 1980;17:824-33.
30. Staneck JL, Allen SD, Harris EE, Tilton RC. Automated reading of MIC microdilution trays containing fluorogenic enzyme substrates with the Sensititre Autoreader. J Clin Microbiol 1985;22:187-91.

31. Steers E, Foltza F, Graves BS, Riden J. An inocula replicating apparatus for routine testing of bacterial susceptibility to antibiotics. Antibiot Chemother 1959;9:307-11.
32. Stubbs KG, Wicher K. Laboratory evaluation of an automated antimicrobial susceptibility system. Am J Clin Pathol 1977;68:769-77.
33. Takatsy G. The use of spiral loops in serological and virological micromethods. Acta Microbiol Acad Sci Hung 1956;3:191-202.
34. Thornsberry C, Anhalt JP, Washington JA II, et al. Clinical laboratory evaluation of the Abbott MS-2 automated antimicrobial susceptibility testing system: report of a collaborative study. J Clin Microbiol 1980;12:375-90.
35. Thornsberry C, Gavan TL, Sherris JC, et al. Laboratory evaluation of a rapid automated susceptibility testing system: report of a collaborative study. Antimicrob Agents Chemother 1975;7:466-80.
36. Tilton RC, Isenberg HD. Evaluation of the performance parameters of a prediluted, quantitative antibiotic susceptibility test device. Antimicrob Agents Chemother 1977;11:272-6.
37. Turner A, Hawkey PM, Pedler SJ. Computer-assisted determination of antibiotic susceptibility in photometer-read microtiter plates. J Clin Microbiol 1983;18:996-8.
38. Waterworth PM. Automated sensitivity tests. J Antimicrob Chemother 1976;2:104-6.
39. Woolfrey BF, Lally RT, Quall CO. Evaluation of the AutoSCAN-3 and Sceptor system s for *Enterobacteriaceae* identification. J Clin Microbiol 1983;17:807-13.

CHAPTER 36

ANAEROBIC PROCEDURES FOR ANTIMICROBIAL SUSCEPTIBILITY TESTING

Ronald J. Zabransky, Ph.D.

INTRODUCTION

Attempts to determine the relative activity of antimicrobial agents against bacteria date back to the early 1940s when broth diluton and disk diffusion tests were first described. The application of such tests to anaerobic bacteria has had a checkered history, limited by the development of anaerobic techniques, the lack of appreciation for the pathogenic significance of anaerobes and the dichotomous approach to standardizing aerobic susceptibility tests. Early attempts to apply the disk procedure as described by Bauer, Kirby, Sherris and Turck[2] to anaerobes were foiled by the nature of that test; i.e., requirements for a controlled inoculum, time and conditions of incubation and media. Dilution tests had an early application to anaerobes when paper disks containing antimicrobial agents were used as a source of drug.[1]

Test Development

In the late 1960s, anaerobic techniques were revolutionized by the development of the self-contained anaerobe jar[3] and the recognition that CO_2 was a necessary ingredient in the atmosphere for anaerobes. Detailed studies for identifying anaerobes described by Smith and Holdeman[12] led to the recognition of anaerobes as significant pathogens. With the ease of application of anaerobic techniques in the clinical laboratory, a concomitant need to determine their resistance to currently used and recently developed antimicrobial agents ensued.

Recognizing that the disk procedure had limitations for a large number of anaerobes because of the nature of their growth and that the basis of a standardized procedure should be a dilution technique, the National Committee for Clinical Laboratory Standards (NCCLS) formed a working group to develop a standard procedure for anaerobic susceptibility testing. That group proposed an agar dilution technique which was accepted as an approved standard in 1985.[10] They concluded that this technique was more reproducible with anaerobes than were any of the other methods. A variety of other methods have been proposed for the susceptibility testing of anaerobic bacteria, including modifications of the standardized agar dilution test, microdilution tests and broth disk or elution procedures. The agar dilution test, however, was conceived as a reference method to be used in evaluating other test procedures. Subsequently, the NCCLS has recommended guidelines for performing susceptibility tests on anaerobes by alternative procedures which provide comparable results and are more useful in the clinical setting.[11]

Susceptibility and Resistance

Early studies that were conducted to determine the activity of antimicrobial agents against a variety of anaerobes showed that certain organisms or groups of organisms had predictable susceptibility patterns. As more data from centers around the country were published, it became obvious that these patterns were not uniform and that the specific identification of the organisms, as well as the variety of techniques used, played a major role in the different patterns observed.[5]

The *Bacteroides fragilis* group was found to be a very active beta-lactamase producer with a varied susceptibility to the newer cephalosporin agents. Members of the *B. melaninogenicus* group were found to carry a plasmid-mediated penicillinase. Several species of the clostridia were found to be resistant to clindamycin and other agents. Consequently, there are substantial reasons for the continued determination of the susceptibility of anaerobic bacteria, particularly at major centers where new drugs are evaluated and a larger variety of isolates can be tested.

It is well known that anaerobes often cause synergistic infections and are isolated frequently with other anaerobes or mixed with aerobic bacteria. In clinical settings where incision and drainage is an important part of therapy, the role of antibiotic therapy is not clear, although a number of studies indicate that antibiotics directed against anaerobes are a necessary part of treatment. The usefulness of susceptibility testing of individual anaerobic species in such situations is not clear, therefore the most prudent approach for doing routine susceptibility testing would be:

1. when the organism is isolated in pure culture from a normally sterile body site, ie. blood, cerebrospinal fluid, etc.;
2. when the organism is isolated from a body site as a predominant strain

or in pure culture, particularly if the organism has a known resistance pattern, i.e., *B. fragilis* group;
3. when specifically requested by an infectious disease physician who has particular ability to interpret the results;
4. when evaluating newer antimicrobial agents; and
5. as part of ongoing surveys to determine the susceptibility patterns for certain drugs or of certain organisms.

General Test Information

It is unrealistic to assume that a single susceptibility technique would serve to test all anaerobic bacteria, but the methods described in this chapter are applicable to the majority of clinically significant anaerobic bacteria. Strain-to-strain variation will exist in certain species of anaerobes, and organisms that grow too poorly to show detectable growth within a 48-hour period should be referred to a reference laboratory for testing. Supplementing the media to permit the growth of these more fastidious organisms may be necessary but must not affect the minimal inhibitory concentrations (MIC) of the specific agents against the control organisms.

For agar dilution testing, Wilkins-Chalgren agar is the medium of choice[15] (see Chapter 45). This medium is relatively defined, but it does not support the growth of all anaerobic organisms and may require additional supplements. Defibrinated sheep blood or lysed blood (5%) is an adequate supplement for many fastidious anaerobes. A similar medium without agar is the recommended choice for broth dilution testing. The medium is available commercially. Additives such as horse serum, Fildes' digest, or yeast extract have been suggested, but such modifications should be undertaken with extreme caution. The recommended medium for preparation of the inoculum is thioglycolate broth (without indicator) supplemented with hemin (5 μg/mL), vitamin K_1 (O.1 μg/mL) and sodium bicarbonate (1 μg/mL), prior to use (see Chapter 45). This medium is also the medium of choice for the broth disk elution technique.

The anaerobic atmosphere for these techniques can be obtained in anaerobic jars equipped with palladium-coated catalyst and disposable hydrogen-carbon dioxide generators. The resultant atmosphere should contain 4-7% CO_2. The catalyst in the jar should be reactivated after each use by heating at 160°C for 1.5-2 hours. Evacuation-replacement and anaerobic chambers are acceptable alternatives for obtaining an adequate atmosphere. All systems that are used should be monitored with appropriate quality control devices to insure anaerobic conditions. Anaerobic incubation for 48 hours is required unless the method (broth disk elution) describes otherwise. Certain organisms, particularly those that are more rapidly growing (some species of the *B. fragilis* group and *Clostridium perfringens*), will have sufficient growth within 24 hours to obtain a reliable test result. It has been found, however, that interrupting the anaerobic atmosphere to examine microdilution trays at an earlier time and subsequent reactivation of the anaerobic system does reduce the reliability of the results.

The inoculum used for anaerobic susceptibility testing is ten times more concentrated than that normally used for aerobic bacteria. Therefore, for each specified test, the standardized stock inoculum should be adjusted to an acceptable colony count. An actively growing culture, either an 8-hour growth of a rapidly growing anaerobe, e.g., *C. perfringens*, or an overnight culture, is adequate for obtaining an inoculum. Alternatively, suspending the growth from an anaerobically incubated culture plate not more than 48 hours old has been shown to produce results comparable to the reference method.[11]

Antimicrobial agents to be tested are those commonly recommended for the therapy of anaerobic infections, i.e., clindamycin, cefoxitin, chloramphenicol, metronidazole and in certain circumstances, penicillin and the newer beta-lactams. Aminoglycosides are inactive against anaerobes, as are a variety of the commonly used urinary tract agents, and therefore, should not be tested.

The control strains to be used for anaerobic susceptibility testing are listed in Table 36:1. Other organisms listed here are recommended as reference strains for evaluating the test conditions and media, or are strains being evaluated as replacement or additional control strains.

THE REFERENCE TEST

The reference test is the approved agar dilution method.[10] Modifications of incubation times or medium may be necessary for slow growing or

Table 36:1. Control and Reference Organisms[10]

Control Organisms:	ATCC #
Clostridium perfringens	13124
Bacteroides fragilis	25285
Bacteroides thetaiotaomicron	29741
Reference Organisms:	
Bacteroides vulgatus	29327
Bacteroides thetaiotaomicron	29742
Peptococcus magnus	29328
Peptococcus magnus	14956
Peptococcus asaccharolyticus	29743
Alternate Organisms:	
Fusobacterium nucleatum	10953
Eubacterium lentum	43055

nutritionally fastidious organisms. When modifications are incorporated, the recommended control strains must give the results shown in Table 36:2.

Antimicrobial Agents and Preparation of Plates

Laboratory standard powders available from the manufacturer should be used. These powders should be stored, diluted and maintained according to the specifications of the manufacturer or as described in the NCCLS dilution standard for aerobic bacteria.[9] Antibiotic powders should be weighed, and dilutions in water or other appropriate diluents should be prepared with adjustment for activity or potency. Melt the medium, previously distributed in 18 mL amounts in screwcapped tubes, and add 2 mL of each of the concentrations of antimicrobial agents, mix thoroughly, and pour into standard round petri dishes. After solidification, allow the plates to dry for up to one hour with the tops of the plates slightly ajar. If conducting the reference method, the agar plates containing antimicrobial agents should be prepared on the day of use. It has been determined that most antimicrobial agents will remain stable in agar plates for up to two weeks if stored at 4°C, however, frequent quality control should be conducted to verify stability.[18]

Table 36:2. Acceptable Ranges of MICs* for Control Strains

Antimicrobial Agent	Control Strains: *Bacteroides fragilis* ATCC 25285	*Bacteroides thetaiotaomicron* ATCC 29741	*Clostridium perfringens* ATCC 13124
Carbenicillin	16–64*	16–64	0.25–1
Cefamandole	32–128	32–128	0.06–0.25
Cefoperazone	16–128†	32–128	NR‡
Cefotaxime	8–32	16–64	0.06—0.25
Cefotetan	4–16	32–128	0.016–0.06
Cefoxitin	4–16	8–32	0.25–1
Chloramphenicol	2–8	4–16	2–8
Clindamycin	0.5–2	2–8	0.03–0.12
Imipenem	0.03–0.12	0.06–0.25	0.03–0.12
Metronidazole	0.25–1	0.5–2	0.12–0.5
Mezlocillin	16–64	8-32	0.06–0.25
Moxalactam	0.25–1	4–16§	0.03–0.12§
Penicillin*	16–64	16–64	0.06–0.25
Piperacillin	2–8	8–64†	0.06–0.25
Tetracycline	0.12–0.5	8–32	0.03–0.12
Ticarcillin	16–64	16–64	0.25–1

* Minimal Inhibitory concentrations (MICs) in μg/mL except for penicillin which is U/mL.
† Ranges span 4 concentrations due to broad modal value
‡ No MIC is recommended with this organism/antibiotic combination. A range of 0.25 to 1 may be obtained with *Peptococcus magnus* ATCC 14956 if a lower control value range is desired.
§ Values valid for agar reference method only; different results may be obtained with other methods, media, or enrichments. Adapted from NCCLS[10]

Preparation of Inoculum

An enriched blood agar plate (anaerobic) provides a suitable source for the organism. Such plates should not be more than 72 hours old. Inoculate portions of five or more colonies into the recommended thioglycolate medium (boiled and cooled prior to use) and allow to incubate for 6-24 h to obtain visible turbidity. Adjust this inoculum to a McFarland 0.5 standard, using a clear broth medium that has been boiled and cooled prior to use. Alternatively, prepare the inoculum by suspending the growth from the agar plate in a clear medium and adjusting the turbidity. The final inoculum is 1 x 10^5 colony-forming units (CFU)/spot.

Inoculation and Incubation

Use a replicate inoculator to inoculate the standardized cultures onto the antibiotic containing plates, beginning with the lowest concentration, proceeding to the highest. At the beginning and end of each series of tests, inoculate two plates of medium without antimicrobial agent, incubate one set of plates anaerobically and the second set aerobically to detect aerobic contamination. After the inoculum has been absorbed into the agar medium, invert the plates and incubate in an anaerobic atmosphere for up to 48 hours. The MIC of each strain is read as the lowest concentration of antimicrobial showing no growth, one to three colonies, or a fine, barely visible haze as determined with the unaided eye. This is best observed as a distinct inhibition of growth compared to the growth control. The results with control strains should be consistent with the information presented in Table 36:2.

BROTH DILUTION TESTS

Macrodilution

Conventional broth dilution tests may be performed as described in Chapter 34, under "Conventional Susceptibility Procedures," however, modifications necessary for the growth of anaerobic bacteria must be made. A variety of broth media have been used for this procedure, including brucella broth containing vitamin K_1 and hemin or Fildes' digest, Schaedler's broth, brain heart infusion broth or the broth formulation of Wilkins-Chalgren agar (see Chapter 45).

The inoculum is prepared as described for agar dilution tests except that the final inoculum is approximately 1 x 10^6 CFU/mL. Add an equal volume of inoculum to the antimicrobial agent-containing broth tubes and incubate in anaerobic jars for 48 hours. Include a tube without antibiotic as a growth control. The MIC is the lowest concentration of antimicrobial with no visible growth. This application lends itself satisfactorily to the performance of bactericidal tests where 99.9% of the organisms must be killed at the bactericidal concentration. This requires plate counts of the inoculum at the time of inoculation of the antimicrobial agent-containing tubes.

Microdilution

Tests may be conducted in microdilution trays as described in Chapter 34, with modifications to accommodate the growth requirements of anaerobic bacteria. This procedure is described in detail in the NCCLS alternative methods document,[11] where the broth formulation of Wilkins-Chalgren agar is recommended as the medium of choice. Microdilution tests have also been conducted in a variety of other broth media including Schaedler's, brain heart infusion, Eugon and Wilkins-West broths.[14] Not all species of anaerobes will grow in these media, therefore, supplements such as horse serum may be necessary to improve growth. The results with quality control strains must be the same as the accepted reference values (Table 36:2).

Microdilution trays containing broth may be made in the laboratory using commercially available equipment. Dilute the antimicrobial agent in water prior to inclusion in the broth media. Each well of the microdilution tray should contain 0.1 mL as a final volume. Lesser volumes are not recommended for anaerobes because of evaporation with resulting concentration of antimicrobial agents during prolonged incubation and because the higher inoculum size in small volumes adversely affects results. Seal laboratory-prepared plates in plastic bags and freeze at -60°C or lower until required. Such trays are usually stable for up to 6 months. Do not store frozen microdilution trays in self-defrosting freezers or refreeze them after thawing because of the degradation of certain antimicrobial agents. Lyophylized plates, usually available commercially, last much longer; however, appropriate quality control must be performed to monitor shelf life. At least one well in the microdilution tray should serve as a growth control and an uninoculated well as a sterility control. Thaw frozen trays either in an anaerobic environment or in oxygen-free CO_2 for at least an hour prior to inoculating. The inoculum for microdilution testing is critical, because the inoculum density significantly affects endpoints. The final inoculum in each well should be approximately 1 x 10^5 CFU (1 x 10^6 CFU/mL).

Incubate the inoculated trays in an anaerobic atmosphere for up to 48 hours. Do not stack microdilution trays more than 4 high, to allow an even distribution of incubation temperature and diffusion of environmental gases. Cover trays to prevent evaporation during incubation.

The MIC is the lowest concentration of agent which completely inhibits the growth of the organism. Trailing endpoints may be observed with some antimicrobial agents or antimicrobial agent-organism combinations.[13] This phenomonon appears as a gradually diminishing amount of growth at successively higher concentrations of drug and therefore a sharp endpoint is difficult to determine. In such cases, an agar dilution test is recommended. The concentration where the most significant reduction of growth is observed should be chosen as the endpoint.

For quality control purposes, each new lot of microdilution trays should be tested: 1) at least twice with the set of quality control organisms to verify that the wells contain the appropriate concentrations of antimicrobial agent, and 2) at subsequent regular intervals to ascertain that the agents have not degraded during storage.

LIMITED AGAR DILUTION

Since the reference agar dilution technique may be too time consuming or too cumbersome for routine use, an application which simplifies the procedure by limiting the range and number of antimicrobial concentrations relevant to clinical situations has been described. This technique, originally described by Hauser, Johnston and Zabransky,[4] combines the advantages of agar dilution with economy and clinical utility. Two concentrations of each drug are tested in divided plates. As many as 16 organisms may be tested against 12 antimicrobial agents on quadrant plates incubated in one anaerobe jar. The concentration of agents are chosen to represent specific breakpoints for the interpretation of susceptible, moderately susceptible and resistant.

As with the reference agar method, Wilkins-Chalgren agar is the medium of choice. If quadrant plates are used, distribute the prepared medium in 4.5 mL volumes prior to sterilization. If a medium additive is required, then this volume needs to be adjusted. Add dilutions of antimicrobial agents (0.5 mL) to the previously melted tubes of agar and pour the molten agar into quadrant plates. Table 36:3 lists the concentrations recommended for the selected agents. Other concentrations, if desired, may be added to include MICs at midrange. Plates may be stored for up to two weeks in a refrigerator in a closed plastic bag.

Prepare the inoculum as described for the reference agar dilution technique. The inoculation pattern should be specifically laid out so that each quadrant of the plate receives an exact duplicate. Specific positions should be reserved for control organisms, and at the end of each series of tests, two plates of Wilkins-Chalgren agar without drug should be inoculated, one incubated aerobically and the other incubated anaerobically. All anaerobic incubations should be for up to 48 hours in an anaerobic atmosphere at 35°C. The MIC of the organism is read as the lowest concentration of drug which inhibits the growth of the organism, one to three discreet colonies, or a fine, barely visible haze as determined with the unaided eye.

Table 36:3. Recommended Antimicrobial Concentration for the Limited Agar Dilution and the Disk Elution Methods

Antimicrobial Agent	Agar Dilution Concentration*		Disk Elution Method		
	Low	High	Disk Concentration	Disks/5ml	MIC†
carbenicillin	32	128	100 μg	6	120
penicillin	0.12	16	10 U	8	16
mezlocillin, ticarcillin	16	64	75 μg	4	60
piperacillin	16	64	100 μg	3	60
cefoperazone	16	32	75 μg	2	30
cefotaxime, moxalactam	8.0	32	30 μg	5	30
cefoxitin, cefamandole	8.0	16	30 μg	3	18
chloramphenicol	8.0	16	30 μg	3	18
clindamycin	0.5	4.0	2 μg	10	4
metronidazole	2.0	8.0	80 μg	1	16
tetracycline	1.0	8.0	30 μg	1	6

* Concentration in μg/mL or U/mL. The listed value approximates the moderately susceptible/resistant breakpoint as described by NCCLS[8].
† Minimal Inhibitory Concentration
Adapted from NCCLS[11]

An interpretation of the degree of susceptibility may be made from the MIC endpoint utilizing the interpretive categories described by NCCLS for aerobic organisms.[9] If an organism is inhibited at both high and low concentrations, the organism is considered susceptible; if the organism grows only in the presence of the low concentration, it is considered moderately susceptible; and if it grows in the presence of both concentrations, the organism is considered resistant.

BROTH DISK ELUTION

The frequency of testing anaerobic bacteria in a small laboratory may be relatively low, therefore, a procedure that is easy to perform provides results when clinical utility is necessary. Such procedures and modifications have been described for aerobic and anaerobic organisms. A procedure described by Wilkins and Thiel[16] is carried out in pre-reduced, anaerobically-sterilized media in gassed-out tubes with rubber stoppered seals under an atmosphere of oxygen-free CO_2, with supplemented brain heart infusion broth as the medium. In a subsequent modification, West and Wilkins[14] used a broth modification of Wilkins-Chalgren agar and sealed the tubes with paraffin to maintain an anaerobic environment. An easier-to-use modification, described by Kurzynski et al,[7] incorporated the use of enriched thioglycolate broth and aerobic incubation. The disk elution procedure described by NCCLS[11] and adapted from previous methods, uses thioglycolate broth, a single concentration of drug and works well for rapidly growing anaerobes.

The antimicrobial disks added to the broth serve as the source for the antimicrobial agents. As the drug elutes from the disk, it diffuses uniformly throughout the broth, yielding the appropriate test concentration. Prepare the thioglycolate medium according to manufacturer's recommendations, dispense in 5 mL volumes in screwcapped tubes, sterilize and store for up to two weeks at room temperature. If fastidious anaerobes are being tested, supplements may be included. Store antimicrobial disks according the manufacturers' instructions. Disks used for disk diffusion testing as described by NCCLS[8] are suitable for this procedure, but disks specified by the manufacturer for identification protocols or automated systems are not. Add the appropriate number of disks to the broth medium prior to inoculation. The number of disks to be added to each tube depends upon the volume of the broth, the final breakpoint concentration desired and the concentration in the disk. Table 36:3 lists the recommended number of disks for each antimicrobial agent.

An actively growing broth culture of the organism less than 48 hours old serves as the inoculum for the procedure. Add the culture (0.1 mL) to each tube, cap tightly, invert gently, and incubate aerobically for 24 hours. If the organism is a particularly slow-growing one, 48 hours of incubation may be necessary; do not incubate longer. Susceptibility is defined as the absence of growth, or less than 50% of growth as compared to the control tube. No MIC value is reported, only an indication of susceptible or resistant. The value chosen as the breakpoint for each drug is between the moderately susceptible and resistant categories as described for aerobic organisms.[9]

At present, no user quality control procedures have been developed for disks manufactured specifically for this disk elution method; however, if the disks are the same as those used for diffusion testing of aerobic organisms, quality control procedures as described for that technique should be used.[8]

OTHER CONSIDERATIONS

A number of anaerobes are active beta lactamase producers. Members of the *B. fragilis* group are known to produce the TEM type of beta-lactamase and members of the *B. melaninogenicus* group possess a plasmid-mediated penicillinase. Both these beta-lactamases may be detected by the iodometric and chromogenic cephalosporin techniques. When used on members of the *B. melaninogenicus* group, a positive test would dictate the use of an agent other than penicillin for the treatment of infections with the organism; however, because of the broad activity of the *B. fragilis* group beta-lactamases, tests for these enzymes cannot be used to determine susceptibility to the broad range of cephalosporins.

FACTORS AFFECTING SUSCEPTIBILITY TEST RESULTS

Results of broth tests for both aerobes and anaerobes are very susceptible to inoculum size. The larger inoculum required of anaerobes is necessary for two reasons: first, to insure that these slower growing organisms will reach a detectable level within a limited period of time, and secondly, to bring the results in line with the agar dilution method for the same drugs. It must be appreciated that organisms tested by these methods have different sizes and shapes which limit the use of a turbidity standard. Organisms such as *C. perfringens*, which are quite large, may not reach the higher inoculum sizes required for this procedure, therefore in certain circumstances actual plate counts should be performed. Direct suspension of the organism sometimes provides a more acceptable method for reaching the desired inoculum size.

Certain organism-drug combinations have been found to produce unreproducible results. This can be seen with very susceptible organisms such as *C. perfringens* at exceedingly low concentrations of the drug. Similarly, some organisms such as *Bacteroides thetaiotaomicron* which are active beta-lactamase producers, may produce trailing endpoints with some cephalosporins, particularly those that are more susceptible to these enzymes.[13]

The incubation conditions, described as 48 hours in an anaerobic atmosphere for agar dilution and microdilution, and 24 hours for the broth disk procedure when using the Kurzynski modification, have been determined to be optimal. Varying from these standards should be done only under limited circumstances. Interrupting the 48 hour incubation period for microdilution testing has a marked effect on endpoints with some drugs, and increasing the incubation time for the broth disk procedure may significantly affect the results with some cephalosporins.[6,17]

The disk elution procedure has excellent correlation with interpretation of the MIC procedures for organisms that are very susceptible or very resistant. Reproducibility is poor when the MIC of the antibiotic is near the selected test concentration and with organisms that are active beta-lactamase producers when tested against some cephalosporins.[6,17] In the absence of specific interpretations of MICs for anaerobic organisms it is the recommendation of workers in the field that the breakpoints of susceptibility as developed for aerobic organisms be used. There is no evidence to indicate that these standards will or will not apply to the therapy of anaerobic infections. Drug manufacturers are compiling data that may indicate the usefulness of susceptibility testing of anaerobes in relation to the treatment of specific infections.

REFERENCES

1. Alvarez JP. A simplified sensitivity procedure for anaerobic microorganisms. Am J Med Tech 1955;21:249-53.

2. Bauer AW, Kirby WM, Sherris JC, Turck M. Antibiotic susceptibility testing by a standardized single disk method. Am J Pathol 1966;45:493-6.
3. Brewer JH, Allgeier DL. Safe self-contained carbon dioxide-hydrogen anaerobic system. Appl Microbiol 1966;14:985-8.
4. Hauser KJ, Johnston JA, Zabransky RJ. Economical agar dilution technique for susceptibility testing of anaerobes. Antimicrob Agents Chemother 1975;7:712-14.
5. Jenkins SG, Birk RJ, Zabransky RJ. Difference in susceptibilities of species of the *Bacteroides fragilis* group to several β-lactam antibiotics: indole production as an indicator of resistance. Antimicrob Agents Chemother 1982;22:628-34.
6. Jorgensen JH, Redding JS, Howell AW. Evaluation of broth disk elution methods for susceptibility testing of anaerobic bacteria with the newer β-lactam antibiotics. J Clin Microbiol 1986;23:545-50.
7. Kurzynski TA, Yrios JW, Hestad AG, Field CR. Aerobically incubated thioglycollate broth disk method for antibiotic susceptibility testing of anaerobes. Antimicrob Agents Chemother 1976;10:727-32.
8. National Committee for Clinical Laboratory Standards: Performance standards for antimicrobial disk susceptibility tests. 3rd ed. Approved standard, M2-A3. Villanova, PA: National Committee for Clinical Laboratory Standards, 1984.
9. National Committee for Clinical Laboratory Standards: Methods for dilution antimicrobial susceptibility tests for bacteria that grow aerobically. Approved standard, M7-A. Villanova, PA: National Committee for Clinical Laboratory Standards, 1985.
10. National Committee for Clinical Laboratory Standards: Reference agar dilution procedure for antimicrobial susceptibility testing of anaerobic bacteria. Approved standard, M11A. Villanova, PA: National Committee for Clinical Laboratory Standards, 1985.
11. National Committee for Clinical Laboratory Standards: Alternative methods for antimicrobial susceptibility testing of anaerobic bacteria. Proposed guideline, M17-P. Villanova, PA: National Committee for Clinical Laboratory Standards, 1986.
12. Smith LDS, Holderman LV. The pathogenic anaerobic bacteria. Springfield, IL: Charles C Thomas, 1968:423.
13. Sutter VL, Emmerman J, Randall E, Zabransky RJ, Birk, RJ. Establishment of MICs of moxalactam for control and reference anaerobic organisms in agar dilution and microdilution techniques. Antimicrob Agents Chemother 1985;27:424-6.
14. West SEH, Wilkins TD. Vaspar broth procedure for antibiotic susceptibility testing of anaerobic bacteria. Antimicrob Agents Chemother 1980;17:288-91.
15. Wilkins TD, Chalgren S. Medium for use in antibiotic susceptibility testing of anaerobic bacteria. Antimicrob Agents Chemother 1976;10:926-8.
16. Wilkins TD, Thiel T. Modified broth disk method for testing the antibiotic susceptibility of anaerobic bacteria. Antimicrob Agents Chemother 1973;3:350-6.
17. Zabransky RJ, Birk RJ, Kurzynski TA, Toohey KL. Predicting the susceptibility of anaerobes to cefoperazone, cefotaxime, and cefoxitin with the thioglycolate broth disk procedure. J Clin Microbiol 1986;24:181-5.
18. Zabransky RJ, Hauser KJ. Stability of antibiotics in Wilkins-Chalgren anaerobic susceptibility testing media after prolonged storage. Antimicrob Agents Chemother 1977;12:440-1.

CHAPTER 37

ANTIMICROBIAL SUSCEPTIBILITY TEST PROCEDURES FOR MYCOBACTERIA

Frederick S. Nolte, Ph.D.

DRUG RESISTANCE IN *M. TUBERCULOSIS*

Resistance and susceptibility are relative terms and practically all naturally occurring populations of *M. tuberculosis* will contain a certain proportion of spontaneously resistant mutants. Approximately 1 in 10^5 bacilli is resistant to isoniazid and 1 in 10^6 bacilli is resistant to streptomycin. The probability that a single mycobacterium, not previously exposed to antituberculosis drugs, is resistant to both isoniazid and streptomycin is assumed to be equal to the product of the probabilities of resistance to each drug alone, 10^{-11}. Theoretically, the likelihood that a lesion contains a resistant bacillus increases with an increasing titer of organisms. However, the number of organisms in an active cavitary lesion rarely exceed 10^9 mycobacteria, so that two drugs are usually adequate to prevent the selection of resistant mutants.

Canetti et al[4] determined the significant proportions of resistant bacilli above which the antituberculosis drugs are not clinically useful. The critical proportions are 1% for isoniazid, *p*-aminosalicylic acid and rifampin and 10% for the remaining antituberculosis drugs. However, in the United States, 1% is accepted as the critical level of resistance for all drugs. When the proportion of resistant bacilli in the population exceeds the critical level, the resistant cells soon become the predominant form and the drug fails.

Primary drug resistance occurs in previously untreated tuberculosis patients, presumably as a result of an exogenous infection with a resistant strain. The incidence of primary drug resistance varies among patients in different areas of the United States and among ethnic groups.[7] The primary drug resistance rate for all ethnic and racial groups in 1982 was 6.9%. Much higher rates are found in Hispanics and Asians.

Acquired drug resistance occurs in patients who initially had drug-susceptible bacilli which later became resistant as a result of inadequate or inappropriate chemotherapy. Acquired drug resistance in patients with disease due to endogenous reactivation of infections that had occurred years previously, possibly at a time when treatment with a single drug was practiced, is also a concern.

ANTITUBERCULOSIS THERAPY

Currently, 10 antibiotics are used in the United States to treat tuberculosis. More than one drug is used to decrease the risk of development of resistant organisms. Isoniazid and rifampin in combination with either ethambutol, *p*-aminosalicylic acid, pyrazinamide or streptomycin are generally used during the first 6-8 weeks of therapy for pulmonary tuberculosis. Therapy is continued with two drugs, isoniazid and rifampin to complete a 9 month course in the standard protocol.[6] Capreomycin, cycloserine, ethionamide and kanamycin are often called second line drugs and used only when the other drugs are unsuitable because of toxicity or drug resistance. Recommendations for the therapy of mycobacterial diseases have been recently summarized by the American Thoracic Society.[2]

ANTIBIOTIC SUSCEPTIBILITY TESTS

The conventional disk diffusion techniques widely used in clinical microbiology laboratories for antibiotic susceptibiliy tests are not applicable to the mycobacteria. Most organisms grow so slowly that the drug diffuses throughout the medium and sharp zones of inhibition are not seen. Over the years, several principal methods have been used for drug susceptibility testing of mycobacteria, each of which has many variations. These include the absolute concentration,[5] resistance ratio,[4] proportion and radiometric methods.[21] The lack of uniformity in drug susceptibility testing procedures led to disagreement between laboratories over the results of these tests. The proportion method, originally described by Middlebrook and Cohn[17] and later revised by Canetti et al[4] has been adopted with slight modification as the standard procedure in the United States.

Kubica and Dye[13] recommended the ''level concept'' for mycobacteriology laboratories, in which only experienced and qualified laboratories perform drug susceptibility tests. This proposal was endorsed by the American Thoracic Society.[1] Under this plan, drug susceptibility tests are performed only by Level II and III laboratories, with the secondary drug susceptibility tests restricted to Level III or reference laboratories.

In the U.S., routine susceptibility tests are not usually required for previously untreated patients with tuberculosis, since greater than 96% of the *M. tuberculosis* isolates from these patients are susceptible to all antituberculosis drugs.[11] However, considering that the incidence of primary drug resistance is much higher in many parts of the country and in certain ethnic groups,[7] the decision whether or not to test all initial isolates should be based on local community data for primary drug resistance. In communities where the rate of primary drug resistance is low, McClatchy[15] suggests several circumstances in which susceptibility tests are of considerable value (Table 37:1).

Proportion Method

With the proportion method, equal quantities of two dilutions of an adjusted inoculum are plated on both drug-free and drug-containing medium. Resistance or susceptibility is determined by comparing the number of colonies that grow on the drug-containing medium with the number that grow on the drug-free medium. Thus, the percentage of resistant organisms in a population of mycobacteria is determined.

The proportion method takes into account the critical concentration of the drug as well as the critical proportion of drug-resistant mutants. The critical concentration of the drug is the level which inhibits the growth of the wildtype parental organism but not resistant mutants. The critical drug concentrations for the proportion method, using various culture media, are given in Table 37:2. These concentrations do not have any direct relationship to peak serum levels in patients treated with conventional doses or minimum inhibitory concentrations determined against pure cultures.

Table 37:1. Criteria for Performing Mycobacterial Antibiotic Susceptibility Tests*

1. May not be indicated for previously untreated patients in areas where the prevalence of primary drug resistant is low.
2. Should be performed under the following circumstances:
   A. Relapse or retreatment cases.
   B. Patients on therapy whose sputum reverts to positive.
   C. Patients whose sputum smears do not convert to negative within 2–3 months of treatment.
   D. Patients whose sputum culture does not convert to negative within 4–6 months of treatment.
   E. Patients with increasing numbers of tubercle bacilli seen in smears after an initial decrease.
   F. Patients suspected of having primary resistance.
      (1) Tuberculosis patients who have lived in areas of the world with high primary drug resistance rates.
      (2) Persons possibly infected by contact with a patient with drug-resistant tuberculosis.

* After McClatchy[15]

Table 37:2. Critical Drug Concentrations for the Proportion Method Using Various Culture Media

Drug	Drug concentration (μg/mL)		
	7H10*	7H11†	Lowenstein-Jensen‡
Isoniazid	0.2, 1.0	0.2, 1.0	0.2, 1.0
Rifampin	1.0	1.0	40.0
Streptomycin	2.0	2.0	4.0
Ethambutol	2.0	7.5	2.0
p-Aminosalicylic acid	2.0	8.0	0.5
Ethionamide	5.0	10.0	20.0
Kanamycin	5.0	6.0	20.0
Capreomycin	10.0	10.0	20.0
Cycloserine	30.0	30.0	30.0
Pyrazinamide	25.0§	—	—

* Reference 9.
† Reference 15.
‡ Reference 4.
§ Reference 3.

Table 37:3. Dilution of Sputum Concentrate for Inocula

No. AFB/oil immersion field	Control quadrant 1	Control quadrant 2	Drug quadrants
<1	Undiluted	10^{-2}	Undiluted
1–10	10^{-1}	10^{-3}	10^{-1}
10	10^{-2}	10^{-4}	10^{2}

Inoculum Preparation

The size of the inoculum for the proportion method does not need to be precisely controlled and the test may be inoculated directly from a decontaminated clinical specimen (direct test) or from a pure culture (indirect test). The inoculum is adjusted such that it will yield from 200-300 colonies on the drug-free medium.

The direct test is performed only on smear-positive specimens. Dilutions of the specimen concentrate are made in sterile water according to the number of organisms seen upon microscopic examination. Table 37:3 shows a suggested dilution scheme for inoculum preparation for the direct test.

The indirect test is usually performed on pure cultures growing on solid medium. Suspend approximately 2-5 mg of growth in a tube containing 3.0 mL of 7H9 broth and 3-4 glass beads. Place the tube on a vortex mixer for 1-2 min. Allow the large particles to settle and remove the supernatant. Adjust the suspension with water to the density of a McFarland No. 1 standard and dilute this suspension 10^{-2} and 10^{-4} in sterile water. If the culture is old, prepare an inoculum from a broth culture. Subculture the organism in 7H9 broth and incubate on a tissue culture roller apparatus until the turbidity is that of a McFarland No. 1 standard. Dilute this culture as described above.

Inoculate 3 drops (0.1 mL) of properly prepared and diluted inocula onto each quadrant of drug and control medium for both the direct and indirect tests. Two plates are used for each organism to be tested.

Since culture of mycobacteria in vitro can influence the proportion of susceptible to resistant cells in the population, direct susceptibility tests are preferred with smear-positive specimens. The direct test also has the advantage over the indirect test in terms of earlier results.

Preparation of Susceptibility Test Media

The proportion method compares the amount of growth on drug-containing medium with that on drug-free medium. A solid medium is employed so that colony count estimates can be made. The choice of medium is important since the activity of the drug varies considerably from one medium to another. Most susceptibility tests are performed with Middlebrook 7H10 or 7H11 rather than egg-based media. The stability of antituberculosis drugs also varies with exposure to extremes of temperature, pH, prolonged storage, dessication or daylight. Therefore, drug-containing media should be stored at 4°C, shielded from daylight and kept in plastic bags to reduce evaporation.

In 1966, Wayne and Krasnow[26] described a practical procedure for mycobacterial susceptibility tests that incorporates paper disks containing standardized amounts of drugs into agar contained in individual quadrants of four-section petri plates. This method compares favorably with reference methods and is recommended for use in diagnostic laboratories.

Drug-containing disks (Baltimore Biological Laboratories) are dispensed to individual quadrants of the petri plates according to the scheme shown in Table 37:4. The disks are centered in the quadrants and held in place

Table 37:4. Distribution of Antibiotic Disks and Final Antibiotic Concentrations for Quadrant Plate Susceptibility Tests*

Plate No.	Quadrant No.	Drug	μg/disk	μg/mL
I	1	Control no. 1	—	—
	2	Isoniazid	1	0.2
	3	Isoniazid	5	1.0
	4	Ethambutol	25	5.0
II	1	Control no. 2	—	—
	2	Streptomycin	10	2.0
	3	Streptomycin	50	10.0
	4	Rifampin	5	1.0

* Reference 26.

with a drop of 7H10 medium. Dispense 5 mL of molten 7H10 medium (50-52°C) to each quadrant. Incubate the plates at 4°C overnight to allow the drug to diffuse uniformly throughout the agar. The plates are used immediately or stored for a maximum of 4 weeks. This procedure allows laboratories to conveniently prepare only the number of plates required for immediate use.

At present, the concentrations of isonazid and streptomycin currently used represent both a lower screening and a higher screening concentration, which may serve to monitor increases in resistance to these drugs. The higher concentrations of each drug may also be useful in establishing the suitability of isoniazid and streptomycin for treatment of infections with nontuberculous mycobacteria.

Incubation and Interpretation

Plates are incubated at 35-37°C in air supplemented with 5-10% CO_2 and examined weekly for 3 weeks. For many strains of *M. tuberculosis*, growth is evident within 2 weeks. However, test results should not be reported at this time because drug-resistant mutants may grow more slowly than their susceptible counterparts and early reading of the susceptibility tests may underestimate the number of resistant cells in the population. Reading the plates after 4 weeks of incubation may overestimate drug resistance, especially with ethionamide, ethambutol and cycloserine.

Although cultures with greater than 1% resistant mutants are considered clinically resistant to the drug, in practice it is seldom necessary to apply this criterion strictly. In most cases, the proportion of resistant colonies is estimated as greater or less than 1% by simple visual inspection of the plates. Laboratories may record the amount of growth on the drug-containing and control quadrants as shown in Table 37:5 or record the actual number of colonies. Laboratories may report the amount of growth (1+ to 4+) obtained on the control and drug quadrants or the actual percentage of drug-resistant bacilli. If the number of colonies on the drug-containing quadrants inoculated with the lower dilution (e.g., 10^{-1}) exceeds the number of colonies

Table 37:5. Reading and Reporting of Proportion Method Susceptibility Tests*

Amount of Growth	Report
Confluent (>500 colonies)	4+
Almost confluent (200–500 colonies)	3+
100–200 colonies	2+
50–100 colonies	1+
<50 colonies	Actual Number

* After McClatchy[16]

seen on the control quadrant inoculated with the higher dilution (e.g., 10^{-3}), the culture contains greater than 1% resistance cells. When the level of resistant mutants is approximately 1% the test should be repeated or the results reported as questionable.

Quality Control

Test mycobacterial strains of known susceptibility patterns each time a new batch of medium is prepared and at least weekly while the medium is in use to ensure that the drugs maintain their activity with storage. Include one susceptible strain and one strain resistant to several of the first-line drugs as controls. Appropriate strains may be obtained from the Curator, Trudeau Mycobacterial Culture Collection, National Jewish Hospital and Research Center/National Asthma Center, Denver, CO 80206. Grow strains in liquid medium, dilute appropriately, dispense in 1 mL samples and freeze at -70°C. For use in quality control, thaw these samples, dilute them in the same manner as the clinical specimens to yield 200-300 colonies.

Radiometric Method

Several susceptibility testing methods for mycobacteria using radiometric techniques have been described. In 1977, Middlebrook et al[18] introduced a special medium (7H12) which contained the basic ingredients of 7H11 medium plus ^{14}C palmitic acid. The BACTEC (Johnston Laboratories) radiometric method detects $^{14}CO_2$ liberated from metabolism of the palmitic acid in an automated ion chamber system. The amount of radioactivity in the gas phase of the culture vial is measured and converted into growth index (GI) units. This method is used for the detection of *M. tuberculosis* in clinical specimens and for performing susceptibility tests.

M. tuberculosis is detected rapidly by inoculation of decontaminated clinical specimens into 7H12 medium containing polymyxin B, amphotericin B, carbenicillin and trimethoprim. Average detection times of 5-8 days are reported with the radiometric technique, compared to 21 days with conventional techniques.[8,19] In addition, rapid identification of *M. tuberculosis* is accomplished by determining the susceptibility of isolates to *p*-nitro-acetylamino-β-hydroxypropiophenone.[14]

Several studies[19,21,22] show that the radiometric method of susceptibility testing correlates with reference methods at a 90-98% level for isoniazid, rifampin, streptomycin and ethambutol. Results are usually obtained in 4-5 days with the radiometric method and 21 days with the reference methods. The radiometric method for mycobacteria deserves serious consideration by diagnostic laboratories because of its speed and relative simplicity.

Inocula for the susceptibility tests are obtained either from a positive BACTEC isolation vial (GI>500) or a suspension prepared from bacteria grown on conventional media. If growth from conventional media is used, prepare a suspension that approximates the turbidity of a McFarland No. 1 standard. Inoculate each of 4 vials containing the test drugs (isoniazid, 0.2 μg/mL; rifampin, 1.0 μg/mL; streptomycin, 2.0 μg/mL and ethambutol, 2.0 μg/mL) with 0.1 mL of the bacterial suspension. A drug-free control vial is inoculated with 0.1 mL of a 10^{-2} dilution of the inoculum.

All vials are tested immediately on the BACTEC instrument which establishes a 5-10% CO_2 atmosphere within the vials. The vials are incubated in the dark, without shaking, at 37°C and tested daily. The GI readings are recorded and the test is interpreted when the GI of the control reads at least 30. If the increase in GI of the drug-containing medium is greater than the GI of the control, the culture is considered resistant to that drug. If there is no clear difference in GIs between the control and drug vials, read the vials an additional 1-2 days to establish the GI differences.

Test mycobacterial cultures of known susceptibility patterns regularly as part of a quality control program. Also, special care should be taken to ensure that the cultures used in the radiometric susceptibility tests are pure because contaminants will rapidly overgrow the mycobacteria.

SUSCEPTIBILITY TESTING WITH NONTUBERCULOUS MYCOBACTERIA

Mycobacteria other than *M. tuberculosis* are often resistant to antituberculosis drugs in vitro. However, the validity of using the same critical drug concentrations and the same critical proportion of resistant cells for both *M. tuberculosis* and the nontuberculous mycobacteria has not been established. The results of in vitro single drug susceptibility tests do not always correlate with the in vivo efficacy of the drugs in the therapy of nontuberculous mycobacterial infections. Better correlation with clinical response is obtained when combined drug testing is done, particularly with *M. kansasii*[23] and *M. avium-intracellulare*.[10]

M. kansasii can produce a pulmonary disease that resembles tuberculosis. Most strains of *M. kansasii* are susceptible to isoniazid, streptomycin, ethambutol and rifampin, and resistant to the other antituberculosis drugs.[23]

M. avium-intracellulare has assumed increased importance with the advent of the acquired immunodeficiency syndrome (AIDS). Disseminated infections in AIDS patients have proved difficult to treat because the organisms are resistant to most of the antituberculosis drugs. However, clofazimine, cycloserine and ansamycin have excellent activity in vitro.[12]

M. marinum can produce subcutaneous infections, including a slowly evolving, nodular skin lesion in swimmers (swimming pool granuloma). The organism is susceptible to rifampin, ethambutol, amikacin, kanamycin, tetracycline, doxycycline and minocycline, but somewhat resistant to isoniazid and streptomycin.[20]

The rapidly growing mycobacteria, *M. chelonae* and *M. fortuitum*, have been associated with skin and soft-tissue infections, especially following surgical procedures.[28] Both *M. chelonae* and *M. fortuitum* are resistant to the standard antituberculosis drugs. Doxycycline, minocycline, amikacin, gentamicin, trimethoprim-sulfamethoxazole, sulfa drugs and some of the cephalosporins all have good in vitro activity. [24,25,27] The method for susceptibility testing employs Mueller-Hinton medium containing 10% oleic acid-albumin-dextrose supplement. Antibiotics are incorporated directly into the medium for agar dilution testing,[25] or a disk diffusion method[24] is used. In the disk diffusion test, plates are inoculated with a broth suspension of bacteria equivalent to one-half of a McFarland No. 1 standard and incubated at 37°C for 48 hours for *M. fortuitum* and 72 hours for *M. chelonae*. Zone diameters and their minimum inhibitory concentration correlates for these organisms are available.[24,25,27]

REFERENCES

1. American Thoracic Society. Official statement on quality of laboratory services for mycobacterial diseases. Am Rev Respir Dis 1974;110:376-7.
2. Bailey WC, Albert RK, Davidson PT, et al. Treatment of tuberculosis and other mycobacterial diseases. Ann Rev Respir Dis 1983;127:790-6.
3. Butler WR, Kilburn JO. Improved method for testing susceptibility of *Mycobacterium tuberculosis* to pyrazinamide. J Clin Microbiol 1982;16:1106-9.
4. Canetti G, Fox W, Khomenk A, et al. Advances in techniques of testing mycobacterial drug sensitivity, and the use of sensitivity tests in tuberculosis control programs. Bull WHO 1969;41:21-43.
5. Canetti G, Froman S, Grosset JH, et al. Mycobacteria: Laboratory methods for testing drug sensitivity and resistance. Bull WHO 1963;29:565-78.
6. Centers for Disease Control. Guidelines for short-course tuberculosis chemotherapy. Morbid Mortal Weekly Rep 1980;29:97-105.
7. Centers for Disease Control. Primary resistance to antituberculosis drugs-United States. Morbid Mortal Weekly Rep 1983;32:521-3.
8. Damato JJ, Collins MT, Rothlauf MV, McClatchy JK. Detection of mycobacteria by radiometric and standard plate procedures. J Clin Microbiol 1983;17:1066-73.
9. David HL. Bacteriology of the mycobacterioses. Washington, DC: US Government Printing Office, 1976; DHEW publication no. (CDC)76-8316.
10. Heifets LB. Synergistic effect of rifampin, streptomycin, ethionamide and ethambutol in *Mycobacterium intracellulare*. Am Rev Resp Dis 1982;125:43-8.
11. Hobby GL, Johnson PM, Boytar-Papirnyik V. Primary drug resistance: A continuing study of drug resistance in tuberculosis in a veteran population within the United States. X. September 1970 to 1973. Am Rev Respir Dis 1973;110:95-8.
12. Kiehn TE, Edwards FF, Brannon P, et al. Infections caused by *Mycobacterium avium* complex in immunocompromised patients: diagnosis by blood culture and fecal examination, antimicrobial susceptibility tests and morphological and seroagglutination characteristics. J Clin Microbiol 1985;21:168-73.
13. Kubica GP, Dye WE. Laboratory methods for clinical and public health mycobacteriology. Washington, DC: US Government Printing Office, 1967; DHEW publication no. (PHS)67-1547.

14. Laszlo A, Siddiqi SH. Evaluation of a rapid radiometric differentiation test for the *Mycobacterium tuberculosis* complex by selective inhibition with p-nitro-α-acetylamino-β-hydroxypropiophenone. J Clin Microbiol 1984;19:694-8.
15. McClatchy JK. Susceptibility testing of mycobacteria. Lab Med 1978;9:47-52.
16. McClatchy JK. Antimycobacterial drugs: Mechanisms of action, drug resistance, susceptibility testing and assays of activity in biological fluids. In: Lorian V, ed. Antibiotics in laboratory medicine. Baltimore: Williams and Wilkins, 1986:187.
17. Middlebrook G, Cohn ML. Bacteriology of tuberculosis. Laboratory methods. Am J Public Health 1958;48:844-53.
18. Middlebrook G, Reggiardo Z, Tigertt WD. Automatable radiometric detection of growth of *Mycobacterium tuberculosis* in selective media. Am Rev Respir Dis 1977;115:1067-9.
19. Roberts GD, Goodman NL, Heifets L, et al. Evaluation of the BACTEC radiometric method for recovery of mycobacteria and drug susceptibility testing of *Mycobacterium tuberculosis* from acid-fast smear positive specimens. J Clin Microbiol 1983;18:689-96.
20. Sanders WJ, Wolinsky E. In vitro susceptibility of *Mycobacterium marinum* to eight antimicrobial agents. Antimicrob Agents Chemother 1980;18:528-31.
21. Siddiqi SH, Libonati JP, Middlebrook G. Evaluation of a rapid radiometric method for drug susceptibility testing of *Mycobacterium tuberculosis*. J Clin Microbiol 1981;13:908-12.
22. Snider DE Jr, Good RC, Kilburn JO, et al. Rapid drug-susceptibility testing of *Mycobacterium tuberculosis*. Am Rev Respir Dis 1981;123:402-6.
23. Tsang A, Bentz RR, Schork MA, Sodeman TM. Combined vs single-drug studies of susceptibilities of *Mycobacterium kansasii* to isoniazid, streptomycin and ethambutol. Am J Clin Pathol 1978;70:816-20.
24. Wallace RJ Jr, Dalovisio JR, Pankey GA. Disk diffusion testing of susceptibility of *Mycobacterium fortuitum* and *Mycobacterium chelonei* to antibacterial agents. Antimicrob Agents Chemother 1979;16:611-14.
25. Wallace RJ Jr, Jones DB, Wiss K. Sulfonamide activity against *Mycobacterium fortuitum* and *Mycobacterium chelonei*. Rev Infect Dis 1981;3:898-904.
26. Wayne LG, Krasnow I. Preparation of tuberculosis susceptibility testing mediums by means of impregnated discs. Am J Clin Pathol 1966;45:769-71.
27. Welch DF, Kelly MT. Antimicrobial susceptibility testing of *Mycobacterium fortuitum* complex. Antimicrob Agents Chemother 1979;15:754-7.
28. Wolinsky E. Nontuberculous mycobacteria and associated diseases. Am Rev Respir Dis 1979:107-59.

Section 4: Direct Detection Methods

CHAPTER 38

MICROSCOPY

Patrick R. Murray, Ph.D.

INTRODUCTION

The microscopic examination of clinical specimens is a rapid and, when carefully performed, precise method for the diagnosis of infection. Microscopy can assist in assessing the quality of submitted specimens and aid in the interpretation of the culture result. Specimens can be examined by phase-contrast or darkfield microscopy; or examined after they have been prepared by methods such as the Gram, acridine orange or acidfast staining procedures. Staining of the specimen is frequently unnecessary for some purposes, such as assessing the quality of a specimen[32,37] or when the organisms are too thin to be seen even with staining (e.g., *Treponema*).

MICROSCOPY-METHODS

Gram Stain

Although Hans Christian Gram originally described the Gram stain in 1884, the precise chemical basis of the differential staining procedure is still not known. The most common explanation is that the structure of bacterial cell walls is responsible for the observed permeability differences. The cell wall of gram-positive bacteria consists of a relatively thick (15-80 nm) peptidoglycan layer with the cytoplasmic membrane adherent to the inner surface. In contrast, gram-negative bacteria have a cell wall composed of an outer membrane covalently linked by lipoprotein to a thin (1-3 nm) peptidoglycan layer and an inner cytoplasmic membrane of phospholipid and protein. The cell walls of gram-positive bacteria, in comparison with those of gram-negative bacteria, are less permeable to small molecules.

Additionally, the rate of dye release from stained cell wall fragments correlates with the Gram staining properties of the intact cell. Dye is released slowly from gram-positive cells and more rapidly from gram-negative cells.

Many variations of the Gram stain have been suggested since the staining method was first introduced; however, the basic staining procedures have remained as originally described. Although some latitude exists with the staining method,[30] a number of cautions must be observed for reproducible, reliable stains.[2] The microscopic slide must be clean and free of fingerprints, oil and lint. Microorganisms introduced with a casually misplaced fingerprint have more than once created confusion when the stained slide was examined. The specimen should be spread onto the slide in a thin, even manner to ensure uniform staining of the material and a thickness that will allow adequate light transmission for examination of the stained specimen. The specimen should be dried completely before it is gently heat fixed. Excessive heating to dry the specimen for fixation to the glass slide will denature the bacterial proteins, disrupting the morphology and staining properties of the organisms. Proper heating can be performed by holding the edge of the slide by hand and passing it through a flame 2 or 3 times. The slide should be warm but not hot. Specimens can also be fixed by immersion in methanol. The following staining procedure (with the reagents described in Chapter 45, "Media, Reagents and Stains,") is recommended:

1. Flood the heat-fixed smear with crystal violet. Stain for a minimum of 10-15 s.
2. Gently rinse the slide with running water for 5 s.
3. Immediately flood the slide with the iodine-iodide solution and apply for a minimum of 15 s.
4. Rinse the slide with running water for 5 s or more.
5. Shake off the excess water and decolorize the slide with 95% ethyl alcohol. Treat the smear 20-30 s. If acetone is used, the slide should be decolorized for 10-15 s.
6. Rinse the slide with running water for 5 s or more.
7. Flood the slide with safranin. Stain for a minimum of 10-15 s.
8. Gently wash the slide with running water for 5 s.

Basic stains, such as crystal violet, are taken up rapidly by bacteria and the staining time for this step is not important. However, the timing of the subsequent rinse step is critical because the dyes are water-soluble and excessive rinsing will remove the stain from gram-positive and gram-negative bacteria. This rinsing step should not exceed 10 s even when water-filled stained jars or automated Gram staining devices are used.

The iodine-iodide solution is a mordant that forms a complex with the intracellular crystal violet. Iodine concentrations as low as 0.1% can be used but this will be rapidly removed during the subsequent decolorization step. A 1% iodine concentration is recommended. When using staining jars and automated stainers, ensure that the mordant solution is not diluted excessively with water carried over from the previous rinse step.

After the mordant solution is removed, the timing of the rinsing step is not critical. However, decolorization should be carefully performed. The rate of decolorization is a function of the intracellular concentration of the crystal violet-iodine complex, the solubility of the complex in the decolorizing agent and the time of decolorization. The most commonly used agents are 95% ethyl alcohol and acetone. Properly prepared slides can be safely decolorized from 15 s to 3 min with 95% ethyl alcohol and from 5 s to 2 min with acetone. The exact length of decolorization time is affected by the density of the prepared specimen and has to be determined by practical experience. A control slide with a mixture of known gram-positive and gram-negative organisms (e.g., *Staphylococcus* and *Escherichia*) should be stained simultaneously. The speed of decolorization can be increased if 95% alcohol is diluted in water; therefore, dilution of the alcohol with rinse water should be carefully avoided. Methyl alcohol cannot be used as a decolorizing agent because decolorization is too rapid.

After the slide is decolorized, it is rinsed with water. The timing of this step is not critical because the intracellular stain-iodine complex cannot be easily removed. The slide is then counterstained with safranin. Safranin, at a concentration of 0.25%, can be used safely if applied up to 60 s. Safranin can replace crystal violet, so the slide should not be counterstained for a prolonged period. The rinse step after counterstaining must be carefully controlled because the secondary dye can be easily washed from the cell, leaving the gram-negative bacteria either faintly stained or colorless. Other basic dyes, such as Bismarck Brown, can be used for colorblind microscopists. Freshly prepared 1:1000 watery basic fuchsin has also been used for counterstaining slides when anaerobes are expected. Basic fuchsin stains gram-negative anaerobes more intensely than does safranin.

Acridine Orange Stain

Another stain proven valuable for the detection of bacteria in clinical specimens is the acridine orange stain.[22] At pH 4.0, bacteria will stain red-orange while nonbacterial cells, such as squamous cells and polymorphonuclear leukocytes, will stain green-yellow. The staining procedure is simple to perform and specimens can be rapidly examined under low power magnification. The following procedure can be used for this stain:

1. Spread the specimen onto a clean glass slide, air-dry and fix by immersion in absolute methanol for 2 min.
2. Flood the slide with a solution of 0.5% acridine orange in 0.15 M acetate buffer, pH 4.0, and stain for 2 min.
3. Rinse the slide with water, air dry and examine at 400–1,000 X magnification under ultraviolet light.

Acidfast Stains

Acidfast stains have been used traditionally to visualize mycobacteria and *Nocardia*. These organisms have unique staining properties. They are very difficult to stain with aniline dyes and, once stained, are resistant to decolorization with acids or alcohols. This acidfast property has been useful for classifying mycobacteria and other acidfast organisms.

Mycobacteria are refractory to staining with water-soluble dyes because their lipid-rich cell wall is hydrophobic. The dyes can penetrate the cells if the staining period is long (12-24 h) or if phenol is added to the dye solution and the specimen is heated during the staining procedure. Once the stain penetrates the cell, it can either remain free or be bound to acidic molecules. Mycolic acids are the major component of the mycobacterial cell wall and are acidfast. However, this is not the only factor responsible for the acidfastness of these organisms,[10] because mechanical injury to the cells following grinding or sonication causes loss of acidfastness. Thus, an intact cell wall and plasma membrane are required for stain retention.

The lipid component of the cell wall provides an effective barrier to decolorization with dilute mineral acids in alcohol. Weak acid solutions and 70% ethanol are poor solvents for mycobacterial lipids so the lipid cell wall in mycobacteria forms a barrier preventing the extraction of the intracellular dye. In contrast, acid-alcohol solutions readily penetrate the cell walls of other bacteria and easily extract the stain.

Three acidfast staining techniques are commonly used: Ziehl-Neelsen, Kinyoun and Truant fluorochrome. With use of the Ziehl-Neelsen stain, the prepared specimen must be gently heated for the primary stain (carbolfuchsin) to penetrate the cell. Kinyoun[21] avoided this problem by increasing the concentration of dye and of phenol in the primary staining solution. For this reason the Kinyoun procedure is called a cold acidfast stain. The use of phenolated fluorescent dyes as primary stains permits examination of the smears under low power magnification because fluorescent bacilli are easily seen against a black background. The use of strong oxidizing agents (e.g., potassium permanganate) denatures the extracellular dye, producing a dark background. It is important to differentiate between stained bacilli and fluorescent debris by examining carefully the morphology of the stained particles.

For each staining procedure, a loopful of the specimen is spread over a 2-3 cm area on a clean glass slide. The smear is then heat-fixed by passing the slide over a flame or preferably by heating the slide at 65°C for a minimum of 2 h on a warming tray. Specimens can also be heated safely overnight at 65°C. The following is a description of these staining procedures. Formulae for all reagents can be found in Chapter 45, "Media, Reagents and Stains."

Ziehl-Neelsen Acidfast Stain

1. Cover the prepared slide with filter paper and saturate with carbolfuchsin.

2. Slowly heat the slide to steaming and maintain the temperature for 5 min. Other temperatures can be used but the staining time must be proportionally adjusted (e.g., 90°C for 5 min, 70°C for 10 min, 55°C for 30 min, 25°C overnight).
3. Discard the filter paper and rinse the slide with water until excess dye is removed.
4. Decolorize with acid-alcohol until free dye is removed.
5. Rinse with water. Counterstain with methylene blue for 30-60 s.
6. Carefully rinse the slide with water for 5 s, blot dry and examine at 1,000 X magnification. Acidfast bacilli stain red; the background and other organisms stain blue.

Excessive heating during the initial staining step must be avoided and additional carbolfuchsin should be added as needed. Decolorization with acid-alcohol should be for a period sufficient to remove all stain from nonspecifically stained material and organisms. The timing of this step will depend upon the thickness of the smear. Overdecolorization is difficult, due to the chemical structure of the mycobacterial cell wall. The time required for application of the counterstain is not critical because the stain rapidly penetrates the nonacidfast organisms and background material.

Kinyoun Stain[21]

1. Flood the prepared slide with carbolfuchsin and stain for 5 min.
2. Rinse the slide with water until the excess dye is removed and then decolorize with acid-alcohol until all free dye is removed.
3. Rinse with water and then counterstain with methylene blue for 30-60 s.
4. Carefully rinse the slide for 5 s, blot dry and examine at 1,000 X magnification. Acidfast bacilli will stain red; the background and other organisms will stain blue.

The increased concentration of carbolfuchsin and phenol used in this staining procedure eliminates the need to heat the specimen.

Truant Fluorochrome (Auramine-Rhodamine) Stain[36]

1. Flood the prepared specimen with the auramine-rhodamine solution. Stain for 20 min. This time can be reduced if the temperature is increased (e.g., 15 min at 37°C, 10 min at 60°C).
2. Rinse the prepared slide with water until the excess dye is removed. Decolorize with acid-alcohol until all free dye is removed (approximately 2-3 min).
3. Rinse with water and counterstain with potassium permanganate for 2-4 min.

4. Rinse the slide with water, blot dry and examine with a fluorescent microscope equipped with the Zeiss BG-12 or Corning 5113 excitation filter and Corning OG-1 barrier filter. Acidfast organisms will appear yellow-green against a dark background.

The principle of the fluorochrome stain is essentially the same as the two carbolfuchsin stains: acidfast organisms are resistant to decolorization with weak acid-alcohol solutions. One special precaution with the fluorochrome stain is the timing of the potassium permanganate step. This compound is a strong oxidizing agent that inactivates free dye. Insufficient treatment produces a background fluorescence that makes examination of the stained specimen difficult. Likewise, if the treatment is longer than 4-5 min, intracellular fluorescence in mycobacteria will be reduced. The stained specimens should be initially examined at low power magnification (e.g., 250 X). All fluorescent particles should then be examined at higher magnification to confirm the morphology of the organisms. If the stained specimens are examined carefully, this stain is very sensitive and specific.

MICROSCOPY-APPLICATIONS

Although bacterial stains are useful for many different types of clinical specimens, the limitations of microscopy must be appreciated. The sensitivity of the examination is directly related to the number of organisms present. Although fluorescent stains permit detection of small numbers of organisms, approximately 10^4-10^5 organisms/mL must be present for detection. The microscopic examination is generally valuable for infections where large numbers of organims are routinely encountered, whereas a negative microscopy report must be cautiously interpreted for infections where only small numbers of organisms are present.

Septicemia

The majority of bacteremic patients have fewer than one organism per mL of blood.[33] Thus, microscopic examination of whole blood is usually unrewarding. Similarly, the examination of buffy coat smears from peripheral blood has been shown to have limited value,[4,8,16] with positive smears observed only in patients with overwhelming bacteremias (e.g., greater than 100 organisms per mL). After blood has been inoculated into culture media and the organisms allowed to grow, Gram and acridine orange stains have proved useful for the rapid detection and preliminary identification of isolates.[3,27] As an example, Agger and Maki[1] reported that the Gram stain was a very accurate method for differentiating between *Staphylococcus* and *Streptococcus*.

Meningitis

The frequency with which positive bacterial stains are observed in patients with bacterial meningitis is directly related to the number of organisms present in cerebrospinal fluid; which in turn is a function of the phase of the infection (early versus late and uncontrolled), the infecting pathogen and previous antimicrobial therapy. The most common pathogens (e.g., *Haemophilus influenzae, Streptococcus pneumoniae, Neisseria meningitidis*) are generally present in concentrations greater than 10^5 organisms per mL of cerebrospinal fluid[9,23] in untreated patients. Gram or acridine orange stains are positive on specimens from 80% or more of these patients. However, the number of organisms can be reduced to visually undetectable levels in previously treated patients or in infections with fastidious organisms such as *Listeria monocytogenes*.[6,14]

Respiratory Infections

Microscopy is invaluable for assessing the quality of lower respiratory specimens.[29] The presence of polymorphonuclear leukocytes in an immunocompetent patient is presumptive evidence that lower respiratory tract secretions were collected, while squamous epithelial cells indicate that the specimen is contaminated with oral secretions and should not be processed. An unstained sputum specimen can be examined rapidly by the physician or laboratory technologist or the specimen can be stained and examined for evidence of contamination as well as to identify the organisms associated with purulence.[32,37] The Gram stain examination of the specimen can also be used to guide interpretation of culture results. Heineman[13] reported that microscopic examination of sputum was responsible for identifying one-half the etiologic agents that would have been missed by nondirected culture procedures.

Gastrointestinal Infections

Examination of fecal specimens has limited value. Observation of fecal leukocytes is indicative that the patient is infected with an invasive organism, but this does not discriminate among *Shigella, Salmonella, Campylobacter* or other bacterial and parasitic pathogens. Furthermore, most bacterial pathogens cannot be specifically identified on a Gram stain smear. Although *Campylobacter* has the characteristic thin curved morphology similar to a *Vibrio* and is frequently seen in pairs like the wings of a sea gull, other intestinal organisms can resemble these organisms and stains have a limited sensitivity. Thus, a Gram stain or an unstained preparation of fecal material may be useful in confirming a clinical impression. However, microscopy has a very limited diagnostic role in gastrointestinal infections.

Urinary Tract Infections

Urinary tract infections have been defined traditionally by the presence of 10^5 or more uropathogens per mL of urine.[18,31] For infections at this level, the Gram stain has a sensitivity between 80-90%.[15,17,25,35] However, as many as one-half of some populations of patients (e.g., women with acute dysuria) have low numbers of organisms responsible for their infections.[34] The microscopic examination of urine from these patients is insensitive. Thus, a positive Gram stain can be useful in the medical management of patients with urinary tract infections, but a negative Gram stain must be interpreted cautiously. Furthermore, Gram stains should not be used to screen urine specimens for further processing because infections with small numbers of organisms cannot be reliably detected.

Genital Infections

A Gram stained smear of urethral exudates from men with symptomatic urethritis is diagnostic for gonococcal urethritis if polymorphonuclear leukocytes with typical intracellular gram-negative diplococci are seen. Under these conditions, the Gram stain has a specificity of 98% and a sensitivity of 90% in comparison with culture. However, the sensitivity is low in asymptomatic infected males. Likewise, the specificity of the Gram stained smear performed by experienced personnel is 97% for women with genital gonococcal infection, but the sensitivity of stained endocervical exudates is only between 45-55%.[7,12,19,26]

Mycobacterial Infections

The acidfast smear is valuable for making a rapid diagnosis of mycobacterial infection. Approximately 40-50% of all specimens with positive cultures are associated with positive acidfast smears, although this is influenced by the staining technique, infecting organism, nature of infection, previous or concurrent therapy and quality of the specimen submitted.[5,20,24] The fluorochrome stain is more sensitive than carbolfuchsin stains because the specimens can be examined under low power magnification and the fluorescent bacilli are readily seen against a black background. Positive smears are associated more commonly with *Mycobacterium tuberculosis* than with other mycobacteria, with culture-positive sputa and bronchial brushings than with other specimen types, and with specimens from which many rather than a few organisms are cultured.[11] For example, sputum specimens from patients with cavitary tuberculosis are more frequently positive than are specimens from patients with noncavitary disease or specimens from a small biopsy. It is important that the morphology of the bacilli be carefully examined to ensure the specificity of the stain.[28] Fewer than 1% of all positive smears should be false-positives if the technique is properly performed and quality controlled.

Conclusion

In conclusion, the following guidelines can be used for the microscopic examination of clinical specimens.

Specimens that should be routinely examined microscopically:

Abscess
Ear aspirate
Eye aspirate
Abdominal fluid
Amniotic fluid
Bone marrow
Cerebrospinal fluid
Culdocentesis fluid
Pericardial fluid
Synovial fluid
Thoracentesis fluid
Bronchial washing
Lung aspirate
Nasal sinus aspirate
Sputum
Tracheal secretions
Transtracheal aspirate
Suprapubic aspirate

Specimens that should be routinely examined microscopically if requested:

External ear
Conjunctiva
Feces
Endocervical secretions
Urethral discharge
Vaginal discharge
Mouth swab
Wound
Autopsy tissue
Burn tissue
Urine

Specimens that should not be routinely examined microscopically:

Catheter tip
Blood
Gastric washings
Rectal swabs

REFERENCES

1. Agger WA, Maki DG. Efficacy of direct Gram stain in differentiating staphylococci from streptococci in blood cultures positive for gram-positive cocci. J Clin Microbiol 1978;7:111-13.
2. Bartholomew JW. Variables influencing results and the precise definition of steps in Gram staining as a means of standardizing the results obtained. Stain Technol 1962;37:139-55.
3. Blazevic DJ, Stemper JF, Matsen JM. Comparison of macroscopic examination, routine Gram stains, and routine subcultures in the initial detection of positive blood cultures. Appl Microbiol 1974;27:537-9.

4. Brooks GF, Pribble AH, Beaty HN. Early diagnosis of bacteremia by buffy-coat examinations. Arch Intern Med 1973;132:673-5.
5. Burdash NM, Manos JP, Ross D, Bannister ER. Evaluation of the acid-fast smear. J Clin Microbiol 1976;4:190-1.
6. Dalton HP, Allison MJ. Modification of laboratory results by partial treatment of bacterial meningitis. Am J Clin Pathol 1968;49:410-13.
7. Dans PE, Judson F. The establishment of a venereal disease clinic: II. An appraisal of current diagnostic methods in uncomplicated urogenital and rectal gonorrhea. J Am Vener Dis Assoc 1975;1:107-12.
8. Fadden HS. Early diagnosis of neonatal bacteremia by buffy-coat examination. J Pediatr 1976;88:1032-4.
9. Feldman WE. Concentration of bacteria in cerebrospinal fluid of patients with bacterial meningitis. J Pediatr 1976;88:549-52.
10. Goren MB, Cernich M, Broki O. Some observations on mycobacterial acid-fastness. Am Rev Respir Dis 1978;118:151-4.
11. Greenbaum M, Beyt BE Jr, Murray PR. The accuracy of diagnosing pulmonary tuberculosis at a teaching hospital. Am Rev Respir Dis 1980;121:477-81.
12. Handsfield HH, Lipman TO, Harnisch JP, Tronca E, Holmes KK. Asymptomatic gonorrhea in men: diagnosis, natural course, prevalence and significance. N Engl J Med 1974;290:117-23.
13. Heineman HS, Chawla JK, Lofton WM. Misinformation from sputum cultures without microscopic examination. J Clin Microbiol 1977;6:518-27.
14. Hodges GR, Perkins RL. Acute bacterial meningitis. Analysis of factors influencing prognosis. Am J Med Sci 1977;270:427-35.
15. Hoff RG, Newman DE, Staneck JL. Bacteriuria screening by use of acridine orange-stained smears. J Clin Microbiol 1985;21:513-16.
16. Humphrey A. Use of the buffy coat layer in the rapid diagnosis of septicemia. Am J Clin Pathol 1944;14:358-62.
17. Jenkins RD, Fenn JP, Matsen JM. Review of urine microscopy for bacteriuria. JAMA 1986;255:3397-403.
18. Kass EH. Asymptomatic infections of the urinary tract. Trans Assoc Am Physic 1956;69:56-63.
19. Kellogg DS, Holmes KK, Hill GA. Cumitech 4: Laboratory diagnosis of gonorrhea. Washington, DC: American Society for Microbiology, 1976.
20. Kim TC, Blackman RS, Heatwole KM, Kim T, Rochester DF. Acid-fast bacilli in sputum smears of patients with pulmonary tuberculosis: prevalence and significance of negative smears pretreatment and positive smears posttreatment. Am Rev Respir Dis 1984;129:264-8.
21. Kinyoun JJ. A note on Uhlenhuth's method for sputum examination for tubercle bacilli. Am J Public Health 1915;5:867-9.
22. Kronvall G, Myhre E. Differential staining of bacteria in clinical specimens using acridine orange buffered at low pH. Acta Pathol Microbiol Scand 1977;85:249-54.
23. Lauer BA, Reller LB, Mirrett S. Comparison of acridine orange and Gram stains for detection of microorganisms in cerebrospinal fluid and other clinical specimens. J Clin Microbiol 1981;14:201-5.
24. Lipsky BA, Gates J, Tenover FC, Plorde JJ. Factors affecting the clinical value of microscopy for acid-fast bacilli. Rev Infect Dis 1984;6:214-22.
25. Lipsky BA, Plorde JJ, Tenover FC, Brancato FP. Comparison of the Auto-Microbic System, acridine orange stained smears, and gram-stained smears in detecting bacteriuria. J Clin Microbiol 1985;22:176-81.
26. Lossick JG, Smeltzer MP, Curran JW. The value of the cervical Gram stain in the diagnosis and treatment of gonorrhea in women in a venereal disease clinic. Sex Transm Dis 1982;9:124-7.
27. McCarthy LR, Senne JE. Evaluation of acridine orange stain for detection of microorganisms in blood cultures. J Clin Microbiol 1980;11:281-5.
28. Murray PR, Elmore C, Krogstad DJ. The acid-fast stain: a specific and predictive test for mycobacterial disease. Ann Intern Med 1980;92:512-13.

29. Murray PR, Washington JA II. Microscopic and bacteriological analysis of expectorated sputum. Mayo Clin Proc 1975;50:339-44.
30. Paine TF. Gram staining without the clock. N Engl J Med 1963;268:941-2.
31. Platt R. Quantitative definition of bacteriuria. Am J Med 1983;(July suppl):44-52.
32. Reimer LG, Kepas A. Comparison of Gram stain and Nomarski optics for screening sputum specimens before culture. J Clin Microbiol 1986;23:377-8.
33. Reller LB, Murray PR, MacLowry JD. Cumitech 1A: Blood cultures II. Washington, DC: American Society for Microbiology, 1982.
34. Stamm WE, Counts GW, Running KR, Fihn S, Turck M, Holmes KK. Diagnosis of coliform infection in acutely dysuric women. N Engl J Med 1982;307:463-8.
35. Thysell H. Evaluation of chemical and microscopical methods for mass detection of bacteriuria. Acta Med Scand 1969;185:393-400.
36. Truant JP, Brett WA, Thomas W Jr. Fluorescence microscopy of tubercle bacilli stained with auramine and rhodamine. Henry Ford Hosp Med Bull 1962;10:287-96.
37. Wetterau LM, Zeimis RT, Hollick GE. Direct examination of unstained smears for the evaluation of sputum specimens. J Clin Microbiol 1986;24:143-4.

CHAPTER 39

MICROBIAL ANTIGEN DETECTION

Richard C. Tilton, Ph.D

INTRODUCTION

Clinical microbiology has lagged far behind other laboratory specialties in being able to report timely and clinically relevant data. Isolation, identification and antimicrobial susceptibility testing of isolates has involved an obligatory 48-72 hours of testing, so that most results have been retrospective. There was obviously a need for a more rapid method of diagnosis and a number of different technologies have been applied, ranging from gas chromatography to mass spectrophotometry. However, only two general methodologies have the potential for routine use: these are the detection of antigen by the use of specific antibodies or the application of DNA probes. This chapter will explore the application of antigen detection methods.

In many laboratories, microbial antigen detection has become a routine procedure. Virtually any body fluid may be analyzed. The initial work on microbial antigen detection focused on the rapid diagnosis of meningitis caused by *Neisseria meningitidis, Streptococcus pneumoniae* and *Haemophilus influenzae*. In the 1970s, laboratories that performed these tests usually used counterimmunoelectrophoresis (CIE). As CIE requires technical competence and is not amenable to routine use, it has been largely replaced by latex agglutination and coagglutination tests. Commercially available reagents in kits detect *S. pneumoniae, H. influenzae, N. meningitidis* and group B streptococcal antigens in cerebrospinal fluid (CSF), urine and blood. Although these kits are readily available and widely used, there is increasing agreement that the detection of antigens in spinal fluid may not be as clinically relevant as once thought. In most cases, the sensitivity of such antigen detection is about the same as the sensitivity of the Gram stain, providing similar information. The real value of antigen detection may be for diagnosis in the antibiotic-treated patient, where several studies have reported up to a 15% diagnostic advantage over Gram or other stains.[1,16]

During the 1980s, there was further development of methods for detection of antigens from organisms other than those responsible for meningitis. These methods included detection of antigens of viral hepatitis, group A and group B streptococcus, agents of sexually transmitted diseases such as *Chlamydia* and *Neisseria gonorrhoeae* and detection of viral antigens such as respiratory syncytial virus and herpesvirus.

IMMUNOASSAYS: SENSITIVITY AND SPECIFICITY

A wide range of antibody-mediated immunoassays have been devised. In general, of the antigen detection methods, CIE is the least sensitive followed by coagglutination, latex agglutination, enzyme and fluoroimmunoassay, and radioimmunoassay. In the past, immunoassays have suffered from lack of sensitivity and specificity but the development of high-quality polyclonal and monoclonal antibodies has solved many of these problems. The production of highly specific polyclonal sera is possible but time-consuming and expensive. It is often advantageous to produce monoclonal antibodies which allow the standardization of extremely reproducible immunoassays.

Much of the published work on the sensitivity of antigen detection systems has dealt with kits for detection of microbial antigens in spinal fluid. Table 39:1 describes minimum bacterial antigen concentrations detected by CIE, coagglutination and latex agglutination.[8] It can also be noted that different investigators have observed a wide range of sensitivities. Several factors may interfere with sensitivity. For example, types 7 and 14 *S. pneumoniae* antigens do not migrate in an electric field, being electrically neutral. CIE,

Table 39:1. Minimum Bacterial Antigen Concentration Detected by CIE, CoA and LA*

Antigen	Minimum antigen concentration (ng/mL) detected by		
	CIE	CoA	LA
Group B *Streptococcus* (type and group antigens)	500–14,000	—	63
S. pneumoniae	25–1,000	6–50	0.2–50
H. influenzae type b	1–30	2–25	0.1–5
N. meningitidis groups A, C, D, and Y	12–75	1.5–12	0.75–50

* CIE = Counterimmunoelectrophoresis; CoA = Coagglutination; LA = Latex Agglutination. Modified from Fung and Tilton.[9]

then, cannot detect these pneumococcal antigens, although enzyme immunoassays and agglutination procedures do.

Table 39:2 presents the sensitivity of microbial antigen detection in CSF and blood. Similarly, a wide range of sensitivity is observed and various factors influence detection. These include bacterial concentration in the CSF, a prozone effect due to antigen excess and the particular phase of the disease process during which the sample was taken. In the early stages of disease, there may be an undetectable threshold level of antigen or there may be such a concentration of antigen that the undiluted specimen will be negative by CIE as well as by agglutination techniques. Dilution of the specimen will be required to demonstrate positivity.

Urine is often a usable and easily obtainable source for detecting bacterial antigens. If urine is concentrated 20- to 50-fold, bacterial antigen will be found in 83-100% of concentrated urines from patients with bacterial meningitis.[8] Concentrated urine may also be the most suitable fluid for antigen detection in group B streptococcal disease. In infants, where CSF and blood specimens may be difficult to obtain, urine is the fluid of choice.

Currently available tests for cryptococcal antigen, herpes simplex virus, respiratory syncytial virus, adenovirus, hepatitis B infection and rotavirus are quite specific. There are few, if any, known crossreactions that occur. However, the Rotazyme II kit (Abbott Laboratories), which contains polyclonal antiserum for the detection of rotavirus, has been shown to be unreliable in infants. The origin of such "false positive" results are unknown.

There have been a number of bacterial crossreactivities encountered in

Table 39:2. Sensitivity of Detection of Bacterial Antigens in CSF and Blood

		% Positive reaction		
Infection	Body fluid	CIE*	CoA*	LA*
Group B *Streptococcus*				
Meningitis	CSF	63–100	83	79–92
	Serum	27–63		27
Bacteremia	CSF	0		
	Serum	88		
S. pneumoniae				
Meningitis	CSF	44–100	67–100	61–88
	Serum	35–75		
N. meningitidis				
Meningitis	CSF	30–92	33–49	71–88
	Serum	14–67		
H. influenzae tybe b				
Meningitis	CSF	63–100	57–100	78–100
	Serum	70–83		

* CIE = Counterimmunoelectrophoresis; CoA = Coagglutination; LA = Latex Agglutination.
Modified from Fung and Tilton.[9]

CIE, coagglutination and latex agglutination: they are listed in Table 39:3.[8] Although such crossreactions may occur, they rarely occur with clinical specimens. Crossreaction between *N. meningitidis* group B and *Escherichia coli* K1 occurs frequently, suggesting that an antigen of *E. coli* K1 is identical to one of *N. meningitidis* B.

There may also be nonspecific crossreactions, particularly in urine and serum. Agglutination tests often show spontaneous nonspecific agglutination. Treatment of these body fluids with heat, EDTA, proteinase or a reducing agent such as n-acetyl cysteine may eliminate this nonspecificity.[8] Each of the commercial kit vendors provides instructions for the elimination of nonspecific agglutination and these should be followed closely.

METHODS

Counterimmunoelectrophoresis (CIE)[18]

CIE was originally described by Boussard in 1959 and was first used clinically for the detection of Hepatitis B surface antigen (HBsAg). CIE is a rapid precipitin reaction in which the reactants are driven by an electric current. The traditional precipitin reaction, which is a function of the precipitation of antibody and soluble antigen at the equivalence point, may take up to 24 hours. CIE, on the other hand, is much faster and combines the advantages of both immunodiffusion and electrophoresis. The antigen

Table 39:3. Antigenic Crossreactivity in CIE, CoA and LA*

Antiserum	Crossreacting strain
S. pneumoniae	Alpha hemolytic *Steptococcus* (certain strains) *H. influenzae* types a, b *N. meningitidis* group B *Klebsiella* species
Group B *Streptococcus*	Beta hemolytic *Streptococcus* groups A, B, C, D, G *S. pneumoniae* *Proteus mirabilis*
N. meningitidis	*H. influenzae* *S. pneumoniae* *E. coli*
H. influenzae	*N. meningitidis* *E. coli* *S. pneumoniae* Group B *Streptococcus* *Staphylococcus aureus*

* CIE = Counterimmunoelectrophoresis; CoA = Coagglutination; LA = Latex Agglutination. Modified from Fung and Tilton.[9]

is placed in a well on the cathodic side of a solid matrix and the antibody is placed on the anodic side. The negatively charged antigen migrates toward the anode. The weakly negative antibody also migrates toward the anode while buffer ions, which are positively charged, tend to sweep the antibody molecule in the opposite direction towards the cathode. This latter phenomenon is known as endoosmotic flow. If conditions of current, voltage, pH, buffer, antigen/antibody concentration and quality of antisera are optimal, a precipitin line appears between the two wells after as little as 30 min of electrophoresis. For specific instructions regarding CIE methods, the reader is referred to a review by Tilton.[18]

Coagglutination (CoA)

The coagglutination technique for the detection of pneumococcal antigens was first introduced by Kronvall.[15] Certain strains of *Staphylococcus aureus*, including Cowan strain I, contain a cell surface protein called Protein A. Antibodies (IgG) adhere to protein A by their Fc portion, leaving the Fab ends free to react with the homologous antigen. The presence of antigen results in the visible agglutination of the staphylococcal particles. The agglutination of sensitized Protein A containing-staphylococci may be less distinct than latex agglutination. The procedure, like latex agglutination, is also subject to nonspecific agglutination in body fluids such as CSF, serum and urine. The preparation of coagglutination reagents is technically simple, and once prepared, the sensitized staphylococci are more stable than latex reagents.

Latex Agglutination (LA)

Latex polystyrene beads were first used to detect rheumatoid factor in serum. Antibody (IgG) is nonspecifically absorbed to the surface of latex polystyrene beads of uniform diameter (0.8 μm). Addition of specific antigen agglutinates the milky white latex suspension. Although latex agglutination tests can be done in test tubes, they are usually performed on slides where various colored latex particles provide easy reading. Latex particles may be sensitized in the laboratory or purchased commercially.

Sedgwick and Tilton[17] described the preparation of a latex suspension for the identification of *Legionella pneumophila*, a method generally applicable to most bacterial systems. One tenth (0.1) mL of antiserum was added to a tube containing 1.0 mL of a 10% solution of Dow latex polystyrene and incubated at 37°C for 2 h. The reagent was diluted 1:20 with glycine buffered saline containing 0.1% bovine serum albumin. The diluted latex reagent was filtered through a thin layer of absorbent cotton to remove any clumped particles, washed and then used.

The procedure for the detection of antigen or antibody by latex agglutination is quite simple. A drop or two of the latex reagent is mixed with a suspension of the colony or the body fluid to be tested. The suspension is mixed and incubated at room temperature with occasional rocking of the slide. Agglutination is a positive test. For some applications, such as the detection of group A streptococci, the antigen may have to be extracted from the clinical material by autoclaving, protease or nitrous acid.

Enzyme Immunoassay (EIA)[6]

There are two major types of enzyme immunoassays, the homogeneous assay and the heterogeneous assay. Heterogeneous immunoassays usually require physical separation of bound and unbound antigen while homogeneous assays do not. Enzyme-multiplied immunoassays (EMIT) are homogeneous assays while enzyme-linked immunosorbent assays (ELISA) are heterogeneous.

The enzyme-multiplied immunoassay is competitive. The substance to be detected, usually a low molecular weight antigen such as an aminoglycoside antibiotic, is attached to an enzyme. This attachment occurs in such a way that binding of antibody to the antigen sterically blocks substrate binding. In the clinical test, a body fluid which contains free or unbound antigen is mixed with the enzyme-labelled or bound antigen. Both free and bound antigen compete for binding sites on the antibody which is added to the mixture. The more free antigen present, the more enzyme will remain unbound and catalytically active upon the addition of substrate. The reaction is read spectrophotometrically; the greater the enzyme activity, the greater the change in absorbance. The absorbance change is directly correlated to the concentration of antigen in the patient's specimen. The rate of change can be read or the reaction can be stopped and a single absorbance value read.

In the ELISA methodology, the solid phase, such as a plastic microtiter plate, may be coated with specific antibody. The antigen-containing body fluid is layered over the sensitized solid phase and is captured by antibody. After appropriate washing to remove unbound material, a second specific antibody is added, and after further washing, an enzyme-labelled antiglobulin and substrate. Here antibody is the "antigen." At other times, antigen is coated on the plate, i.e., this is a capture and tag system.

Although ELISA methodology is not conceptually difficult, there are many variables to control. These include the nature of the solid phase, the washing process, enzyme and substrates used, and the termination of the reaction.

Radioimmunoassay (RIA)[12]

RIA is a technique which, like the the EMIT, is both specific and sensitive when appropriate antibody is available. The principle use of RIA is in endocrinology for the assay of hormones, but all areas of laboratory medicine have found RIA a useful tool. In most applications, labelled antigen (usually ^{125}I) competes with unlabelled antigen for available binding sites on a specified amount of homologous antibody. After equilibrium between the bound and the unbound antigen is reached, the bound fraction is separated from the unbound one by centrifugation and/or precipitation. In some applications, the antibody is coated on tubes and separation of the phase takes place by decanting the fluid in the tube.

Although microbiological research employs RIA widely, it is rarely used routinely in clinical microbiology laboratories except for the determination of Hepatitis A or B antibodies and antigens and aminoglycoside antibiotics.

Solid Phase Immunofluorescence and Fluorescence Polarization Immunoassay (FPIA)

The fluorescent immunoassays[3] are similar to RIA and EIA except that fluorescing compounds are used to tag antibodies. The assays may be competitive or noncompetitive. Solid phases such as beads, discs, tubes or paddles are coated with antibody. If the tests are competitive, then fluorescing, labelled antigens compete with nonlabelled antigens for binding sites. The bound and free components are separated by centrifugation, decanting or by the use of magnetic beads.

An instrument (TDX, Abbott Laboratories) based on fluorescence polarization immunoassay is used in many laboratories. FPIA is a nonseparation immunoassay; that is, the bound and free complexes need not be separated prior to reading the test. FPIA is a competitive assay in that bound and free antigen-antibody complexes generate different signals when fluorescent light is polarized in both horizontal and vertical planes. FPIA combines the specificity of a heterogeneous immunoassay with the speed and convenience of a homogeneous technique. Methods are currently available for the measurement of aminoglycoside antibiotics and vancomycin in serum as well as other substances such as digoxin, cortisol and drugs of abuse.

Antigen Detection Tests

There are many companies offering complete kits or reagents for a wide variety of bacterial, viral, fungal and protozoan antigens. It would be counterproductive to list all of the available kits, as these are changing constantly. Table 39:4 lists those organisms for which antigen detection methods are available. Some are agglutination methods: others are enzyme immunoassays. Comprehensive instrumentation is also available for EIAs. This may include a programmable spectrophotometer so that all calculations are performed automatically, including the construction of a standard curve. Kits are available for diagnosis of infectious diseases, including those for

Table 39:4. Organisms for which Antigen Detection Methods are Available

Adenovirus	*Mycobacterium*
Brucella abortus	*Mycoplasma*
Candida albicans (envelope protein, mannan)	*Neisseria gonorrhoeae*
Chlamydia trachomatis	*Neisseria meningitidis*
Clostridium difficile toxin A, B, D1	Norwalk virus
Cryptococcus neoformans	Parainfluenza virus
Cryptosporidium	Respiratory syncytial virus
Epstein-Barr virus	Rotavirus (human, calf)
Escherichia coli toxin (LT, ST)	*Salmonella typhi*
Haemophilus influenzae	*Schistosoma mansoni*
Hepatitis A antigen	*Staphylococcus* Toxin A (enterotoxin)
Hepatitis B surface antigen, e antigen	*Staphylococcus* toxin (Toxic shock syndrome)
Herpes simplex virus 1 & 2	*Streptococcus,* Group A, B
Human papilloma virus	*Streptococcus pneumoniae*
Influenza virus	*Trichomonas vaginalis*
Legionella pneumophila, other legionellae	*Vibrio cholerae* (enterotoxin)
	Vibrio vulnificus
	Yersinia enterocolitica

antigens of *N. gonorrhoeae*, group A streptococcus, *Chlamydia trachomatis* and rotavirus, as well as those for hepatitis A and B antigens and antibodies, rubella antibodies (IgG, IgM), cytomegalovirus antibodies, herpes simplex virus antigens and antibodies and HIV (HTLV-III/LAV) antibodies.

Clinical Applications of Antigen Detection:

Edwards[4] first demonstrated the polysaccharide capsule of *N. meningitidis* in the serum of patients with meningococcemia. The same polysaccharide was detected by CIE in the CSF of 47/68 patients with meningococcal meningitis. The Gram stain was positive in 17/68 patients and the culture positive in 42/68 patients. Since these early reports, much has been published on the rapid diagnosis of bacterial meningitis by CIE. The most commonly detected antigenic components are those of *H. influenzae, S. pneumoniae, N. meningitidis*, Group B streptococci and *E. coli* K1. The combination of CSF, serum and urine CIE's can identify virtually 100% of children with *H. influenzae* type b meningitis, 60% of patients with pneumococcal meningitis and about 50% of those with meningococcal meningitis.[9]

Feigin et al.[7] emphasized the value of testing urine in a prospective trial of CIE for the diagnosis of bacterial meningitis in children. Spinal fluid CIE was positive in 89.1% and urine CIE in 96.9% of 64 patients with *H. influenzae* meningitis. Of 14 patients with pneumococcal meningitis, 78.5% had positive CSF CIE's and 50% had positive urine CIE's.

The value of CIE for the prospective diagnosis of early onset group B streptococcal (GBS) infection has been reported.[5]

The clinical advantages of CIE also apply to the latex and coagglutination techniques. As agglutination is theoretically more sensitive than CIE, it should offer a greater diagnostic advantage. The ability of LA to detect cryptococcal polysaccharide in serum or CSF has been well documented.[10] It was specific and more sensitive than demonstration of the capsule of *C. neoformans* by India ink.

Prognostic Value of Antigen Detection:

The detection of bacterial antigens in CSF is associated with increased morbidity and mortality. CSF with detectable group A meningococcal antigen by CIE is associated with a greater incidence of petechial and severe neurologic damage.[2] Similarly, CSF specimens with group C meningococcal antigen have been associated with prolonged coma and clinical signs of markedly increased intracranial pressure.[11] The detection of *E. coli* K1 antigen in infants was related to their clinical outcome, being 50% in normal survivors, 86% in those with neurologic damage and 82% in those that died. The mean antigen concentration was higher in infants with a poorer prognosis, as was the mean duration of detection of antigen.[14] Early and permanent neurologic sequelae were noted especially in patients with *H. influenzae* type b meningitis with CSF polyribitol phosphate (PRP) concentrations greater than 1.28 μg/mL.[14] A strong correlation between antigenemia, bacteremia and patient mortality was observed in patients with pneumococcal pneumonia.[13]

The real impact of antigen detection tests is yet to come. Methods are now available for rapid, nongrowth-dependent detection of *Chlamydia*, viruses, fungi and protozoan parasites, as well as a variety of clinically significant bacteria. Many of these microorganisms are difficult or expensive to grow. The ability, then, to use antigen detection in virtually any laboratory setting to diagnose infectious diseases should have a profound effect on patient care.

REFERENCES

1. Baker CJ, Rench MA. Commercial latex agglutination for detection of group B streptococcal antigen in body fluid. J Pediatr 1983;102:393-5.
2. Coonrod JD, Rytel MW. Detection of type specific pneumococcal antigens by counterimmunoelectrophoresis. II. Etiologic diagnosis of pneumococcal pneumonia. J Lab Clin Med 1973;81:770-7.
3. Dandliker WB, Kelly RJ, Dandliker J, et al. Fluorescense polarization immunoassay. Theory and experimental method. Immunochemistry 1973;10:219-27.

4. Edwards EA. Immunologic investigations of meningococcal antigens. I. Group-specific *Neisseria meningitidis* antigens present in the serum of patients with fulminant meningococcemia., J Immunol 1971;106:314-17.
5. Edwards MS, Baker CJ. Prospective diagnosis of early-onset Group B streptococcal infection by countercurrent immunoelectrophoresis. J Pediatr 1979;94:286-8.
6. Engvall E, Pearlmann P. Enzyme-linked immunosorbent assay (ELISA). Quantitative assay of immunoglobulin G. Immunochemistry 1971;8:871-4.
7. Feigin RD, Wong M, Shackelford PG, Stechenberg BW, Dunkle IM, Kaplan S. Countercurrent immunoelectrophoresis of urine as well as of CSF and blood for diagnosis of bacterial meningitis. J Pediatr 1976; 89:773-5.
8. Fung JC, Tilton RC. Bacterial antigen detection by CIE, coagglutination and latex agglutination. In: Lennette EH, Balows A, Hausler WJ Jr, Shadomy JH, eds. Manual of clinical microbiology. 4th ed. Washington, DC: American Society for Microbiology, 1985:883-90.
9. Fung JC, Tilton RC. Detection of bacterial antigens. In: Wicher K, ed. Microbial antigenodiagnosis, CRC Press, Boca Raton, FL: 1987; (in press).
10. Gentry LO, Wilkinson ID, Lea AS, Price MF. Latex agglutination test for detection of *Candida* antigen in patients with disseminated disease. Eur J Clin Microbiol 1983;2:122-8.
11. Hoffman TA, Edwards EA. Group specific polysaccharide antigen and humoral antibody response in disease due to *Neisseria meningitidis*. J Infect Dis 1972;126:636-44.
12. Kayhty H, Makela PH, Ruoslahti E. Radioimmunoassay of capsular polysaccharide antigens of groups A and C meningococci and *Haemophilus influenzae* type b in cerebrospinal fluid. J Clin Pathol 1977;30:831-3.
13. Kenny GE, Wentworth BB, Beasley RP, Foy HM. Correlation of circulating capsular polysaccharide with bacteremia in pneumococcal pneumonia. Infect Immun 1972;6:431-7.
14. McCracken GH, Sarff LD, Clode MD. Relation between *Escherichia coli* K1 capsular polysaccharide antigen and clinical outcome in neonatal meningitis. Lancet 1974;1:246-50.
15. Kronvall G. A rapid slide agglutination method for typing pneumococci by means of specific antibody absorbed to Protein A-containing staphylococci. J Med Microbiol 1973;6:187-9.
16. McGinnis MR. Detection of fungi in cerebrospinal fluid. Am J Med 1983;75:129-38.
17. Sedgwick AK, Tilton RC. Identification of *Legionella pneumophilia* by latex agglutination. J Clin Microbiol 1982;17:365-8.
18. Tilton RC. Counterimmunoelectrophoresis in biology and medicine; Critical Reviews in Laboratory Medicine. Boca Raton, FL: CRC Press, 1978.

CHAPTER 40

CHROMATOGRAPHY FOR THE IDENTIFICATION OF MICROORGANISMS

Robert Martin, Dr.P.H. and William A. Schneider, B.S.

INTRODUCTION

Chromatographic techniques have been used since the 1960s for characterizing microorganisms.[1,17,19,24] Such techniques have provided means for separating and identifying cellular components and products of metabolism as an aid to taxonomic classification of bacteria. In the last ten years, use of gas-liquid chromatography in the clinical microbiology laboratory has increased due to advances in instrumentation. Electronics have become more reliable, vastly improved columns provide the capability for resolving closely related compounds and computerized data systems can store chromatographic patterns for development of data bases.

This chapter will provide information and procedures for use in the identification of anaerobic and aerobic bacteria. Techniques found to be of major value in the identification of microorganisms will be described in detail. Readers are referred to the literature for complete information regarding spent metabolites or fatty acid composition of specific bacteria.

BASIC PRINCIPLES

Gas-Liquid Chromatography (GLC)

The gas chromatograph was introduced in the early 1950s by James and Martin[11] and has been said to be the most important analytical tool developed in this century. The chromatograph (Fig.40:1) consists of injector ports, column, detector, temperature controls and chart recorder. The most

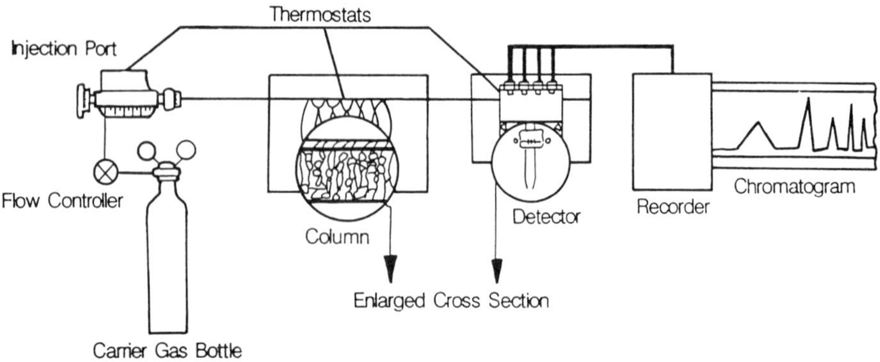

FIGURE 40:1. Schematic of a gas chromatographic system.

important component is the column, since it is here that separation of components in a mixture takes place. The column may be made of metal or glass and may be a packed column or a capillary column. Packed columns utilize an inert material such as diatomaceous earth coated with a liquid phase. Liquid phases are chosen on the basis of the components to be separated. Capillary columns, as the name implies, are very narrow. The liquid phase, rather than being coated on packing material, is coated on the inner walls of the column. The narrow bore and the long length of such columns provide excellent resolution of closely related compounds.[26]

A sample mixture is injected through the injector port where the mixture is heated and converted to vapor. The gaseous mixture then passes through the column where components are partitioned on the basis of their affinity for the liquid phase and on their molecular weight. The compounds with least affinity and of lower molecular weight will elute first, while those with greatest affinity and higher molecular weight will elute last. As each compound elutes from the column and separated components move through the detector, a change in conductivity is detected and recorded. Each component will emerge from a given column at a specific time. This time is known as the retention time and will be constant as long as other conditions are constant (e.g., temperature, flow rate of gases, liquid phase, etc.). Retention times of unknown components of a mixture may be compared to retention times of standards for tentative identification of unknowns.

There are a variety of detectors available. Each type has its particular advantages and the type chosen depends on the application. Thermal conductivity (TC) and flame-ionization detectors (FID) are commonly used in microbiology laboratories.[14,26] A number of manufacturers, including Varian Instruments and Hewlett-Packard, produce chromatographs suitable for both spent metabolite and fatty acid analysis. For anaerobic analysis (spent metabolites), programmable oven temperatures are not required and

TC detectors are sufficient. Manufacturers producing such equipment are Dohrman Environtech, Fisher Scientific and Gow-Mac Instrument Company.

High-pressure Liquid Chromatography (HPLC)

High-pressure liquid chromatography utilizes a liquid rather than a gas as the mobile phase. The liquid mobile phase carries the sample mixture over an immobilized stationary phase on which separation takes place. The liquid phase is pumped at high pressure through the stationary phase in a narrow stainless steel column. As the compounds are eluted from the column, a chromatogram is traced on a chart recorder as in gas-liquid chromatography. Separated compounds are tentatively identified on the basis of retention time and may be quantitated on the basis of height and area under a peak. HPLC has a variety of applications in microbiology, including the measurement of isoprenoid quinones, proteins and nucleotides.[5,27,28,29,30]

Although both GLC and HPLC have applications in clinical microbiology, the former is used frequently in reference and public health laboratories while the latter is primarily a research tool.

BACTERIAL IDENTIFICATION

Historically, clinical microbiology laboratories have relied upon biochemical and morphological features for the identification of bacterial isolates. However, many bacteria are metabolically inert, making identification time-consuming and difficult. Moreover, a great deal of expertise is often necessary for identification, since judgment is required to determine biochemical utilization patterns, to assess morphological appearance of bacterial colonies and to note other morphological features such as flagellar arrangements. GLC analyses of microbial metabolites and of cellular fatty acids provide useful additional information for the identification of both anaerobic and aerobic bacteria.[4,7,20,22,29]

Spent Metabolites

Identification of anaerobic bacteria by GLC has become a routine procedure in many microbiology laboratories. The procedures and equipment are relatively simple and inexpensive. Anaerobic metabolism produces a variety of by-products from fermentation of glucose in broth culture media such as peptone yeast glucose (PYG).[9,12,15,16,18,19,23] Since the metabolic pathways of a given species are usually stable, the products of metabolism are identical within a species. Anaerobic bacterial metabolities include volatile and nonvolatile fatty acids. Volatile acids (acetic, formic, propionic, isobutyric, butyric, isovaleric, valeric, isocaproic, caproic and heptanoic) (Fig.40:2) and nonvolatile acids (pyruvic, lactic, oxalacetic, oxalic, malonic, fumaric, succinic, benzoic, phenylacetic and hydrocinnamic) (Fig.40:3) can be differentiated by using different temperature conditions. These compounds are analyzed after removal from the growth medium by extraction with an organic solvent. The following procedure is used for the extraction of short-chain acids.

Materials and methods:[10,14,19]

All reagents are American Chemical Society (A.C.S.) grade unless otherwise noted. All organic reagents must be analyzed for volatile and nonvolatile acids prior to use.

1. Chloroform
2. Ethyl ether, anhydrous
3. Methanol, anhydrous
4. Non-volatile acid standard (Supelco #4-6985)
5. Peptone-yeast extract broth with glucose (PYG) (see Chapter 45, "Media, Reagents and Stains")-each new lot must be analyzed for volatile and nonvolatile acids.
6. Sodium sulfate, anhydrous, crystalline
7. Sulfuric acid (50% aqueous, v/v)
8. Volatile acid standard (Supelco #4-6975)

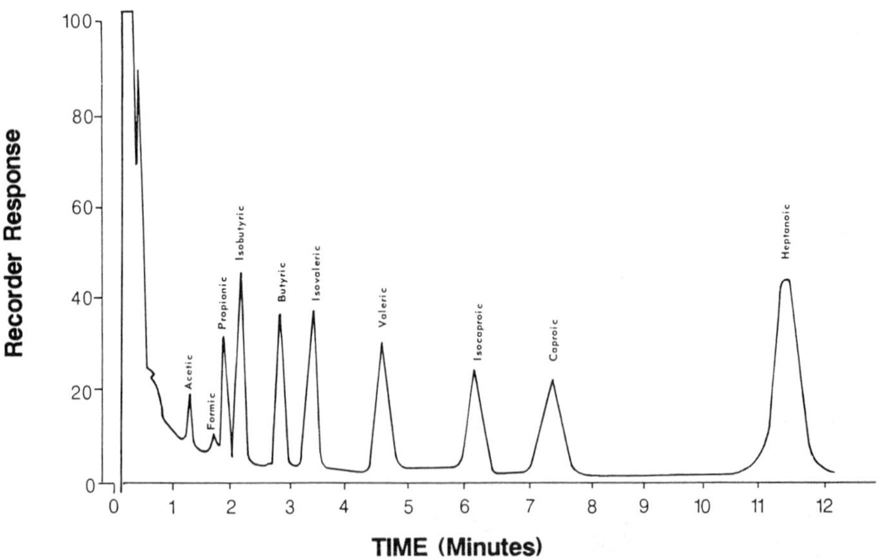

FIGURE 40:2. Gas chromatographic pattern of volatile acids.

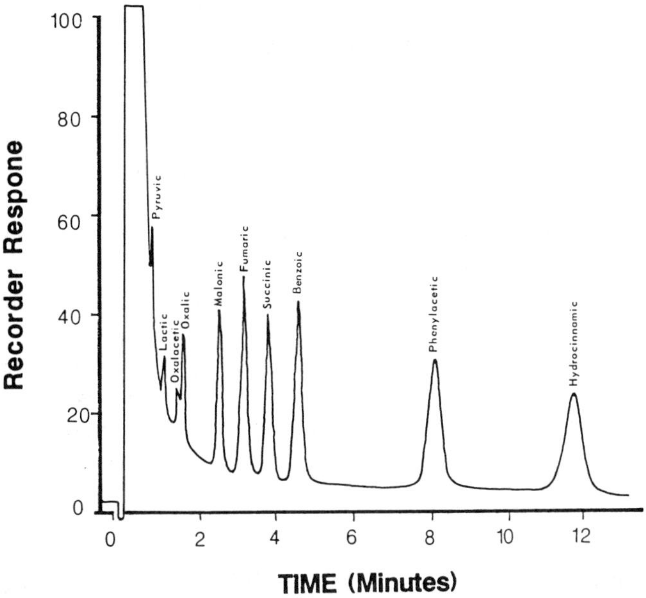

FIGURE 40:3. Gas chromatographic pattern of nonvolatile acids.

9. Chromatographic column (6 ft glass)
10. Packing material-Supelco SP-1000 (SP-1220 may also be used. However, the acid peaks are not resolved as well as with SP-1000).

Preparation of culture:

1. Inoculate a single colony of the organism to be identified into 5 mL of PYG broth. Use one tube for each culture and include one uninoculated tube as a negative control.
2. Incubate anaerobically until turbidity equivalent to a MacFarland #2 (24-48 h) develops.
3. After incubation, examine a Gram stain to determine cultural homogeneity.
4. Add 1.0 mL of the volatile or nonvolatile acid standard to a labeled tube. The standard used will depend on the desired extraction procedure.
5. Acidify the culture to pH 2 or below by adding 0.1 mL 50% (v/v) aqueous sulfuric acid to each 5 mL broth culture, the negative control and the standard.
6. Carry out all extraction procedures in a chemical safety cabinet.

Volatile acids extraction procedure:

1. Transfer 2 mL of each acidified culture, the negative control and the standard into separate sterile 16 X 100 mm screwcapped tubes.

2. Add 1 mL ethyl ether to each tube and replace the cap.
3. Mix each tube by gently inverting 20 times.
4. Centrifuge tubes briefly (5 min at 750-1000 X g) to break the ether-broth emulsion.
5. Carefully remove the ether layer from the aqueous layer with a pasteur pipette and transfer the ether extract to a sterile 4 mL screwcapped vial. Do not contaminate the ether with water.
6. Add anhydrous sodium sulfate equal to approximately one half the volume of ether in the tube and mix. This will ensure that any residual water is removed from the ether extract. Cap the tube and let stand 10 min.
7. Inject 3 μL of the ether extract into the column. Rinse the syringe 4 times with ether after each injection. Each extract will take approximately 15 min to elute from the chromatographic column.

Nonvolatile acid extraction procedure:

1. Place 1 mL of the acidified culture, the negative control and the standard into 16 X 100 mm screwcapped tubes.
2. Add 2 mL methanol and 0.4 mL of 50% sulfuric acid to each tube. Recap each tube and heat at 55°C in a water bath for 30 min or hold overnight at room temperature.
3. To each tube add 1 mL distilled water and 0.5 mL chloroform, recap and mix by gently inverting 20 times. If an emulsion forms, centrifuge for 5 min at 750-1000 X g.
4. Draw the chloroform into the injection syringe directly from under the aqueous layer.
5. Wipe off the injection needle with a tissue and inject 3μL of the chloroform extract into the column. After each injection rinse the syringe 4 times with methanol. Each extract will require approximately 16 min to be eluted from the chromatographic column.
6. After analysis of 20 samples, recondition the column by injecting 4 μL of methanol. Leave the detector on for 10 min to burn any material rinsed from the column by the methanol.

Chromatographic conditions:

1. Injector temperature	200°C
2. Detector temperature	185°C
3. Oven temperature	155°C for volatile acids (135°C for SP1220 packing) 145°C for nonvolatile acids (125°C for SP1220 packing)
4. Flow rate of carrier gas	Helium 20 mL/min

Using these procedures, volatile acids will be found in the ether layer and nonvolatile acids will be found in the chloroform layer.

Bacteroides fragilis is the anaerobe most commonly isolated in the clinical microbiology laboratory. Figures 40:4 and 40:5 show chromatographic patterns of volatile and nonvolatile acids produced by *B. fragilis* grown in PYG.

It is important to be sure that solvents, glassware, reagents and media are free from contaminating acids and that appropriate standards are used. Since products of metabolism depend on the nature of the medium in which the organism is grown, it is important to employ the same medium used in generating data for identification tables. It is also important to use a reagent blank, as both acetic and succinic acids are found in PYG medium. The level of each acid must be determined for comparative purposes before bacterial metabolites are analyzed.

Cellular Fatty Acid Analysis

A number of studies have confirmed that gas-liquid chromatographic analysis of cellular fatty acids provides useful information for characterizing many bacteria.[4,6,7,8,18,22] These lipids are found in the cell wall and cell membrane. After growth on a suitable medium, the cells are saponified and the lipids are extracted with an organic solvent.

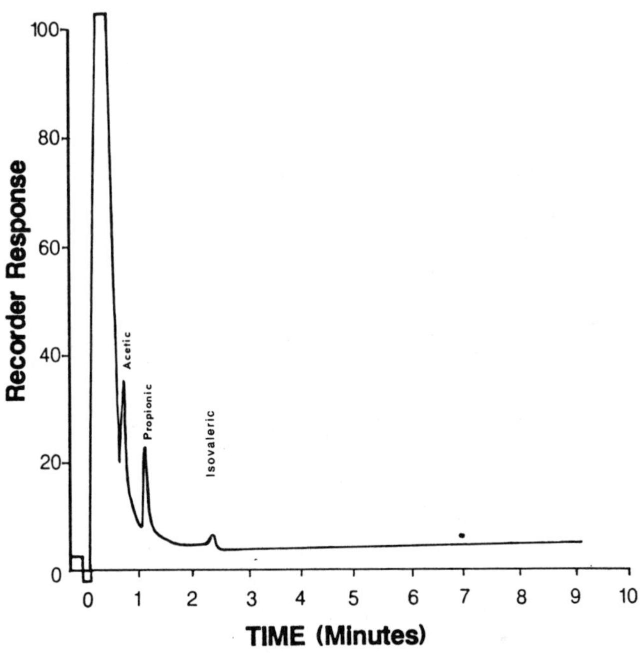

FIGURE 40:4. Volatile acids of *Bacteroides fragilis*.

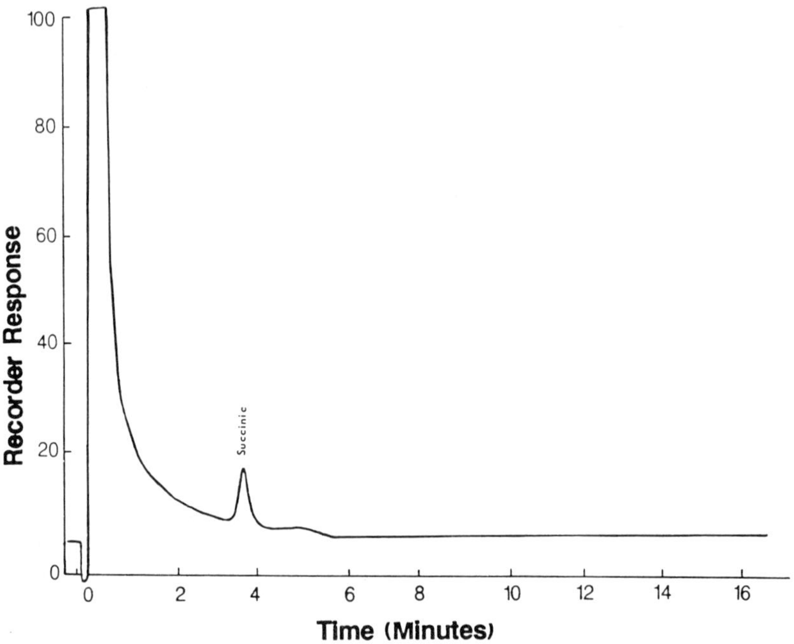

FIGURE 40:5. Nonvolatile acids of *Bacteroides fragilis*.

Materials:

All reagents are A.C.S. grade unless otherwise noted and all organic reagents must be analyzed for fatty acids prior to use.

1. Sodium hydroxide
2. Methanol
3. 20 X 150 mm screwcapped glass tubes with teflon liners in caps (American Scientific Products)
4. Hydrochloric acid
5. Hexane-must be chromatography grade
6. Diethylether
7. Disodium sulfate, anhydrous
8. 2 mL sample vials with teflon-lined septum (Varian Scientific)

Method:

1. Harvest the bacterial growth from an agar plate after 24 h incubation. Add 0.5 mL sterile distilled water to the plate and use a bent glass rod to scrape bacterial growth from the surface of the agar. Perform this twice to ensure maximum collection of cells.
2. Transfer the cell suspension to a clean 20 X 150 mm test tube.

3. Add 4 mL of 5% sodium hydroxide in 50% methanol. Tighten the teflon-lined cap securely.
4. Heat for 30 min in a boiling water bath.
5. Cool the tube with cold water and add 4 mL of 15% hydrochloric acid in methanol. Invert the tubes 8 times. Do not shake since an emulsion may develop that inhibits recovery of the sample. Check the pH with pH paper. If not under pH 2 then add 2 to 3 drops of concentrated hydrochloric acid. Tighten teflon-lined cap.
6. Heat for 15 min in a boiling water bath. Cool to room temperature.
7. Add 8 mL of diethyl ether/hexane (1:1 v/v) Cap the tube and mix by inverting 8 times.
8. Allow the mixture to separate and remove the organic phase (top layer) to a second tube.
9. Repeat the extraction process in steps 7 and 8 and combine the ether layers.
10. Evaporate contents of the second tube under nitrogen to a final volume of approximately 1.0 to 1.5 mL.
11. Add a small amount of disodium sulfate to the tube to absorb traces of water that may have been produced during evaporation. Transfer the remaining liquid to a 2 mL sample vial.
12. Evaporate contents of the vial to a final volume of approximately 0.3 mL.
13. Unless analyzing immediately, label vials and store in freezer at -20°C until samples are analyzed.

Chromatographic Conditions Using a Packed Column:

1. Injector temperature	165°C
2. Detector temperature	250°C
3. Oven temperature	150°C
4. Temperature ramping	4°C per min to 230°C
5. Flow rate of carrier gas	Helium 30 mL/min

Fatty acid methyl esters can be analyzed by packed column or by fused-silica capillary column with this procedure. Most bacterial fatty acid esters can be separated by the use of a flame-ionization detector and a temperature-programmable oven. Tentative identification of peaks can be made by comparing the retention times of unknown samples to those retention times of compounds in the fatty acid standard (Fig.40:6). Using techniques described by Moss et al,[13] it is possible to accurately identify compounds by hydrogenation of unsaturated acids and by acylation of hydroxy acids. Mass spectrometry is used by some laboratories for confirmation of components not identified by retention times.

Lipids found in the cell wall of *Legionella* spp. possess unique charac-

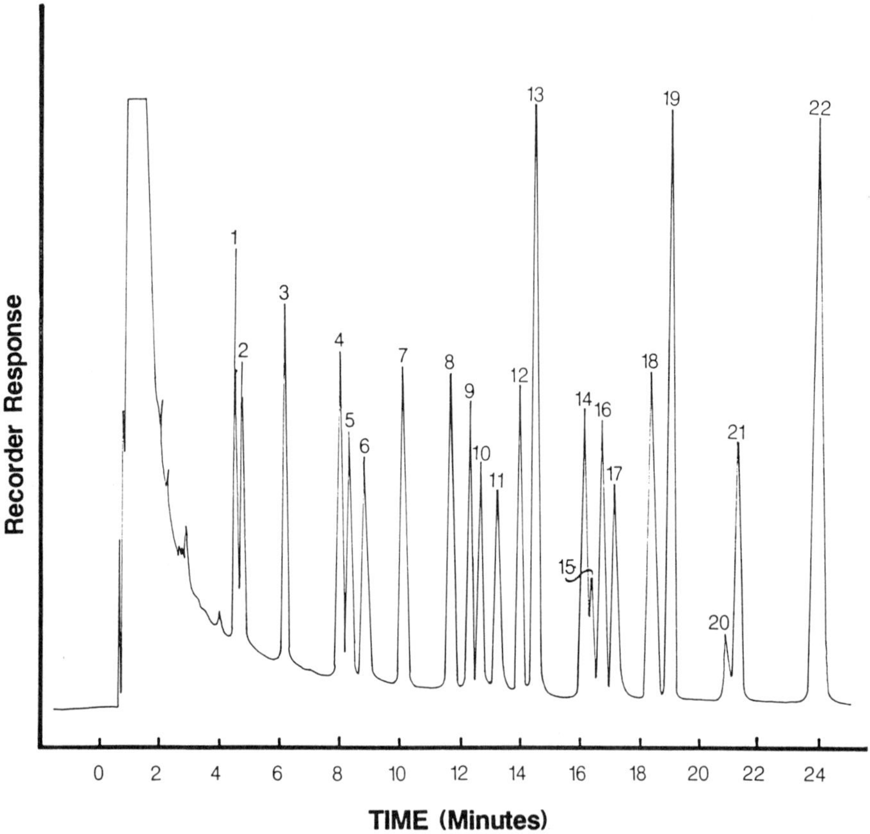

FIGURE 40:6. Bacterial acid methyl ester standard; numbered peaks correspond to the following shorthand designations and names.

Shorthand Designation	Name	Shorthand Designation	Name
1. 11:0	Methyl undecanoate	12. 16:1	Methyl palmitoleate
2. 2-OH 10:0	Methyl 2-hydroxydecanoate	13. 16:0	Methyl palmitate
3. 12:0	Methyl laurate	14. a-17:0	Methyl 14-methylhexadecanoate
4. 13:0	Methyl tridecanoate	15. 17:0c	Methyl dl-cis-9,10-methyl hexadecanoate
5. 2-OH 12:0	Methyl 2-hydroxydodecanoate	16. 17:0	Methyl heptadecanoate
6. 3-OH 12:0	Methyl 3-hydroxydodecanoate	17. 2-OH 16:0	Methyl 2-hydroxyhexadecanoate
7. 14:0	Methyl myristate	18. 18:1	Methyl oleate
8. a-15:0	Methyl 12-methyltetradecanoate	19. 18:0	Methyl stearate
9. 15:0	Methyl pentadecanoate	20. 19:0	Methyl dl-cis-9,10-methylene octadecanoate
10. 2-OH 14:0	Methyl 2-hydroxytetradecanoate	21. 19:0	Methyl nonadecanoate
11. 3-OH 14:0	Methyl 3-hydroxytetradecanoate	22. 20:0	Methyl arachidate

teristics.[8,25] The fatty acid components consist of a number of branched-chain acids, a characteristic not shared by other gram-negative bacteria. New *Legionella* spp. can be tentatively identified on the basis of negative direct fluorescent antibody tests combined with a chromatographic pattern characteristic of *Legionella* spp.

Other Cellular Components

Isoprenoid quinones are involved in electron transport in the plasma membrane. These compounds form two major groups: napthoquinones and benzoquinones. Both thin-layer chromatography and reverse-phase high-pressure liquid chromatography are used for identification of quinones. The taxonomic significance of quinones has been demonstrated for a variety of microorganisms.[5,27,28,30]

Carbohydrate analysis has not met with the same success as the methods previously described due mainly to technical difficulties. However, a number of studies have demonstrated possible taxonomic value of carbohydrate analysis.[2,3,31,32]

GLC, HPLC and other chromatographic techniques have proved to be of value in the clinical microbiology laboratory. Future developments will undoubtedly bring additional applications of these techniques to the diagnosis of infectious disease.

REFERENCES

1. Abbey LE, Highsmith AK, Moran TF, Reiner EJ. Differentiation and characterization of *Klebsiella pneumoniae* strains by pyrolysis-gas-liquid chromatograph-mass spectrometry. J Clin Microbiol 1981;13:313-19.
2. Abuyi HS, Drucker DB. Trimethylsilyl sugar profiles of *Streptococcus milleri* and *Streptococcus mitis*. J Appl Bacteriol 1983;54:391-7.
3. Alvin CL, Larsson L, Magnusson M, Mardh PA, Odham G, Westerdahl G. Determination of fatty acids and carbohydrate monomers in microorganisms by glass capillary gas chromatography,: analysis of *Mycobacterium gordonae* and *Mycobacterium scrofulaceum*. J Gen Microbiol 1983;129:401-5.
4. Braunthal SD, Holt SC, Tanner ACR, Socransky SS. Cellular fatty acid composition of *Actinobacillus actinomycetemcomitans* and *Haemophilus aphrophilus*. J Clin Microbiol 1980;11:625-30.
5. Collins MD, Jones D. Distribution of isoprenoid quinone structural types in bacteria and their taxonomic implications. Microbiol Rev 1981;45:316-54.
6. Dees SB, Moss CW. Cellular fatty acids of *Alcaligenes* and *Pseudomonas* species isolated from clinical specimens. J Clin Microbiol 1975;1:414-19.
7. Dees SB, Moss CW. Identification of *Achromobacter* species by cellular fatty acids and by production of keto acids. J Clin Microbiol 1978;8:61-6.
8. Edelstein PH, Brenner DJ, Moss CW, Steigerwalt AG, Francis EM, George WL. *Legionella wadsworthii* species nova: a cause of human pneumonia. Ann Intern Med 1982;97:809-13.
9. Guerrant GO, Lambert MA, Moss CW. Analysis of short-chain acids from anaerobic bacteria by high-performance liquid chromatography. J Clin Microbiol 1982;16:355-60.

10. Holdeman LV, Cato EP, Moore WEC, eds. Anaerobic laboratory manual. 4th ed. Blacksburg, VA: Virginia Polytechnic Institute and State University, 1977:134-6.
11. James AT, Martin AJP. Gas-liquid partition chromatography: the separation and micro-estimation of volatile fatty acids from formic to dodecanoic acid. Biochem J 1952;50: 679-90.
12. Lambert MA, Moss CW. Production of p-hydroxyhydrocinnamic acid from tyrosine by *Peptostreptococcus anaerobius*. J Clin Microbiol 1980;12:291-3.
13. Lambert MA, Moss CW. Comparison of the effects of acids and base hydrolysis on hydroxy and cyclopropane fatty acids in bacteria. J Clin Microbiol 1983;18:1370-7.
14. Lombard GL, Dowell VR Jr. Gas liquid chromatography analysis of the acid products of bacteria. Atlanta: U.S. Department of Health and Human Services, 1982:1-24.
15. Moore WEC, Cato EP. Synonomy of *Eubacterium limosum* and *Butyribacterium rettgeri. Butyricum limosum* comb nov. Int Bull Bacteriol Nomen and Taxon 1965;15:69-80.
16. Moore WEC, Cato EP, Holdeman LV. Fermentation patterns of some *Clostridium* species. Int J Syst Bacteriol 1966;16:383-415.
17. Morgan MA. Gas-liquid chromatography in the clinical microbiology laboratory. Lab Med 1984;15:544-50.
18. Moss CW, Lewis VJ. Characterization of clostridia by gas chromatography. Appl Microbiol 1967;15:390-7.
19. Moss CW, Dowell VR, Farshtchi D, Raines LJ, Cherry WB. Cultural characteristics and fatty acid composition of propionibacteria. J Bacteriol 1969;97:561-70.
20. Moss CW. Gas-liquid chromatography as an analytical tool in microbiology. Public Health Lab 1975;33:81-103.
21. Moss CW, Dees SB. Identification of microorganisms by gas chromatographic-mass spectrometric analysis of cellular fatty acids. J Chromat 1975;112:595-604.
22. Moss CW, Dees SB. Cellular fatty acids and metabolic products of *Pseudomonas* species obtained from clinical specimens. J Clin Microbiol 1976;4:492-502.
23. Moss CW, Hatheway CL, Lambert MA, McCroskey LM. Production of phenylacetic and hydroxyphenylacetic acids by *Clostridium botulinum* type G. J Clin Microbiol 1980;11:743-5.
24. Moss CW. Gas-liquid chromatography as an analytical tool in microbiology. J Chromat 1981;203:337-47.
25. Moss CW, Karr DE, Dees SB. Cellular fatty acid composition of *Legionella longbeachae* sp. nov. J Clin Microbiol 1981;14:692-4.
26. Moss CW, Nunez-Montiel OI. Analysis of short-chain acids from bacteria by gas-liquid chromatography with fused-silica capillary column. J Clin Microbiol 1982;15:308-11.
27. Moss CW, Bibb WF, Karr DE, Guerrant GO, Lambert MA. Cellular fatty acid composition and ubiquinone content of *Legionella feeleii* sp. nov. J Clin Microbiol 1983;18:917-19.
28. Moss CW, Guerrant GO. Separation of bacterial ubiquinones by reverse-phase high-pressure liquid chromatography. J Clin Microbiol 1983;18:15-17.
29. Moss CW. Uses of gas-liquid chromatography and high-pressure liquid chromatography in clinical microbiology. In: Lennette EH, Balows A, Hausler WJ Jr, eds. Manual of clinical microbiology. 3rd ed. Washington, DC: American Society for Microbiology, 1984:1029-36.
30. Moss CW, Kai A, Lambert MA, Patton C. Isoprenoid quinone content and cellular fatty acid composition of *Campylobacter* species. J Clin Microbiol 1984;19:772-6.
31. Pritchar DG, Coligan JE, Speed SE, Gray BM. Carbohydrate fingerprints of streptococcal cells. J Clin Microbiol 1982;13:89-92.
32. Wilkinson SG, Carby KA. Amino sugars in the cell walls of *Pseudomonas* species. J Gen Microbiol 1971;66:221-7.

CHAPTER 41

NUCLEIC ACID PROBES

Stephen C. Edberg, Ph.D.

INTRODUCTION

Principle of Nucleic Acid Hybridization

Nucleic acids are polymers that may be single- or double-stranded helixes. Whether these associate into double-stranded molecules or not is based upon such physical-chemical parameters as temperature, base-pair composition,[25] ionic strength[33] and the concentration of denaturing agents in the medium.[26]

The physical-chemical parameters under which a particular nucleic acid hybridization reaction occurs are known as the stringency conditions. Under high stringency the amount of base-pair homology to permit single strands to associate into double strands is large. Conversely, at low stringency fewer homologous base pairs are needed for a double-stranded helix to form from two single-stranded polymers. Stringency conditions can, therefore, be manipulated to adjust the specificity of the test. For example, if one wishes to develop a nucleic acid hybridization probe to a microbial genus (e.g., herpesvirus), low stringency conditions may be employed. If the stringency conditions are increased, the same probe would react only with a particular species of the microbe (e.g., herpes simplex virus type 1). Because the physical-chemical conditions of the test have a direct bearing on its sensitivity and specificity, a considerable amount of research in the area of nucleic acid hybridization technology has centered on factors affecting stringency conditions.

Nucleic acid hybridization diagnosis of an infectious disease follows a general strategy regardless of the type of disease investigated: (1) one must open the target microbe to access its nucleic acid; (2) one must react with the target microbe's nucleic acid a labelled probe that binds avidly and specifically with the target; (3) a signal from the combination (i.e., hybridization) of the target with the probe must be generated and interpreted. Most work, and success, to date has been in the second step.

There is currently a large library of specific nucleic acid sequences for virtually all major microbial pathogens. The reactivity of these probes with target microbes has been well studied in vitro. Means for obtaining microbial nucleic acid from clinical specimens are still largely developmental. In the same vein, although significant progress in the generation of a signal has occurred, there is currently no nonradiometric technique amenable to routine laboratory testing.

METHODOLOGY

Synthesis of Nucleic Acid Hybridization Probes

The process of making a nucleic acid hybridization probe is analogous to the production of monoclonal antibodies (Table 41:1). First, a specific nucleic acid fragment from the target microbe is isolated. This fragment must be both specific to the target microbe and exhibit good avidity. Second, this fragment is inserted into a vector that amplifies the microbial pathogen's nucleic acid. The vector must be able to accept foreign DNA and replicate in living cells. Generally, specially constructed plasmids have been utilized for this purpose. Next, the vector is inserted into a suitable host organism. The host must not only have the ability to accept a foreign vector but to replicate it as if the vector were part of itself. Finally, one screens the candidates (i.e., clones) to capture the one that has reproduced the desired nucleic acid. This clone is subsequently utilized to grow large quantities of the nucleic acid,which is harvested and labelled.

Table 41:1. Cloning Protocol

Step	DNA Hybridization	Monoclonal Ab
Selection of template	Restriction endonuclease and capture of DNA fragments	Immunization of animal and capture of B-lymphocytes
Insertion of template	Ligation to a plasmid-insertion in recipient *E. coli*	Fusion with a thymidine kinase-negative myeloma cell
Selection of active template	Successful insertion shown by antibiotic susceptibility	Successful fusion by growth in HAT medium (thymidine kinase activity restored)
Amplification of template product	Growth of vector *E. coli*	Growth of fused B-lymphocyte/myeloma cells
Selection of choice with desired properties	DNA hybridization	Immunoassay

Selection of the Nucleic Acid Fragment

The key finding that opened the field of nucleic acid cloning and permitted the development of hybridization tests was the discovery of restriction endonucleases. These enzymes specifically cut nucleic acid sequences inside the polymer. There are two types of these enzymes. Type I restriction endonucleases are complex proteins of two to eight subunits that require ATP, N-adenosyl-L-methionene and magnesium. These enzymes hydrolyze the polymer molecule randomly. Type II restriction endonucleases are simple proteins that require only magnesium to function. They hydrolyze the double-stranded nucleic acid molecule at defined points. This is the class of restriction endonucleases that is instrumental in nucleic acid hybridization technology.[8,15]

It appears that microbes produce restriction endonucleases to protect themselves against foreign DNA. The microbe methylates its own DNA[38] so it is not attacked by the enzyme. There are many hundred restriction endonucleases available in purified form from a wide variety of sources. Some examples of the most commonly utilized restriction endonucleases are seen in Table 41:2. Because the investigator knows exactly where the restriction endonuclease will cut the nucleic acid polymer, he or she can choose a particular enzyme to produce nucleic acid fragments of known size from the parent DNA molecule.

In practice, the microbial target is grown in large volumes of media to a high density. The nucleic acid is extracted from the target cells by a combination of physical (sonication) and chemical (detergents and sodium hydroxide) means. The harvested nucleic acid is then reacted with a specific restriction endonuclease. After reaction, the small pieces of nucleic acid are separated from each other by gel electrophoresis and column chromatography. The investigator then chooses the desired pieces for insertion into a cloning vector.[8,12] Either DNA or RNA can be chosen as targets for nucleic acid hybridization probes. The first licensed nucleic acid hybridi-

Table 41:2. Restriction Endonucleases Commonly Employed in the Diagnosis of Infectious Diseases

Enzyme Name	Species	Sequence Attacked
EcoRl	*Escherichia coli* (with plasmid Rl)	5′-G-A-A-T-T-C3′
Bam Hl	*Bacillus amyloliquefaciens*	5′-G-G-A-T-C-C-3′
Hing III	*Hemophilus influenzae*	5′-A-A-G-C-T-T-3′
Hpal	*Hemophilus parainfluenzae*	5′-G-T-T-A-A-C-3′
Hae III	*Hemophilus aegypticus*	5′-G-G-C-C-3′
Hinc	*Haemophilus influenzae* R_c	5′-G-T-Py-Pu-A-C-3′
Hinf I	*Haemophilus influenzae* R_f	5′-G-A-N-T-C-3′
Alu I	*Arthrobacter luteus*	5′-A-G-C-T-3′

zation probe for the diagnosis of human infectious diseases (Gen-Probe) utilizes bacterial ribosomal RNA as the probe target.

The nucleic acid from bacteria can be used directly to make probe assays. However, one must make complementary DNA (cDNA) from viruses and eukaryotic pathogens. Also, it is common practice to clone microbial RNA indirectly. To make cDNA, RNA is converted into DNA using a reverse transcriptase enzyme from retroviruses. The RNA serves as a template for this enzyme, producing cDNA. The cDNA is purified using RNAse and absorption columns. Therefore, cDNA is a DNA copy of the original RNA polymer which can be utilized directly to produce nucleic hybridization probes.

Investigators are currently debating the optimum nucleic acid target. Most investigations have been performed with DNA-DNA hybridization, but accumulated data indicates an RNA target may be more useful. DNA has the obvious limitation of being present only once in a given cell whereas ribosomal RNA (rRNA), or messenger RNA (mRNA), may be repeated thousands of times. Therefore, RNA targets should inherently have greater sensitivity than DNA targets.[12] Recently, Edelstein[11] and Wilkinson et al.[41] reported the ability to specifically detect *Legionella* with ribosomal RNA probes. They found these ribosomal probes not only specific but much more rapid than DNA probes.

The means for selection of fragments is also in a state of development. Currently, two techniques are utilized. First is the "shot-gun" cloning method where all fragments from the original target nucleic acid are collected and inserted into vectors. Each vector is cloned and amplified; subsequently, each must be tested for specific utility. Second, pre-selection cloning methods are being developed where the tedious task of testing the extensive library of clones is reduced. This is accomplished by affinity chromotography which removes from the fragment mixture those pieces in which the investigator has no interest. The desired fragments stick to the affinity column while unwanted fragments pass through it. The desired fragments are eluted from the column. The investigator, therefore, has a much smaller library of clones to analyze.

Amplification of the Fragment in a Vector

Specific restriction endonucleases are used to insert a nucleic acid fragment into a vector for amplification. The vector contains recognition sites for one or more of these enzymes; so as the vector multiplies, the nucleic acid fragment increases in number. Common vectors have been completely sequenced and contain sites for the insertion of foreign DNA inside genes that either code for antibiotic resistance or the production of a specific enzyme, such as beta-galactosidase. A successful insertion of the foreign DNA can, therefore, be determined by testing for the loss of antibiotic resistance. Some common cloning vectors and their properties are shown in Table 41:3. For example, a common vector plasmid is pBr322, which contains genes that confer resistance to the antibiotics ampicillin and tetracycline. If one inserts the nucleic acid from the microbe into the tetracycline resistance gene, tetracycline resistance is lost. Accordingly, once this plasmid is transferred to a host bacterium, successful insertions will be observed by resistance only to ampicillin. After the foreign DNA is inserted into the cloning vector, the plasmid is reassociated with a DNA ligase. The cloning vector containing the foreign DNA from the target microbe must then be inserted into a receptive host for multiplication.

Amplification of the Vector

Escherichia coli and particularly *E. coli* K12, is the host most commonly used to amplify the vector. This bacterium is susceptible to all commonly used antibiotics, accepts the vector efficiently and replicates it at least once every time it multiplies. In practice, the host sees two vectors. The first is the plasmid that has accepted foreign DNA (it is a chimera) and the second is a reannealed vector that did not accept a nucleic acid fragment. These vectors are mixed in liquid growth medium with the host with three possible outcomes. First, an *E. coli* may accept no vector at all. Second, *E. coli* can accept a reannealed vector that does not contain the foreign DNA fragment. Third, *E. coli* may accept the chimera. After 24-72 hours, the mixture is spread over the surface of agar media designed to select the host containing the chimera. Colonies of the transformed bacteria are selected and grown in large numbers. The cells are harvested and copies of the original target nucleic acid excised, again using specific restriction endonucleases.[8,12]

Table 41:3. Commonly Utilized Cloning Vectors

Vector Name	Selection Marker	Source	Use
pBR322	Ampicillin tetracycline resistance	Laboratory construct of three naturally found plasmids	Expression in *E. coli* used for constructing new cloning vectors: e.g., pSP64 and pUC
pSP64	Ampicillin resistance	Laboratory construct	For producing RNA hybridization probes in vitro
M13 series	Beta-galactosidase	Natural	DNA sequencing and DNA hybridization probes
pUC series	Ampicillin resistance and beta-galactosidase	Laboratory construct	DNA sequencing and expression in *E. coli*

Generally, subcultures of the clones are frozen to establish a permanent library.

The cloned microbial nucleic acid can now be labelled by a nick translation process.[23,32] Single-stranded nicks are made in the double-stranded DNA, utilizing the specific enzyme DNAse I. Because DNA is repaired in vivo by means of a DNA polymerase, this same enzyme (DNA polymerase I) is used in vitro in the presence of ^{32}P-labelled deoxyribonucleotide triphosphates. The repaired DNA, with incorporated radioactive phosphorus, may have counts in the range of 10^8/min/microgram of DNA. Single-stranded DNA probes capable of detecting 0.1 picogram of target DNA can be obtained.

Its inherent hazard to human health limits use of radioactivity in the clinical laboratory. Accordingly, intensive research has been conducted and is ongoing to generate nonradiolabelled probes. The first system that enjoyed widespread usage was biotin-labelled analogs of uridine and deoxyuridine triphosphate. Biotin is a highly reactive molecule that may react with a number of chemical groupings. For nucleic acid attachment, biotin is covalently linked to the C5 position of the pyrimidine ring through an allylamine linker arm.[19] The attachment of biotin does not affect the association properties of nucleic acid molecules and permits the generation of a readable signal. The signal is generated because the biotinyl moiety of the molecule reacts strongly with the egg white protein avidin. The interaction between avidin and biotin is of the order of $Kd = 10^{-15}$. Avidin has four binding sites for biotin.[19] One or more can be labelled with an enzyme, such as alkaline phosphatase (E.R. Unger, personal communication) or horseradish peroxidase.[17]

In practice, the nucleic acid probe to which biotin is attached is allowed to react with the target nucleic acid under particular stringency conditions. If sufficient homology exists, the probe will associate with the target nucleic acid. Avidin, to which an enzyme has been attached, is added. The avidin will bind to the biotin and coat the hybridized nucleic acids. An enzyme substrate is added, with the subsequent generation of color at the site of nucleic acid hybridization. Recently, the sensitivity of the biotin-avidin system has been increased by the utilization of polymerized alkaline phosphatase.[20] Because avidin binds with such high affinity, it has a propensity to stick nonspecifically to other substances. Strepavidin, which has a lower affinity, has been used to reduce false-positivity.

The attachment of a hapten directly to the probe is an alternative nonradiometric procedure for labelling nucleic acid. High-titered antibody to the hapten is subsequently used to detect the reaction of the probe with its target nucleic acid. [22] It was found that guanine residues in nucleic acids could be labelled with N-acetoxy-N-2-acetylaminofluorene (AAF) and its 7-iodo (AAIF) derivatives. The nucleic acid probe labelled with hapten and reacted with the target nucleic acid could be detected by specific antibody in a manner analogous to fluorescent antibody tests.

Other methods to label nucleic acids include the insertion of nucleic acid analogues directly into the nucleic acid,[19,40] and the employment of glycosylated T4 bacteriophage DNA whose carbohydrate-modified nucleotides act as natural signals.[7] A comparison of the generation of radiometric and nonradiometrically labelled probes is seen in Table 41:4.

RNA may be utilized as a probe in addition to DNA. DNA:RNA hybrids are more temperature stable than DNA:DNA hybrids and therefore, RNA hybridization probes can be utilized under higher stringency conditions than those using DNA. There is evidence to suggest that these RNA probes may be able to detect smaller numbers of pathogens than DNA probes.[14,27,43]

The Assay

After the probe homologous to the nucleic acid of the target microbe has been grown in large numbers and labelled, the assay itself is performed. Currently, it is not possible to conduct the assay directly on the specimen in a liquid medium as immunoassays are performed. Obviously, this is a goal of nucleic acid hybridization research. Current tests utilize solid support methods. In comparison to immunochemical techniques these may be considered heterogeneous methodologies because several washing steps are required to remove bound from unbound reactants. Homogeneous techniques, in which the bound does not have to be removed from the unbound, have not yet been developed for nucleic acid hybridization.

Five basic assay designs have been employed to diagnose infectious diseases directly from clinical specimens. The most extensively used is the dot, or dot-blot, hybridization technique. This method is based on adsorption of target nucleic acid onto a clear filter film, most commonly a nitrocellulose membrane. A patient specimen containing the infecting microbe is disrupted to release its nucleic acid, is adsorbed to the nitrocellulose with a combination of physical (heating) and chemical (salts, detergents) means. The film is then washed to remove extraneous material and the labelled nucleic acid hybridization probe is added under a particular set of stringency conditions.

Table 41:4. Labeling the Nucleic Acid Probe

Step	Radiometric	Non-Radioactive (Biotin)
Choice of signal	^{32}P	Biotin:Avidin:Enzyme
Insertion of signal	Nick translation	Covalent enzymatic linking of biotin to pyrimidine ring
Reading of signal	Direct	Indirect
Developer	None	Avidin to which an enzyme is attached
Measurement	Radioactive counts (generally film exposure)	Detection of enzyme activity by addition of substrate
Stability	^{32}P half-life 14.3 days	−20°C for two years
Precautions	Radioactivity	None

If there is complementary nucleic acid in the patient's sample, the labelled nucleic hybridization probe will bind to it. If there is no homologous nucleic acid on the nitrocellulose paper, the hybridization probe will not bind and will be washed away. A substrate for the label on the probe is added and the released chromogen measured. If the nucleic acid hybridization probe was labelled with ^{32}P, the measurement requires autoradiography. If the label is nonradiometric and is an enzyme, the measurement may be either by densitometry or by direct visualization (E.R. Unger, personal communication).

In the past several years there has been increased utilization of the dot hybridization technique in clinical testing. This assay technique can detect as little as 1-2 picograms of target sequence.[6,20,21] The clinical utility of dot hybridization analysis has been demonstrated for a wide range of microbial pathogens, including many viral and bacterial agents. Both stringency conditions and the factors involved in the adsorption of nucleic acids have been intensively investigated. For example, it was found that NaI was more efficient in binding nucleic acid, especially mRNA, to nitrocellulose than was NaCl. Adding or subtracting detergents such as Brij-35 and DOC allowed one to affix selectively either DNA or mRNA to nitrocellulose.[5,13] Furthermore, there has been a concerted effort to automate membrane dot hybridization. One of the major limiting factors in the use of dot hybridization is the large amount of labor and time required for processing of specimens. Dot hybridization also requires significant time for either colorimetric or radiometric development.

The second assay technique used in nucleic acid hybridization is the sandwich hybridization procedure. This design utilizes two noncomplementary nucleic acid sequence reagents. These reagents are produced from adjacent sites on the microbial pathogen's genome. The first nucleic acid sequence is immobilized onto the solid nitrocellulose support and serves as the target sequence to interact with nucleic acid from the microbial pathogen. The second sequence is labelled and serves as the nucleic acid detector probe. Nucleic acid is first extracted from the clinical sample, then mixed with the probe and hybridized against the target sequence on the nitrocellulose paper. If the microbial pathogen nucleic acid is complementary to both the probe reagent and the filter-bound nucleic acid, a sandwich will be formed and the complex detected by the addition of a developer to the probe label.[31] This method has a published sensitivity in the range of that of radioimmunoassay with a time of detection of approximately 20 hours.[40]

The third method for analyzing specific DNA fragments is the classic Southern Technique,[34] published in 1975. This method has become the standard for establishing the identity of nucleic acid fragments. Nucleic acid is first cut with specific restriction endonuclease(s); the pieces are separated by agarose gel electrophoresis and then transferred to nitrocellulose paper either by blotting or electroelution. Nucleic acid hybridization probes are added to the nitrocellulose paper to establish identity.

The Southern Technique is not currently amenable to routine clinical laboratory testing since it requires relatively large amounts of DNA and restriction endonucleases and is labor-intensive and time-consuming. Modifications of the Southern Technique have been developed to analyze RNA (Northern Technique) and proteins (Western Technique).

A procedure that has been particularly useful in the study of viruses is in situ hybridization. In this procedure, human tissue is treated with a combination of detergents, mild acid and proteases on a nitrocellulose support to both fix the cell and to allow microbial nucleic acid inside the human cell to react with a hybridization probe. This procedure is used to establish the presence of microbial nucleic acid within cells. A probe is added to the cell layer and the signal is detected as described for dot hybridization. Many viruses, including parvovirus, polyomavirus, herpes simplex virus, adenovirus and retroviruses have been studied in this way.[6] This method is especially useful with agents which are difficult to grow. The use of in situ hybridization is limited by the fact that it detects genetic material but generates no information concerning the activity of the particular infectious agent. For example, the detection of Epstein-Barr virus in a cell does not differentiate between latent inactivity and active infection.

Another strategy, which uses an adsorption column to separate bound from unbound nucleic acid, was devised by Kohne and colleagues (Kohne, personal communication). This method utilizes ^{125}I-labelled DNA as the probe and the target is rRNA. The main ingredients in the procedure include the labelled DNA probe, a hydroxyapatite-containing separation solution and phosphate-buffered saline washing reagents. The patient's specimen is mixed with the probe solution and heated for 2 h in a waterbath at 72°C. To this mixture is added the hydroxyapatite solution and after incubation for 5 min, the tube is centrifuged at approximately 1000 X g to sediment the hydroxyapatite. The sediment is washed again and the pellet is counted in a gamma counter. DNA:rRNA will adsorb to hydroxyapatite whereas the single-stranded DNA probe will not. The presence of the target microbe is determined by subtracting background counts from bound counts, with 10% or more hybridization considered a positive result. As of September, 1986, this system has been approved for the direct detection of *Legionella pneumophila* and *Mycoplasma pneumoniae* in human specimens. Limitations of the method include the requirement to analyze gamma-emitting radioactivity and the high costs of the individual tests. Research is underway to develop a nonradiometric label.

CLINICAL UTILITY OF NUCLEIC ACID HYBRIDIZATION PROBES

The routine diagnosis of infectious diseases by nucleic acid hybridization probes should be considered to be in an advanced developmental state. Unlike clinical laboratory serology, which has been routinely performed since the 1920s, the field of clinical laboratory nucleic acid hybridization analysis began with the 1975 description of restriction endonucleases and Southern's technique to establish genetic identity. It is only in the 1980s that basic research data and techniques have been translated into diagnostic methods for detection of infectious agents. This technology is in an early phase of growth, generating new discoveries and techniques, so than any given procedure or method of detection is likely to be superceded.

It is now possible, under conditions not far removed from the routine clinical laboratory, to diagnose many of the pathogens causing human and animal diseases. All major groups of microbes have been examined and successfully analyzed in the research laboratory. Description of the analyses may be found in the published literature.[1,2,3,4,10,11,16,18,24,28,29,30,35,36,37,38,39,40,41,42]

Many active areas of research are directed at the problems now limiting the use of nucleic acid hybridization in routine diagnostic testing. At least five problems need to be solved. First, radioactivity must be replaced with a colorimetric system having rapid color development. Second, nucleic acid hybridization probes must have a sensitivity of approximately 10^3 bacteria/mL. Currently, the average limit of detection is approximately 10 to 100 times this amount. Third, the probe, albeit DNA or RNA, must be broad enough to detect all members of a given species. For example, the hybridization mixture used by Chou and Merrigan[9] to detect cytomegalovirus in human urine contained probes against seven different strains of this virus. Fourth, probes must be developed to detect resistance to antibiotics at the same time as the identity of the pathogen is determined. Because a single probe can detect only one parameter, instruments must be developed to automate the large number of procedures to be performed on each clinical specimen. If, for example, one wishes to examine cerebrospinal fluid, one would have to test simultaneously not only for a large number of bacteria, viruses and yeasts, but also for a variety of antibiotic resistance factors. This large battery of tests virtually precludes manual performance. Fifth and finally, homogeneous assays must be developed to replace currently employed heterogeneous technologies.

REFERENCES

1. Ambinder RF, Charache P, Staal S, et al. The vector homology problem in diagnostic nucleic acid hybridization of clinical specimens. J Clin Microbiol 1986;24:16-20.
2. Berninger M, Hammer M, Hoyer B, Gerin JL. An assay for the detection of the DNA genome of hepatitis B virus in serum. J Med Virol 1982;9:57-68.
3. Brandsma J, Miller G. Nucleic acid spot hybridization: rapid quantitative screening of lymphoid cell lines for Epstein-Barr viral DNA. Proc Natl Acad Sci 1980;77:6851-5.
4. Brechot C, Hadchouel M, Scotto J, et al. Detection of hepatitis B virus DNA in liver and serum; a direct appraisal of the chronic carrier state. Lancet 1981;2:765-8.
5. Bresser J, Doering J, Gillespie D. Laboratory methods: quick-blot: selective mRNA or DNA immobilization from whole cells. DNA 1983;2:243-54.

6. Brigati DJ, Myerson D. Leary JJ, et al. Detection of viral genomes in cultured cells and paraffin-embedded tissue sections using biotin-labeled hybridization probes. Virology 1983;126:32-50.
7. Casna NJ, Shub DA. Bacteriophage T4 as a generalized DNA-cloning vehicle. Gene 1982;18:297-307.
8. Cedarbaum SD. Introduction to recombinant DNA. Pediatrics 1984;74:408-11.
9. Chou S, Merrigan TC. Rapid detection and quantitation of human cytomegalovirus in urine through DNA hybridization. New Engl J Med 1982;308:921-5.
10. Diegutis PS, Keirnan E, Burnett L, Nightingale BN, Cossart YE. False-positive results with hepatitis B virus DNA dot-hybridization in hepatitis B surface antigen-negative specimens. J Clin Microbiol 1986;23:797-9.
11. Edelstein PH. Evaluation of the Gen-Probe DNA probe for the detection of legionellae in culture. J Clin Microbiol 1986;23:481-4.
12. Engleberg NC, Eisenstein BI. The impact of new cloning technique on the diagnosis and treatment of infectious diseases. New Engl J Med 1984;311:892-901.
13. Gillespie D, Bresser J. mRNA immobilization in NaI: quick-blots. BioTechniques 1983:184-92.
14. Green MR, Maniatis T, Melton DA. Human B-globulin pre-mRNA synthesized in vitro is accurately spliced in *Xenopus* oocyte nuclei. Cell 1983;32:681-94.
15. Grimont PAD, Grimont F, Desplaces N, Tchen P. DNA probe specific for *Legionella pneumophila*. J Clin Microbiol 1986;21:431-7.
16. Hill WE, Madden JM, McCardell BA, et al. Foodborne enterotoxigenic *Escherichia coli*; detection and enumeration by DNA colony hybridization. Appl Environ Microbiol 1983;45:1324-30.
17. Hsu SM, Raine L, Fanger H. Use of avidin-biotin-peroxidase complex (ABC) in immunoperoxide techniques: a comparison between ABC and unlabeled (PAP) procedures. J Histochem Cytochem 1981;29:577-80.
18. Kuritza AP, Getty CE, Shaughnessy P, Hesse R, Salyers AA. DNA probes for identification of clinically important *Bacteroides* species. J Clin Microbiol 1986;23:343-9.
19. Langer PR, Waldrop AA, Ward DC. Enzymatic synthesis of biotin-labelled polynucleotides: novel nucleic acid affinity probes. Proc Nat Acad Sci 1981;78:6633-7.
20. Leary JJ, Brigati DJ, Ward DC. A sensitive colorimetric method for visualizing biotin-labeled probes hybridized to DNA or RNA on nitrocellulose filters. Chromosomes Cancer 1983;15:273-90.
21. Leary JJ, Brigati DJ, Ward DC. Rapid and sensitive colorimetric method for visualizing biotin-labeled DNA probes hybridized to DNA or RNA immobilized on nitrocellulose: bioblots. Proc Natl Acad Sci 1983;80:4045-9.
22. Lefevre JF, Fuchs RPP, Daune MP. Comparative studies on the 7-iodo and 7-fluoro derivatives of N-acetoxy-N-2-acetylamino-fluorene: binding sites on DNA and conformational change of modified deoxytrinucleotides. Biochemistry 1978;17:2561-7.
23. Maniatis T, Jeffrey A, Klieg DG. Nucleotide sequence of the rightward operator of phage. Proc Natl Acad Sci 1975;72:1184-8.
24. Marlowe S, Watkins P, Kowalsky P, Hirsch M, Crumpaker C. Rapid detection of CMV infection and replication by DNA-DNA hybridization [Abstract]. Las Vegas: Interscience Conference on Antimicrobial Agents and Chemotherapy, 1983.
25. Marmur J, Doty P. Determination of the base composition of DNA from its thermal denaturation temperature. J Mol Biol 1962;5:109-18.
26. McConoughy JL, Laird CD, McCarthy MJ. Nucleic acid reassociation in formamide. Biochemistry 1969;3289-95.
27. Melton DA, Krieg P, Green MR. Increased sensitivity in Northern and Southern blotting methods using RNA probes synthesized in vitro with SP6 RNA polymerase. Cell 1987; (in press).
28. Moseley SL, Huq I, Alim A, So M, Samadpour-Montelebi M, Falkow S. Detection of enterotoxigenic *Escherichia coli* by DNA colony hybridization. J Infect Dis 1982;142:892-9.

29. Moseley SL, Echeverria P, Seriwatana J, et al. Identification of enterotoxigenic *Escherichia coli* by colony hybridization using three enterotoxin gene probes. J Infect Dis 1982;145:8,63-9.
30. Nishibuchi M, Hill WE, Zon G, Payne WL, Kaper JB. Synthetic oligodeoxyribonucleic probes to detect Kanagawa phenomenon-positive *Vibrio parahaemolyticus*. J Clin Microbiol 1986;23:1091-5.
31. Ranki M, Palva A, Virtanen M, Laaksonen M, Soderlund H. Sandwich hybridization as a convenient method for the detection of nucleic acids in crude samples. Gene 1983;21:76-7.
32. Rigby PW, Dieckman PW, Rhodes C, Berg P. Labelling deoxyribonucleic acids to high specific activity *in vitro* by nick translation with DNA polymerase. J Mol Biol 1977;113:237-51.
33. Schildkraut CL, Lifson S. Dependence of the melting temperature of DNA on salt concentration. Biopolymers 1965;3:195-208.
34. Southern EM. Detection of specific sequences among DNA fragments separated by gel electrophoresis. J Mol Biol 1975;98:503-17.
35. Spector SA, Rus JA, Spector DH, McMillan R. Detection of human cytomegalovirus in clinical specimens by DNA-DNA hybridization. J Infect Dis 1984;150:121-6.
36. Stanhandske P, Hyypia T, Gadler H, Halonene P, Pettersson U. The use of molecular hybridization for demonstration of adenoviruses in human stools. Curr Topics Microbiol Immunol 1983;104:299-306.
37. Stanhandske P, Pettersson U. Identification of DNA viruses by membrane filter hybridization. J Clin Microbiol 1982;15:744-7.
38. Torres AR, Li MK, Ward DC, Edberg SC. Differentiation of *Neisseria gonorrhoeae* from other *Neisseria* species by use of the restriction endonuclease HaeIII. J Clin Microbiol 1985;20:687-90.
39. Totten PA, Holmes KK, Handsfield HH, Knapp JS, Perine PL, Falkow S. DNA hybridization technique for the detection of *Neisseria gonorrhoeae* in men with urethritis. J Infect Dis 1973;148:462-71.
40. Virtanen M, Laaksonen M, Sonderlund H, Palva A, Halonen P, Ranki M. Novel test for rapid viral diagnosis in nasopharyngeal mucus aspirates by means of nucleic-acid sandwich hybridization. Lancet 1983;1:381-3.
41. Wilkinson HW, Sampson JS, Plikaytis BB. Evaluation of a commercial gene probe for identification of *Legionella* cultures. J Clin Microbiol 1986;23:217-20.
42. Wood PK, Morris JG, Small PLC, et al. Comparison of DNA probes and the Sereny test for identification of invasive *Shigella* and *Escherichia coli* strains. J Clin Microbiol 1986;24:,498-500.
43. Zinn K, DeMaio D, Maniatis T. Identification of two distinct regulatory regions adjacent to the human B-interferon gene. Cell 1983;34:865-79.

Section 5: Laboratory Practice

CHAPTER 42

LABORATORY SAFETY

William M. Wagner, Sc.D.

INTRODUCTION

The laboratory can be a hazardous workplace because of the nature of the work and the materials used unless precautions are taken to minimize the risk of inadvertent laboratory exposure or injury. To provide a safe work area, certain objectives must be addressed by management, supervisors and laboratorians. They must recognize that a mishap will happen in the laboratory and take steps to minimize the incidence of personal injury and property damage.[5]

First, employees must understand the hazards and characteristics of the particular materials used in the laboratory and what the absolute and relative hazards are. The absolute hazard deals with a physical or biological fact, whereas the relative hazard deals with the importance of the absolute hazard in relationship to the overall setting.[14] For example, a small amount of alcohol will burn, causing a relatively small fire if controlled, but that amount of alcohol burning in the midst of a cluttered laboratory bench could result in a major blaze. Laboratorians must make knowledgeable risk assessments by considering the characteristics of the material, the condition of the environment and the training of the workers, as well as by using common sense. Most hazards in the laboratory can be reduced to a low level by the use of proper procedures, containment devices and protective equipment. Reductions can be accomplished by "engineering-out" elements that present unnecessary risk and "engineering-in" elements that provide protection against risk.

LABORATORY SAFETY PROGRAM

The responsibilities of management, of the safety officer or safety professional, of the safety committee, of supervisors and of employees are combined to form a working laboratory safety program. Specific safety guidelines describing the manner in which hazardous material should be handled, the type of protective clothing or eyewear that must be worn and when to wear it, and the procedures to follow in case of an inadvertent exposure or injury must be put in writing, either in a safety manual or as part of the procedures manual.

Management Responsibility

Management must establish a safety policy and then enforce it, must provide a safe working environment, and must review inspection and incident reports and reports from the safety officer. The cost of providing safety equipment and personnel resources for a safety program is an extremely good investment. The cost of preventing or limiting injury is far less than the costs incurred from an incident.

Safety Officer Responsibility

It is the safety officer's responsibility to implement safety policy. The safety officer should be knowledgeable about laboratory hazards and ways of alleviating them, familiar with safety equipment and generally well informed about safety matters.[13] Safety inspections of the laboratory should be conducted regularly by the safety officer, preferably at least every three months and not less than once a year. A checklist should be used and every part of the laboratory should be inspected. The safety officer should maintain all records related to safety.

Safety Committee Responsibility

The role of the safety committee is one of advising management in safety-related matters. This committee should have 5-10 members, chosen to represent the various work levels or sections of the laboratory. The creation of a safety subcommittee in larger laboratories, with a representative of the subcommittee being part of an overall safety committee, provides for input and exchange from all levels. The term of service should be specified (usually 2-3 years) and membership should be rotated so that there are always some experienced members on the committee. Recommendations should be forwarded to management for implementation. Meetings should be held regularly and minutes should be recorded. Circulation of minutes to the whole staff will increase awareness and produce good feedback.

Supervisor Responsibility

Supervisors are key persons in the safety program just as they are in the overall operation of the laboratory. They should be responsible for most of the training of new employees in the area of safety and should maintain continual surveillance of safety in the laboratory's daily operation. When violations are observed, supervisors should take steps immediately to correct them. Supervisors should constantly seek ways to identify and reduce hazards.

Employee Responsibility

All employees are responsible for following the specified safety procedures, using safety equipment and reporting incidents. Employees should also be constantly on the alert for hazards in the environment and should report such to a supervisor, suggesting ways to reduce or remove the hazard.

SAFETY HAZARDS

Laboratory hazards can be grouped into four general classes: biological, chemical, radiological and physical or mechanical. Biological hazards include infection or intoxication caused by biological materials. Chemical hazards include contact with toxic, carcinogenic, corrosive and flammable substances. Some chemicals may combine a number of these hazards. A few chemicals, such as perchlorates, peroxides or dry picric acid, are unstable or may form unstable compounds that can explode. Radiological hazards are minimal in the clinical laboratory but include human ingestion. Physical or mechanical hazards include electrocution, falls and slips, needle punctures, cuts from broken glass, burns, eye damage from ultraviolet light and injuries from fire.

Biological Hazards

Recently, the Centers for Disease Control (CDC) and the National Institutes of Health (NIH) jointly developed recommended practices for handling infectious agents based on the hazard of the agent and the laboratory operation performed. These recommendations were published in a monograph entitled "Biosafety in Microbiological and Biomedical Laboratories."[3] This publication gives specific descriptions of microbiological practices, laboratory facilities and safety equipment for use in laboratory operations. The four biosafety levels described in this monograph consist of combinations of laboratory practices, techniques, safety equipment and appropriate facilities. The recommended safety practices and equipment that correspond to the biosafety levels are summarized in Table 42:1.

A combination of practices, facilities and safety equipment described as Biosafety Level 2 can be safely used in the initial processing of clinical

Table 42:1. Summary of Recommended Biosafety Levels for Infectious Agents.*

Biosafety Level	Practices and Techniques	Safety Equipment	Facilities
1	Standard microbiological practices.	None; primary containment provided by adherence to standard laboratory practices during open bench operations.	Basic
2	Level 1 practices plus laboratory coats; decontamination of all infectious wastes; limited access; protective gloves; biohazard warning signs as indicated.	Partial containment equipment (i.e., Class I or II biological safety cabinets) used to conduct mechanical and manipulative procedures that have high aerosol potential, which may increase the risk of exposure to personnel.	Basic
3	Level 2 practices plus special laboratory clothing; controlled access.	Partial containment equipment used for all manipulations of infectious material.	Containment
4	Level 3 practices plus entrance through change room where street clothing removed and laboratory clothing donned; shower on exit; all wastes decontaminated on exit from facility.	Maximum containment equipment (i.e., Class III biological safety cabinet or partial containment equipment in combination with full-body, air-supplied, positive-pressured personnel suit) used for all procedures and activities.	Maximum Containment

* Adapted from reference 3.

specimens and in identifying most isolates. Mycobacterial cultures should be processed at Biosafety Level 3. If the initial processing of an unknown clinical specimen could produce an infectious aerosol, a biological safety cabinet (BSC) should be used. Segregating clinical laboratory functions and limiting or restricting access to hazardous areas are the responsibility of the laboratory director.

Research has shown that most laboratory-associated infections are acquired through infectious aerosols.[12] The incorrect use of laboratory equipment such as pipettes, inoculating loops, needles and syringes can produce droplet aerosols of various sizes. Droplets that have a diameter greater than 5 μm will settle quickly and contaminate only the immediate laboratory area, but droplets that have a smaller diameter can remain suspended and viable for several hours. Centrifuges and blenders can produce large quantities of infectious aerosols. Use blenders designed for the laboratory, which allow removal of the mixture through the opening at the bottom of the chamber rather than at the top. Centrifuge infectious material in safety cups and open the cups in the BSC.

Procedures with a high potential for creating aerosols should be conducted in a BSC, either the Class I negative-pressure cabinet or the Class II vertical, laminar-flow cabinet (Fig. 42:1). The Class I BSC draws air through the frontal opening and exhausts through high-efficiency, particulate air (HEPA) filters designed to remove 99.97% of the particles 0.3 μm in size. A Class I BSC provides protection for the operator but does not protect the work from room contamination, a major drawback. An optimum average, inward face velocity through the work opening should be 75 linear feet per minute (lf/min) to provide adequate personnel protection.

The Class II BSC blows HEPA-filtered air over the work area, providing protection for the product, while the air coming through the frontal opening makes an air barrier that prevents the migration of contaminants in or out of the cabinet. Approximately 70% of the air is recirculated inside the Class II Types A and B3 units after passing through the HEPA filters, whereas 100% is totally exhausted from Type B2 (Fig. 42:1). Since Types A and B3 recirculate a portion of the exhaust air within the cabinet, volatile, toxic chemicals or radionuclides should not be used because of the chance of building up the level of these hazardous materials. A BSC should not be used in place of a chemical fume hood.

The industrial "clean bench," sometimes referred to as a horizontal

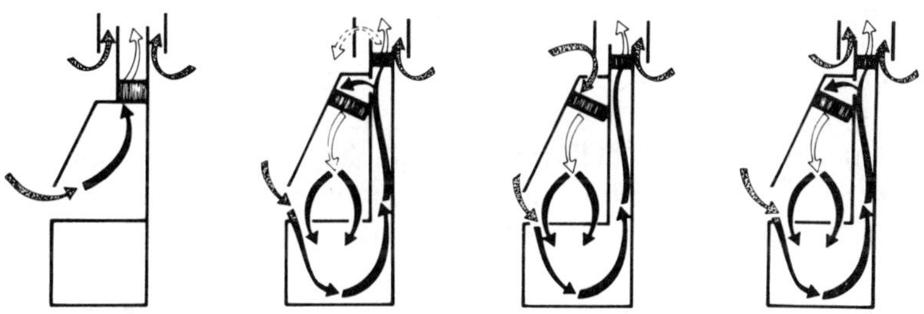

Class	I	II	II	II
Type	–	A	B2	B3
Inflow (lfpm)	75	75	100	100
% Recirculation	0	70	0	70
Downflow (lfpm)	0	75	80	50
Exhaust (cfm/ft)	50	45	65	65
Use: Biohazards	+	+	+	+
Toxic, Volatiles	+	–	+	±
Protection (User/Product)	U	U P	U P	U/P

FIGURE 42:1. Airflow characteristics of various biological safety cabinets (lfpm = linear feet per minute; cfm/ft = cubic feet per minute per width of cabinet opening in feet). Adapted from Kent PT and Kubica GP, "Public Health Mycobacteriology: A Guide for the Level III Laboratory," CDC, Public Health Service, U.S. Department of Health and Human Services, 1985. (CDC 85-3439).

laminar-flow cabinet, has no place in the laboratory and should not be used even for the preparation of sterile media or pharmaceuticals. The airflow in this device blows across the work area into the worker's face, subjecting the worker to fumes and vapors of materials used in media preparation, many of which are sensitizing agents. "Clean benches" are often mistaken for chemical fume hoods or BSCs and therefore used for the manipulation of hazardous materials; when used for this purpose, the "clean bench" creates a far greater danger than the open bench. Laboratorians must understand the design principles of protective equipment so they can use it correctly.

Decontamination of biohazardous material, contaminated work surfaces, instruments or equipment is accomplished by physical or chemical means, including heat, liquid, vapor and gas disinfectants. See Chapter 44, "Sterilization and Disinfection," for these procedures.

Chemical Hazards

Safe handling of chemicals begins with understanding and recognizing the hazards associated with the materials commonly found in the laboratory.[8] Most microbiology laboratories have as much flammable chemical material as the typical chemistry laboratory. Chemicals in the laboratory are of three general types: flammable or combustible chemicals; chemicals that produce acute effects on a worker (e.g., severe burns), lethal effects, or severe internal damage after inhalation, ingestion or absorption; and chemicals that cause damaging effects after long-term, chronic, low-level exposure.

A basic principle to follow in the laboratory is to keep the quantity of flammable chemicals at the lowest volume consistent with efficient operation. The National Fire Protection Association prescribes maximum quantities of flammable substances allowed outside of a flammable-substances storage cabinet in the laboratories of health care facilities.[7] It is acceptable to use a flammable-liquid storage cabinet in the laboratory to store excess stocks of chemicals up to 60 gallons. However, this should not be construed to mean that a flammable-liquid storage cabinet should routinely be used for storing such large volumes. All bulk flammable chemicals should be stored in a flammable-substances storage room constructed to meet the specifications of the Occupational Safety and Health Administration (OSHA) general industry standards.[11]

Understanding the design principles of the flammable-substances storage cabinet is important in using it correctly. The purpose of such a cabinet, as defined in the National Fire Codes, is to keep the temperature of its contents below 325°F for at least 10 minutes during a fire. This amount of time will allow the occupants of the laboratory to either put out the fire or get out of the laboratory. Once the temperature rises above 325°F, some chemicals may ignite. Most flammable-material storage cabinets come with ports for venting the cabinet to the outside. The cabinet should not be vented directly into the laboratory because the hot gases and vapors from a laboratory fire will enter the cabinet and cause autoignition of some of the flammable contents. A flammable-substances storage cabinet for liquids need not be vented at all unless ventilation is required by local fire codes or if a certain quantity of a flammable carcinogen is stored. If ventilation is required, the cabinet must be vented to the outside through galvanized steel piping. Plastic or polyvinyl piping should not be used because it will burn at a temperature of about 200°F.

Careful attention should be given to the storage of all chemicals.[9] Certain chemicals are considered incompatible because of the possible violent reaction resulting from their being spilled or otherwise inadvertently mixed. Chemicals such as perchloric acid, nitric acid and ether should be stored in separate areas to prevent the creation of explosive or highly flammable mixtures. Never store ether in a refrigerator or freezer, even if the unit is of an explosive-proof design. Avoid concentrating ether vapors. Opened cans of ether should be stored only on the open shelf, away from fire or flame. Ether should be discarded after being open for 30 days. In addition, the special precautions listed by OSHA[11] must be taken in handling, storing and disposing of chemical carcinogens.

Strong acids and alkalis should be transported only in a container that shields the bottles to prevent breakage and is large enough to retain the contents of the bottles if they should break. Large containers of such chemicals (5 pounds or more) should be stored in the laboratory only in base cabinets. Never store hazardous chemicals on shelves above eye level or on the floor in open areas. Strong chemicals should be poured or delivered from a burette over a plastic tray that will retain any spillage.

The chemical fume hood should be used for worker protection, whether for removal of vapors, protection from explosion or prevention of fire. It should not be used for routine storage. The hood should be used properly with the front, protective sash in position and the optimum airflow of 100 lf/min moving inward through the frontal opening. Various types of hoods are available, as shown in Fig. 42:2.

The standard chemical fume hood draws conditioned laboratory air through the hood, up the exhaust duct to the outside. The volume of air leaving the laboratory depends on the position of the sash and can cause air supply problems for the laboratory. Since laboratory air has been conditioned to satisfy the occupants, it is expensive to use it as exhaust air. The supplied air hood is more economical to operate because unconditioned outside air is supplied to the front of the hood. This supplied air, however, usually blows directly on the worker, causing some discomfort. The constant volume hood draws a constant amount of laboratory air, regardless of the position of the sash, and eliminates the need for special adjustment in the air supply to the laboratory. However, this hood also exhausts expensive conditioned laboratory air.

The direction of air flow in a hood or BSC should be checked frequently

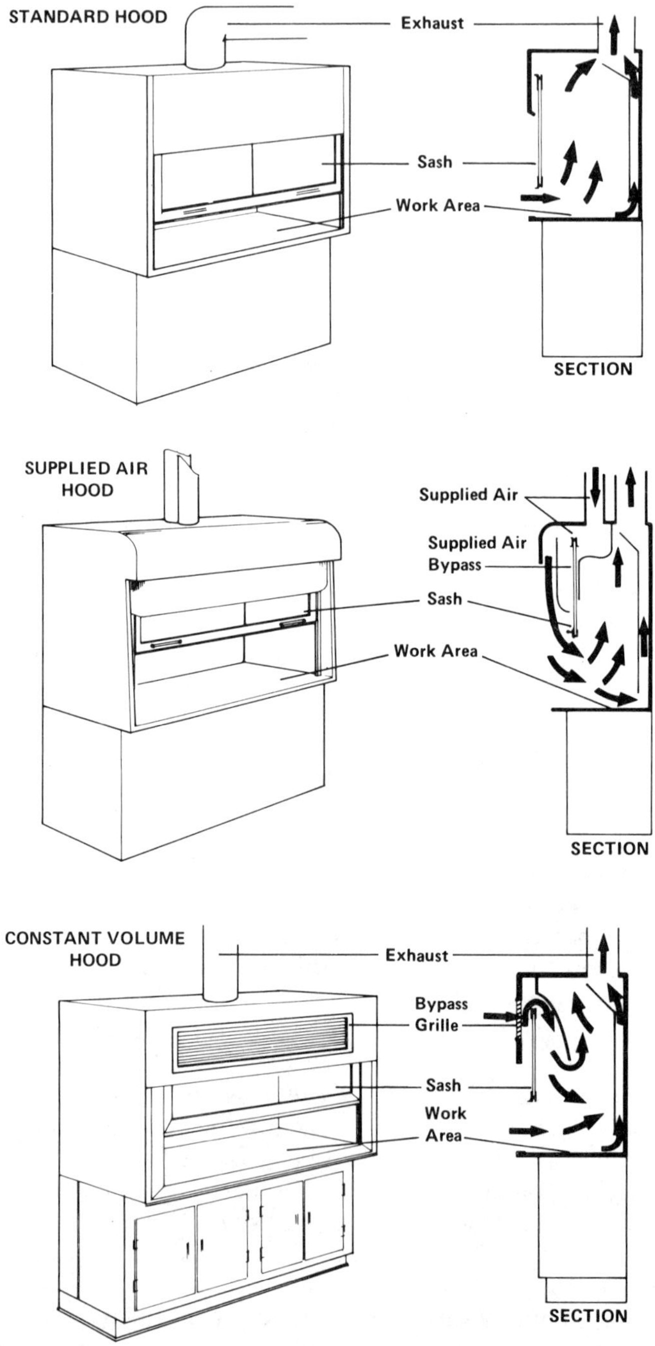

FIGURE 42:2. Chemical fume hoods protect workers from fumes.

to ensure that fumes remain in the hood or cabinet. Restrict the storage of material or equipment in a hood or BSC, because they cause turbulence, resulting in flow back into the room. Known carcinogenic material should be handled in a properly designed chemical fume hood or glove box. Take additional precautions by wearing and using specific safety equipment for carcinogens. Always wear gloves, a laboratory coat and face or eye protection when handling hazardous chemicals.

The disposal of chemicals is a serious problem for the laboratory. Incineration of flammable liquids and combustibles is a practical solution if done in properly designed incinerators. Some chemicals can be neutralized, while others must be disposed of by a professional hazardous waste company. Do not mix waste chemicals; some are incompatible and violent reactions may occur. Disposal must be done in accordance with the Environmental Protection Agency Resource Conservation and Recovery Act regulations.

Pressurized gas storage cylinders present a number of hazards. The properties of the gas will determine how the gas should be stored and what to do in case of an incident. Further, the physical mass of a cylinder can cause extensive personal injury and property damage. If the valve is inadvertently broken, the pressurized cylinder could become a rocket. Cylinders must be properly secured at all times. When a cylinder is not in use, the safety cap should be in place.

Gas cylinders should be clearly labeled with content identification and date of filling. The color of the cylinder does not indicate the contents. Dates stamped on the neck of the cylinder indicate the last hydrostatic test of the cylinder. Cylinders containing flammable gas must be hydrostatically tested every 5 years; other gases, every 10 years. If the cylinder has not been tested in accordance with this criterion, DO NOT USE IT. Call the vendor for a replacement.

Pressure regulators are designed to meet the requirements of specific gases. The threads of a connection nut on an oxygen regulator will only match the threads of an oxygen cylinder. Never force the connection nut onto the valve threads; it may be the wrong regulator. Tighten the nut with your fingers first; then use a special regulator wrench to tighten firmly. Never use oils or any other lubricant on the threads or regulator. Such substances may react with the gas. Test all connections for leaks with a soap and water solution; tighten loose connections and replace broken tubing.

When a pressurized cylinder drops to 25 pounds of gas per square inch, replace it. Label the spent tank "Empty." The small amount of gas pressure remaining will prevent ambient air from entering and damaging the cylinder. Store extra cylinders, full or empty, in a well-ventilated, fire-resistant area away from sources of ignition, outside the laboratory. The bottoms may corrode if cylinders are set directly on concrete; place cylinders on a piece of wood or similar material. Oxidizing and flammable gases (e.g., oxygen and hydrogen) should be stored at least 50 feet apart or separated by a fire-resistant barrier.

Care must be taken in handling the small cylinders of propane used on some equipment. Full cylinders should be stored outside the laboratory, preferably in a flammable-substance storage room. All the gas should be purged from spent cylinders. Dispose of these empty, purged cylinders so they will not be placed in an incinerator or compactor. Some commercial manufacturers will recycle these cylinders.

Radiological Hazards

The hazard from radiation sources in a typical laboratory is relatively low. However, the recent introduction into the clinical environment of radioimmunoassay (RIA) procedures involving the use of radioiodine-125 (^{125}I) requires that radiation safety precautions be considered.[1] The inhalation or ingestion of radioactive material presents a greater hazard than external radiation exposure. Though precautions for external radiation exposure cannot be neglected, the greatest concern should be the control and reduction of internal radiocontamination.

The use of proper laboratory techniques can reduce the potential for contamination, but a surveillance program is also needed. Two monitoring techniques are available: the survey meter and the wipe-sample analysis. The survey meter can use various detection probes for measuring radiation levels and fixed contamination from ^{125}I; however, some radionuclides, such as Carbon-14 or tritium (^{3}H), cannot be detected by the survey meter. The wipe-sample analysis technique is recommended for measuring low-level contamination of radionuclides. The best surveillance program combines both of these techniques. At completion of daily work with radioactive material, a survey of the immediate work area should be conducted. A complete laboratory survey should be done weekly.

The disposal of radioactive waste has become an expensive political and social problem. One vial containing 10 microcuries of radioactive material can produce enough waste to fill a 55-gallon barrel unless waste management methods are used. All materials used under the Nuclear Regulatory Commission's "general license criteria" (which includes Bactec systems) may be disposed of as ordinary waste if all radiation labels are removed. Sink disposal is an acceptable method if allowed by local environmental disposal regulations. Be sure to place all needles, glass pipettes and other sharp objects in a closed, solid container for disposal into waste containers, and disinfect or neutralize all biological or chemical waste to protect the workers who handle waste.

A plan for handling an inadvertent spill or injury involving radioactive material should be prepared. If biohazardous material containing a radionuclide is spilled, the material should be covered with a towel and disinfectant or neutralizing solution should be poured on top. A dike should be formed around the spill to avoid spread of the liquid; then the spill should be decontaminated. If a spill contaminates a person or if personal injury is involved, the person should be protected from further contamination. A safety shower should be used without hesitation if chemical or biological materials are spilled on a person; the person is assumed to be contaminated until a survey shows differently. A safety blanket should be used to cover an injured person being transported to a medical facility. The attending medical personnel should be advised of contamination problems. With proper precautions, most inadvertent spills will not be health-threatening.

Physical or Mechanical Hazards

Many physical laboratory hazards are not unique to the laboratory situation. These include light, heat, noise and electricity. Many of these hazards are taken for granted in the laboratory. For example, an employee working in a hot environment has a higher risk of a mishap than one working in a cooler room. The same is true for employees working in a room with a low light level (less than 80 foot-candles). Ultraviolet light presents a real eye hazard and protective eyewear must be worn. The noise level in a working laboratory should not exceed 75 decibels over an extended period.

All new electrical equipment should be checked for correct grounding before it is used, and electrical wiring should be inspected routinely at least semiannually for short circuits and unsafe materials. Employees should know the location of the electrical panels and should have access to the circuit breakers. The area supported by each breaker should be identified, and equipment, switches and outlets should be labeled with the location of the appropriate circuit breaker.

Mechanical hazards include obstructed aisles and corridors, unsafe chairs and stools that may tip, heavy objects placed on overhead shelves and hazards related to broken glassware. Probably the biggest single hazard in a laboratory is an unintentional skin puncture with a hypodermic needle. Syringes and needles should not be used as pipetting devices. Never attempt to recap a needle. Needles should be discarded into containers that cannot be penetrated by needle points, then autoclaved and discarded with solid waste material. Blunted needles or cannulas should be used when possible.

FIRE PROTECTION

A fire is probably the most disastrous event that can occur in a laboratory. Not only does a fire endanger personnel, disrupt work and cause the direct destruction of property, it also frequently results in extensive smoke and water damage. Personnel should be educated in a continous and ongoing program in the prevention and control of fire. Everyone should be familiar with the location of fire alarms and fire extinguishers. Every person in the laboratory should be trained in the proper use of fire extinguishers, actually discharging one to practice putting out a fire. Fire evacuation routes and procedures should be posted in every laboratory. Unannounced fire drills, involving all personnel, should be scheduled at least quarterly.

At the first indication of a fire, nearby workers should be notified. Then the fire department should be called, regardless of the size of the fire. Do not delegate the task of making the call to someone else, it may not get done. Assess the situation, keeping a clear path between yourself and the exit, and decide whether you can put out the fire with available equipment. If you feel confident in your ability to fight the fire, do so; if not, evacuate. By calling the fire department initially, you give them time to respond while you are making your decision. The proper fire extinguishers for the appropriate burning material are listed in Table 42:2. Each laboratory should be equipped with the proper class extinguisher for the materials used in the laboratory; usually an ABC dry chemical unit with a capacity of 10 pounds[6] is appropriate. For areas with computers or computer-based equipment, the new Halon fire extinguisher should be considered. The Halon system leaves no residue after being discharged as do the dry chemical units. Locate the fire extinguisher near an exit, not in the back area of the laboratory.

Should a person catch fire, have that person stop, drop to the floor and

Table 42:2. Recommended Classes of Extinguishers for Different Types of Fires

Type of Fire	Class of Extinguishers	Comments
Ordinary combustibles (paper, wood, cloth, plastics)	A — pressurized water A,B — multipurpose dry chemical	Soak fire site with water after extinguishing with dry chemical to prevent flashback
Flammable liquids and gases (greases, oils, and other combustible organic materials)	B — dry chemicals or carbon dioxide (CO_2) A,B — multipurpose dry chemical	Never use water! Do not hold nozzle when using CO_2 extinguisher because of possibility of frostbite.
Electrical equipment or outlets	A,B — Halon gas C — dry chemical B,C — multipurpose dry chemical A,B,C — multipurpose dry chemical	Deenergize burning equipment; then use A or B extinguisher
Combustible metal (magnesium, titanium, zirconium, sodium, potassium, etc.)	D — dry powder	Do not use dry chemical or water

roll (STOP-DROP-ROLL). Do not wrap the person in a blanket to smother the fire because many synthetic garments, when smothered, increase in temperature and burn the skin to a greater extent than when burning uncovered. Wrapping the person in a blanket can also result in the "chimney effect," burning the face. Once the fire is out, use the safety blanket to lessen shock or as a modesty blanket to cover the person. The blanket can also be used as a shield to enable one to run through a fire.

ENVIRONMENTAL CONTROLS

Proper ventilation in a laboratory provides more personnel protection than perhaps any other single safety system. Although ventilation will not help contain the fragments from an exploding flask, it will remove hazardous vapors or infectious aerosols. An appropriate fume hood or BSC should be used for primary containment of infectious aerosols, chemical fumes, dust, vapors or other airborne hazards. The laboratory ventilation system is a secondary containment system and should provide 6 to 10 room air changes each hour. Those areas designed for manipulation of more hazardous material (e.g., mycobacterial cultures or carcinogenic chemicals) should have higher ventilation rates. Air from hazardous laboratories like the mycobacteriology suite should be exhausted directly to the outside and not recirculated to other areas. Workers should know whether air is recirculated or not ("single-pass" air). In case of a spill, a recirculation system should be shut down or the exhaust ducts in the room with the spill should be blocked to prevent the spread of contaminated air. Single-pass air should remain on to remove contaminated air.

In controlling airborne hazards, the direction the air moves throughout the laboratory is as important as the amount of air moved. The air pressure of the laboratory should be negative with respect to that of corridors and other public areas; i.e., air should flow from corridors into the laboratory. To check the direction of airflow, place a thin strip (1/2 x 4 inches) of tissue paper in the doorway with the door 1-2 inches ajar. The strip will move in the direction of the airflow. Within the laboratory, the air should flow from the area of least hazard to an area of greater hazard. A small strip of tissue paper attached at the face of a hood or BSC will indicate the direction of airflow and whether the hood is operating properly. Use of a smoke stick will graphically demonstrate airflow patterns. The fact that a fan is operating does not mean the system is providing adequate protection. There have been instances in which fume hood fans or even entire air handling system fans were wired in reverse, thus blowing air out of hoods or out of a laboratory suite. Do not take anything for granted. Check to be sure.

Special exhaust vents may be required to remove organic vapors from the staining areas in a histology or similar laboratory. Since these vapors are usually heavier than air and tend to settle to counter tops and floors, they should be removed at the bench and floor levels to provide adequate personnel protection. A face velocity of 200 lf/min should be required for these units. A canopy hood, which is the type often installed, cannot raise these heavy vapors unless it has a hurricane-like force. In addition, the canopy hood draws the vapors up past the worker's breathing zone, adding to the possibility of inhalation of hazardous materials.

PERSONNEL PROTECTION

Personnel protection begins with understanding the hazards and is followed by training in good laboratory techniques and the correct use of safety equipment. Responsibility for raising the level of awareness lies with the supervisor or laboratory director. Training should be an ongoing commitment.

Protective clothing provides an essential barrier between the person and the work, and must be worn properly. The front-button coat offers minimum protection and provides even less protection when worn unbuttoned. Coats worn in the laboratory should not be worn into public areas nor into areas with patients. Neither the public nor immunologically compromised patients should be exposed to possible contamination from a dirty laboratory coat. Always wear gloves when handling blood specimens and radioactive or carcinogenic material and change gloves frequently because they develop small holes and tears with use. However, frequent handwashing is most important and the best defense against contamination entering the body.[2]

Protective eyewear should be required for procedures that could result in hazardous liquid or debris entering the eye. Supervisors, safety professionals and laboratorians should decide when eye protection is required and enforce this requirement. Automatic analyzers present an extremely hazardous situation, since the chemicals are under pressure in small "spaghetti tubing." If the tubing should pop off, liquid could spray into eyes. Protective eyewear should always be worn when servicing or filling automatic analyzers. Available eye protection equipment varies from eyeglasses to full-face shields, and includes glasses with solid or perforated side shields, goggles and partial face masks. All eye protection equipment should meet the quality standards established by the American National Standards Institute. Discourage the wearing of contact lens (even under goggles or glasses) in the laboratory. Since osmotic pressure holds the contact lens over the eye lens, this pressure will also draw any liquid or vapor under the contact lens, resulting in severe pain and possible eye damage. Some organic solvents make the lens very slick and difficult to remove.

Eyewash fountains and safety showers provide additional personnel protection. Locate shower or eye-and-body-wash combinations near each work area. Laboratory safety showers are designed to deliver approximately 200-400 L of water when activated by a pull chain or ring. Test this unit at least every 6 months to remove sediment or rust. Instruct all laboratorians to use these showers in an emergency, even though the water makes a mess. No one should try to wash off acid spills in sinks if showers are available. Workers should practice discharging a safety shower in a simulated emergency situation.

Eyewash fountains or facilities are of several types. Locate these systems strategically in the laboratory, preferably at a sink, a location all personnel use frequently and "can find with their eyes closed." The eye should be irrigated for at least 30 minutes; thus, the eyewashing squirt bottles frequently found on laboratory walls are not suitable. One highly recommended model on a long rubber hose discharges a soft, foamy spray. This model can be used to wash an arm, a face or even a body in those institutions without safety showers. This eyewash system located at the sink can be used for routine laboratory operations like washing out a container. If no eyewash facility is available, hold the eye open while submerging it in a pan of water. This procedure may be uncomfortable, but it can prevent severe eye damage. After irrigating the eye by any of these procedures, seek prompt medical treatment.

SPILL CLEANUP

Spilling hazardous material is a common incident in the laboratory and if not handled promptly can lead to severe injury or infection. Being prepared can limit the impact of such an incident. Contain spills by working over absorbent paper and carrying specimens or reagents in safety carriers. The action for a spill depends on the quantity and hazard level of the material. Assess the greatest hazard and treat it first, trying not to spread contamination.

If a large quantity of concentrated, hazardous material is spilled, avoid breathing its vapors or aerosol. Cover the spill if it can be done quickly, then leave the room. Warn fellow workers and go directly to a wash or change room if clothing is contaminated. Remove clothing carefully to avoid contaminating other areas of the body or environs and wash all potentially contaminated areas with soap and water. If a biological agent was present, use a germicidal soap. Do not abrade the skin; that opens the skin's protective barrier and allows invasion. Seek medical attention from personnel trained in treating laboratory injuries.

Wear protective clothing when entering the laboratory to clean up a spill. Gloves, laboratory coats, shoe covers and a face mask or respirator should be worn. A "spill kit" with leakproof containers, paper towels, sponges, disinfectant or neutralizing agent, respirator or face mask and rubber gloves should be available. For a biological spill, immediately cover the spill with a towel or laboratory coat, pour on the appropriate disinfectant and allow it to stand for 30 minutes. Neutralize chemical spills with appropriate agents. Commercially available spill kits contain neutralizing, absorbent and indicator materials to show how well the chemicals are neutralized. After the spill is neutralized, the material can be discarded in the proper manner.

Immediately cover radioactive spills with absorbent paper towels or laboratory coats to absorb the liquid; remove the absorbing material and, while wearing gloves, scour the area with dry powder on a moist paper towel. Check for residual contamination by appropriate survey means and repeat the procedure if contamination persists. Stubborn areas may be covered with plastic and allowed to decay to background radiation levels. If radioactive material is combined with a biohazardous material like blood, cover the spill and apply an effective chemical disinfectant. Allow the mixture to stand for 30 minutes, then proceed as for a radioactive spill. Be sure to wear gloves throughout the entire process.

WASTE MANAGEMENT

Laboratory waste must be rendered safe before it leaves the laboratory. It must be the responsibility of the microbiologist, chemist or other knowledgeable generator to prepare the waste for safe transportation to the point of decontamination or disposal.

Laboratories must comply with local, state and federal regulations for proper waste management. Waste should be placed in strong, leak-proof containers or sturdy plastic bags. Sharp objects, especially needles, should be placed in puncture-proof containers; needles should NOT be recapped. Biologically hazardous material can be autoclaved, incinerated, or in some instances, poured down the drain (bloods, urines, other excreta).[4] Materials to be autoclaved should have a high water content; otherwise, a cup of liquid should be added. Autoclave bags should be left open to allow steam to enter. Incinerators are a viable option for disposal of contaminated biological material and some chemical and radioactive substances. Materials to be incinerated should be placed in strong, sealed containers or plastic bags, and the entire container should be burned. Commercial disposal may be the only method for some chemicals or radioactive material, but one should investigate the reputation of a commercial firm before signing a contract with them.[10]

SUMMARY

A laboratory can be made a safe place to work through the efforts of all those involved, management, supervisors and employees. An effective safety program requires a sincere management effort and employee support. Good laboratory practices and the use of common sense, however, are 90% of a good safety program.

Use of trade names is for identification only and does not constitute endorsement by the Public Health Service or by the United States Department of Health and Human Services.

REFERENCES

1. Centers for Disease Control. Radiation safety in the radioimmunoassay laboratory. In: Principles of radioimmunoassay. Atlanta: Centers for Disease Control, 1984:23-34.
2. Centers for Disease Control. Guidelines in handwashing and hospital environmental control. Atlanta: Centers for Disease Control, 1985.
3. Centers for Disease Control-National Institutes of Health. Biosafety in microbiological and biomedical laboratories. Atlanta: Centers for Disease Control, 1984.
4. Environmental Protection Agency. Guide to infectious waste management. Washington, DC: Environmental Protection Agency, 1986.
5. Fuscaldo AJ, Erlick BS, Hindman BA, eds. Laboratory safety: theory and practice. New York: Academic Press, 1980.
6. National Fire Protection Association. Fire Protection Handbook. 14th ed. Quincy, MA: National Fire Protection Association, 1975.
7. National Fire Protection Association. Health care facilities (NFPA Standard 99). Quincy, MA: National Fire Protection Association, 1985.
8. National Institute of Occupational Safety and Health. Pocket guide to chemical hazards. Atlanta: Centers for Disease Control, 1985.
9. National Research Council. Prudent practices for handling hazardous chemicals in laboratories. Washington, DC: National Academic Press, 1981.
10. National Research Council. Prudent practices for the disposal of chemicals from laboratories. Washington, DC: National Academic Press, 1983.
11. Occupational Safety and Health Administration. OSHA general industry standards. Washington, DC: Occupational Safety and Health Administration, 1980.
12. Pike RM. Laboratory associated infections: summary and analysis of 3921 cases. Health Lab Sci 1975;13:105-14.
13. United States Code of Federal Regulations, Title 10, Part 1-179: Part 19: Requirements for providing worker information and inspection; Part 20: Standards for protection against radiation; Part 30: Requirements for licensing radioactive material; Part 31: General licensure requirements.
14. Wagner WM, Landon GG. Laboratory safety. In: Miller JM, Wentworth BB, eds. Methods for quality control in diagnostic microbiology. Washington, DC: American Public Health Association, 1985:323-47.

CHAPTER 43

TRANSPORTATION OF CLINICAL SPECIMENS AND ETIOLOGIC AGENTS

John H. Richardson, D.V.M.

REGULATIONS

Clinical specimens and etiologic agents must be transported in the process of obtaining diagnostic services, confirmatory testing, exchange of research materials, proficiency testing and other activities that are in the national and individual health interests. Inherent in the shipment of these materials is the potential for damage or leakage in transit, resulting in contamination or exposure of personnel and materials. Commonsense packaging procedures, which provide containment of infectious materials that may leak or be damaged in shipment, also provide the best assurance that transported specimens arrive at their destination in a satisfactory and usable condition. Records maintained at the Office of Biosafety, Centers for Disease Control (CDC), indicate that, although transportation personnel have occasionally been exposed to damaged or leaking shipments of etiologic agents, there is no recorded nor anecdotal evidence that infections have occurred as a result of such exposures.

Three federal agencies (Public Health Service, United States Department of Transportation, United States Postal Service) and at least one transportation organization (Air Transport Association) have direct responsibility for regulating or specifying conditions under which etiologic agents, diagnostic specimens and biological products are shipped.

The Public Health Service (PHS) has been involved in establishing requirements for shipping infectious materials for more than two decades. In 1959, the Interstate Quarantine Regulations administered by the Food and Drug Administration (FDA) were amended to provide for containment packaging and other shipping requirements for etiologic agents. The regulations (42 CFR, Section 72.25) specified 31 etiologic agents for which the following requirements were applicable: that airtight and watertight primary and secondary specimen containers be used; that a maximum volume of 500 mL be allowed in each primary container and an aggregate volume of 4 L in a single shipping container; that shipments have "appropriate labeling;" and that the Surgeon General be notified in the event of damage or leakage of specimens in transit. These 31 infectious agents were the agents of anthrax, botulism, brucellosis, cholera, Colorado tick fever, Coxsackie viral disease, diphtheria, arthropodborne encephalitis, glanders, leptospirosis, lymphocytic choriomeningitis, melioidosis, meningococcal meningitis, paratyphoid fever, plague, poliomyelitis, Q fever, rabies, relapsing fever, rickettsialpox, Rift Valley fever, Rocky Mountain spotted fever, schistosomiasis, scrub typhus, smallpox, tetanus, tuberculosis, tularemia, typhoid fever, typhus fever and yellow fever.

In 1971, the FDA's authority for regulating the interstate shipment of etiologic agents was delegated to the CDC and the regulation was amended, effective July 31, 1972, to incorporate packaging, labeling, volume limitations and shipping procedures for etiologic agents, diagnostic specimens and biological products; to expand the list of etiologic agents for which regulations are applicable; to establish additional procedures for reporting damage or leakage of etiologic agents in transit; and to require notification of receipt of certain agents. This regulation was subsequently amended in July, 1980, further expanding the list of etiologic agents and increasing the maximum allowable volume of an agent in a primary container from 500-1,000 mL.

The U.S. Department of Transportation (DOT) concurrently developed companion regulations (49 CFR, Section 173.386-7) governing all modes of shipment of etiologic agents, diagnostic specimens and biological products (i.e., air carriers, motor carriers, rail carriers and water carriers). The DOT regulations differ from those of the PHS in two principal areas:

1. Section 173.387 specifies environmental conditions, test conditions (water spray, free drop amd penetration) and testing procedures applicable to packages containing etiologic agents; and
2. The authority of the DOT expands the application of their regulations to include the transport of etiologic agents by carriers licensed in interstate commerce regardless of whether material is shipped intrastate or interstate.

The U.S. Postal Service also has requirements applicable to mailing "diseased tissues, blood, serum and cultures of pathogenic microorganisms." These requirements, compiled in the "Postal Service Manual" available from the Superintendent of Documents, Government Printing Office, Washington, DC 20402, are, in general, compatible with those of the PHS and the DOT.

The Air Transport Association (ATA), an organization of domestic carriers, publishes and periodically revises Restricted Articles Tariff 6-D

(Airlines Tariff Publishing Co., Dulles International Airport, Post Office Box 17415, Washington, DC 20041), which further specifies conditions for air-shipping etiologic agents, diagnostic specimens and biological products.

The ATA Restricted Articles Tariff incorporates the pertinent requirements of the PHS and DOT regulations. It also requires documentation (shippers' certificates) to further identify air-shipped etiologic agents and allows volumes of agents of less than 50 mL to be transported on passenger-carrying aircraft. Volumes of more than 50 mL are relegated to cargo-only aircraft.

PACKAGING REQUIREMENTS

Diagnostic specimens and biological products are subject to the minimum packaging requirements described in Section 72.2 of the PHS Interstate Quarantine Regulation (Table 43:1) and must "withstand leakage of contents, shocks, pressure changes and other conditions incident to ordinary handling in transportation." Because of the wide spectrum of materials included in the definition of "diagnostic specimen," a precise definition of the variety of packagings that may be needed is impractical. The sender is, however, responsible for assuring that packaging will withstand the rigors of "ordinary handling in transit." One packaging system that has proved satisfactory for shipping diagnostic specimens involves commercially available molded polystyrene containers which are taped or enclosed in cardboard sleeves or containers for shipment. These molded containers are available in various sizes and shapes for single or multiple specimens. Several other commercially available packaging systems are equally effective for shipping diagnostic specimens. Organizations such as the National Committee for Clinical Laboratory Standards have also developed standards that include shipping procedures for diagnostic specimens and other clinical materials.

Diagnostic specimens and biological products are not subject to volume limitations of the primary specimen containers or to limitations of the aggregate volume of single shipping containers, regardless of the mode of shipment. Special markings and improved hazard warnings or other labels are not required. "ETIOLOGIC AGENT/BIOMEDICAL MATERIALS" labels should not be affixed to shipments of diagnostic specimens or biological products. If dry ice is used as a refrigerant for air shipments, the applicable labeling requirements of the ATA Restricted Articles Tariff 6-D apply. Shippers should contact commercial air carriers for current requirements.

ETIOLOGIC AGENTS

Materials known or presumed to contain an etiologic agent or its toxin, which causes or may cause human disease, are subject to additional

Table 43.1.

DEPARTMENT OF HEALTH, EDUCATION, AND WELFARE
PUBLIC HEALTH SERVICE
CENTERS FOR DISEASE CONTROL
ATLANTA, GEORGIA 30333
Telephone: (404) 329-3883 (Commercial)
236-3883 (FTS)

42 CFR Part 72—Interstate Shipment of Etiologic Agents[1]

Sec.
72.1 Definitions.
72.2 Transportation of diagnostic specimens, biological products, and other materials; minimum packaging requirements.
72.3 Transportation of materials containing certain etiologic agents; minimum packaging requirements.
72.4 Notice of delivery; failure to receive.
72.5 Requirements; variations.

Authority; Sec. 215, 58 Stat. 690, as amended, 42 U.S.C. 216; sec. 361, 58 Stat. 703, (42 U.S.C. 264)

§72.1 *Definitions.*

As used in this part:

"Biological product" means a biological product prepared and manufactured in accordance with the provisions of 9 CFR Parts 102–104 and 21 CFR Parts 312 and 600–680 and which, in accordance with such provisions, may be shipped in interstate traffic.

"Diagnostic specimen" means any human or animal material including, but not limited to, excreta, secreta, blood and its components, tissue, and tissue fluids being shipped for purposes of diagnosis.

"Etiologic agent" means a viable microorganism or its toxin which causes, or may cause, human disease.

"Interstate traffic" means the movement of any conveyance or the transportation of persons or property, including any portion of such movement or transportation which is entirely within a State or possession, (a) from a point of origin in any State or possession to a point of destination in any other State or possession, or (b) between a point of origin and a point of destination in the same State or possession but through any other State, possession, or contiguous foreign country.

§72.2 *Transportation of diagnostic specimens, biological products, and other materials; minimum packaging requirements.*

No person may knowingly transport or cause to be transported in interstate traffic, directly or indirectly, any material including, but

[1] The requirements of this part are in addition to and not in lieu of any other packaging or other requirements for the transportation of etiologic agents in interstate traffic prescribed by the Department of Transportation and other agencies of the Federal Government.

Table 43.1. (Continued)

not limited to, diagnostic specimens and biological products which such person reasonably believes may contain an etiologic agent unless such material is packaged to withstand leakage of contents, shocks, pressure changes, and other conditions incident to ordinary handling in transportation.

§72.3 Transportation of materials containing certain etiologic agents; minimum packaging requirements.

Notwithstanding the provisions of §72.2, no person may knowingly transport or cause to be transported in interstate traffic, directly or indirectly, any material (other than biological products) known to contain, or reasonably believed by such person to contain, one or more of the following etiologic agents unless such material is packaged, labeled, and shipped in accordance with the requirements specified in paragraphs (a)–(f) of this section:

BACTERIAL AGENTS

Acinetobacter calcoaceticus.
Actinobacillus—all species.
Actinomycetaceae—all members.
Aeromonas hydrophila.
Arachnia propionica.
Arizona hinshawii—all serotypes.
Bacillus anthracis.
Bacteroides spp.
Bartonella—all species.
Bordetella—all species.
Borrelia recurrentis, B. vincenti.
Brucella—all species.
Campylobacter (Vibrio) foetus, C. (Vibrio) jejuni.
Chlamydia psittaci, C. trachomatis.
Clostridium botulinum, Cl. chauvoei, Cl. haemolyticum, Cl. histolyticum, Cl. novyi, Cl. septicum, Cl. tetani.
Corynebacterium diphtheriae, C. equi, C. haemolyticum, C. pseudotuberculosis, C. pyogenes, C. renale.
Edwardsiella tarda.
Erysipelothrix insidiosa.
Escherichia coli, all enteropathogenic serotypes.
Francisella (Pasteurella) tularensis.
Haemophilus ducreyi, H. influenzae.
Klebsiella—all species and all serotypes.
Legionella—all species and all *Legionella*-like organisms.
Leptospira interrogans—all serovars.
Listeria—all species.
Mimae polymorpha.
Moraxella—all species.
Mycobacterium—all species.
Mycoplasma—all species.
Neisseria gonorrhoeae, N. meningitidis.
Nocardia asteroides.
Pasteurella—all species.
Plesiomonas shigelloides.
Proteus—all species.
Pseudomonas mallei.
Pseudomonas pseudomallei.
Salmonella—all species and all serotypes.
Shigella—all species and all serotypes.
Sphaerophorus necrophorus.
Staphylococcus aureus.

Table 43.1. (Continued)

Streptobacillus moniliformis.
Streptococcus pneumoniae.
Streptococcus pyogenes.
Treponema careteum, T. pallidum, and *T. pertenue.*
Vibrio cholerae, V. parahemolyticus.
Yersinia (Pasteurella) pestis, Y. enterocolitica.

FUNGAL AGENTS

Blastomyces dermatitidis.
Coccidioides immitis.
Cryptococcus neoformans.
Histoplasma capsulatum.
Paracoccidioides brasiliensis.

VIRAL AND RICKETTSIAL AGENTS

Adenoviruses—human—all types.
Arboviruses—all types.
Coxiella burnetii.
Coxsackie A and B viruses—all types.
Creutzfeldt—Jacob agent.
Cytomegaloviruses.
Dengue viruses—all types.
Ebola virus.
Echoviruses—all types.
Encephalomyocarditis virus.
Hemorrhagic fever agents including, but not limited to, Crimean hemorrhagic fever (Congo), Junin, Machupo viruses, and Korean hemorrhagic fever viruses.
Hepatitis associated materials (hepatitis A, hepatitis B, hepatitis nonA-nonB).
Herpesvirus—all members.
Infectious bronchitis-like virus.
Influenza viruses—all types.
Kuru agent.
Lassa virus.
Lymphocytic choriomeningitis virus.
Marburg virus.
Measles virus.
Mumps virus.
Parainfluenza viruses—all types.
Polioviruses—all types.
Poxviruses—all members.
Rabies virus—all strains.
Reoviruses—all types.
Respiratory syncytial virus.
Rhinoviruses—all types.
Rickettsia—all species.
Rochalimaea quintana.
Rotaviruses—all types.
Rubella virus.
Simian virus 40.
Tick-borne encephalitis virus complex, including Russian spring-summer encephalitis, Kyasanur forest disease, Omsk hemorrhagic fever, and Central European encephalitis viruses.
Vaccinia virus.
Varicella virus.
Variola major and Variola minor viruses.
Vesicular stomatis viruses—all types.
White pox viruses.
Yellow fever virus.[2]

(a) *Volume not exceeding 50 ml.* Material shall be placed in a securely closed, watertight container (primary container (test tube, vial, etc.) which shall be enclosed in a

[2] This list may be revised from time to time by Notice published in the Federal Register to identify additional agents which must be packaged in accordance with the requirements contained in this part.

Table 43.1. (Continued)

second, durable watertight container (secondary container). Several primary containers may be enclosed in a single secondary container, if the total volume of all the primary containers so enclosed does not exceed 50 ml. The space at the top, bottom, and sides between the primary and secondary containers shall contain sufficient nonparticulate absorbent material (e.g., paper towel) to absorb the entire contents of the primary container(s) in case of breakage or leakage. Each set of primary and secondary containers shall then be enclosed in an outer shipping container constructed of corrugated fiberboard, cardboard, wood, or other material of equivalent strength.

(b) *Volume greater than 50 ml.* Packaging of material in volumes of 50 ml. or more shall comply with requirements specified in paragraph (a) of this section. In addition, a shock absorbent material, in volume at least equal to that of the absorbent material between the primary and secondary containers, shall be placed at the top, bottom, and sides between the secondary container and the outer shipping container. Single primary containers shall not contain more than 1,000 ml of material. However, two or more primary containers whose combined volumes do not exceed 1,000 ml may be placed in a single, secondary container. The maximum amount of etiologic agent which may be enclosed within a single outer shipping container shall not exceed 4,000 ml.

(c) *Dry ice.* If dry ice is used as a refrigerant, it must be placed outside the secondary container(s). If dry ice is used between the secondary container and the outer shipping container, the shock absorbent material shall be placed so that the secondary container does not become loose inside the outer shipping container as the dry ice sublimates.

(d)(1) The outer shipping container of all materials containing etiologic agents transported in interstate traffic must bear a label as illustrated and described on page 65.

(2) The color of material on which the label is printed must be white, the symbol red, and the printing in red or white as illustrated.

(3) The label must be a rectangle measuring 51 millimeters (mm) (2 inches) high by 102.5 mm (4 inches) long.

(4) The red symbol measuring 38 mm (1½ inches) in diameter must be centered in a white square measuring 51 mm (2 inches) on each side.

(5) Type size of the letters of label shall be as follows:

ETIOLOGIC AGENTS—10 pt. rev.
BIOMEDICAL MATERIAL—14 pt.
IN CASE OF DAMAGE OR LEAKAGE—10 pt. rev.
NOTIFY DIRECTOR CDC, ATLANTA, GEORGIA—8 pt. rev.
404-633-5313—10 pt. rev.

(e) *Damaged packages.* The car

Table 43.1. (Continued)

rier shall promptly, upon discovery of evidence of leakage or any other damage to packages bearing an Etiologic Agents/Biomedical Material label, isolate the package and notify the Director, Center for Disease Control, 1600 Clifton Road, NE, Atlanta, GA 30333, by telephone: (404) 633-5313. The carrier shall also notify the sender.

(f) *Registered mail or equivalent system.* Transportation of the following etiologic agents shall be by registered mail or an equivalent system which requires or provides for sending notification of receipt to the sender immediately upon delivery:

Coccidioides immitis.
Ebola virus.
Francisella (Pasteurella) tularensis.
Hemorrhagic fever agents including, but not limited to, Crimean hemorrhagic fever (Congo), Junin, Machupo viruses, and Korean hemorrhagic fever viruses.
Herpesvirus simiae (B virus).
Histoplasma capsulatum.
Lassa virus.
Marburg virus.
Pseudomonas mallei.
Pseudomonas pseudomallei.
Tick-borne encephalitis virus complex including, but not limited to, Russian spring-summer encephalitis, Kyasanur forest disease, Omsk Hemorrhagic fever, and Central European encephalitis viruses, Variola minor, and Variola major.
Variola major, Variola minor, and Whitepox viruses.
Yersinia (Pasteurella) pestis.

§*72.4 Notice of delivery; failure to receive.*

When notice of delivery of materials known to contain or reasonably believed to contain etiologic agents listed in §72.3(f) is not received by the sender within 5 days following anticipated delivery of the package, the sender shall notify the Director, Center for Disease Control, 1600 Clifton Road, NE, Atlanta, GA 30333 (telephone (404) 633-5313).

§*72.5 Requirements; variations.*

The Director, Center for Disease Control, may approve variations from the requirements of this section if, upon review and evaluation, it is found that such variations provide protection at least equivalent to that provided by compliance with the requirements specified in this section and such findings are made a matter of official record.

[FR Doc 80-21757 Filed 7-18-80; 8:45 am]

BILLING CODE 4110-86-m

Effective August 20, 1980

packaging and shipping requirements. Section 72.3 of the Interstate Quarantine Regulations (Table 43:1) lists those etiologic agents for which the requirements are applicable and describes packaging, labeling and shipping requirements.

Packaging requirements for etiologic agents are described in Section 72.3(a)-(d) and are based on the volume of material in the primary container (i.e., volumes of less than 50 mL and volumes of more than 50 mL). The commercially available two-part shipping containers illustrated in Fig. 43:1 are satisfactory.

Cultures or suspensions of etiologic agents should be placed in a securely closed, watertight, primary container, such as a sealed plastic or glass ampoule, a taped, gasketed, screwcapped vial, or a wheaton bottle. Screwcaps should be secured with tape to prevent loosening during shipment. Petri dishes and other primary containers that cannot be securely closed should never be used for transporting cultures.

The space between the primary and secondary containers should contain enough nonparticulate absorbent material (e.g., paper toweling) to absorb the entire contents of the primary container in the event of breakage or leakage. The screwcap of the secondary container should be tightly secured and can be taped to prevent loosening in transit. Patient and laboratory data forms should be placed between the primary and secondary containers. A label indicating the name and address of the sender and the receiving laboratory should be affixed securely to the outer shipping container. In addition, a label reading "ETIOLOGIC AGENT/BIOMEDICAL MATERIALS," described in Section 72.3(d), must be affixed to all shipments of etiologic agents. The label must be of the size and color specified in the regulation and must not be altered or amended by including the shipper's name, shipping instructions nor other markings. Small specimens shipped by airmail or first class mail are acceptable to the Postal Service and are handled with other letter mail. Affixing the "NOTICE TO CARRIER" label, illustrated in Table 43:2, may facilitate the handling of etiologic agents sent by first class mail. This label is applicable only to domestic shipments of etiologic agents of less than 50 mL that meet all other regulatory requirements and is used instead of the "SHIPPER'S DECLARATION FOR DANGEROUS GOODS" (Fig. 43:2) specified in the ATA Restricted Articles Tariff 6-D. Specimens so packaged and labeled meet all applicable federal regulations and carrier tariffs for shipment by all modes, including transport on passenger-carrying aircraft.

For shipment of etiologic agents in volumes of 50 mL or more,the requirements for the primary container, absorbent material and secondary container are the same as for those for smaller volumes. In addition, shock-absorbent material must be placed between the secondary container and the outer shipping container. Individual primary containers shall not exceed 1,000 mL in volume and the aggregate volume of all primary containers in a single outer shipping container shall not exceed 4,000 mL.

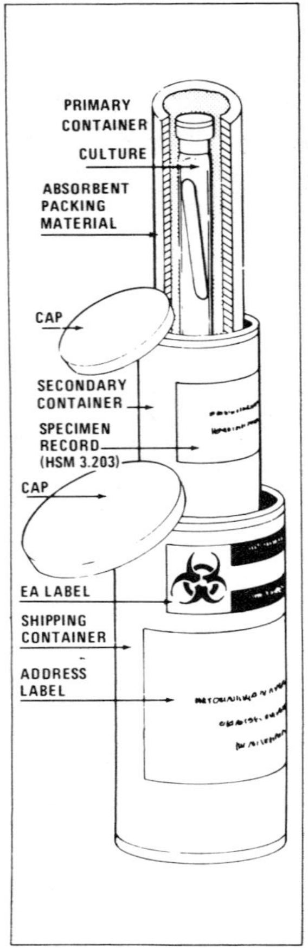

PACKAGING AND LABELING OF ETIOLOGIC AGENTS

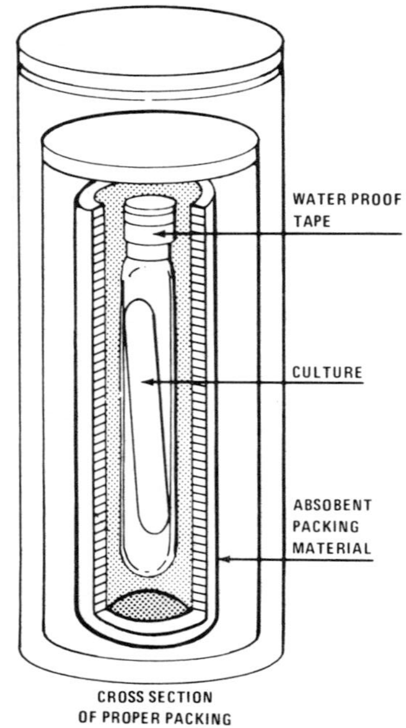

The Interstate Quarantine Regulations (Code of Federal Regulations, Title 42, Part 72.25, Etiologic Agents) was revised July 30, 1972, to provide for packaging and labeling requirements for etiologic agents and certain other materials shipped in interstate traffic.

The figure diagrams packaging and labeling of etiologic agents in volumes less than 50 ml in accordance with the provisions of subparagraph (C) (1) of the cited regulation.

The Etiologic Agents—Biomedical Material label (see subparagraph (C) (4) of regulations) which must be placed on all shipments of etiologic agents is depicted below. The label must be 2 inches high by 4 inches long and printed in red ink on white stock. For further information on any provision of this regulation contact:

Center for Disease Control
Attn: Office of Biosafety
1600 Clifton Road
Atlanta, Georgia 30333

Telephone: (404) 633-3311

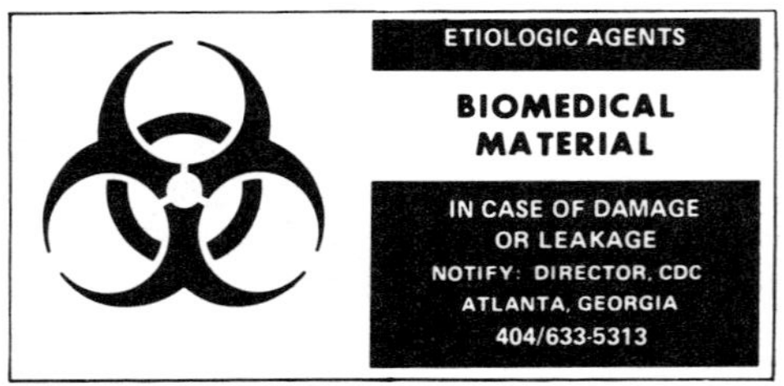
ETIOLOGIC AGENTS
BIOMEDICAL MATERIAL
IN CASE OF DAMAGE OR LEAKAGE
NOTIFY: DIRECTOR, CDC
ATLANTA, GEORGIA
404/633-5313

FIGURE 43:1. Packaging and labeling.

Table 43:2

SHIPMENT OF ETIOLOGIC AGENTS

The Air Transport Association's (ATA's) Restricted Articles Tariff 6-D, which specifies transportation requirements for hazardous materials shipped by air, was amended June 25, 1977. One of the provisions of this amended tariff, effective September 1, 1977, is that a large shipper's certificate must be used on domestic as well as international air shipments of etiologic agents and other hazardous materials.

This new requirement has prompted a review of applicable regulations and tariffs for alternatives to the use of this large shipper's certificate on small (less than 50-ml) shipments of etiologic agents sent by mail and airmail. The following statement has been reviewed with the U.S. Department of Transportation, the U.S. Postal Service, and the ATA, and it is consistent with the requirements of each of these agencies. In place of the large certificate, the Center for Disease Control (CDC) will use this statement on all domestic shipments of etiologic agents less than 50 ml in volume. Other shippers should consider using the statement in lieu of the large certificate:

NOTICE TO CARRIER

This package contains LESS THAN 50 ml OF AN ETIOLOGIC AGENT, N.O.S., is packaged and labeled in accordance with the U.S. Public Health Service Interstate Quarantine Regulations (42 CFR, Section 72.25 (c) (1) and (4)), and MEETS ALL REQUIREMENTS FOR SHIPMENT BY MAIL AND ON PASSENGER AIRCRAFT.

This shipment is EXEMPTED FROM ATA RESTRICTED ARTICLES TARIFF 6-d (see General Requirements 386 (d) (1) and from DOT HAZARDOUS MATERIALS REGULATIONS (see 49 CFR, Section 173.386 (d) (3)). SHIPPER'S CERTIFICATES, SHIPPING PAPERS, AND OTHER DOCUMENTATION OR LABELING ARE NOT REQUIRED.

____________________ ____________________

Date Signature of shipper

____

Address

____

SHIPPER'S CERTIFICATION FOR RESTRICTED ARTICLES
(excluding radioactive materials)
Two completed and signed copies of this certification shall be handed to the carrier. (Use block letters.)

WARNING: Failure to comply in all respects with the applicable regulations of the Department of Transportation, 49-CFR, CAB 82 and, for international shipments, the IATA Restricted Articles Regulations may be a breach of the applicable law, subject to legal penalties. This certification shall in no circumstance be signed by an IATA Cargo Agent or a consolidator for international shipments.

This shipment is within the limitations prescribed for: *(mark one)*

☐ passenger aircraft ☐ cargo-only aircraft

Number of Packages	Article Number (int'l only See Section IV IATA RAR)	Proper Shipping Name of Articles as shown in Title 49 CFR, CAB 82 Tariff 6-D and (for int'l shipments) the IATA Restricted Articles Regulations. Specify each article separately. Technical name must follow in parenthesis, the proper shipping name for N.O.S. items.	Class	IATA Packing Note No. Applied (int'l only)	Net Quantity per Package	Flash Point (Closed cup) For Flammable Liquids	
						°C	°F

Special Handling Information:

I hereby certify that the contents of this consignment are fully and accurately described above by Proper Shipping Name and are classified, packed, marked, labelled and in proper condition for carriage by air according to applicable national governmental regulations, and for International Shipments the current IATA Restricted Articles Regulations.

Name and full address of Shipper	Name and title of person signing Certification
Date	Signature of the Shipper (see WARNING above)

Air Waybill No.*	Airport of Departure*	Airport of Destination*

*This box is iptional for completion by issuing carrier.

[illegible].776

FIGURE 43:2. Shipper's certificate.

Shipments of etiologic agents exceeding 50 mL in one or more primary containers are relegated to cargo-only aircraft in accordance with the ATA Restricted Articles Tariff 6-D. In addition to carrying the "ETIOLOGIC AGENT" label previously described, such containers to be shipped by air must also have affixed, or be accompanied by, two copies of the completed and signed "SHIPPER'S DECLARATION FOR DANGEROUS GOODS" form (Fig. 43:2), as specified in Tariff 6-D. If dry ice is used as a refrigerant in shipments, appropriate marking and labels should be used in accordance with carrier requirements.

Comment

The International Civil Aviation Organization (ICAO), affiliated with the United Nations, has promulgated technical instructions for the packaging, labeling, documentation and shipment by air of a variety of dangerous goods, including "Infectious Substances—Human" and "Infectious Substances—Nonhuman." These technical instructions have been incorporated in the Dangerous Goods Regulations of the International Air Transport Association (IATA) and are applicable to all member carriers. Other than the documentation required for international shipment of "Infectious Substances—Human," the packaging, labeling and shipping provisions of the ICAO instructions and the IATA regulations parallel those of the ATA and the regulations of the PHS and DOT for shipment within the United States.

For international shipments of "Infectious Substances—Human" (etiologic agents), all quantities (including those less than 50 mL) must be accompanied by a completed "SHIPPER'S DECLARATION FOR DANGEROUS GOODS" form (Fig. 43:2). It has been the interpretation of many international carriers that the "scientific name" of the "Infectious Substance—Human" must follow this shipping designation (e.g., Infectious Substance—Human n.o.s. (*Mycobacterium tuberculosis*).

It is the responsibility of the shipper or of the receiver to verify the need for, and to obtain if necessary, authorization from national health authorities of the country of destination for transporting etiologic agents into their jurisdiction.

RECOMBINANT DNA MOLECULES - SPECIAL REQUIREMENTS

Appendix H of the "Guidelines for Research Involving Recombinant DNA Molecules"[1] specifies packaging, labeling and shipping requirements for recombinant DNA materials. Under the provisions of these Guidelines, recombinant DNA molecules in any organism or virus, irrespective of the potential of the organism, virus or recombinant DNA molecule to cause human disease, shall be shipped only as an "etiologic agent." As such, these materials are subject to the provisions of the PHS and DOT regulations indicated in the following guidelines:

"When transported or offered for transportation, recombinant DNA molecules contained in any organism or virus requiring biosafety level 1, 2 or 3 physical containment[2] are subject to all packaging, labeling and shipping requirements specified in Section 72.3(a)-(e), Part 72, Title 42 CFR and Sections 173.386-.388, Part 173, Title 49 CFR" (Table 43:1). Recombinant DNA molecules contained in any organism or virus requiring biosafety level 4 physical containment are, in addition to the requirements specified for lower levels, required to be transported by registered mail or an equivalent system that provides for sending notification of receipt to the sender immediately upon delivery, in accordance with Section 62.3(f) of the cited regulation.

REFERENCES

1. U.S. Department of Health and Human Services. NIH guidelines for research involving recombinant DNA molecules. Washington, DC: Federal Register 49, no. 227, Part IV, Nov. 23, 1984;46226-46285.
2. Centers for Disease Control-National Institutes of Health. Biosafety in microbiological and biomedical laboratories. Atlanta: Centers for Disease Control, U.S. Department of Health and Human Services, 1984; HHS publication no. (CDC)84-8395.

CHAPTER 44

STERILIZATION AND DISINFECTION

Martin S. Favero, Ph.D.

INTRODUCTION

The purpose of this section is to discuss the various procedures used for sterilization, disinfection and decontamination in the public health laboratory, as well as the basic rationale behind the optimal selection of each procedure. [3] Emphasis will be placed on correct terminology and general recommendations for procedures which can be applied to a large variety of laboratory situations. Because sterilization and disinfection procedures are used daily in modern laboratories, laboratorians should be familiar with the general principles that are involved.

TERMINOLOGY

Sterilization is the process by which all living forms are inactivated. An item or solution is considered sterile only if no viable microorganisms are present. The classic definition of sterility is the complete absence of all living microorganisms; however, the operational definition of sterilization is: a process, that when challenged with a relatively high number (usually about 1×10^6) of resistant bacterial spores, will provide an inactivation rate such that there will be less than one chance in a million of a bacterial spore surviving. This concept is used to set standard dry and wet heat sterilization cycles of commercially available sterilization devices. In the laboratory, sterilization procedures are used for sterilizing clean wrapped items, microbiologic culture media and reagents, as well as for a quick means of decontamination for contaminated items or infective wastes.

Disinfection is a less lethal procedure than sterilization, and one that is used to inactivate recognized pathogenic microorganisms but not necessarily all forms of microorganisms (e.g., bacterial endospores) on inanimate objects.

Disinfection procedures inherently do not have an extensive safety margin, thus the element of "overkill" which is a basic part of sterilization is not present. Disinfection can be the result of heat (e.g., heat pasteurization), or more commonly of the use of chemical germicides.

A decontamination procedure is one where the primary consideration is safety; safety for laboratory personnel as well as safety for other individuals who are associated with laboratory operations and the community.[4] Decontamination is defined as the destruction or removal of microorganisms to a low level but not necessarily to zero. The objective of decontamination is to render material safe for handling, whether it be items that need to be washed and subsequently sterilized, or liquid and solid wastes that require disposal. It is quite common for sterilization procedures, such as steam autoclaving, to be used for purposes of decontamination. On the other hand, the principles of chemical disinfection can be applied in the case of blood or culture spills in the laboratory environment.

An antiseptic is an antimicrobial substance that is used on or in living tissue to inhibit or destroy microorganisms. Often the distinction between an antiseptic and a disinfectant is not made; a disinfectant is a chemical germicide that is used solely for destroying microorganisms on inanimate objects, whereas an antiseptic is used on or in living tissue. Some chemical agents, for example iodophors, are used as active ingredients in chemical germicides that can be formulated as either disinfectants or as antiseptics. However, the precise formulations are significantly different, depending on the intended use, and germicidal efficacy differs substantially. Disinfectants should never be used as antiseptics nor vice versa. Antiseptic procedures in laboratories range from swabbing injection sites on experimental animals to personnel handwashing with antimicrobial soaps.

REGULATION OF CHEMICAL GERMICIDES IN THE UNITED STATES

Chemical germicides that are formulated as disinfectants and sterilants are regulated and registered by the Environmental Protection Agency (EPA). The authority for this responsibility comes under the Federal Insecticide, Fungicide, and Rodenticide Act (FIFRA). The EPA requires manufacturers of chemical germicides formulated as general disinfectants, hospital disinfectants and disinfectants applied in other environments, such as in the food industry, to test these formulations by using specific protocols for microbicidal efficiency, stability and toxicity to humans. The decision to register a disinfectant is based on data provided to the EPA by the manufacturer. Although in past years the EPA has reserved the right to independently test and verify formulations of chemical gemicides for their specified efficacy, in practice only those formulations registered as sterilants or sporicides were actually tested. In 1982, the EPA discontinued this testing. Formulations of chemical germicides currently are registered by the EPA on the basis of data obtained from the manufacturer, without independent verification except as these formulations are tested by investigators who report findings in the scientific literature. This lack of independent verification has caused concern among health professionals who believe that EPA verification of sporicidal or sterilant claims was a significant consideration in the selection of a sterilant or high-level disinfectant.

Users should keep in mind that the field of chemical germicides is highly competitive and that exaggerated claims are often made about the germicidal efficiency of specific formulations. New formulations of chemical germicides that become commercially available should be scrutinized by health professionals. It may also be necessary to consult with the Disinfectants Branch, Registration Division, Office of Pesticides, EPA, when questions regarding specific claims or use arise. Studies published in the scientific literature and presented at scientific meetings also provide important information on the efficacy of these formulations.

Chemical germicides that are formulated as antiseptics, preservatives, drugs to be used on or in the human body, or as preparations to be used to inhibit or kill organisms on the skin are regulated by the Food and Drug Administration (FDA). However, the FDA method of regulating these formulations is significantly different from that of EPA. FDA has an advisory review panel on nonprescription, antimicrobial drug products. Manufacturers of such formulations voluntarily submit data to the panel, which in turn categorizes the products for their intended use, i.e., antimicrobial soaps, health care personnel handwashes, patient preoperative skin preparations, skin antiseptics, skin wound cleansers, skin wound protectants and surgical hand scrubs. Generic chemical germicides for each use are further divided into Category I, safe and efficacious; Category II, not safe or efficacious; and Category III, insufficient data to categorize. Consequently, chemical germicides formulated as antiseptics and regulated by the FDA are categorized basically by use and efficacy and are not regulated or registered in the same fashion as are disinfectants and sterilants by EPA.

STERILIZATION PROCEDURES

Sterilization by Heat

Dry heat is used to sterilize articles which are corrosively attacked by steam: glassware such as flasks, bottles and pipettes packed in sealed cans; and anhydrous, dehydrated or hydrophobic materials that cannot tolerate moist heat. Common examples of materials that are dry-heat sterilized include instruments with cutting edges, surgical gut, groundglass surfaces, dry chemicals, grease, oil and glycerol. The primary limitation of dry heat is the time necessary for sterilization. If higher temperatures are used to shorten the sterilization period, fabrics, rubber goods, plastics and chemicals can be degraded or destroyed. In a dry-heat sterilizer, the hot air should be mechanically circulated to prevent stratification and to insure uniformity of temperature.

The recommended time-temperature relationships for dry heat in Table 44:1 refer to actual load temperature and NOT to chamber temperature. Consequently, a recommendation of 170°C for 1 hour does not allow for the time required for the materials being sterilized to reach that temperature. Variations in the load and equipment necessitate that a temperature-sensing device be placed in the center of the load, or in that part of the load that is assumed to be the most difficult for heat penetration, to confirm the time when the material reaches the sterilization temperature. Once the cycle has been established, thermocouples need not be used daily, but it is recommended that the cycle be checked once each month. In addition, commercially available bacterial spores (*Bacillus subtilis* subsp. *niger*) should periodically be placed in the centers of loads or into those areas considered to be the most difficult for heat penetration to check the sterilization process. Table 44:1 lists time-temperature ratios as guidelines for dry-heat sterilization in a laboratory. These times represent the length of exposure needed after the recommended temperature is reached.

Moist heat saturated steam under pressure is most frequently used for sterilization. The procedure is based on direct contact with saturated steam, which is a physical entity with properties that can be measured conveniently. All living microorganisms can be rapidly destroyed by pressurized steam. The time-temperature relationships applicable to this type of sterilization are generally agreed upon. Steam is a readily available store of latent energy liberated simply by change of state, which carries the advantage of rapid heating. When it comes in contact with cold objects, saturated steam condenses, simultaneously heating and wetting the object, and thus provides two requisites for the rapid thermal destruction of microorganisms.

If this sterilization method is to be effective, air and moisture present in the sterilizing chamber must be removed, preferably automatically. Air can be removed from the sterilization chamber by being displaced downward with steam or by being suctioned with a high-vacuum pump. The high-

Table 44:1. Dry Heat Time-Temperature Ratios

170° C (340° F)	1 hour
160° C (320° F)	2 hours
150° C (300° F)	2.5 hours
140° C (285° F)	3 hours
121° C (250° F)	6 hours

vacuum method is much more effective because it removes approximately 98% of the air from the chamber and load before the steam is introduced. Steam penetration after air evacuation is almost instantaneous, and the absence of air during heating eliminates the risk of damage to textiles and rubber by oxidation at high temperatures. The time-temperature-pressure relationships in Table 44:2 are recommended for steam sterilization. These times relate only to the period after the materials reach the designated temperature and moisture levels of saturated steam and do not include penetration or heat-up lag. Steam-sterilizer manufacturers have recently developed automatic sterilizers which incorporate new concepts in process and equipment design. Consequently, the modern-day autoclave has progressed from manually operated units to fully automatic, gravity-displacement and high-vacuum, high-pressure sterilizers with integrated time-temperature controls on steam-jacketed vessels with motorized doors. Tables 43:3, 4 and 5 illustrate the effects of the type of load on the total length of a steam sterilization cycle. These data are guidelines only; actual sterilization cycles should be determined for each autoclave (with thermocouples and commercially available indicator spores such as *Bacillus stearothermophilus*).

Sterilization by Filtration

The two basic systems for filtering microorganisms from liquid media are depth filtration and screen or membrane filtration.

Table 44:2. Time-Temperature-Pressure for Steam Sterilization

15 minutes at 121° C, 15 psig
10 minutes at 126° C, 20 psig
3 minutes at 134° C, 29.4 psig

Table 44:3. Sterilization Times

Sterilizer Type	Temperature (°C)	Article Being Sterilized	Penetration	Sterilization Time (Minutes)* Holding	Safety	Total
Downward displacement	121	Instruments	3	12	0	15
		Gloves	5	12	3	20
		Packs	12	12	6	30
High prevacuum	132	Instruments	1	2	1	4
		Gloves	1	2	1	4
		Packs	1	2	1	4

* Measured from the time the autoclave gauge reaches the temperature selected.

Table 44:4. Steam Sterilization of Liquids—Effect of Volume/Container (Erlenmeyer Flasks) on Time Required to Reach 121°C (Single Container Load)

Size of Container (mL)	Volume of Liquid/ Container (mL)	Liquid Temp. at Initiation of Cycle (°C)	Time Needed for Chamber to Reach 121°C (Min)	Time Needed for Center of Liquid to Reach 121°C (Min)	Total Time of Cycle (Min)
50	25	25	2	4	14
125	75	25	2	5	15
200	150	25	3	7	17
500	400	25	3	10	20
1000	800	25	3	14	24
2000	1500	25	6	19	29
3000	2500	25	7	25	35
5000	4500	25	8	33	43
6000	5500	25	8	44	54

Table 44:5. Steam Sterilization of Liquids—Effect of Volume/Container and Number of Containers on Time Required for Liquid to Reach 121°C

Liquid per Container (Liter)	Containers per Load (No.)	Liquid Temp. at Initiation of Cycle (°C)	Time Needed for Chamber to Reach 121°C (Min)	Time Needed for Liquid to Reach 121°C (Min)	Total Time of Cycle (Min)
0.5	30	29	10	19	29
1.0	20	26	12	34	44
1.5	15	26	12	36	46
2.0	10	27	13	37	47
2.5	10	26	15	40	50
3.0	8	26	15	43	53
3.5	6	26	12	50	60
4.0	5	26	12	52	62
4.5	5	26	14	58	68
5.0	5	26	15	60	70
5.5	5	26	17	60	70
6.0	4	26	15	62	72

Depth Filtration: Depth filters can be asbestos pads, porcelain candles or diatomaceous earth. The surface portion of the filter removes large particles, and the center or matrix portion removes small particles to a rated degree, although never completely. Several factors determine the ability of a depth filter to perform its prescribed function: particle geometry, pore size, surface characteristics, medium velocity, pressure changes, particle migration and filter-medium migration. The depth filter has a distinct advantage over others in that it can retain a large volume of particulate matter before becoming plugged. Generally speaking, it is best not to reuse depth filters.

Screen or Membrane Filters: Screen filters are classified by pore size, usually restricted to at least 20 μm. Their usefulness is limited because particles accumulate rapidly. This type of filter is often used to clarify liquids rather than in sterilization.

Membrane filters can be used to sterilize various aqueous media, including serum, water, culture broth, etc. Membrane filters with a rated pore size of 0.22 μm or less should be used for sterilization. This is especially true for reagents or media prepared with water containing high levels of gram-negative bacteria. The membrane filter offers the advantage that pores are of uniform size and that the filtration rate is faster than with other types of filtration equipment.

Chemical Sterilization

If the more reliable physical methods are not available or cannot be used, materials can be sterilized with gaseous and liquid germicides. Chemical sterilization, commonly referred to as "cold sterilization," is used primarily for treating heat-sensitive items. Relatively high concentrations of germicides and prolonged exposure are necessary to assure that all microorganisms are destroyed -- particularly the more resistant bacterial endospores.

Aqueous formaldehyde is used as a chemical sterilizing agent. Usually alcohol is added to the solution to retard polymerization of the formaldehyde. An 8%-70% (formaldehyde-alcohol) solution is satisfactory for sterilizing purposes (18 h of exposure at 25°C).

Glutaraldehyde-based chemical germicides are broad-spectrum germicides used widely in chemical sterilization. Glutaraldehyde is preferable to formaldehyde for certain items such as instruments with lens because the former is less corrosive. Although glutaraldehyde solutions are relatively stable at low temperatures (4°C), they are effective for only 2-4 weeks when stored at room temperature (20-25°C). Glutaraldehyde sterilization usually consists of exposing cleaned items to a 2% solution for 6-10 hours at 25°C.

When using chemical sterilizing agents, it is important to determine whether the concentration of the active materials is adequate to destroy the entire microbial population - especially the more resistant bacterial spores. The time required for sterilization can vary significantly. The types of organisms and their physical and chemical states determine the length of time necessary for the germicide to destroy them. Such factors as pH, size of the microbial population, surface activity and the presence of extraneous matter affect the final results obtained. Since proteinaceous material and grease can interfere with the action of a germicidal solution, items being treated must be scrupulously clean, with minimal soil or bacterial contamination. The sterilizing chemical must completely penetrate any interstices or small bores of complex pieces to assure sterilization.

Because heat-sensitive materials are increasingly being used as components of scientific and medical equipment, gas sterilization is now more widely used. Currently, the biocidal agent of most gas sterilizers is ethylene oxide (EO). Many items damaged by heat can be sterilized with gaseous EO, which is effective against all types of microorganisms. It has excellent penetrating properties and can be used at moderate temperatures and pressures in the closed chamber which confines it. The optimal relative humidity of the gaseous atmosphere is about 50%, and the temperature should be kept between 40-60°C. With nonexplosive mixtures of EO and CO_2, or freon, concentrations of 450-760 mg EO/L are readily attainable. For concentrations equal to or greater than 1,000 mg/L, EO without a carrier gas is used. Length of exposure depends on the type of load and the contaminating microbial population.

Users of EO sterilization are cautioned that the chemical is toxic to the skin and when inhaled. The gas is highly penetrating; such materials as rubber and plastic can absorb the chemical while being sterilized. Ample time must be allowed for dissipation of the EO after the sterilization cycle is completed. Some sensitive materials must be stored at room temperature in a well-ventilated area for a week after sterilization before they can be safely used. Several manufacturers now produce aeration cabinets designed to increase the rate at which gas is dissipated from sterilized items.

Such factors as temperature, time, concentration and relative humidity must be precisely controlled to insure an effective sterilization. Although EO is effective against all types of organisms, the physical state of the microorganisms is an important determining factor in the sterilization process. Extremely dry organisms, particularly bacterial endospores, can be comparatively resistant to the action of EO. Even with a preconditioning period of relatively high humidity before exposure to the gas, some bacterial endospores may not rehydrate to the level necessary for effective EO action. As with heat sterilization, commercially available spores should be placed in the center of loads, or in those areas where the least gas penetration is expected, to monitor sterilization.

Although formaldehyde gas was once used for sterilization, it is now used primarily for fumigation and decontamination. Formaldehyde vapors can be obtained by heating flaked paraformaldehyde in a relative humidity of at least 70% and at a minimum temperature of 20°C. Generally, this gas kills bacterial cells within a few hours, but it takes longer to destroy bacterial endospores.

Although the pharmaceutical industry currently sterilizes various medical equipment such as needles, syringes, disposable rubber gloves and plastic equipment by ionizing radiation, this technique is not practical in the average public health or clinical laboratory. The cost of a cobalt-60 (gamma source) installation or of an electron accelerator for sterilization is prohibitive for all except largescale commercial applications.

DISINFECTION PROCEDURES[2]

Disinfection refers to the destruction of disease-producing vegetative microorganisms. The term is generally used to indicate a reduction in the level of microbial contamination in a particular environment. Contamination in the laboratory can be minimized or eliminated by good cleaning procedures. Restricting the presence of microbes on inanimate surfaces or physically removing all or a major portion of the microbial population from objects is usually not difficult. As an adjunct to physical cleanliness, chemical agents are also widely used in disinfecting procedures. Since it is difficult to disinfect large objects or surfaces by heat, disinfection is most often carried out with chemical substances which have antimicrobial properties.

Chemical germicides are more often effective against vegetative microbial cells than against bacterial and fungal spores, tubercle bacilli or the more resistant viruses. The ultimate action of chemical agents may be either biocidal (the microorganism is killed) or biostatic (growth and multiplication of the microorganism are inhibited).

Chemical Disinfectants

Inorganic and organic mercurials, which are among the oldest types of disinfectants, are not widely used. At present, they are used primarily as fungicides in industrial preservatives. The mercurials are essentially biostatic rather than biocidal, with poor biostatic properties even when highly concentrated. The presence of organic matter markedly reduces their effectiveness as disinfectants.

Quaternary ammonium compounds are widely used as germicides and are effective primarily against vegetative cells. They are relatively ineffective against tubercle bacilli and bacterial spores. These compounds are good wetting agents because of their strong surface tension-reducing properties. Because cationic quaternaries are not compatible with soaps, surfaces and objects to be treated should be free of soap films. Organic matter such as serum, proteins, cork and cotton fibers also inactivate these compounds. The quaternaries should be diluted carefully, because substances in certain natural waters may affect their germicidal activity adversely. In addition, gram-negative water bacteria can grow in dilute or aged solutions. Thus, freshly prepared solutions are the most effective .

Chlorine, iodine and bromine have been widely used as disinfectants. The chlorine-type germicides (sodium hypochlorite, calcium hypochlorite, dichloro-trichloro-isocyanuric acid and chlorine dioxide) can be used for various decontamination procedures. The presence of organic matter reduces the effectiveness of chlorine disinfectants. They are effective against vegetative cells but may not be effective against tubercle bacilli and bacterial spores at commonly used concentrations, i.e., 500-5000 ppm. Disinfectants which contain chlorine are generally corrosive to inanimate objects and surfaces and are irritating to live tissues.

Tincture of iodine or aqueous iodine preparations are generally used as antiseptics but can also be formulated as disinfectants. Iodophors contain iodine and a solubilizing agent and are applied as general disinfectants. The iodophors are stable, relatively stain- and odor-free, and have the antimicrobial properties of iodine. They are effective against vegetative cells and tubercle bacilli but not against bacterial spores.

Phenol or carbolic acid is infrequently used as a disinfectant in laboratories. The compound is effective against vegetative bacterial cells, but it has several drawbacks. It is irritating and destructive to skin and tissues, particularly at high concentrations and it smells unpleasant. Phenol's primary use is as a standard against which other types of phenolic preparations can be compared in laboratory tests. Synthetic phenols have replaced the original compound as disinfectants. These compounds are similar to phenol but lack its undesirable characteristics. The phenolic derivatives are effective germicides against vegetative bacterial cells and tubercle bacilli but are not very effective against bacterial spores. The compounds are stable, but can be inactivated by organic matter though not by soap. Many of the synthetic phenols are odorless. Since the formulations are compatible with detergents, the synthetic phenols are widely used for general sanitation purposes as disinfectant-detergents.

Factors Influencing Activity of Chemical Disinfectants

In general, the higher the concentration of a chemical disinfectant, the greater its germicidal activity. To assure lethal action, the chemical agent must be allowed enough time to be absorbed by and to destroy the microorganisms. Elevated temperatures may increase the agent's biocidal activity, although some formulations are not stable at higher temperatures. The presence of organic matter interferes with the action of most chemical disinfectants.

The level of contamination must be physically reduced before a disinfectant is applied. No known disinfectant is completely effective against all types of microorganisms and, obviously, some agents are more effective than others against particular microbes. Usually, the effectiveness of a chemical disinfectant is stated in terms of selected strains of microorganisms against which it is most effective.

Selecting a Chemical Disinfectant

A primary consideration in selecting a suitable chemical disinfectant is the purpose for which it is intended. An ideal disinfectant is one with the following characteristics:

a. It should have a wide range of activity, i.e., it should be effective against viral, rickettsial, fungal, protozoan and bacterial species;
b. It should be stable: prolonged storage or exposure to moderate temperatures should not decrease its activity;
c. It should not be adversely affected by salts, organic matter, pH or the hardness of water used to dilute it;
d. It should not stain or corrode surfaces or objects;
e. It should not be toxic nor irritating to tissues or skin.

REFERENCES

1. Favero MS. Chemical disinfection of medical and surgical materials. In: Block SS, ed. Disinfection, sterilization and preservation. 3rd. ed. Philadelphia: Lee and Febinger, 1983:469-92
2. Favero MS. Sterilization, disinfection and antisepsis in the hospital. In: Lennette EH, Balows A, Hausler WJ Jr, Shadomy HJ, eds. Manual of clinical microbiology. 4th ed. Washington, DC: American Society for Microbiology, 1985:129-37.
3. Vesley D, Lauer J. Decontamination, sterilization, disinfection and antisepsis in the microbiology laboratory. In: Groschel DH, Richardson JH, Vesley D, Songer JR, Housewright RD, Barkley WE, eds. Laboratory safety: principles and practices. Washington, DC: American Society for Microbiology, 1986:182-98.
4. Favero MS, Petersen NJ, Bond W. Transmission and control of laboratory-acquired hepatitis infection. In: Groschel DH, Richardson JH, Vesley D, Songer JR, Housewright RD, Barkley WE, eds. Laboratory safety: principles and practices. Washington, DC: American Society for Microbiology, 1986:49-58.

CHAPTER 45

MEDIA, REAGENTS AND STAINS

Richard H. Bell, Ph.D.

BACTERIOLOGICAL CULTURE MEDIA

Alkaline Peptone Broth[16]

Intended use: An enrichment broth medium for *Vibrio cholerae* isolation.

Formula:	*Ingredients per Liter*
Peptone	10.0 g
Sodium chloride	10.0 g

Final pH 8.4-8.5 at 25°C

Method of preparation:

1. Suspend ingredients in 1 L of distilled or deionized water and adjust pH to 8.4-8.5 with 1N sodium hydroxide.
2. Dispense in 10 mL amounts in test tubes.
3. Sterilize in the autoclave for 15 min at 121°C.

Appearance of uninoculated medium: Light amber, clear liquid medium.

Storage:

1. Prepared medium: 2-8°C
2. Shelf life: Approximately 6 months

Quality control: Organism	*Growth*
Positive *Vibrio cholerae* (delicate membrane on surface in 6-9 h)	+
Negative Uninoculated	–

Arylsulfatase Test Medium and Reagent[45,62]

Intended use: A medium and test for detecting sulfatase enzyme activity by mycobacteria.

Formula:	*Ingredients per Liter*
Middlebrook 7H9 broth (with glycerol)	100.0 mL
Phenolphthalein disulfate tripotassium salt (PDTS)	0.2 g

Final pH 6.6 ±0.2 at 25°C

Reagent:

Sodium carbonate solution (1M):	
Sodium carbonate	10.6 g
Distilled or deionized water	100.0 mL

Method of Preparation:

1. Suspend 0.47 g of Middlebrook 7H9 Broth in 90 mL distilled or deionized water containing 0.2 mL glycerol and heat to boiling to dissolve completely.
2. Sterilize in the autoclave for 10-15 min at 121°C. Cool.
3. Add 10 mL of a 2% filter-sterilized PDTS solution.
4. Dispense in 16 x 125 mm sterile screwcapped tubes in 3 mL amounts.
5. Inoculate tube of substrate with 0.1 mL of a 7-day Tween-Albumin or Middlebrook 7H9 broth culture of organism to be tested. One drop of a barely turbid suspension of organism in sterile water may be used as inoculum.
6. Incubate aerobically at 35°C for 3 days. Add 4-5 drops of 1 M sodium carbonate solution to each tube and observe for a color change. A pink to deep red color is a positive reaction.

Appearance of uninoculated medium: Light amber, clear liquid medium.

Storage:

1. Prepared medium: 2-8°C
2. Shelf life: Approximately 6-8 weeks

Quality Control: Organism		*Growth*
Positive	*Mycobacterium fortuitum* (pink-red)	+
Negative	*Mycobacterium phlei* (no color change)	+
	Uninoculated	−

Bordet-Gengou (BG) Agar Without Peptone[1]

Intended use: A primary isolation medium for the characterization of *Bordetella pertussis* and *Bordetella parapertussis*.

Formula:	*Ingredients per Liter*
Peeled, diced potatoes	187.5 g
Distilled water	1500.0 mL
Glycerol	15.0 mL
Sodium chloride, reagent grade	10.0 g
Agar	30.0 g
Sterile defibrinated sheep blood	300.0 mL

Final pH 6.7 ±0.2 at 25°C

Method of preparation:

1. Boil the potatoes in water for about 30 min until soft and filter through several layers of gauze.
2. Add glycerol, NaCl and agar to 1,000 mL of the filtrate, adjust the pH to 7.0 and bring to a boil.
3. Dispense 100 mL amounts into screwcapped bottles or 20 mL amounts into screwcapped tubes.
4. Autoclave for 15 min at 121°C, cool, seal and store refrigerated.
5. Just before use, melt the base and hold it at 50-60°C. Add 30 mL of sterile defibrinated sheep blood to 100 mL, mix well and pour 5-6 plates (or add 6 mL blood to 20 mL of agar for a single plate).

Comments:

Home-made BG base is superior to commercially prepared dehydrated medium. If commercial BG base is used, it should contain 125 g/L potato extract, and it should not contain added peptone. Added peptone is inhibitory to clinical isolates of *B. pertussis*. Difco Bordet-Gengou Agar Base (0048) prepared according to the manufacturer's directions except using 30 mL blood per 100 mL base has been satisfactory. Antibiotics may be added to molten medium prior to pouring plates. Recommended antibiotics include methicillin (at a final concentration of 2.5 μg per mL) or cephalexin (final concentration 40 μg per mL). If RL transport medium is used with specimens plated on BG, cephalexin should be used rather than methicillin.

Appearance of uninoculated medium: Base Medium; colorless to straw, may have a slight precipitate. Base with blood; cherry red, opaque, moist and free from bubbles.

Storage:

1. Prepared medium without blood: 2-8°C
2. Shelf life: Approximately 1 year for base without blood. Approximately 1 week, tightly sealed at 2-8°C for plates used in subculturing. Freshly poured plates (within 4 h) should be used for primary isolation.

Quality control:	*Organism*	*Growth*
Positive	Properly maintained clinical isolates of *Bordetella pertussis* and	+
	optionally, properly maintained clinical isolates of *B. parapertussis*	+
Negative	Uninoculated	−

Buffered Charcoal-Yeast Extract Agar With α-Ketoglutarate (BCYE-α)[8]

Intended use: For primary isolation and cultivation of *Legionella* spp.

Formula:	*Ingredients per Liter*
ACES [N-(2-acetamido)-2-aminoethanesulfonic acid] buffer	10.00 g
KOH pellets (85% KOH, reagent grade)	2.80 g
Activated charcoal (Norit A)	1.50 g
Yeast extract	10.00 g
Agar	17.00 g
α-ketoglutarate, monopotassium salt (Sigma)	1.00 g
L-cysteine hydrochloride (ICN) in 10 mL distilled water	0.40 g
Ferric pyrophosphate (Sigma) in 10 mL distilled water	0.25 g

Final pH 6.9 ±0.05 at 40°C

Method of preparation:

1. Dissolve ACES buffer in 900 mL distilled water by heating in a water bath at 50°C for about 1.5 h or until buffer is dissolved.

2. Add KOH pellets to buffer solution.
3. Add dry charcoal, yeast extract, agar and α-ketoglutarate. Mix well. Use 80 mL distilled water to rinse into flask.
4. Autoclave for 15 min at 121°C.
5. Cool to 50°C in water bath.
6. Add filter-sterilized (0.2 μm filter) ferric pyrophosphate and L-cysteine hydrochloride.
7. Check pH, which should be between 6.85-6.95 at 40°C. Correct with 1N HCl or KOH pellets.
8. Cool to 40°C and pour plates.
9. Preincubate the entire batch for 1 day at 35°C to detect contaminants.
10. Cool to room temperature and store non-contaminated plates.

Appearance of uninoculated medium: Black, opaque, solid medium.

Storage:

1. Prepared medium: 2-8°C
2. Shelf life: Approximately 2 months in plastic sleeves

Quality control:	*Organism*	*Growth*
Positive	*Legionella pneumophila*	+
Negative	Uninoculated	−

Buffered Charcoal-Yeast Extract Agar with Cefamandole, Polymyxin B, Anisomycin and α-ketoglutarate (BMPA-α medium)[8]

Intended use: A selective medium for the isolation of *Leqionella* spp.

Formula:	*Ingredients per Liter*
ACES [N-(2-acetamido)-2-aminoethanesulfonic acid] buffer	10.00 g
KOH pellets (85% KOH, reagent grade)	2.80 g
Activated charcoal (Norit A)	1.50 g
Yeast Extract	10.00 g
Agar	17.00 g
α-ketoglutarate, monopotassium salt (Sigma)	1.00 g
L-cysteine hydrochloride (ICN) in 10 mL distilled water	0.40 g
Ferric pyrophosphate (Sigma) in 10 mL distilled water	0.25 g
Polymyxin B sulfate (Pfizer or Sigma) as base	80,000 U
Cefamandole lithium (Lilly) as base	4.00 mg
Anisomycin (General Diagnostics)	80.00 g

Final pH 6.9 ±0.05 at 40°C

Method of preparation:

1. Prepare BCYE-α medium and cool to 50°C in a water bath. Do not check pH until after antimicrobial agents have been added.
2. Add filter-sterilized antimicrobial agents and mix by swirling.
3. Check pH, which should be 6.85-6.95 at 40°C.
4. Pour into petri dishes, each containing approximately 24 mL.
5. Pre-incubate one plate from batch at 35°C for 24 h to detect contamination.
6. Store non-contaminated plates.

Appearance of uninoculated medium: Black, opaque, solid medium.

Storage:

1. Prepared medium: 2-8°C
2. Shelf life: Approximately 3-4 weeks in plastic sleeves.

Quality control:	*Organism*	*Growth*
Positive	*Legionella pneumophila*	+
Negative	*Escherichia coli*	−

Cary-Blair Transport Medium[3]

Intended Use: A medium for the transport of microorganisms.

Formula:	*Ingredients per Liter*
Sodium thioglycolate	1.5 g
Sodium phosphate, dibasic	1.1 g
Sodium chloride	5.0 g
Agar	5.0 g
Calcium chloride, dihydrate (1% solution)	9.0 mL

Final pH 8.4 ±0.2 at 25°C

Method of preparation:

1. Suspend the ingredients in 991.0 mL of distilled or deionized water and heat medium only until clear.
2. Cool to 50°C, add 9 mL of freshly prepared aqueous 1% calcium chloride and adjust the pH to 8.4.
3. Dispense 7 mL into chemically-clean 9 mL screwcapped vials rinsed with Sorensen 0.067M buffer (pH 8.1) that have been sterilized.
4. Steam vials for 15 min, cool and tighten the caps.

Appearance of uninoculated medium: Light amber, clear to slightly opalescent, semi-solid medium.

Storage:

1. Prepared medium: 2-8°C
2. Shelf life: Approximately 1.5 years

Quality control:	*Organism*	*Growth*
Positive	*Vibrio cholerae* (on subculture after transport)	+
Negative	Uninoculated	–

Cation Supplemented Mueller Hinton Broth (CSMHB)[40]

Intended use: A modified Mueller Hinton broth for antibiotic susceptibility tests.

Formula:	*Ingredients per Liter*
Mueller Hinton broth	21.0 g
MG^{++} ions	25.0 mg
Ca^{++} ions	50.0 mg

Final pH 7.3 ±0.1 at 25°C

Method of preparation:

1. Magnesium stock solution: Dissolve 8.36 gm of magnesium chloride ($MgCl_2 \cdot 6H_20$) in 100 mL of deionized water. This solution will contain 10 mg of Mg^{++}/mL. Sterilize by membrane filtration and store at 4°C.
2. Calcium stock solution: Dissolve 3.68 gm of calcium chloride ($CaCl_2 \cdot 2H_20$) in 100 mL of deionized water. This solution will contain 10 mg of Ca^{++}/mL. Sterilized by membrane filtration and store at 4°C.
3. Prepare Mueller Hinton broth as the manufacturer directs, autoclave and chill overnight at 4°C or in an ice bath if it is to be used the same day. With stirring, add 2.5 mL of chilled Mg^{++} stock solution to each liter of broth. The concentration of Mg^{++} will be 25 mg/L. With stirring, add 5.0 mL of chilled Ca^{++} stock solution to each liter of broth. The concentration of Ca^{++} will be 50 mg/L. This medium is called Cation Supplemented Mueller Hinton Broth (CSMHB). (These recommendations are valid only for broth with essentially no cations.)

Appearance of uninoculated medium: Very light amber, clear liquid with no significant precipitate.

Storage:

1. Prepared medium: 2-8°C
2. Shelf life: Approximately 1 year

Quality control:	*Organism*	*Growth*
Positive	*Pseudomonas aeruginosa* (ATCC 27853)	+
	Streptococcus faecalis (ATCC 29212 or 33186)	+
Negative	Uninoculated	−

The MIC for gentamicin for *P. aeruginosa* must be between 1.0 and 4.0 and the MIC for sulfisoxazole for *S. faecalis* should be within one 2-fold dilution, 1:32-1:128.

Cetrimide Agar,[2,25,32]

Intended use: A selective medium for the isolation and identification of *Pseudomonas aeruginosa*.

Formula:	*Ingredients per Liter*
Pancreatic digest of gelatin	20.0 g
Magnesium chloride·$6H_20$	1.4 g
Potassium sulfate	10.0 g
Cetrimide (cetyltrimethyl ammonium bromide)	0.3 g
Agar	13.6 g

Final pH 7.2 ±0.2 at 25°C

Method of Preparation:

1. Suspend ingredients in 1 L of distilled or deionized water. Add 10 mL glycerol and heat to boiling to dissolve.
2. Dispense into tubes or flasks prior to autoclaving (if making plates, pour 20 mL per plate after sterilization).
3. Sterilize in the autoclave for 15 min at 121°C.

Appearance of uninoculated medium: Light amber, opalescent, solid medium, which may have a precipitate.

Storage:

1. Prepared medium: 2-8°C
2. Shelf life: Approximately 6-8 weeks

Quality control: Organism		*Growth*
Positive	*Pseudomonas aeruginosa* (production of blue green pigments)	+
Negative	*Escherichia coli*	−
	Uninoculated	−

Chocolate Agar[55]

Intended use: For isolation of fastidious organisms, such as *Haemophilus* and *Neisseria* species.

Formula:	*Ingredients per Liter*
GC agar base (BBL)	7.2 g
Distilled water	100.0 mL
IsoVitaleX (BBL)	2.0 mL
Hemoglobin Solution:	
Hemoglobin	2.0 g
Distilled water	100.0 mL

Method of preparation:

1. Mix GC agar base and water, boil for 1 min. Autoclave for 15 min at 121°C. Cool to 50°C.
2. Mix the hemoglobin with 2-3 mL of the distilled water to form a smooth paste. Continue mixing and gradually add the balance of the water.
3. Autoclave for 15 min at 121°C. Cool to 50°C.
4. Aseptically combine cooled base and hemoglobin solution.
5. Add 2 mL IsoVitaleX (BBL). Mix and pour 20-25 mL per petri plate.

Supplements:

Thayer-Martin Agar, modified: Add 1 mL VCN inhibitor containing 300 μg/mL of vancomycin, 750μg/mL of colistin, and 1250 units/mL of nystatin to cooled medium.

Trimethoprim lactate can be added to Thayer-Martin agar at a final concentration of 5μg/mL.

Appearance of uninoculated medium: Dark brown, opaque, solid medium.

Storage:

1. Prepared medium: 2-8°C
2. Shelf life: Approximately 1 month, plates sealed in plastic sleeves.

Quality control for Chocolate agar:	*Organism*	*Growth*
Positive	*Haemophilus influenzae*	+
	Neisseria gonorrhoeae	+
Negative	Uninoculated	–

Quality Control for Thayer-Martin medium:	*Organism*	*Growth*
Positive	*Neisseria gonorrhoeae*	+
Negative	*Neisseria sicca*	–
	Candida albicans	–
	Staphylococcus epidermidis	–
	Proteus mirabilis	–

Colistin-Nalidixic Acid

See Columbia CNA Agar

Columbia CNA (Colistin-Nalidixic Acid) Agar[10]

Intended use: A selective basal medium to which blood is added for the selective isolation of gram-positive cocci; particularly when gram-negative bacilli are present and tend to overgrow on conventional blood agar plates.

Formula:	*Ingredients per Liter*
Casein/meat (50/50) peptone	10.0 g
Polypeptone (BBL) or Pantone (Difco)	
Casein/yeast (50/50) peptone	10.0 g
Biosate (BBL) or Bitone (Difco)	
Heart peptone	3.0 g
Myosate (BBL) or Tryptic digest of Beef Heart (Difco)	
Corn starch	1.0 g
Sodium chloride	5.0 g
Agar	13.5 g
Colistin sulfate	10.0 g
Nalidixic acid	10.0–15.0 mg

Final pH 7.3 ±0.2 at 25°C

Method of preparation:

1. Suspend ingredients in 1 L of distilled or deionized water and heat to boiling to dissolve completely.

2. Sterilize in the autoclave for 15 min at 121°C. Avoid overheating. Cool to 45-50°C.
3. Aseptically add 5% sterile, defibrinated, room temperature blood (v/v).
4. Dispense 20 mL per petri dish.

Appearance of uninoculated medium: Cherry red, opaque, solid medium.

Storage:

1. Prepared medium: 2-8°C
2. Shelf life: 2 days

Quality control:	*Organism*	*Growth*
Positive	*Streptococcus pyogenes* (beta hemolysis)	+
Negative	*Escherichia coli*	–

Cystine Glucose Blood Agar (CGBA) or Cystine Heart Agar[13,44]

Intended use: A medium enriched with hemoglobin used for the cultivation of *Francisella tularensis*.

Formula:	*Ingredients per Liter*
Beef heart infusion	500.0 g
Proteose peptone	10.0 g
Dextrose	10.0 g
Sodium chloride	5.0 g
L-cystine	1.0 g
Agar	15.0 g

Final pH 6.8 ±0.2 at 25°C

Method of preparation:

1. Suspend 51.0 g of ingredients in 500 mL of distilled or deionized water and heat to boiling to dissolve completely.
2. Sterilize in the autoclave for 15 min at 121°C.
3. Place 2 g of hemoglobin powder in a dry flask and add 500 mL cold distilled or deionized water, while the flask is being agitated vigorously. The hemoglobin suspension is shaken intermittently for 10-15 min to break up all aggregates and effect complete solution.
4. Sterilize in the autoclave for 15 min at 121°C.
5. Cool both solutions to 50-60°C, mix and pour into sterile petri dishes or tubes.

Appearance of uninoculated medium: Light to medium brown, opaque, solid medium.

Storage:

1. Prepared medium: 2-8°C
2. Shelf life: Approximately 6-8 weeks

Quality control:	*Organism*	*Growth*
Positive	*Francisella tularensis*	+
Negative	Uninoculated	–

Cystine Tellurite Blood Agar[14]

Intended use: A selective and differential medium for the isolation of *Corynebacterium diphtheriae*.

Formula:	*Ingredients per Liter*
Heart infusion agar	20.0 g
Potassium tellurite, 0.3% solution	150.0 mL
L-cystine	3.0–5.0 mg
Sheep blood, defibrinated	50.0 mL

Final pH 7.4 ±0.2 at 25°C

Method of preparation:

1. Dissolve heart infusion agar in 1 L of distilled or deionized water, heat to boiling to dissolve completely.
2. Sterilize in the autoclave for 15 min at 121°C.
3. Cool to 45-50°C and maintain this temperature throughout the procedure.
4. Add aseptically 150 mL of sterile 0.3% (w/v) solution of potassium tellurite in distilled or deionized water.
5. Add aseptically 50 mL sterile, defibrinated sheep blood.
6. Add 3-5 mg of L-cystine. Dry powder may be used and need not be sterilized. Depending upon the lot of cystine, the precise amount required for optimal propagation of *Corynebacterium diphtheriae* may vary.
7. Thoroughly mix the medium and pour into sterile petri dishes with frequent shaking of the contents of the flask to insure even distribution of the cystine.

Appearance of uninoculated medium: Cherry red, opaque, solid medium.

Storage:

1. Prepared medium: 2-8°C
2. Shelf life: Approximately 1 month

Quality control: Organism		*Growth*
Positive	*Corynebacterium diphtheriae* (gray-black colony)	+
Negative	*Streptococcus pyogenes* (pin point black colonies)	±
	Uninoculated	−

Decarboxylase Broth, Moeller[35]

Intended use: A biochemical test medium for the differentiation of bacteria based on their ability to decarboxylate various amino acids to form amines and resultant alkalinity.

Formula:	*Ingredients per Liter*
Peptic digest of animal tissue, USP	5.0 g
Beef extract	5.0 g
Dextrose	0.5 g
Pyridoxal	0.005 g
Cresol red	0.005 g
Bromocresol purple	0.1 g

Final pH 6.0 ±0.2 at 25°C

Method of preparation:

1. Suspend the ingredients in 1 L of distilled or deionized water, heat to boiling to dissolve completely.
2. Divide into 4 parts, with tube 1 as a control, tube 2 as 1% L-arginine monohydrochloride, tube 3 as 1% L-lysine dihydrochloride, and tube 4 as 1% L-ornithine dihydrochloride. Alternatively, add 2% DL-amino acids.
3. Readjust the pH of the ornithine portion.
4. Dispense in 3-4 mL amounts into 13 x 100 mm screwcapped tubes and sterilize in the autoclave for 15 min at 121°C. A small amount of floccular precipitate in the ornthine does not interfere with its use.
5. Cool and inoculate test and control portions lightly from a young agar slant culture.
6. Aseptically overlay the inoculated broth tubes and controls with 4-5 mm sterile mineral oil.
7. Incubate tubes at 35°C for up to 4 days. Tubes must be read daily after 24 h incubation and observed for a change in color. Positive reactions are indicated by alkaline (purple) reactions. The media turns yellow first due to acid production from glucose.

Appearance of uninoculated medium: Yellowish to purple, slightly opalescent, liquid medium.

Storage:

1. Prepared medium: 2-8°C
2. Shelf life: Approximately 6-8 weeks

Quality control:	*Organism*	*Growth*
Positive	*Salmonella arizonae* (positive reaction purple or yellow-purple color)	+
Negative	*Proteus vulgaris* (negative reaction yellow color)	+
	Uninoculated	−

DNase Test Agar[29]

Intended use: A medium for the isolation and differentiation of bacteria based upon their deoxyribonuclease activity.

Formula:	*Ingredients per Liter*
DNA	2.0 g
Pancreatic digest of casein, USP	15.0 g
Papaic digest of soy meal, USP	5.0 g
Sodium chloride	5.0 g
Agar	15.0 g

Final pH 7.3 ±0.2 at 25°C

Method of preparation:

1. Dissolve ingredients in 1 L of distilled or deionized water. Heat to boiling to dissolve completely.
2. Sterilize in the autoclave for 15 min at 121°C.
3. Dispense 20 mL in petri dishes. Allow to solidify.
4. Plates are inoculated heavily over a 1 cm^2 area. Several cultures may be tested on the same plate.
5. Incubate for 18–24 h at 35°C and flood with 1N HCl. A zone of clearing around the colony indicates a positive DNase test.

Appearance of uninoculated medium: Light to medium amber, slightly opalescent, solid medium.

Storage:

1. Prepared medium: 2-8°C
2. Shelf life: Approximately 4-8 weeks

Quality control: Organism		*Growth*
Positive	*Serratia marcescens*	+ (zone)
Negative	*Klebsiella pneumoniae*	+ (no zone)
	Uninoculated	−

Alternate method of Gilardi:

DNase test agar	1.0 L
Toluidine blue	0.1 g

Inoculate as described above, and observe for a change in the indicator to pink around the growth.

Enriched Gonococcal Agar (GcHbS, see Gonococcal Agar, Enriched)

Farrell's Medium[11]

Intended use: A medium for the selective isolation of *Brucella abortus* from contaminated sources.

Formula:	*Ingredients per Liter*
Serum dextrose agar base	35.0 g
Sterile, inactivated horse serum	50.0 mL (v/v)
Sterile dextrose	10.0 g
Bacitracin	25,000 units
Vancomycin	20,000 μg
Polymyxin B	5,000 units
Nalidixic acid	100,000 units
Nystatin	100,000 units
Cycloheximide	100,000 units

Method of preparation:

1. Dissolve ingredients of base in 1 L of distilled or deionized water, heat to boiling to dissolve completely.
2. Sterilize in the autoclave for 15 min at 121°C.
3. Cool to 45-50°C.
4. Aseptically add 5% sterile, inactivated horse serum, mix.
5. Aseptically add 1% sterile dextrose, mix.
6. Aseptically add sterile antibiotics, mix.
7. Dispense 20 mL per petri dish.

Appearance of uninoculated medium: Light amber, slightly opalescent solid medium.

Storage:

1. Prepared medium: 2-8°C
2. Shelf life: Approximately 2-4 weeks

Quality control: Organism		*Growth*
Positive	*Brucella abortus*	+
Negative	*Escherichia coli*	–
	Uninoculated	–

Fletcher's Medium[12]

Intended use: A medium for the isolation, cultivation and maintenance of cultures of *Leptospira*.

Formula:	*Ingredients per Liter*
Peptone	0.3 g
Beef extract	0.2 g
Sodium chloride	0.5 g
Agar	1.5 g
Rabbit serum (filter-sterilized, inactivated)	8–10% v/v

Final pH 7.8 ±0.2 at 25°C

Method of preparation:

1. Dissolve basal ingredients in 920 mL of distilled or deionized water.
2. Heat to boiling to dissolve completely.
3. Sterilize in the autoclave for 15 min at 121°C.
4. Allow the medium to cool to 50-55°C and add 80 mL of sterile rabbit serum.
5. Aseptically dispense into sterile screwcapped tubes in 5-7 mL amounts. Store at room temperature overnight.
6. Inactivate the whole medium the day following its preparation by placing the tubes in a water bath at 56°C for one hour.
7. Allow to cool before inoculating.

Appearance of uninoculated medium: Very light amber, very slightly opalescent, solid medium.

Storage:

1. Prepared medium: Below 30°C
2. Shelf life: Approximately 6-8 weeks

Quality control: Organism		*Growth*
Positive	*Leptospira interrogans*	+
Negative	Uninoculated	−

Gelatin Agar[53]

Intended use: A nonselective medium for the cultivation of *Vibrio cholerae* and other pathogenic *Vibrio* species.

Formula:	*Ingredients per Liter*
Peptone	4.0 g
Yeast extract	1.0 g
Gelatin	15.0 g
Sodium chloride	30.0 g
Agar	15.0 g

Final pH 7.2 ±0.2 at 25°C

Method of preparation:

1. Suspend ingredients in 1 L of distilled or deionized water and heat to boiling to dissolve completely (Delete NaCl for selective isolation of *Vibrio cholerae*).
2. Sterilize in the autoclave for 15 min at 121°C.
3. Dispense 20 mL in petri dish.

Appearance of uninoculated medium: Light amber, cloudy, solid medium.

Storage:

1. Prepared medium: 2-8°C
2. Shelf life: Approximately 6-8 weeks

Quality control: Organism		*Growth*
Positive	*Vibrio cholerae*	+ (clear zone)
Negative	Uninoculated	−

Gelatin-Cysteine-Thiosulfate (GCF) Medium

Intended use: Detection of H_2S formation by selected *Enterobacteriaceae*.

Formula:	*Ingredients per Liter*
Lab lemco (Oxoid)	3.0 g
Tryptone (Oxoid)	10.0 g
Potassium chloride	4.0 g
L-cysteine hydrochloride	0.1 g
Sodium thiosufate	0.1 g
Ferric ammonium citrate	0.4 g
Agar (Difco Bacto)	12.0 g

Final pH 7.4 ±0.2 at 25°C

Method of preparation:

1. Suspend ingredients in 1 L of distilled or deionized water and heat to boiling to dissolve agar completely.
2. Dispense in tubes that can be used for stab culturing.
3. Sterilize in the autoclave for 15 min at 121°C.

Appearance of uninoculated medium: Light amber, clear to slightly opalescent, no significant precipitate.

Storage:

1. Prepared medium: 2-8°C
2. Shelf life: Approximately 6-8 weeks

Quality control: Organism		*Growth*
Positive	*Aeromonas hydrophila* (ATCC 7965)	+
Negative	*Aeromonas caviae* (ATCC 15468)	–

Gelatin, Nutrient[6]

Intended use: A medium used for determining gelatin liquefaction (gelatinase production) by proteolytic microorganisms.

Formula:	*Ingredients per liter*
Nutrient broth	8.0 g
Gelatin	120.0 g

Final pH 6.8 ±0.2 at 25°C

Method of preparation:

1. Suspend ingredients in 1 L of distilled or deionized water.
2. Warm to 50°C to dissolve completely.

3. Distribute into tubes.
4. Sterilize in the autoclave for 15 min at 121°C.
5. Inoculate by stabbing with a wire and incubate at 20°C for 30 days.

Appearance of uninoculated medium: Medium amber, clear to slightly opalescent, solid medium.

Storage:

1. Prepared medium: 2-8°C
2. Shelf life: Approximately 6 months

Quality control:	*Organism*	*Growth*
Positive	*Proteus vulgaris* (liquefication)	+
Negative	*Escherichia coli* (no liquefication)	+
	Uninoculated	−

Gonococcal Agar, Enriched (GcHbS)[7]

Intended use: For isolation of fastidious organisms, in particular, *Haemophilus ducreyi.*

Formula:	*Ingredients per Liter*
Gc agar base, Gibco	36.0
Distilled water	600.0 mL
CVA (Gibco)	10.0 mL
Fetal calf or sheep serum	50.0 mL
Vancomycin	3.0 mg
Hemoglobin, bovine	10.0 g
Distilled water	440.0 mL

Method of preparation:

1. Mix Gc agar and 600 mL water and boil for 1 min. Autoclave at 121 °C for 15 min. Cool to 50°C.
2. Mix the hemoglobin with 20-30 mL of the distilled water to form a smooth paste. Continue mixing and gradually add the balance of the water.
3. Aseptically combine the base and the hemoglobin solution.
4. Add 10 mL CVA, 50 mL fetal calf or sheep serum and 3 mg vancomycin. Mix and pour 20-25 mL per petri plate.

Appearance of uninoculated medium: Dark brown, opaque, solid medium.

Storage:

1. Prepared medium: 2-8°C
2. Shelf life: 2 weeks

Quality control:	*Organism*	*Growth*
Positive	*Haemophilus ducreyi*	+
Negative	Uninoculated	–

7H11 Agar, Middlebrook, see Middlebrook 7H11 Agar

Inositol-Brilliant Green-Bile Salts Agar[50,60]

Intended use: A selective and differential medium for the isolation of *Plesiomonas shigelloides* and *Aeromonas* from feces.

Formula:	*Ingredients per Liter*
Proteose peptone (Difco)	10.0 g
Lab lemco extract (Oxoid)	5.0 g
Meso-inositol	10.0 g
Sodium chloride	5.0 g
Bile salts no. 3 (Difco)	8.5 g
Agar	15.0 g
Brilliant green	0.33 mg
Neutral red	25.0 mg

Final pH 7.2 ±0.2 at 25°C

Method of preparation:

1. Suspend ingredients in 1 L of distilled or deionized water and heat to boiling to dissolve agar completely.
2. Sterilize in the autoclave for 15 min at 121°C.
3. Dispense 20 mL per petri dish.

Appearance of uninoculated medium: Reddish-green colored solid medium.

Storage:

1. Prepared medium: 2-8°C
2. Shelf life: Approximately 6-8 weeks

Quality control:	*Organism*	*Growth*
Positive	*Plesiomonas shigelloides* (reddish pink colored colonies or white colonies with a reddish coloration)	+
	Aeromonas spp. (no reddish coloration)	+
Negative	*Staphylococcus* spp. (Acid reaction from inositol utilization)	−

Johnson's Medium[21]

Intended use: A medium for the cultivation and maintenance of the *Leptospira*. The basal medium and the enrichment are prepared according to the formulations described by Ellinghausen and McCullough as modified by Johnson and Harris.

Formula:	*Ingredients per Liter*
Basal Medium:	
10% Sodium phosphate, dibasic	10.0 mL
3% Potassium phosphate, monobasic	10.0 mL
10% Sodium chloride	10.0 mL
25% Ammonium chloride	1.0 mL
0.5% Thiamine	1.0 mL
10% w/v glycerol (8% v/v)	1.0 mL
Final pH 7.15 at 25°C	
Albumin Enrichment:	
Bovine albumin fraction V	20.0 g
Sterile distilled or deionized water	100.0 mL
1.0% Calcium chloride, anhydrous	2.0 mL
1.0% Magnesium chloride ($MgCl_2 \cdot 6H_2O$)	2.0 mL
0.4% Zinc sulfate ($ZnSO_4 \cdot 7H_2O$)	2.0 mL
0.3% Copper sulfate ($CuSO_4 \cdot 5H_2O$)	2.0 mL
0.5% Ferrous sulfate ($FeSO_4 \cdot 7H_2O$)	20.0 mL
0.02% Vitamin B_{12}	2.0 mL
10% Tween 80	25.0 mL
Final pH 7.4 at 25°C	
Complete Medium:	
Sterile basal medium	900 mL
Sterile albumin enrichment	100 mL
Final pH 7.2 at 25°C	

Method of preparation:

1. Mix the ingredients of basal medium in 940 mL of distilled or deionized water. Swirl to dissolve completely.

2. Sterilize in the autoclave for 15 min at 121°C.
3. Allow to cool to room temperature.
4. For the albumin enrichment, add the albumin slowly to the distilled or deionized water, stirring gently to avoid foaming.
5. After the albumin is completely dissolved, slowly add the remaining components. Mix continuously. Add 1.6 mL 1N sodium hydroxide and adjust to a total volume of 200 mL. Filter sterilize.
6. Aseptically mix 100 mL of sterile albumin enrichment with 900 mL of sterile basal medium.
7. Aseptically dispense into sterile tubes or bottles as desired.

Appearance of uninoculated medium: Colorless, clear liquid medium.

Storage:

1. Prepared medium: 2-8°C
2. Shelf life: Approximately 6-8 weeks

Quality control:	*Organism*	*Growth*
Positive	*Leptospira interrogans* (after 2-7 days at 29-30°C)	+
Negative	Uninoculated	–

Loeffler's Serum Medium

Intended use: A medium for the recovery of *C. diphtheriae* from clinical specimens. Because of its serum content, the medium may also be used more generally to determine the proteolytic activity of various microorganisms.

Formula:	*Ingredients per Liter*
Beef serum	70.0 g
Infusion dextrose broth (dry powder)	2.5 g
Egg (whole, dried)	7.5 g

Final pH 7.6

Method of preparation:

1. To rehydrate the medium, dissolve 80 g of the above Loeffler's medium (BBL) in one liter of distilled water and warm to 42-45°C.
2. Gradually add the powder while gently rotating the flask to minimize mixing air into the suspension.
3. Dispense in tubes when the suspension is uniform.

4. Arrange the tubes in a slant position not more than four deep with several layers of newspaper or paper towels below and above the tubes to prevent rapid coagulation.
5. Tightly close the autoclave, turn on the steam, and allow pressure to remain at 10 ppi for 20 min.
6. During this time allow no air or steam to escape.
7. Adjust the steam-inlet valve and open the air-escape valve so as to maintain a pressure of 10 ppi. Abrupt changes in pressure may cause the medium to bubble.
8. Close the outlet valve when all air has been replaced by steam and allow the pressure to reach 15 ppi and hold there for 15 min.
9. Allow the autoclave to cool slowly. The slants should be incubated before inoculation for 24 hours at 35°C as a sterility check.

Appearance of uninoculated medium: Smooth, gray-white solid slanted medium.

Storage:

1. Prepared medium: 2-8°C
2. Shelf life: Sealed tubes, approximately 1 month

Quality Control:	*Organism*	*Growth*
Positive	*C. diphtheriae*	+
Negative	Uninoculated	−

MacConkey Agar[30]

Intended use: A selective and differential medium for the isolation of lactose- and nonlactose-fermenting organisms.

Formula:	*Ingredients per Liter*
Bacto peptone (Difco) or Gelysate (BBL)	17.0 g
Proteose peptone (Difco) or Polypeptone (BBL)	3.0 g
Lactose	10.0 g
Bile salts	1.5 g
Sodium chloride	5.0 g
Agar	13.5 g
Neutral red	0.03 g
Crystal violet	0.001 g

Final pH 7.1 ±0.2 at 25°C

Method of preparation:

1. Suspend the ingredients in 1 L distilled or deionized water. Heat to boiling with gentle swirling to dissolve completely.

2. Sterilize in the autoclave for 15 min at 121°C. Avoid over-heating of the medium. If inoculated the same day as prepared the medium may be used without autoclave sterilization after it has been boiled for 2-3 min. Sucrose may be added to give a final concentration of 1%.
3. Cool to 45-50°C and dispense in approximately 20 mL amounts into sterile petri dishes or as slants in tubes.
4. The surface of the medium should be dry when inoculated. Drying may be accomplished by allowing the medium to stand after dispensing for 1-2 h with lids slightly ajar.

Appearance of uninoculated medium: Reddish-purple, slightly opalescent, solid medium.

Storage:

1. Prepared medium: 2-8°C
2. Shelf life: Approximately 6-8 weeks

Quality control:	*Organism*	*Growth*
Positive	*Escherichia coli* (pink-red with some bile precipitation)	+
Negative	*Enterococcus* species	–
	Uninoculated	–

Middlebrook 7H11 Agar[33]

Intended use: A nonselective medium for the isolation, cultivation and antimicrobial susceptibility testing of *Mycobacterium.*

Formula:	*Ingredients per Liter*
Middlebrook 7H11 agar (Difco)	21.0 g
OADC enrichment (Difco)	100.0 mL
Glycerol	5.0 g

Final pH 6.6 ±0.2 at 25°C

Method of preparation:

1. Suspend the dehydrated powder in 900 mL of distilled or deionized water containing 5 mL glycerol and heat to boiling to dissolve completely.
2. Sterilize in the autoclave for 10-15 min at 121°C. Cool to 50-55°C.
3. Aseptically add 100 mL OADC enrichment and mix thoroughly.
4. If preparing the medium for sensitivity testing, add drugs at this point.

5. Dispense as desired within 1 h of sterilization and allow to solidify at room temperature in the dark.

Appearance of uninoculated medium: Light amber, very slightly opalescent, solid medium.

Storage:

1. Prepared medium: 2-8°C, protected from light
2. Shelf life: Approximately 4 weeks

Quality control:	*Organism*	*Growth*
Positive	*Mycobacterium tuberculosis*	+
Negative	Uninoculated	−

Modified Wadowsky-Yee (MWY) Medium[8]

Intended use: A selective medium for the isolation of *Legionella pneumophila*.

Formula:	*Ingredients per Liter*
Yeast extract	10.0 g
Agar (Difco)	17.0 g
Activated charcoal (Norit A)	1.5 g
ACES [N-(2-acetamido)-2-aminoethanesul fonic acid] buffer	10.0 g
KOH pellets (reagent grade, 85% KOH)	2.9 g
α-ketoglutarate, monopotassium (Sigma)	1.0 g
Glycine (Sigma)	3.0 g

Final pH 6.9 ±0.05 at 40°C

Method of preparation:

1. Prepare as for BCYE-α medium, except that 2.9 g of KOH and glycine are added to this medium.
2. Autoclave for 15 min at 121°C. Cool to 50°C in a water bath.
3. Add filter-sterilized supplements and antimicrobial agents separately.

L-cysteine hydrochloride (ICN)	0.4 g
Ferric pyrophosphate (Sigma)	0.25 g
Polymyxin B sulfate (Pfizer or Sigma) (as base)	80,000 U
Vancomycin hydrochloride (Lilly) (as base)	1.0 mg
Anisomycin (General Diagnostics)	80.0 mg

4. If differential medium is desired, add 1.0 mL of filter-sterilized dyes separately. Dissolve each dye in 0.1N potassium hydroxide in amounts that will yield 10 mg/mL.

Bromothymol blue (Sigma)	10.0 mg
Bromocresol purple (Sigma)	10.0 mg

5. Check pH, which should be between 6.85-6.95 at 40°C. Correct pH with 1N hydrochloric acid or potassium hydroxide pellets.
6. Cool to 40°C and pour into petri dishes.
7. Preincubate the entire batch for 24 h at 35°C to detect contaminants.
8. Cool to room temperature and store non-contaminated plates.

Appearance of uninoculated medium: Black, opaque, solid medium. With bromothymol blue or bromocresol purple added, the plates are purplish-black, opaque, solid medium.

Storage:

1. Prepared medium: 2-8°C
2. Shelf life: Approximately 1 month in plastic sleeves

Quality control:	*Organism*	*Growth*
Positive	*Legionella pneumophila* (white to pale green colonies)	+
Negative	*Legionella micdadei* (blue colonies)	+
	Escherichia coli	−

Moeller Decarboxylase Broth, see Decarboxylase Broth.

Motility Test Medium[15]

Intended use: A differential medium use to demonstrate motility particularly among the nonfermenting gram negative bacteria.

Formula:	*Ingredients per Liter*
Pancreatic digest of casein, USP	100.0 g
Yeast extract	3.0 g
Sodium chloride	5.0 g
Agar	3.0 g

Final pH 7.2 ±0.2 at 25°C

Method of preparation:

1. Suspend ingredients in 1 L of distilled or deionized water and heat to boiling to dissolve completely.

2. Dispense 3.5 mL per 13 x 100 mm tubes and sterilize in the autoclave for 15 min at 121°C.
3. Allow the medium to cool quickly with tubes in the upright position. Place tubes in cold water for best results.
4. Inoculate sterile medium by stabbing through the center of the medium.
5. Incubate at the proper temperature for organism under consideration and examine at 18-40 h.
6. Motility is manifested macroscopically by a diffuse zone of growth spreading from the line of inoculation. Certain species of motile bacteria will show diffuse growth throughout the entire medium, while others may show diffusion from one or two points only, appearing as modular growths along the line of the stab.

Appearance of uninoculated medium: Light amber, clear to slightly opalescent, semi-solid medium.

Storage:

1. Prepared medium: 2-8°C
2. Shelf life: Approximately 6 months

Quality control:	*Organism*	*Growth*
Positive	*Pseudomonas aeruginosa*	+ (motility)
Negative	*Flavobacterium*	+ (no motility)
	Uninoculated	–

Mueller-Hinton Agar[38,64]

Intended use: A standardized medium for testing the susceptibility of microorganisms to antimicrobial agents as described in the disk-diffusion techniques of The World Health Organization and The National Committee for Clinical Laboratory Standards.

Formula:	*Ingredients per Liter*
Beef, Infusion	300.0 g
Acid hydrolysate of casein	17.5 g
Starch	1.5 g
Agar	17.0 g

Final pH 7.3 ±0.1 at 25°C

Method of preparation:

1. Suspend the ingredients in 1 L of distilled or deionized water and heat to boiling to dissolve completely.

2. Sterilize in the autoclave for 15 min at 121°C.
3. Cool to 45-50°C and add blood, if necessary.
4. Dispense as desired.

Appearance of uninoculated medium: Light amber, slightly opalescent, solid medium.

Storage:

1. Prepared medium: 2-8°C
2. Shelf life: Approximately 6-8 weeks

Quality control:	*Organism*	*Growth*
Positive	*Escherichia coli* (ATCC 2522)	+
	Staphylococcus aureus (ATCC 25923)	+
	Pseudomonas aeruginosa (ATCC 27853)	+
Negative	Uninoculated	–

Mueller-Hinton Agar (MHHB), Enriched[7]

Intended use: For isolation of fastidious organisms, particularly, *Haemophilus ducreyi*.

Formula:	*Ingredients per Liter*
Mueller-Hinton agar (BBL)	38.0 g
Horse blood	50.0 mL
CVA (Gibco)	10.0
Vancomycin	3.0 mg

Method of preparation:

1. Prepare base as described for Mueller-Hinton agar. Cool after autoclaving and aseptically add horse blood.
2. Heat medium to 80°C for 15 min (to chocolatize horse blood) until the medium is a chocolate brown color.
3. Aseptically add CVA and vancomycin. Mix and dispense as desired.

Appearance of uninoculated medium: Brown, opaque, solid medium.

Storage:

1. Prepared medium: 2-8°C
2. Shelf life: 2 weeks

Quality control:	*Organism*	*Growth*
Positive	*Haemophilus ducreyi*	+
Negative	Uninoculated	−

Mueller Hinton Broth, Cation Supplemented, see Cation Supplemented Mueller Hinton Broth (CSMHB)

Mycoplasma Agar Medium[9,17]

Intended use: A medium for the selective isolation of *Mycoplasma*.

Formula:	*Ingredients per Liter*
Basal Medium:	
Mycoplasma broth base (1)	21.0 g
Purified agar (Noble) (2)	8.5 g
Water (3)	700.0 mL
Supplements:	
Horse serum (1)(4)	200.0 mL
Yeast extract (1)(5)	100.0 mL
Optional Supplements:	
Antibiotics (6)	
Penicillin G sodium	1,000,000 units
Ampicillin sodium	1.0 g
Polymyxin B sulfate	500,000 units
Amphotericin B	0.5 g
Nystatin USP	50,000 units
Metabolic Indicators (7)	
Dextrose (8)	20.0 mL
Arginine·HCl (9)	4.0 mL
Phenol red sodium (10)	2.0 mL

Final pH 7.8 ±0.1 at 25°C

(1) Lots must be pretested for ability to support optimum growth of *M. pneumoniae*.
(2) Crude agars inhibitory: ultra-pure agar at equivalent density may be used. Omit for broth medium.

(3) Glass-distilled or high-quality deionized.
(4) IgG-free serum may be substituted.
(5) Active dry baker's yeast 25% w/v in distilled water. Autoclave at 121°C for 5 min. Clarify by filtration/centrifugation. Sterilize in the autoclave for 15 min at 121°C. Store at −20°C.
(6) For primary isolation, select according to specimen source: penicillin usually adequate for respiratory tract specimens, broader spectrum antibiotics may be needed for genitourinary samples. Amphotericin contains desoxycholate as a solubilizer which may be deleterious to mycoplasmas.
(7) Broth only.
(8) Sterile 50% solution, USP.
(9) Filter-sterilized 50% stock solution. Store at -20°C.
(10) Autoclave-sterilized 1% stock solution.

Method of preparation:

1. Heat the basal medium to dissolve.
2. Sterilize in the autoclave for 15 min at 121°C.
3. Cool to 56°C, then aseptically add supplements and/or optional supplements.
4. Dispense 20 mL in petri dishes or desired amount into sterile culture vessels.

Appearance of uninoculated medium: Amber, slightly opalescent, solid medium.

Storage:

1. Prepared base and completed media: room temperature, 2-8°C
2. Shelf life: With additives and supplements, not longer than 2 weeks: base only, approximately 6-8 weeks.

Quality control:	*Organism*	*Growth*
Positive	*Mycoplasma pneumoniae*	+
Negative	Uninoculated	−

Mycoplasma Broth Medium SP-4[9,58]

Intended use: A medium used for the cultivation of fastidious, classic *Mycoplasma*.

Formula:	*Ingredients per Liter*
Basal Medium:	
Mycoplasma broth base	3.5 g
Tryptone	10.0 g
Peptone	5.0 g
Dextrose (1)	10.0 mL
Water (2)	615.0 mL
Supplements:	
CMRL 1066 tissue culture medium (3)	50.0 mL
Yeast extract (4)	35.0 mL
Yeastolate (5)	100.0 mL
Fetal bovine serum (6)	170.0 mL
Optional Supplements:	see Mycoplasma Agar Medium

Final pH 7.5 ±0.1 at 25°C

(1) Sterile 50% solution, USP
(2) Glass-distilled or deionized
(3) 10X concentration, with glutamine, without sodium bicarbonate (Gibco or equivalent)
(4) Lots must be pretested for ability to support optimum growth of *M. pneumoniae*. Active dry baker's yeast 25% w/v in distilled water. Autoclave at 121°C for 5 min; clarify by filtration/centrifugation. Autoclave for 5 min at 121°C. Store at −20°C.
(5) 2% solution
(6) Heat at 56°C for 45 min

Method of preparation:

1. Dissolve basal medium ingredients, adjust to pH 7.5.
2. Sterilize in the autoclave for 15 min at 121°C.
3. Cool to 45-50°C and aseptically add supplements.
4. Dispense in tubes or bottles.

Appearance of uninoculated medium: Medium amber, slightly opalescent, liquid medium.

Storage:

1. Prepared base and completed media: 2-8°C
2. Shelf life: With additives and supplements, approximately 3-4 weeks. Base only, approximately 6-8 weeks.

Quality control: Organism		*Growth*
Positive	*Mycoplasma pneumoniae*	+
Negative	Uninoculated	–

Nitrate Reduction Broth[15]

Intended use: A medium for the determination of nitrate reduction by bacteria.

Formula:	*Ingredients per Liter*
Pancreatic digest of casein	10.0 g
Yeast extract	3.0 g
Potassium nitrate	2.0 g

Final pH 7.1 ±0.2 at 25°C

Method of preparation:

1. Suspend ingredients in 1 L of distilled or deionized water and heat to boiling to dissolve completely.
2. Dispense 4 mL into 13 × 100 mm test tubes containing Durham vials.
3. Sterilize in the autoclave for 15 min at 121°C.
4. For *Pseudomonas* and other gram-negative bacteria, inoculate and incubate at 30°C (or 35°C). Examine after 24 and 48 h for reduction of nitrate to nitrogen gas which accumulates in the Durham tube. After 48 h test for nitrite by the addition of 0.5 mL each of reagents A and B. A red color indicates a positive test, provided the uninoculated control medium is negative. Negative tests should be confirmed by the addition of zinc dust to convert unreduced nitrate to nitrite.

See Reagent section for reagents A and B formulae.

Appearance of uninoculated medium: Light amber, clear liquid medium.

Storage:

1. Prepared medium: 2-8°C
2. Shelf life: Approximately 6 months

Quality control:	*Organism*	*Growth*
Positive	*Pseudomonas aeruginosa* (nitrate positive, gas positive)	+
Negative	*Acinetobacter calcoaceticus* (nitrate negative, gas negative)	+
	Uninoculated	−

Nutrient Gelatin, see Gelatin, Nutrient

Oxidation-Fermentation (OF) Test Medium (OF Basal Medium)[19]

Intended use: A differential medium used for the classification of gram-negative microorganisms on the basis of fermentative and oxidative metabolism of carbohydrates, especially for the *Corynebacterium, Enterobacteriaceae, Aeromonas, Pseudomonas* and nonfermenting gram-negative bacteria.

Formula:	*Ingredients per Liter*
Peptone (pancreatic digest of casein)	2.0 g
Sodium chloride	5.0 g
Dipotassium phosphate	0.3 g
Bromothymol blue	0.03 g
Agar	3.0 g

Final pH 7.1 ±0.2 at 25°C

Method of preparation:

1. Suspend ingredients in 1 L of distilled or deionized water and heat to boiling to dissolve completely.
2. Distribute in appropriate amounts and sterilize in the autoclave for 15 min at 121°C.
3. To 90 mL of sterile base medium add 10 mL of sterile 10% carbohydrate solution.
4. Mix thoroughly and aseptically dispense in 5 mL amounts into sterile 13 x 100 mm culture tubes.
5. Inoculate (stab) lightly two tubes of medium from a young agar slant culture. Cover one of the tubes with a layer (about 5 mm) of sterile melted petrolatum or sterile paraffin oil.
6. Incubate at 35°C and observe daily for 3-4 days. Acid formation only in the open tube indicates oxidative utilization of carbohydrate. Acid formation in both the open and the sealed tube is indicative of a

fermentative reaction. Lack of acid production in both tubes indicates that the organism does not utilize carbohydrate by either method.

Appearance of uninoculated medium: Green, clear to very slightly opalescent, liquid medium.

Storage:

1. Prepared medium: 2-8°C
2. Shelf life: Approximately 6 months

Quality control: Organism (in dextrose)		*Growth*
Positive	*Escherichia coli* (acid = yellow and gas open and closed)	+
Negative	*Alcaligenes faecalis* (alkaline = green open and closed)	+
	Uninoculated	–

Peptone-Yeast Extract Glucose Broth (PYG)[18,36]

Intended use: A medium for the cultivation of anaerobes.

Formula:	*Ingredients per Liter*
Peptone (Difco)	20.0 g
Yeast extract (Difco)	10.0 g
L-cysteine hydrochloride·H_2O	0.5 g
Resazurin solution (1)	4.0 mL
D-glucose (sterile) (2)	10.0 g
Salt solution (3)	40.0 mL

Final pH 7.0 ±0.2 at 25°C

(1) 11 mg resazurin in 44 mL distilled or deionized water.
(2) Add D-glucose to 100 mL distilled or deionized water and sterilize though a 0.45 μm membrane filter.
(3) Salt solution

Calcium chloride ($CaCl_2 \cdot 2H_2O$)	0.2 g
Magnesium sulfate ($MgSO_4 \cdot 7H_2O$)	0.2 g
Potassium phosphate, dibasic	1.0 g
Sodium bicarbonate	10.0 g
Sodium chloride	2.0 g

Add calcium chloride and magnesium sulfate to 300 mL of distilled or deionized water and stir until dissolved. Add 500 mL distilled or deionized water and remaining salts, while mixing. After all salts have dissolved, add

200 mL distilled or deionized water, stir and store at 4°C. Each new lot must be analyzed for volatile and nonvolatile acids.

Method of preparation:

1. Suspend ingredients, except glucose, in 900 mL of distilled or deionized water and heat to dissolve completely. Adjust pH to 6.95–7.0 with a 0.1N Hydrochloric acid or 0.1N Sodium hydroxide.
2. Dispense in 5 mL amounts into 10 x 125 mm screwcapped tubes.
3. Autoclave for 15 min at 121°C.
4. Cool and add filter-sterilized glucose.

Appearance of uninoculated medium: Light amber, clear liquid medium.

Storage:

1. Prepared medium: 2-8°C
2. Shelf life: Approximately 6-12 months

Quality control: Organism		*Growth*
Positive	*Bacteroides fragilis*	+
Negative	Uninoculated	−

Pril-Xylose-Ampicillin Agar[49,60]

Intended use: A selective and differential medium for the isolation and differentiation of oxidase-positive *Aeromonas hydrophila* from other oxidase-positive organisms found in feces.

Formula:	*Ingredients per Liter*
Nutrient agar	23.0 g
Xylose	10.0 g
Phenol red	25.0 mg
Ampicillin, sterile	30.0 mg
Pril, 0.02% (Quaternary ammonium detergent: mixture of primary alkyl-sulfate, alkyl-benzyl sulfonate and salts which prevent the swarming of *Proteus*.)	0.2 g

Method of preparation:

1. Suspend 23 g of nutrient agar in 1 L distilled or deionized water and heat to boiling to dissolve completely.

2. Sterilize in the autoclave for 15 min at 121°C.
3. Add aseptically the xylose, phenol red, Pril and ampicillin; mix thoroughly.
4. Dispense 20 mL per petri dish.

Appearance of uninoculated medium: Pinkish-yellow solid medium.

Storage:

1. Prepared medium: 2-8°C
2. Shelf life: Approximately 6-8 weeks

Quality control: Organism		*Growth*
Positive	*Aeromonas hydrophila* (colorless colonies)	+
Negative	*E. coli* (yellow colonies or inhibited)	±
	Uninoculated	−

Pyrazinamidase Test Medium and Reagent[59,61]

Intended use: A medium for the detection of pyrazinamidase in mycobacteria.

Formula:	*Ingredients per Liter*
Medium:	
Dubose broth base	6.5 g
Pyrazinamide	0.1 g
Pyruvic acid, sodium salt	2.0 g
Agar	15.0 g

Final pH 6.6 ±0.2 at 25°C

Reagent:
Ferrous ammonium sulfate, 1% aqueous. Prepare fresh before each use.

Method of preparation:

1. Suspend ingredients in 1 L of distilled or deionized water and heat to boiling to dissolve completely.
2. Dispense in 5 mL amounts in 16 x 125 mm screwcapped tubes.
3. Sterilize in the autoclave for 15 min at 121°C.
4. Allow to harden upright, not slanted.

Appearance of uninoculated medium: Very light amber, clear solid medium.

Storage:

1. Prepared medium: 2-8°C; Reagent: prepared fresh before each use
2. Shelf life: Approximately 4-8 weeks

Quality control:	*Organism*	*Growth*
Positive	*Mycobacterium tuberulosis* (pink color)	+
Negative	*Mycobacterium bovis* (no change in color)	+
	Uninoculated	–

Regan-Lowe (RL) Medium[43]

Intended use: A medium for the primary isolation of *Bordetella pertussis* and *Bordetella parapertussis*.

Formula:	*Ingredients per Liter*
Charcoal agar (Oxoid CM 119)	51.0 g
Horse blood, defibrinated	100.0 mL
Cephalexin	0.04 g
Amphotericin B (optional)	0.05 g

Final pH 7.4 ±0.2 at 25°C

Method of preparation:

1. Suspend charcoal agar dehydrated powder in 1 L of deionized or distilled water, and bring to a boil to dissolve completely.
2. Sterilize in the autoclave for 15 min at 121°C.
3. Cool to 50°C and add defibrinated horse blood (to 10% v/v) and cephalexin (to 40 µg/mL final concentration), and optionally add amphotericin B (50 µg/mL final concentration).
4. Mix gently and dispense into sterile petri plates.

Appearance of uninoculated medium : Base: grayish-black, opaque, solid medium. Base with blood: reddish-black, opaque, solid medium.

Storage:

1. Prepared medium with blood: 2-8°C
2. Shelf life: With blood, approximately 1-2 weeks
   Without blood, approximately 1 year

Quality control: Organism		*Growth*
Positive	Properly maintained clinical isolates of *Bordetella pertussis* and optionally, properly maintained clinical isolates of *B. parapertussis*	+
Negative	Uninoculated	–

Regan-Lowe Semisolid Transport Medium[43]

Intended use: A transport medium for *Bordetella pertussis* and *Bordetella parapertussis*.

Formula:

(See Regan-Lowe Medium)

Method of preparation:

1. Prepare Regan-Lowe agar as for plates, but use only 25.5 g of Oxoid CM 119 charcoal agar. After adding the blood and both antibiotic supplements, aseptically dispense into small screwcapped vials to fill them half full.
2. Seal tightly.

Comments:

The use of Oxoid CM 119 agar base is necessary for good results. The components of CM 119 in g/L are as follows: Lab-Lemco powder - 10; peptone - 10; starch - 10; bacteriological charcoal - 4; NaCl - 5; nicotinic acid - 0.001; agar - 12. Amphotericin B is not routinely added to RL plates. Some American workers have successfully substituted defibrinated sheep blood for the horse blood in plates. However, use of sheep blood in transport medium is untested.

Appearance of uninoculated medium: Base with blood: reddish-black, opaque, solid medium.

Storage:

1. Prepared medium with blood: 2-8°C
2. Shelf life: Approximately 2 months

Quality control: Organism		*Growth*
Positive	Properly maintained clinical isolates of *Bordetella pertussis* and optionally, properly maintained clinical isolates of *B. parapertussis*	+
Negative	Uninoculated	−

Serum Dextrose Agar[22]

Intended use: A medium for the cultivation of *Brucella.*

Formula:	*Ingredients per Liter*
Peptone	10.0 g
Meat extract	5.0 g
Sodium chloride	5.0 g
Agar	15.0 g

Final pH 7.5 ±0.2 at 25°C

Method of preparation:

1. Dissolve ingredients in 1 L of distilled or deionized water, heat to boiling to dissolve completely.
2. Sterilize in the autoclave for 15 min at 121°C.
3. Cool to 45-50°C.
4. Aseptically add 5% sterile, inactivated horse serum.
5. Aseptically add 1% sterile dextrose.
6. Mix thoroughly then pour 20mL per petri plate.

Appearance of uninoculated medium: Light amber, slightly opalescent, solid medium.

Storage:

1. Prepared medium: 2-8°C
2. Shelf life: Approximately 6-8 weeks

Quality control: Organism		*Growth*
Positive	*Brucella abortus*	+
Negative	Uninoculated	−

Serum Potato Infusion Agar[4]

Intended use: A medium used for the cultivation of *Brucella.*

Formula:	*Ingredients per Liter*
Sliced potato	250.0 g
Peptone	10.0 g
Beef extract	5.0 g
Sodium chloride	5.0 g
Glycerin	20.0 mL
Agar	25.0 g

Final pH 6.9 ±0.1 at 25°C

Method of preparation:

1. Submerge 250 g of cleaned, peeled, sliced potato in 1 L of distilled or deionized water and infuse for 24 h in a covered container at 60°C.
2. Filter through gauze and readjust volume to 1 L as necessary.
3. Add other ingredients, heat to boiling to dissolve completely, then adjust pH to 6.9 ±0.2 at 25°C.
4. Sterilize in the autoclave for 30 min at 121°C.
5. After sedimentation, separate supernate aseptically.
6. Add 10% (v/v) sterile horse serum to supernate.
7. Dispense 20 mL per petri plate.

Appearance of uninoculated medium: Light amber, slightly opalescent, solid medium.

Storage:

1. Prepared medium: 2-8°C
2. Shelf life: Approximately 6-8 weeks

Quality control: Organism		*Growth*
Positive	*Brucella abortus*	+
Negative	Uninoculated	–

Stuart's Medium[54]

Intended use: A medium for the cultivation of *Leptospira*.

Formula:	*Ingredients per Liter*
Basal Medium:	
Disodium phosphate	0.666 g
Monopotassium phosphate	0.087 g
Sodium chloride	1.925 g
Ammonium chloride	0.268 g

Magnesium chloride·$6H_2O$	0.190 g
L-asparagine	0.132 g
Glycerol (optional)	5.0 mL
Enrichment:	
Rabbit serum (filter-sterilized, heat inactivated)	8-10% v/v

Final pH 7.5 ±0.1 at 25°C

Method of preparation:

1. Dissolve ingredients in 995 ml of distilled or deionized water. Add 5 mL of glycerol if desired.
2. Sterilize in the autoclave for 15 min at 121°C.
3. Allow the medium to cool to room temperature.
4. Aseptically add 8-10% rabbit serum. Mix well.
5. Dispense aseptically into sterile screwcapped test tubes in 8-10 mL amounts.

Appearance of uninoculated medium: Very light amber, clear to slightly opalescent, without precipitate, liquid medium.

Storage:

1. Prepared medium: 2-8°C
2. Shelf life: Approximately 6-8 weeks

Quality control: Organism		*Growth*
Positive	*Leptospira interrogans*	+
Negative	Uninoculated	−

Tellurite Test Medium and Reagent[24,47,59]

Intended use: A medium and test for detecting tellurite reduction by mycobacteria.

Formula:	*Ingredients per Liter*
Medium:	
Middlebrook 7H9 broth (without glycerol)	4.7 g
Tween 80 (10% filter sterilized)	0.5 mL
ADC enrichment (Difco or BBL)	100.0 mL

Final pH 6.6 ±0.2 at 25°C

Reagent:

Tellurite solution:	Ingredients per 100 mL
Potassium tellurite	0.1 g

Method of preparation: Medium:

1. Suspend 4.7 g of Middlebrook 7H9 broth in 900 ml of distilled or deionized water.
2. Sterilize in the autoclave for 15 min at 121°C.
3. Cool to 55°C, and add aseptically 100 mL ADC enrichment and 0.5 mL Tween 80.
4. Dispense aseptically in 5 mL amounts in 16 x 125 mm screwcapped tubes.

Method of preparation: Reagent:

1. Dissolve 0.1 g of potassium tellurite in 50 mL of distilled or deionized water.
2. Sterilize in the autoclave for 15 min at 121°C.
3. Store at 2-8°C. Just prior to use, dispense in 2-5 mL amounts in sterile 16 X 125 mm screwcapped tubes.

Appearance of uninoculated medium: Light amber, clear liquid medium.

Storage:

1. Prepared medium and reagent: 2-8°C
2. Shelf life: Approximately 6 months

Quality control:	*Organism*	*Growth*
Positive	*Mycobacterium avium-intracellulare* (black ppt.)	+
Negative	*Mycobacterium kansasii* (no color change)	+
	Uninoculated	–

Thioglycolate Broth (Without Indicator, Supplemented)[39]

Intended use: A general purpose medium for the cultivation of anaerobes and for use in susceptibility testing of anaerobes.

Formula:	*Ingredients per Liter*
Thioglycolate broth without indicator, BBL 135c	quantity stated by manufacturer
Hemin	5.0 mg

Vitamin K_1	0.1 mg
Sodium bicarbonate	1.0 mg

Final pH 7.2 ±0.2 at 25°C

Method of preparation:

1. Suspend all ingredients except sodium bicarbonate in 1 L of distilled or deionized water and heat to boiling to dissolve completely.
2. Dispense in 5-6 mL volumes in 13 x 100 mm screwcapped tubes.
3. Steam sterilize for 15 min.
4. Cool and store. Before use, place medium once in boiling water or steam bath to drive off absorbed oxygen and cool to room temperature.
5. Add sodium bicarbonate (1 μg/mL) to each tube.

Appearance of uninoculated medium: Light amber, very slightly opalescent, thick, liquid medium.

Storage:

1. Prepared medium: 15-30°C in the dark for immediate use; or 2-8°C for prolonged storage.
2. Shelf life: Approximately 6 months

Quality control:	*Organism*	*Growth*
Positive	*Bacteroides fragilis* (ATCC 25285)	+
	Bacteroides thetaiotaomicron (ATCC 29741)	+
	Clostridium perfringens (ATCC 13124)	+
Negative	Uninoculated	−

Thiosulfate Citrate Bile Sucrose (TCBS) Agar[26,37]

Intended use: A selective medium for the isolation and cultivation of *Vibrio cholerae* and other enteropathogenic vibrios.

Formula:	*Ingredients per Liter*
Peptone	10.0 g
Yeast extract	5.0 g
Sodium thiosulfate	10.0 g
Sodium citrate	10.0 g
Oxgall	8.0 g

Sucrose	20.0 g
Sodium chloride	10.0 g
Ferric citrate	1.0 g
Brom thymol blue	0.04 g
Thymol blue	0.04 g
Agar	15.0 g

Final pH 8.6 ±0.2 at 25°C

Method of preparation:

1. Suspend ingredients in 1 L of distilled or deionized water and heat to boiling to dissolve completely. DO NOT AUTOCLAVE.
2. Dispense 20 mL into sterile petri plates as desired.

Appearance of uninoculated medium: Forest green, slightly opalescent, without precipitation or surface scum, solid medium.

Storage:

1. Prepared medium: 2-8°C
2. Shelf life: Approximately 6-8 weeks

Quality control:	*Organism*	*Growth*
Positive	*Vibrio cholerae* (yellow)	+
Negative	*Escherichia coli* (translucent if present)	–
	Uninoculated	–

Tinsdale's Agar, Moore and Parsons Modified[42]

Intended use: A medium that supports the growth of all species of *Corynebacterium* while inhibiting the growth of most of the normal flora of the upper respiratory tract. Moore and Parsons modified the original Tinsdale formula, simplifying the composition but retaining the specificity for the recovery of *C. diphtheriae* and *C. ulcerans.*

Formula:	*Ingredients per Liter*
Modified Base:	
Thiotone peptone	20.0 g
Sodium chloride	5.0 g
Agar	14.0 g
L-cystine	0.24 g

Sodium thiosulfate	0.24 g
Sterile bovine serum	100.0 mL
Tellurite solution, 1%	30.0 mL

Final pH 7.4 ±0.2 at 25°C

Method of preparation:

1. Suspend 39 g of powder in 1 liter of distilled or deionized water and heat with agitation.
2. Boil for 1 min. Autoclave for 15 min at 121°C.
3. Cool the modified base to 50°C and add the sterile bovine serum and the 1% tellurite solution.
4. Pour 15-20 mL into petri plates and allow to harden.

Appearance of uninoculated medium: Clear, light amber solid medium.

Storage:

1. Prepared medium: 2-8°C
2. Shelf life: Base, in sealed screwcapped tubes, indefinitely; Completed medium, 2-3 days

Quality Control: Organism		*Growth*
Positive	*C. diphtheriae* (brown halo)	+
	Staphylococcus aureus (no halo)	+
Negative	Uninoculated	–

Ureaplasma Agar Medium (A8, Shepard)[51]

Intended use: A special agar medium for isolation and specific identification of ureaplasmas in primary cultures of clinical material from human and animal sources.

Formula:	*Ingredients per Liter*
Trypticase soy broth (TSB)	24.0 g
Calcium chloride ($CaCl_2 \cdot 2H_2O$) (1)	0.14 g
Putrescine dihydrochloride	1.66 g
Water (2)	800.0 mL
Agar	10.5 g
Horse serum, unheated (normal)	200.0 mL
CVA enrichment (3)	5.0 mL

Yeast extract	10.0 mL
Urea (4)	10.0 mL
L-cysteine·HCl (5)	5.0 mL
GHL tripeptide (6)	1.0 mL
Antibiotics	see Mycoplasma Agar Medium

Final pH 5.5 ±0.1 at 25°C

(1) Calcium chloride dihydrate alternative: omit, apply drop of spot test reagent to colonies (urea, 1%, Magnesium chloride [$MgCl_2 \cdot 4H_2O$], 0.8%).
(2) Glass-distilled or deionized
(3) Gibco Diagnostics cat. no. D-1000 and D-1500 (restoring solution); a chemically defined enrichment containing cofactors, vitamins and amino acids.
(4) Filter-sterilized 10% solution
(5) Filter-sterilized 2% solution
(6) 20 μg/mL solution, glycyl-L-histidyl-L-lysine acetate (Calbiochem-Behring cat. no. 36395)

Method of preparation:

1. Dissolve TSB, calcium chloride and putrescine in water, adjust pH to 5.5 with 2N hydrochloric acid.
2. Add agar, heat to boiling to dissolve completely.
3. Sterilize in the autoclave for 15 min at 121°C.
4. Cool to 56°C then aseptically add remaining ingredients combined separately in a sterile bottle.
5. Dispense 20 mL in petri plates.

Appearance of uninoculated medium: Medium amber, slightly opalescent, solid medium.

Storage:

1. Prepared medium: 2-8°C
2. Shelf life: Undetermined

Quality control:	*Organism*	*Growth*
Positive	*Ureaplasma urealyticum* (deep brown or brown black colonies)	+
Negative	*Mycoplasma hominis* (no color change)	+
	Uninoculated	–

Ureaplasma Broth Medium (U10C, Shepard)[52]

Intended use: A selective and differential broth medium for the primary isolation of *Ureaplasma*.

Formula:	*Ingredients per Liter*
Mycoplasma broth base (MBB) (1)	14.7 g
Water (2)	700.0 mL
Horse serum (3)	200.0 mL
Yeast extract (4)	100.0 mL
L-cysteine·HCl (5)	5.0 mL
Urea (6)	4.0 mL
CVA enrichment (7)	5.0 mL
GHL tripeptide (8)	1.0 mL
Phenol red (9)	1.0 mL
Antibiotics	see Mycoplasma Agar Medium

Final pH 5.5 ±0.1 at 25°C

(1) PPLO broth without CV (Difco or equivalent)
(2) Glass-distilled or deionized
(3) Pooled, unheated
(4) Active dry baker's yeast 25% w/v in distilled water, autoclave at 121°C for 5 min, clarify by filtration/centrifugation. Sterilize in the autoclave for 15 min at 121°C. Store at -20°C.
(5) Sterile 2% solution.
(6) Sterile 10% solution.
(7) Gibco Diagnostics cat. no. D-1000 and D-1500 (restoring solution); a chemically defined enrichment containintg cofactors, vitamins and amino acids.
(8) 20 μg/mL solution. (Calbiochem-Behring cat. no. 363951).
(9) 1% autoclaved solution.

Method of preparation:

1. Dissolve MBB in water with heating, adjust pH to 5.5 with 2N hydrochloric acid.
2. Sterilize in the autoclave for 15 min at 121°C.
3. Cool to 50-56°C.
4. Aseptically add remaining ingredients.
5. Dispense 1.8 mL volumes aseptically into sterile 4.0 mL Wheaton screwcapped culture vials.

Appearance of uninoculated medium: Yellow, slightly opalescent, liquid medium.

Storage:

1. Prepared medium: −20°C
2. Shelf life: Undetermined

Quality control: Organism		*Growth*
Positive	*Ureaplasma urealyticum* (color change from yellow to orange red, a clear broth)	+
Negative	Uninoculated (yellow)	–

Urease Production Test Broth[47,56,59,61]

Intended use: A medium for detecting urease-producing bacteria, particularly among the members of the genus *Mycobacterium*.

Formula:	*Ingredients per Liter*
Bacto-Urea broth concentrate (Difco Laboratories)	10 mL
Sterile distilled or deionized water	90 mL

Final pH 6.8 ±0.1 at 25°C

Method of preparation:

1. To prepare 100 mL of final medium, sterilize 90 mL distilled or deionized water in autoclave for 15 min at 121°C.
2. Cool to 40-50°C and aseptically add the contents of one 10 mL tube of Bacto-Urea broth concentrate. Mix thoroughly (avoid temperature above 50°C).
3. Distribute in 4 mL amounts in 16 × 125 mm screwcapped tubes.
4. Should crystals form in the concentrate before preparing the final medium, place the tubes of sterile concentrate in a water bath at 40-50°C for a few moments with agitation to effect complete solution of the crystals.

Appearance of uninoculated medium: Reddish orange, clear liquid medium.

Storage:

1. Prepared medium: 2-8°C
2. Shelf life: Approximately 6-8 weeks

Quality control: Organism		*Growth*
Positive	*Mycobacterium kansasii* (pink red color, pH 8.1 or more)	+
Negative	*Mycobacterium avium* (yellow color, pH 6.8 or more)	+

Uninoculated (no color change)	–

Wadowsky-Yee Medium, Modified, see Modified Wadowsky-Yee (MWY) Medium

Wilkins-Chalgren Agar[63]

Intended use: A medium for the cultivation and susceptibility testing of anaerobic bacteria by the agar dilution procedure.

Formula:	*Ingredients per Liter*
Pancreatic digest of casein	10.0 g
Pancreatic digest of gelatin	10.0 g
Yeast extract	5.0 g
D-glucose, anhydrous, ACS certified	1.0 g
Sodium chloride, crystal, ACS certified	5.0 g
L-arginine, free base	1.0 g
Sodium pyruvate	1.0 g
Hemin (equine, type III, crystalline)	5.0 mg
Vitamin K_1	0.5 mg
Agar	15.0 g

Final pH 7.1 ±0.1 at 25°C

Method of preparation:

1. Suspend ingredients in 1 L of distilled or deionized water and heat to boiling to dissolve completely.
2. Dispense as desired into tubes or flasks and steam sterilize for 15 min.
3. Cool to 50-56°C before adding antibiotics.
4. Mix gently and dispense 20 mL into petri plates.

Alternate Procedure: Use prepared powder, Difco 1805-17-6.

Appearance of uninoculated medium: Light to medium amber, slightly opalescent, solid medium.

Storage:

1. Prepared medium: 2-8°C
2. Shelf life: Approximately 6-8 weeks, without antibiotics

Quality control: Organism		*Growth*
Positive	*Clostridium perfringens* (ATCC 13124)	+
	Bacteroides thetaiotaomicron (ATCC 29741)	+
	Bacteroides fragilis (ATCC 25285)	+
Negative	Uninoculated	–

Xylose-Deoxycholate-Citrate Agar[34,60]

Intended use: For the selective and differential isolation of *Aeromonas* spp.

Formula:	*Ingredients per Liter*
Nutrient broth (Oxoid)	12.5 g
Sodium citrate (Oxoid)	5.0 g
Sodium thiosulfate	5.0 g
Ferric ammonium citrate	1.0 g
Sodium deoxycholate	2.5 g
Agar	12.0 g
Xylose	10.0 g
Neutral red (1% in DDW)	2.5 mL

Method of preparation:

1. Dissolve ingredients in 997.5 mL of distilled or deionized water, heat to boiling to dissolve completely. Add 2.5 mL of neutral red, simmer for 20 min, cool.
2. Dispense 20 mL into petri dishes.

Storage:

1. Prepared medium: 2-8°C
2. Shelf life: Approximately 1 month, plates sealed in plastic sleeves

Quality control: Organism		*Growth*
Positive	*Aeromonas hydrophila* (ATCC 7965) (colorless colonies)	+

Negative	*E. coli* (NCTC 9111) (red colonies or inhibited)	+
	Uninoculated	−

REAGENTS

Bovine Albumin Fraction V, 0.2%[59]

1. Dissolve 0.85 g sodium chloride in 100 mL distilled water.
2. Add 2.0 g bovine albumin fraction V (2% solution) and dissolve by swirling the flask or by gently stirring on a magnetic stirrer.
3. Adjust pH to 6.8 with 4% sodium hydroxide.
4. To make a 0.2% solution, dilute 1:10 with sterile saline.

Catalase Test Reagents[28]

Hydrogen peroxide, 3%

Catalase Test:

The organism to be tested should be grown on an agar slant heavily inoculated from a colony of the organism. The slant is usually incubated for 18-25 h at optimal temperature. To test for catalase, set the slant in an inclined position and pour 1 mL of a 3% solution of hydrogen peroxide over the growth. The appearance of gas bubbles indicates a positive test.

An alternative to conducting the test with a slant culture is to emulsify a colony in one drop of 30% hydrogen peroxide (superoxol) on a glass slide. Immediate bubbling indicates a positive catalase test. Extreme care must be exercised if a colony is taken from a blood agar plate. The enzyme catalase is present in erythrocytes, and the carry-over of blood cells with the colony can give a false-positive reaction.

Catalase Test, Tween-hydrogen peroxide, 30%[48]

Semiquantitative test to detect catalase production by mycobacteria.

1. Tween 80 solution:

Distilled or deionized water, sterile	90 mL
Tween 80, sterile	10 mL

   Equal parts of Tween 80 solution and hydrogen peroxide (30%) should be added together just before performing the catalase test.
2. Catalase inactivation at 68°C:
   Phosphate buffer, M/15, pH 7.0
   (See Tween hydrolysis reagent)

FA Mounting Fluid[41]

For preparation of mounting fluid for examination of slides in fluorescent antibody tests.

Carbonate buffer:

Solution 1:	
Sodium carbonate	5.3 g
Water, qs to	100.0 mL
Solution 2:	
Sodium bicarbonate	4.2 g
Water, qs to	100.0 mL

1. Measure 100 mL of Solution 2 and add 4-17 mL of Solution 1 so as to adjust pH to 9.0.
2. Mix one part carbonate buffer with 9 parts neutral glycerol.

Hydrochloric Acid Solution with Bromcresol Purple Indicator Solution[49]

Bromcresol purple indicator solution:

Bromcresol purple	1.2 g
Ethyl alcohol, 95%	50.0 mL
Sterile distilled water	50.0 mL

Acid solution with indicator:

Sterile distilled water	1835.0 mL
Concentrated hydrochloric acid	165.0 mL
Bromcresol purple indicator solution	9.0 mL

Method of preparation: Add acid to water followed by indicator solution.

MacFarland 0.5 Turbidity Standard

Prepare this turbidity standard by adding 0.5 mL of 0.048M barium chloride (1.175% $BaCl_2 \cdot H_2O$ w/v to 99.5 mL of 0.36N sulfuric acid [1% v/v]). Distribute 4-6 mL into screwcapped tubes of the same size as those used in growing the broth culture inoculum. Tightly seal these tubes and store them in the dark at room temperature. Vigorously agitate this turbidity standard on a mechanical vortex mixer just before use.

N-Acetyl-L-Cysteine-Sodium Hydroxide (NALC-NaOH)[59]

2.9% Sodium citrate (0.1M):

1. Dissolve 29.4 g of anhydrous sodium citrate in 1 liter of distilled water.
2. Sterilize in the autoclave for 15 min at 121°C.
3. Store at room temperature.
4. Do not use if a precipitate forms.

4% Sodium hydroxide (1N):

1. Dissolve 40 g NaOH in 1 liter of distilled water.
2. Sterilize in the autoclave for 15 min at 121°C.
3. Store at room temperature.
4. Do not use if a precipitate forms.

To make the NALC-NaOH, combine 50 mL sterile 2.9% sodium citrate, 50 mL sterile NaOH and 0.5 g N-acetyl-L-cysteine powder. The solution should be used within 24 h of preparation (dissolved NALC is unstable when exposed to air and loses its mucolytic activity). It can be stoppered tightly, refrigerated and used within 48 h if necessary.

Niacin Test Reagents[46]

1. Aniline reagent (4%):

Ethanol, 95%	96.0 mL
Aniline	4.0 mL

Store refrigerated in a brown bottle. Discard solution when a yellow color develops.

2. Cyanogen bromide (10%):

Cyanogen bromide	5.0 g
Distilled water	50.0 mL

Prepare only in a well-ventilated safety cabinet. Store in a tightly-capped brown bottle at 4°C. If a precipitate forms, warm to room temperature to dissolve. Prepare in small quantities to prevent volatilization and loss of potency.

Nitrate Reductase Test for Mycobacteria; Rapid Reagents[48]

Nitrate solution:

Sodium nitrate	5.0 g
Tween 80 (20%)	1.0 mL

Saline	100.0 mL

1. Heat gently to dissolve.
2. Filter sterilize.
3. Aliquot 0.5 mL amounts into sterile 15 X 100 mm screwcapped tubes.
4. Refrigerate until used.
5. Prepare a new reagent every three months.

Reagent-impregnated disks:

Glacial acetic acid	10.0 mL
Distilled water	25.0 mL
Sulfanilic acid	0.14 g
N-(1-naphthyl) ethylenediamine·HCl	0.105 g

1. Stir to dissolve.
2. Lyophilize 0.03 mL of reagent on 1/4 inch analytical paper disk.
3. Store in dark at room temperature.
4. Prepare new reagent every 2 months.

Nitrate Reduction Test Reagents[48]

1. Solution A:	
Sulfanilic acid	8.0.g
Acetic acid, 5N	1.0 L
2. Solution B:	
N,N-dimethyl-1-naphthylamine	6.0 mL
Acetic acid, 5N	1.0 L

(The 5N acetic acid consists of 1 part glacial acetic acid to 2.5 parts distilled water.) Although N,N-dimethyl-1-naphthylamine, unlike α-naphthylamine, has not been listed as a carcinogen by the Occupational Safety and Health Administration, Department of Labor, its structural similarity to α-naphthylamine would indicate that such safety precautions as the avoidance of aerosols, mouth pipetting, and contact with the skin should be followed.

Nitrate Reduction Test for Mycobacteria: Reagents[48]

1. Sodium nitrate phosphate buffer:	
Sodium nitrate	0.085 g
Sodium phosphate, dibasic·12 H_2O	0.485 g
Potassium phosphate, monobasic	0.117 g
Distilled water	100.0 mL
pH to 7.0	

2. Hydrochloric acid solution:

Hydrochloric acid, concentrated	10.0	mL
Distilled water	10.0	mL
Add acid to water		

3. Sulfanilic acid:

Sulfanilamide	0.2	g
Distilled water	100.0	mL

4. N-Naphthylethylenediamine dihydrochloride:

N-Naphthylethylenediamine dihydrochloride	0.1	g
Distilled water	100.0	mL

Oxalic Acid, 5%[23]

1. Dissolve 50 g oxalic acid in 950 mL distilled water.
2. Sterilize in the autoclave for 15 min at 121°C.

Oxidase (Kovacs' Reagent)[27]

1% Tetramethyl-*p*-phenylenediamine dihydrochloride (TPD)

Kovacs' Oxidase Test: The Kovacs' Oxidase Test is recommended for nonfermenters and miscellaneous gram-negative bacteria.

1. Place filter paper in a petri disk and saturate it with 0.5% tetramethyl-*p*-phenylenediamine hydrochloride.
2. With a platinum wire, pick a portion of the colony to be tested and rub the colony on the filter paper.

A positive reaction is indicated by the appearance of a dark-purple color within ten seconds. With this technique, there should be enough of the colony left for subculturing.

Alternate Procedure: Place a few drops of the oxidase reagent directly onto colonies on a plate. Colonies producing oxidase become pink and then purple. The reagent does not interfere with the Gram stain, so purple colonies may be stained even though they are not viable. The oxidase reagent may be divided into small aliquots and stored at −20°C. Thaw one aliquot as needed, and do not use it for more than one day. Check the reagent daily with a known oxidase-positive organism. The Kovacs' oxidase is more sensitive than the indophenol method.

Phosphate Buffer, M/15, pH 6.6 – 7.0[59]

Prepare stock solutions 1 and 2.

1. M/15 Sodium phosphate dibasic: In a volumetric flask, dissolve 9.47 g of anydrous Na_2HPO_4 in distilled water to make one liter.

2. M/15 Potassium phosphate monobasic: In a volumetric flask, dissolve 9.07 g of KH_2PO_4 in distilled water to make one liter.

To prepare buffers with specific pH values, mix volumes of Solutions A and B as follows:

pH	Solution A	Solution B
6.6	37.5 mL	62.5 mL
6.8	50.0 mL	50.0 mL
7.0	61.1 mL	38.9 mL

Confirm final values with a pH meter.

Phosphate-Buffered Saline

For use in fluorescent antibody staining.

Sodium phosphate, dibasic	1.24 g
Sodium phosphate, monobasic, monohydrate	0.18 g
Sodium chloride	8.50 g
Water, qs to	1.0 L

1. Dissolve reagents in distilled or deionized water in order given.
2. If necessary, adjust pH to 7.6.

Sodium Chloride, 0.85%

Dissolve 8.5 g NaCl in one liter of distilled water.

Sodium Hydroxide, 2%

1. Dissolve 20 g of NaOH in one liter of distilled water.
2. Sterilize in the autoclave for 15 min at 121°C.
3. Store at room temperature.
4. Do not use if a precipitate forms.

Tween 80 Hydrolysis Reagent[46,48]

Substrate:

M/15 Phosphate buffer, pH 7.0	100.0 mL
Polysorbate 80	0.5 mL
Aqueous neutral red solution, 0.1% (adjust available dye content to 100%)	2.0 mL

1. Combine the above reagents.
2. Dispense in 2.0 mL amounts and autoclave 10 min at 121°C.

3. Color of liquid should be amber.
4. Let cool and store in the dark at 4°C for a maximum of two weeks.

Vibriostatic Reagent 0/129[20]

Reagent:

2, 4-diamino-6, 7-diisopropyl pteridine
Acetone soluble, available from Calbiochem - Behring, San Diego, CA. Water soluble potassium salt, available from Sigma Chemical Co., St. Louis, MO.

Disks:

Use disks containing 10 and 150 μg 0/129 on non-selective medium containing 0.5% sodium chloride (NaCl concentrations greater than 1% will inactivate the reagent, producing false resistance).

Zephiran-Trisodium Phosphate[59]

1. Dissolve 1 kg trisodium phosphate ($Na_3PO_4 \cdot 12H_2O$) in 4 L hot distilled water and add 7.5 mL Zephiran concentrate (17% benzalkonium chloride, Winthrop Laboratories, New York, NY).
2. Mix and store at room temperature.

STAINS

Acridine Orange Stain[31]

The acridine orange stain is a stain for the detection of bacteria in clinical specimens. At pH 4.0, bacteria will stain red-orange while nonbacterial cells such as squamous cells and polymorphonuclear leukocytes will stain green-yellow.

1. Spread the specimen onto a clean glass slide, air dry and fix by immersion in absolute methanol for 2 min.
2. Flood the slide with a solution of 0.5% acridine orange in 0.15M acetate buffer, pH 4.0, and stain for 2 min.
3. Rinse the slide with water, air dry and examine at 400–1,000X magnification under ultraviolet light.

Auramine-Rhodamine Stain (Truant's) Reagents[57]

A. Auramine O - Rhodamine B Solution:
Combine 1.5 g auramine O and 0.75 g rhodamine B with 10 mL phenol (melted) and 25 mL distilled water. Mix. Add 75 mL glycerol and 25 mL distilled water. Mix well and clarify by filtration. Store as solution in a tightly-stoppered brown bottle away from heat and bright light at 4°C or room temperature.. Shelf life is one year.

B. Acid-alcohol:
0.5% (Concentrated) Hydrochloric acid in 70% ethyl alcohol. Mix well.

C. Counterstain
0.5% Aqueous solution of potassium permanganate in distilled water.

Flagellar stain[5]

1. Solution A:

Basic fuchsin (certified for flagellar stain)	0.6 g
Ethyl alcohol, 95%	50.0 mL

Shake and let stand overnight to dissolve the fuchsin.

2. Solution B:

Sodium chloride	0.37 g
Tannic acid	0.75 g
Distilled water	50.0 mL

Combine solutions A and B and mix thoroughly. Adjust the pH to 5.0 with 1N sodium hydroxide. If the solution is more acidic, flagella stain slowly and are difficult to detect. The stain may be used immediately, but it works better if held 2-3 days at 4°C. Store in a tightly stoppered bottle. At 4°C the stain is stable for about one month; in the freezer, it will keep indefinitely. The stain deteriorates rapidly if held at room temperature. Allow any precipitate which forms to remain undisturbed. Use only the clear supernatant solution.

Test procedure:

Make a slightly cloudy suspension in distilled water (not saline) from 18-24 h growth on agar plates or slants. Do not carry over any agar. Growth equivalent to a 1 mm colony is mixed with 3 mL of sterile distilled water. Emulsify the growth in a drop of water against the side of the tube and then mix it with the remaining water.

Slides must be clean and free of grease. Soak the slides 4 days in 3% concentrated HCl in 95% ethyl alcohol or in acid dichromate solution. Rinse in 10 changes of tap water and 2 changes of distilled water, then air dry. Pick up a clean slide with forceps and hold it for a few seconds in a blue gas bunsen flame. When the slide has cooled, draw thick wax pencil lines on it to contain the stain in an area about 1 by 1.75 inches (ca. 2.5 by 4.4 cm).

Put a loopful of the suspension on one end of the slide. Tilt the slide and allow the suspension to flow to the opposite end of the slide. Air dry on a level surface. Do not fix with heat. Apply 1 mL of stain, warmed to room temperature, to the smear. Do not move the slide. A fine precipitate forms over the entire slide in 5-15 min. Once the precipitate has formed, wash the slide in a gentle stream of tap water. Do not tilt to rinse. Air dry and examine under oil immersion.

For a control suspension, inoculate flagella broth with an actively motile bacterium and incubate overnight at 25°C. Add 0.25 mL of formalin to 5 mL of broth culture. Mix and allow the mixture to stand for 15 min. Wash twice in distilled water. Resuspend the packed cells in enough distilled water to obtain a faintly turbid suspension.

Giemsa Stain

1. Giemsa stain stock solution:
   Dissolve 0.75 g Giemsa stain, powdered (certified), in 65.0 mL of pure absolute methanol. Add 35 mL of pure glycerol, and mix well by shaking the mixture with glass beads. Keep tightly stoppered at all times. Filter if necessary.
2. Phosphate buffer, pH 6.4:
   Prepare by combining 6.63 g anhydrous monobasic potassium phosphate (KH_2PO_4) and 2.56 g of anhydrous dibasic sodium phosphate (Na_2HPO_4) and diluting the mixture to one liter.

Prepare a thin film of blood, and let it dry. Fix the film by flooding with absolute methanol, draining, and permitting the film to dry. Flood slide with dilute Giemsa stain (1 part stain to 50 parts phosphate buffer at pH 6.4), and stain for 30-60 min. Wash the stain off the slide using large quantities of phosphate buffer. Dry the smear and examine.

Gram Stain

A. Crystal violet:
   Solution A - 10% crystal violet in 95% ethyl alcohol
   Solution B - 0.8 g ammonium oxalate dissolved in 80 mL distilled water
   Mix solutions A and B together; filter after overnight storage.

B. Gram's iodine:
   1 g iodine and 2 g potassium iodide dissolved in 300 mL distilled water

C. Decolorizers:
   1. Ethyl alcohol (slowest), 95%
   2. Equal mixture of 95% ethyl alcohol and acetone (intermediate)
   3. Acetone (fastest)

D. Counterstain:
Stock solution - 2.5% safranin O in 95% ethyl alcohol
Working solution - 10 mL of stock solution in 90 mL of distilled water

Procedure: See Chapter 38, "Microscopy"

Kinyoun Stain[46]

A. Carbol-fuchsin:
Solution A - Dissolve 4 g of basic fuchsin in 20 mL ethyl alchohol
Solution B - Dissolve 8 g phenol (melted) in 100 mL of distilled water
Mix solution A and B together and allow to stand for a few days.
B. Acid-alcohol decolorizing agent:
Mix 97 mL of 95% ethyl alcohol with 3 mL hydrochloric acid
C. Methylene blue counterstain:
Dissolve 4.0 g methylene blue in 400 mL distilled water, dissolve by shaking.

Truant Auramine-Rhodamine Stain, see Auramine-Rhodamine Stain, Truant

Ziehl-Neelsen Acidfast Stain[46]

A. Carbolfuchsin:
Solution A - 0.3 g basic fuchsin dissolved in 10 mL of 95% ethyl alcohol.
Solution B - 5 mL phenol (melted) dissolved in 95 mL of distilled water.
Mix solutions A and B together; allow to stand for 2-3 days before use.
B. Acid-alcohol decolorizing agent:
97 mL of 95% ethyl alcohol mixed with 3 mL of concentrated hydrochloric acid.
C. Methylene blue counterstain:
0.3 g dissolved in 100 mL distilled water, dissolve by shaking.

REFERENCES

1. Bordet J, Gengou D. Le microbe de la coqueluche. Ann Inst Pasteur 1906;731-41.
2. Brown VI, Lowbury EJL. Use of an approved cetrimide agar medium and of culture methods for *Pseudomonas aeruginosa*. J Clin Pathol 1965;18:752-6.
3. Cary SG, Blair EB. New transport medium for shipment of clinical specimens. I. Fecal specimens. J. Bacteriol 1964;88:96-8.
4. Castaneda MR. Laboratory diagnosis of brucellosis in man. Bull WHO 1961;24:73-84.
5. Clark WA. A simplified Leifson flagella stain. J Clin Microbiol 1976;3:632-4.
6. Difco Manual, 5th ed. Detroit: Difco Laboratories, 1935;65-6.
7. Dylewski J, Nsanze H, Martha G, Ronald A. Laboratory diagnosis of *Haemophilus ducreyi*: sensitivity of culture media. Diag Microbiol Infect Dis 1986;4:241-5.

8. Edelstein PH. Legionnaires. In: Disease laboratory manual. Springfield, VA: National Technical Service, U.S. Department of Commerce, Document PB83-213571, 1983.
9. Edward DG. A selective medium for pleuropneumonia-like organisms. J Gen Microbiol 1947;1:238-43.
10. Ellner PD, Stossel CI, Drakeford E, Vasi F. A new culture medium for medical bacteriology. Am J Clin Pathol 1966;45:502-4.
11. Farrell ID. The development of a new selective medium for the isolation of *Brucella abortus* from contaminated sources. Res Vet Sci 1974;16:280-6.
12. Fletcher W. Recent work on leptospirosis, Tsutsugamuchi disease and tropical typhus in the Federated Malay States. Trans Roy Soc Trop Med Hyg 1928;21:265-88.
13. Francis E. Symptoms, diagnosis and pathology of tularemia. JAMA 1928;91:1155-61.
14. Frobisher M Jr. Cystine-tellurite agar for *Corynebacterium diphtheriae*. J Infect Dis 1937;60:99-105.
15. Gilardi GL, ed. Glucose non-fermenting gram-negative bacteria in clinical microbiology. West Palm Beach, FL: CRC Press, 1978.
16. Han GK, Khie TD. A new method for the differentiation of *Vibrio comma* and *Vibrio* El Tor. Am J Hyg 1963;77:184-6.
17. Hayflick L. Tissue cultures and mycoplasmas. Tex Rep Biol Med 1965;231:285-303.
18. Holdeman LV, Cato EP, Moore WEC, eds. Anaerobe laboratory manual. 4th ed. Blacksburg, VA: Virginia Polytechnic Institute and State University, 1977:134-6.
19. Hugh R, Leifson E. The taxonomic significance of fermentative vs. oxidative metabolism of carbohydrates by various Gram negative bacteria. J Bacteriol 1953;66:24-6.
20. Janda JM. Biochemical and exoenzymatic properties of *Aeromonas* species. Diagn Microbiol Infect Dis 1985;3:223-32.
21. Johnson RC, Harris VG. Differentiation of pathogenic and saprophytic leptospires. I. Growth at low temperatures. J. Bacteriol 1967;94:27-31.
22. Jones LM, Morgan WHB. A preliminary report on a selective medium for the culture of *Brucella*, including fastidious types. Bull WHO 1958;19:200-3.
23. Karandanis D, Schulman JA. Recent survey of infectious meningitis in adults: review of laboratory findings in bacterial, tuberculous and aseptic meningitis, South Med J 1976;69:449-57.
24. Kilburn JO, Silcox VA, Kubica GP. Differential identification of mycobacteria. V. The tellurite reduction test. Am Rev Respir Dis 1969;99:94-100.
25. King EO, Ward MK, Raney DE. Two simple media for the demonstration of pyocyanin and fluorescein. J Lab Clin Med 1954;44:301-7.
26. Kobayashi T, Enomoto S, Sakazaki R, Kuwahara S. A new selective medium for pathogenic vibrios, TCBS (modified Nakanishi's agar). Jap J Bacteriol 1963;18:387-91.
27. Kovacs N. Identification of *Pseudomonas pyocyanea* by the oxidase reaction. Nature 1956;178;703.
28. Kulczycki LL, Murphy TM, Bellanti JA. *Pseudomonas* colonization in cystic fibrosis. JAMA 1978;240:30-4.
29. Martin WJ, Ewing WH. The desoxyribonuclease test as applied to certain gram negative bacteria. Can J Microbiol 1967;13:616-18.
30. MacConkey AT. Bile salt media and their advantages in some bacteriological examinations. J Hyg 1908;8:322-34.
31. McCarthy LR, Senne JE. Evaluation of acridine orange stain for detection of microorganisms in blood cultures. J Clin Microbiol 1980;11:281-5.
32. Microbial limits test. Buffer solution and media. In: The United States pharmacopeia, 20th rev. Rockville, MD: United States Pharmacopeial Convention, 1980:875.
33. Middlebrook G, Cohn ML, Dye WE, Russel WF, Levy D. Microbiologic procedures of value in tuberculosis. Acta Tuberc Scand 1960;38:66-81.
34. Millership SE, Curnow SR, Chattopadhyay B. Fecal carriage rate of *Aeromonas hydrophila*. J Clin Pathol 1983;36:920-3.
35. Moeller V. Simplified tests for some amino acid decarboxylases and for the arginine dihydrolase system. Acta Pathol Microbiol Scand 1955;36:158-72.

36. Moore WEC, Cato EP. Synonomy of *Eubacterium limosum* and *Butyribacterium rettgeri. Butyricum limosum* comb nov. Int Bull Bacteriol Nomen Taxon 1965;15:69-80.
37. Nakanishi Y. An isolation agar medium for cholerae and enteropathogenic halophilic vibrios. Modern Media 1963;9:246.
38. National Committee for Clinical Laboratory Standards. Performance standards for antimicrobial disc susceptibility tests. Approved standard, ASM-2. Villanova, PA: National Committee for Clinical Laboratory Standards, 2nd informational supplement, March, 1982.
39. National Committee for Clinical Laboratory Standards. Alternate method for antimicrobial susceptibility testing of anaerobic bacteria. Proposed guideline, M17-P. Villanova, PA: National Committee for Clinical Laboratory Standards, 1985.
40. National Commitee for Clinical Laboratory Standards. Methods for dilution antimicrobial susceptibility tests for bacteria that grow aerobically. Approved standard M7-A. Villanova, PA: National Committee for Clinical Laboratory Standards, 1985.
41. Parker CD, Payne BJ. *Bordetella*. In: Lennette EH, Balows A, Hausler WJ Jr, Shadomy HJ, eds. Manual of clinical microbiology. 4th ed. Washington, DC: American Society for Microbiology, 1985:394-9.
42. Phillips E, Nash P. Culture media. In: Lennette EH, Balows A, Hausler WJ Jr, Shadomy HJ, eds. Manual of clinical microbiology. 4th ed. Washington, DC: American Society for Microbiology, 1985:1086.
43. Regan J, Lowe F. Enrichment medium for the isolation of *Bordetella*. J Clin Microbiol 1977;6:303-8.
44. Rhamy BW. A new and simplified medium for *Pasteurella tularensis* and other delicate organisms. J Clin Pathol 1933;3:121-4.
45. Roberts GD. Mycobacteria and nocardia. In: Washington JA II, ed. Laboratory procedures in clinical microbiology. New York: Springer Verlag, 1981:384-5.
46. Roberts GD. Mycobacteria and nocardia. In: Washington JA II, ed. Laboratory procedures in clinical microbiology. New York: Springer-Verlag, 1985:379-418.
47. Roberts GD. Mycobacteria and nocardia. In: Washington JA II, ed. Laboratory procedures in clinical microbiology. New York: Springer Verlag, 1981:389-90.
48. Roberts GD. Mayo Clinic mycobacteriology laboratory procedure manual. Rochester, MN: Mayo Foundation, 1985.
49. Rogol M, Sechter I, Grinberg L, Gerichter CHB. Pril-xylose-ampicillin agar, a new selective medium for the isolation of *Aeromonas hydrophilia*. J Med Microbiol 1979;12:229-31.
50. Schubert RHW. Ueber den Nachweis von *Plesiomonas shigelloides* Habs und Schubert, 1962, und ein Elektivmedium, den Inositol-Brillantgrun-Gallesalz-Agar. E. Rodenwaldt-Arch 1977;4:97-103.
51. Shepard MC. Culture media for ureaplasmas. In: Razin S, Tully JG, eds. Methods in mycoplasmology I: Mycoplasma characterization. New York: Academic Press, 1983:137-46.
52. Shepard MC, Lunceford CD. Serological typing of *Ureaplasma urealyticum* isolates from urethritis patients by an agar growth inhibition method. J Clin Microbiol 1978;8:566-74.
53. Smith HL Jr, Goodner K. Detection of bacterial gelatinases by gelatin-agar plate methods. J Bacteriol 1958;76:662-5.
54. Stuart RD. The preparation and use of a simple culture medium for leptospirae. J Pathol Bacteriol 1946;58:343-9.
55. Thayer JD, Martin JE Jr. Improved medium selective for cultivation of *Neisseria gonorrhoeae* and *Neisseria meningitidis*. Public Health Rep 1966;81:559-62.
56. Toda T, Hagihara Y, Takeya K. A simple urease test for the classification of mycobacteria. Am Rev Respir Dis 1960;83:757-61.
57. Truant JP, Brett WA, Thomas W Jr. Fluorescence microscopy of tubercle bacilli stained with auramine and rhodamine. Henry Ford Hosp Med Bull 1962;10:287-96.
58. Tully JG, Whitcomb RF, Wenzel RP. Enhanced isolation of *Mycoplasma pneumoniae* from throat washings with a newly modified culture medium. J Infect Dis 1979;139:478-82.
59. Vestal AL. Procedures for the isolation and identification of mycobacteria. Atlanta: Centers for Disease Control; U.S. Public Health Service Publication 76-8230, 1975.

60. Von Graevenitz A, Bucher C. Evaluation of differential and selective media for isolation of *Aeromonas* and *Plesiomonas* spp. from human feces. J. Clin Microbiol 1983;17:16-21.
61. Wayne LG. Simple pyrazinamidase and urease tests for routine identification of mycobacteria. Am Rev Respir Dis 1974;109:147-51.
62. Whitehead JEM, Wildy R, Emgback HC. Arylsulfatase activity of mycobacteria. J Pathol Bacteriol 1953;65:451-60.
63. Wilkins TD, Chalgren S. Medium for use in antibiotic susceptibility testing of anaerobic bacteria. Antimicrob Agents Chemother 1976;10:926-8.
64. World Health Organization. Standardization of methods for conducting microbic sensitivity tests. Geneva: World Health Organization, Technical Report Series No. 210, 1961.

MANUFACTURERS CITED IN CHAPTERS

Abbott Laboratories, Analytical Systems
P.O. Box 152020
Irving, TX 75015

American MicroScan
200 Corporate Drive
Mahwah, NJ 07430

American Microscan, Inc.
1584 Enterprise Boulevard
Sacramento, CA 95691

Analytab Products
200 Express Street
Plainview, NY 11803

Austin Biological Laboratories
6620 Manor Road
Austin, TX 78723

BBL Microbiology Systems
P.O. Box 243
Cockeysville, MD 21030

Beckman Instruments, Inc.
Micro-Media Systems
6200 El Camino Real
Carlsbad, CA 92008

Bellco Glass, Inc.
340 Edrudo Road
Vineland, NJ 08360

Carr-Scarborough Microbiologicals, Inc.
P.O. Box 1328
Stone Mountain, GA 30086

Carr-Scarborough Microbiologicals, Inc.
5342 Panola Industrial Boulevard
Decatur, GA 30035

Coy Laboratory Products, Inc.
P.O. Box 1108
Ann Arbor, MI 48106

Difco Laboratories, Inc.
P.O. Box 1058A
Detroit, MI 48232

DMS Laboratories, Inc.
White House, NJ 08889

Dohrman Environtech
Mountain View, CA 94040

Dynatech Laboratories, Inc.
900 Slaters Lane
Alexandria, VA 22314

Fisher Scientific
711 Forbes Avenue
Pittsburgh, PA 15219

Flow Laboratories, Inc.
7655 Old Springhouse Road
McLean, VA 22102

General Diagnostics
201 Tabor Road
Morris Plains, NJ 07950

Gen-Probe, Inc.
9620 Chesapeake Drive
San Diego, CA 92123

Gibco Laboratories
231 Sutton Street
North Andover, MA 01845

Gibco Laboratories
421 Merrimack Street
Lawrence, MA 01843

Gow-Mac Instrument Co.
P.O. Box 32
Bound Brook, NJ 00805

Hewlett Packard
3000 Hanover Street
Palo Alto, CA 94304-1181

Innovative Diagnostic Systems
3404 Oakcliff Road, Suite C1
Atlanta, GA 30340

MCT Diagnostics
1997 Slan Pl., Suite 26
St. Paul, MN 55117

Marion Scientific
Division of Marion Laboratories
P.O. Box 8480
Kansas City, MO 64114

Meridian Diagnostics
3471 River Hills Drive
Cincinnati, OH 45244

Micro-Media Systems
6200 El Camino Real
Carlsbad, CA 92008

Organon Teknika Corp.
800 Capitola Drive
Durham, NC 27713

Oxoid U.S.A., Inc.
9107 Red Branch Road
Columbia, MD 21045

Pasco, Inc.
12750 West 42nd Avenue
Wheatridge, CO 80033

Remel (Regional Medical
Laboratories)
12076 Santa Fe Drive
P.O. Box 14428
Lenexa, KS 66215

Roche Diagnostic Systems
340 Kingsland Street
Nutley, NJ 07110

Scott Laboratories, Inc.
771 Main Street
Fiskeville, RI 02823

Toxin Technology, Inc.
Food Research Institute
Department of Microbiology and
Toxicology
University of Wisconsin
1925 Willow Drive
Madison, WI 53706

Varian Instruments
505 Julie Rivers Road, Suite 150
Sugar Land, TX 77478

Virion International Ltd
Ruschliken CH8803
Zurich, Switzerland

Vitek Systems, Inc.
595 Anglum Drive
Hazelwood, MO 63042

Wellcome Diagnostics Division
3030 Cornwallis Rd.
Research Triangle Park, NC 27709

COLOR PLATES

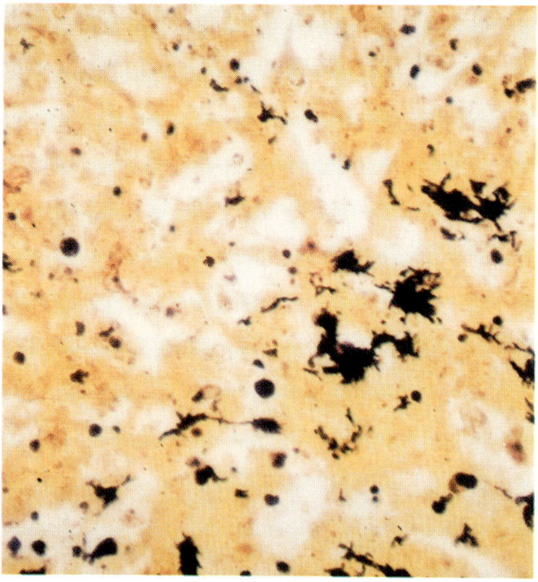

FIGURE 7:1 Warthin-Starry stain of lymph node. Silver stained bacteria are in clusters around vessel walls and in lymphoid sinuses.

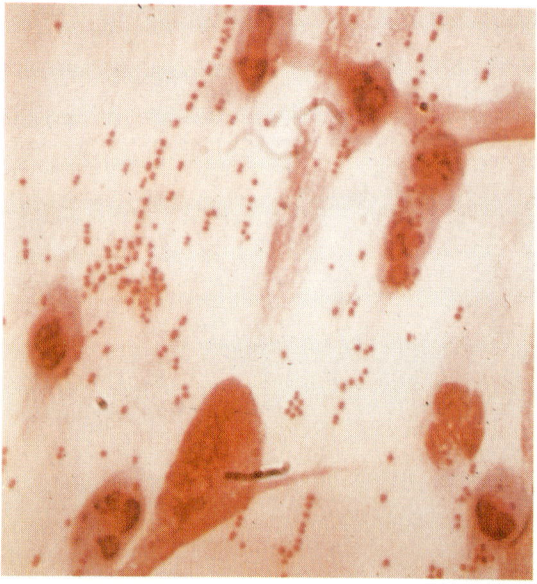

FIGURE 10:1. Gram-stained smear of expectorated sputum from a patient with *Branhamella catarrhalis* pneumonia revealing numerous polymorphonuclear leukocytes and large numbers of intracellular and extracellular gram-negative diplococci.

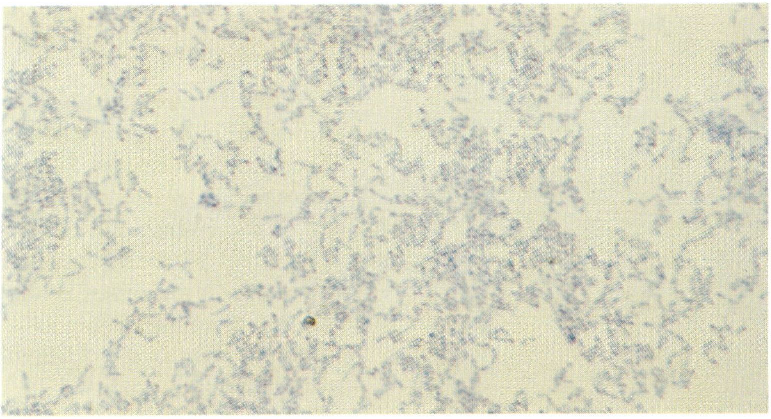

FIGURE 13:1. *Corynebactarium diphtheriae.*

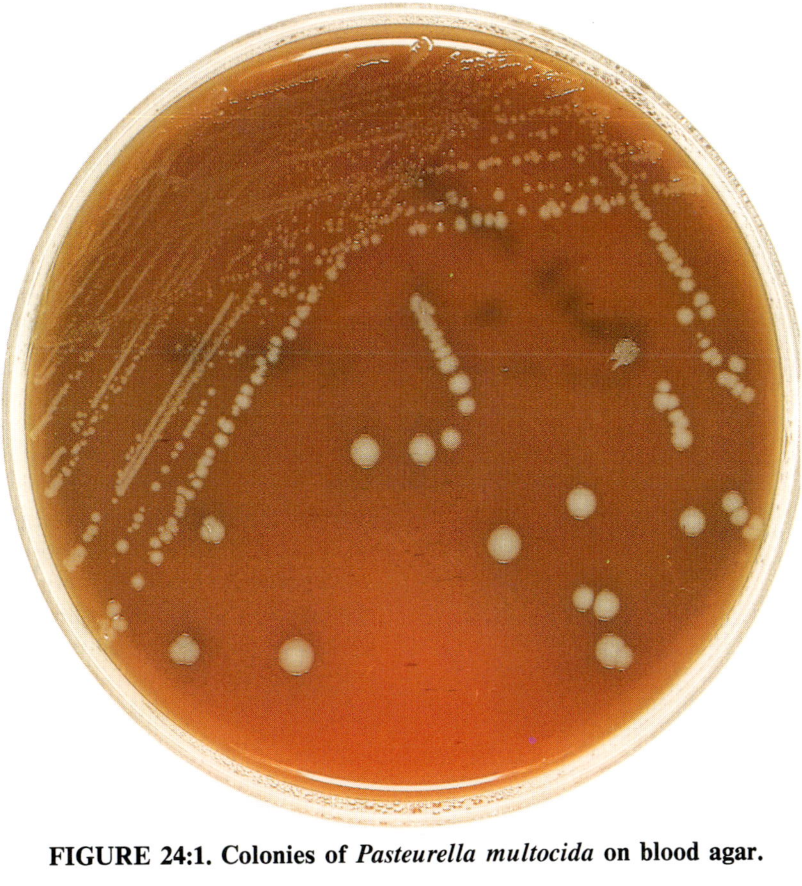

FIGURE 24:1. Colonies of *Pasteurella multocida* on blood agar.

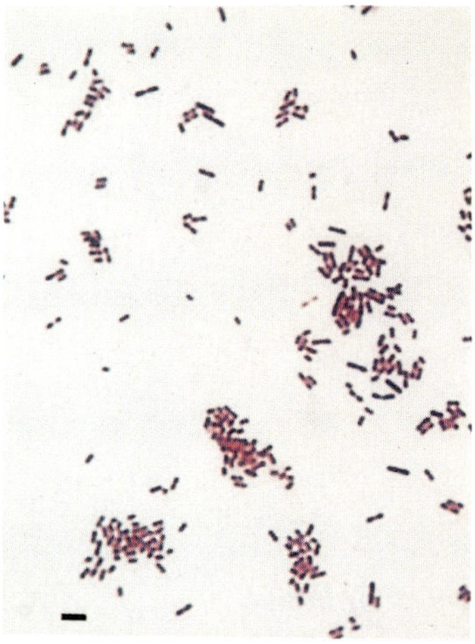

FIGURE 19:1A Gram Stain Morphology of *Listeria monocytogenes.* When grown in culture, *Listeria* is increasingly gram-variable with age of the culture. Cell morphology is that of cocci, coccobacilli or bacilli. Organisms may appear in pairs, short chains or in palisade layers, resembling diptheroids. Bar = 2 μm.

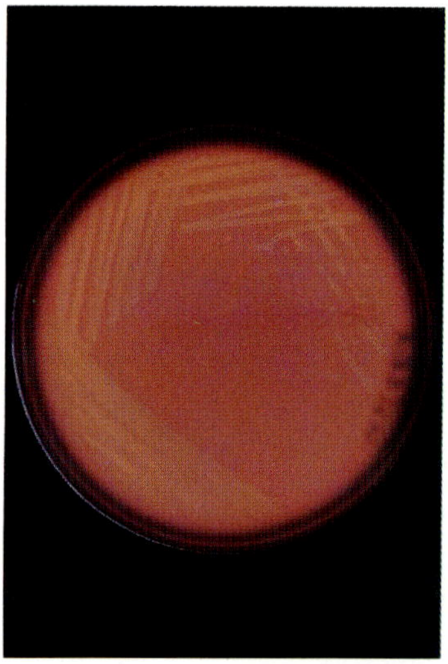

FIGURE 19:1B Hemolytic Reaction of *Listeria monocytogenes.* When grown on sheep, rabbit or horse blood agar, the organism is generally beta hemolytic. On sheep blood agar, the hemolytic zone may be very narrow; in some cases it may be necessary to scrape off the colony to reveal the hemolysis underneath it. Plate shows the faint hemolysis characteristic at 24 h; after 48 h, hemolysis is often more pronounced.

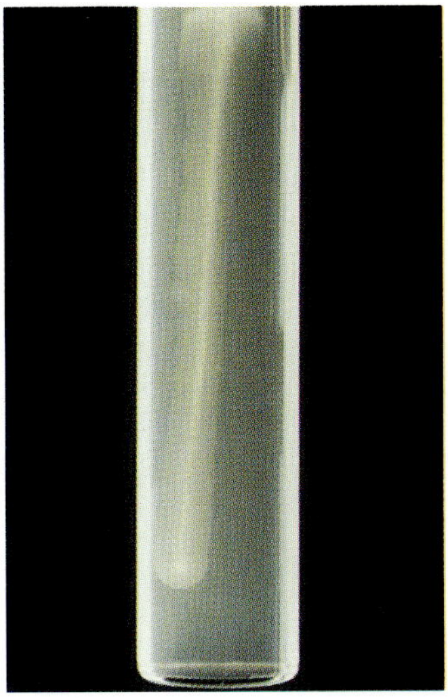

FIGURE 19:1C Motility of *Listeria monocytogenes* in Semi-Solid Agar. When grown at room temperature, the organisms are motile, forming an umbrella shape a few millimeters below the surface of the agar.

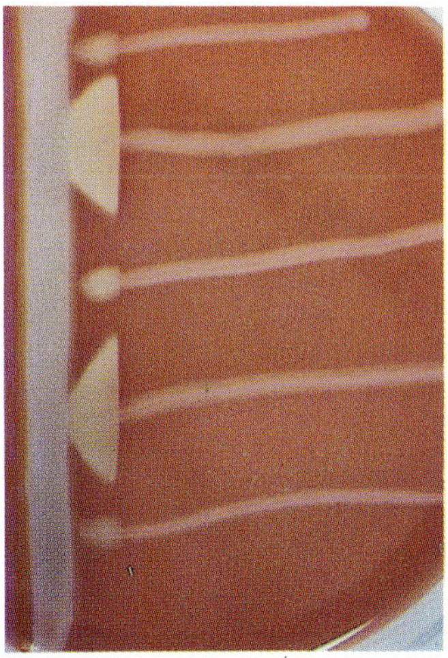

FIGURE 19:1D CAMP Reactions of *L. monocytogenes* and Group B Streptococci. When streaked perpendicularly to *Staphylococcus aureus,* the zone of hemolysis of the group B streptococci takes the form of an arrowhead at the juncture between the two streaks. For *Listeria monocytogenes*, the zone of the hemolysis at the juncture is more rounded. Two group B streptococcal streaks are shown flanked by three *Listeria* streaks.

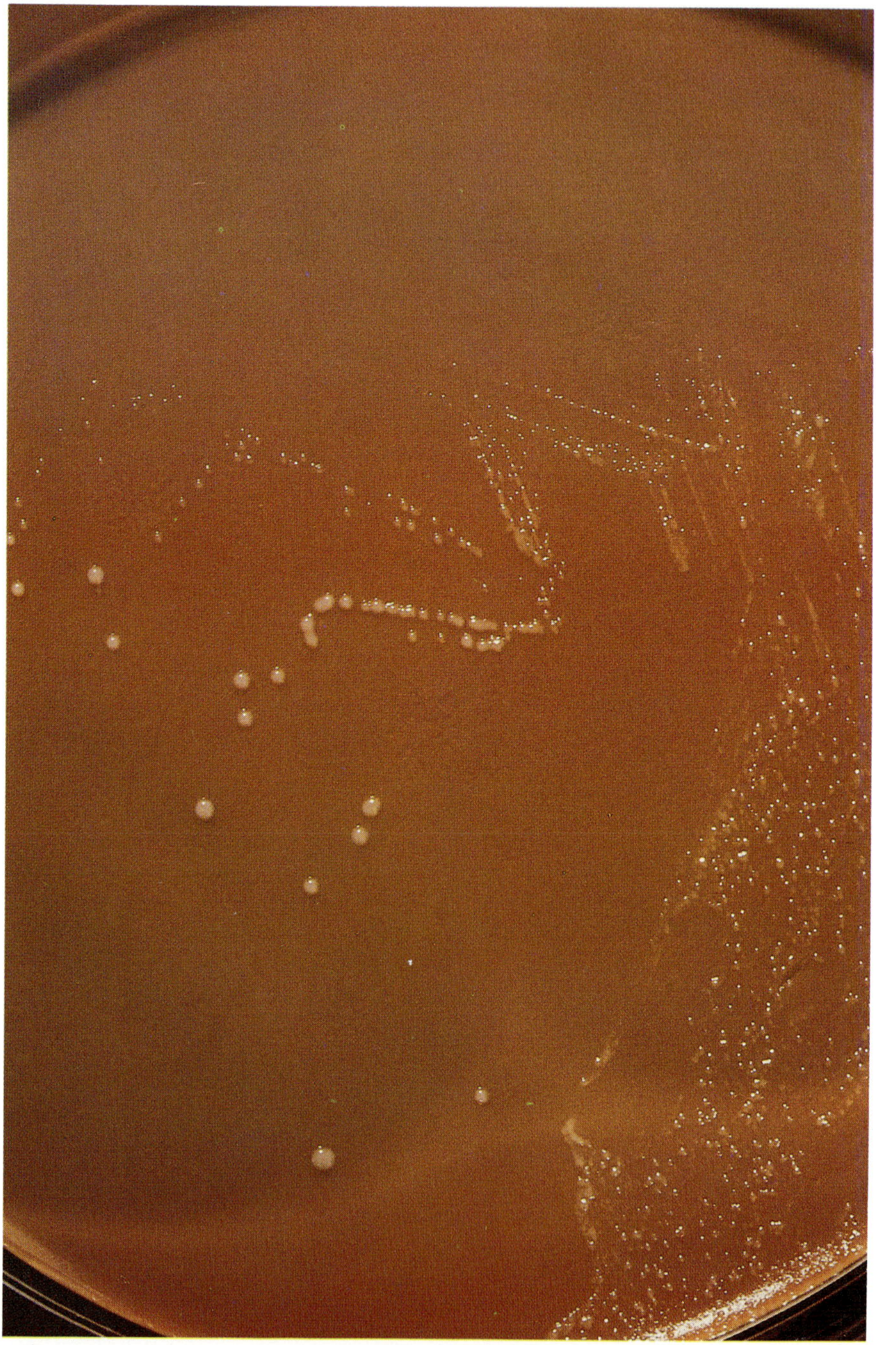

FIGURE 31:1. *Francisella tularensis* **blood culture isolate on chocolate agar supplemented with 1% Isovitalex and 1% hemin.**

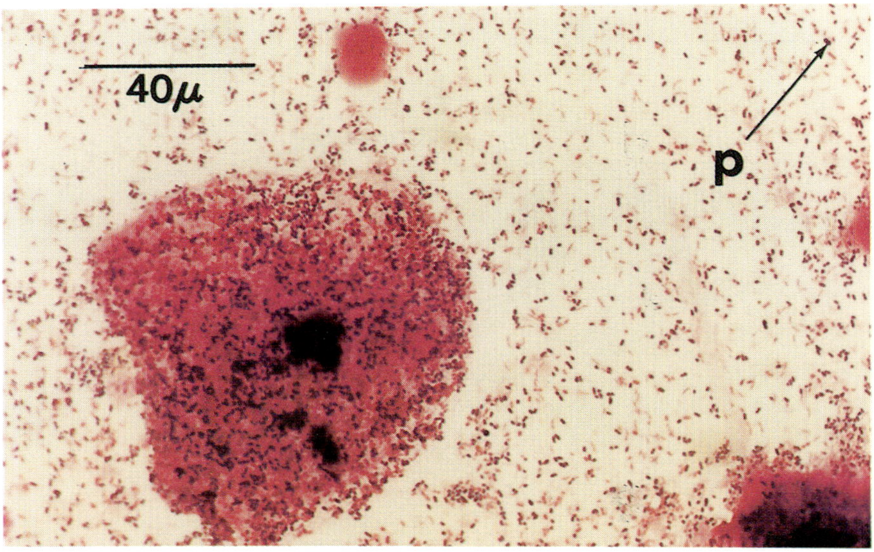

FIGURE 32:1. Clue cell and mixed flora, including few Gram-positive cocci, 800 ×.

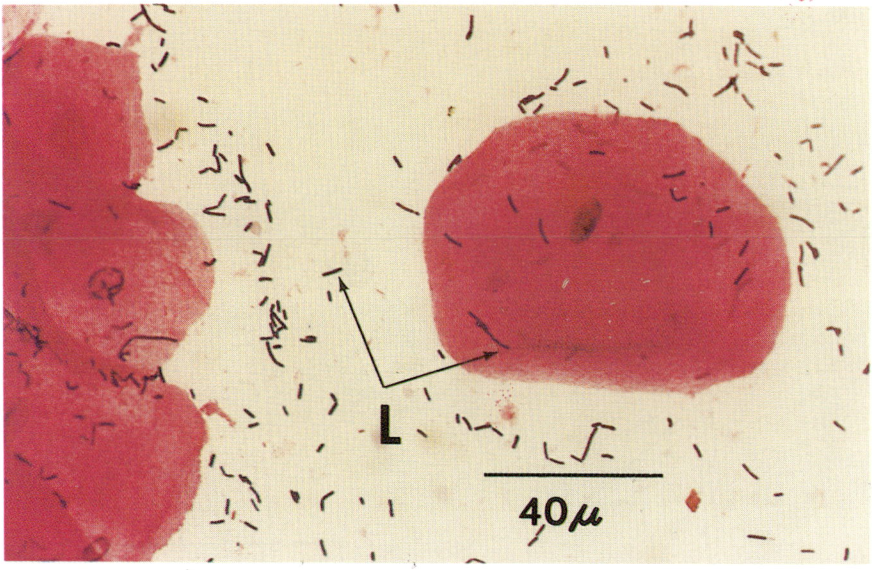

FIGURE 32.2A. Vaginal fluid smears stained by the Kopeloff modification of the Gram stain. L. *Lactobacillus* morphotype; g. *Gardnerella* morphotype; p. Gram-positive cocci; b. small Gram-negative rods; c. curved rods (Courtesy of Spiegel, et al.[7]).

(A) Vaginal squamous epithelial cells and many large Gram-positive rods (*Lactobacillus* morphotype). No. *G. vaginalis* was isolated. Clinical examination was normal, 800 ×.

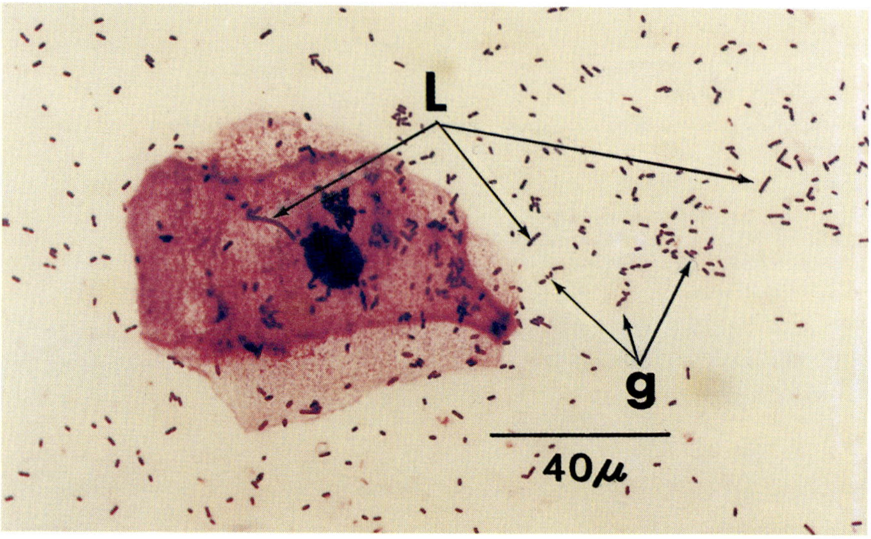

FIGURE 32.2B. Vaginal squamous epithelial cell, numerous large Gram-positive rods (*Lactobacillus* morphotype) and many small Gram-positive rods (*Gardnerella* morphotype). *G. vaginalis* was isolated. Clinical examination was normal, 800 ×.

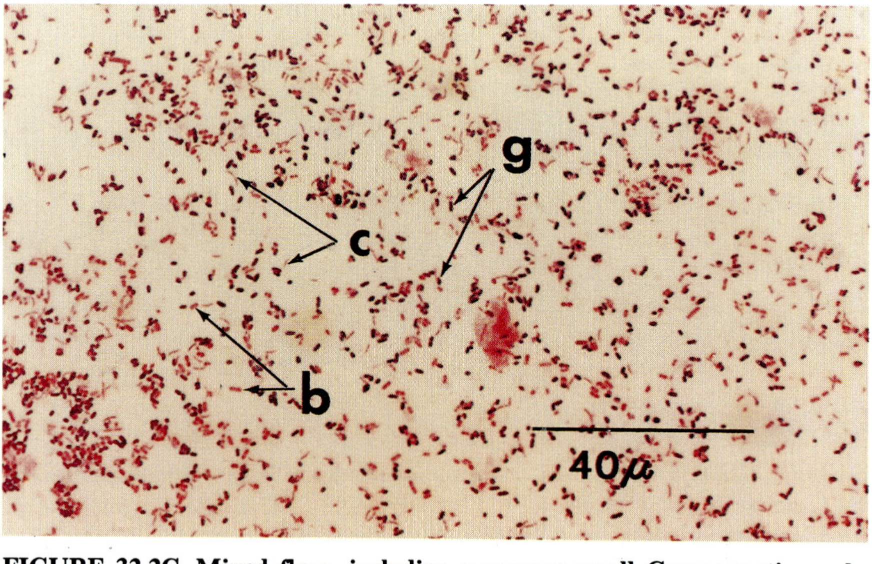

FIGURE 32.2C. Mixed flora, including numerous small Gram-negative rods, many *Gardnerella* morphotype and curved rods. No *Lactobacillus* morphotype was present. Clinical diagnosis of BV. *G. vaginalis* was isolated, 1000 ×.

INDEX

A

C

F

G

H

I

J

K

L

M

N

Q

R

S

T

U

V

W

X

Y

Z

U

V